Emergency Nursing

made Incredibly Easy!®

Third Edition

T0176450

Emergency Nursing

made
Incredibly
Easy!®

Third Edition

Clinical Editors

Nicole M. Heimgartner, DNP, RN, COI

Cherie R. Rebar, PhD, MBA, RN, COI

Carolyn J. Gersch, PhD, RN, CNE

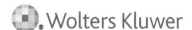 Wolters Kluwer

Philadelphia • Baltimore • New York • London
Buenos Aires • Hong Kong • Sydney • Tokyo

Executive Editor: Nicole Dernoski
Development Editor: Maria M. McAvey
Editorial Coordinator: Ashley Pfeiffer
Production Project Manager: Kim Cox
Design Coordinator: Elaine Kasmer
Manufacturing Coordinator: Kathleen Brown
Marketing Manager: Linda Wetmore
Prepress Vendor: Absolute Service, Inc.

3rd edition

9 8 7 6 5 4

Printed in the United States of America

Library of Congress Cataloging-in-Publication Data

Library of Congress Control Number:2019944146

shop.lww.com

Dedication

For Jeremy, Alayna, and Addison—my sunshine and inspiration.
For my sweet momma—I know you love me "more." Until we meet again.

Nicole

For Michael, always my one and only.
For Gillian, forever my reason.
For Flash, my faithful assistant.
For Kim, until we meet again.

Cherie

Dedicated with love and appreciation to my family and in memory of Jerry.

Carolyn

Contributors

Andrea Borchers, PhD, RN
Assistant Professor
School of Nursing
Northern Arizona University
Flagstaff, AZ

Adair Carroll, DNP, MSN, RN
Associate Professor
Department of Nursing
Shawnee State University
Portsmouth, OH

Beverly J. Cobb, PhD, MSN, PMHNP-BC
Nurse Practitioner
Department of Behavioral Medicine
Kettering Health Network
Kettering, OH

Keelin C. Cromar, MSN, RN
Adjunct Faculty
Nursing Department
Mississippi Gulf Coast Community College
Biloxi, MS

Deva Ellis, MSN, RN, C-EFM, CBC
Faculty
Department of Nursing
Keiser University
Fort Lauderdale, FL

Carolyn J. Gersch, PhD, RN, CNE
Vice President for Operations and
    Procedures
Connect: RN2ED
Beavercreek, OH
Ohio Institute of Allied Health
Dayton, OH

Darla Green, DNP, RN, FNP-C
Associate Professor
Department of Nurse Education
Del Mar College
Medical Staff Member
Corpus Christi, TX

Charity Hacker, MSN-Ed, RN
Assistant Professor
Department of Nursing
Ivy Tech Community College
Madison, IN

Nicole M. Heimgartner, DNP, RN, COI
Vice President for Business and Finance
Connect: RN2ED
Beavercreek, OH
Adjunct Faculty
Mercy College of Ohio
Toledo, OH
Adjunct Faculty
American Sentinel University
Aurora, CO

Christopher M. Kyer, BS, EMT-P
Manager of Network Emergency Disaster
    Preparedness
Department of Emergency Outreach
Kettering Health Network
Dayton, OH

Tara Latimore, MSN, RN, CMSRN
Registered Nurse
Kaiser Medical Corporation
Middletown, OH

Casey Moebius, DNP, RN
Assistant Professor
Department of Nurse Education
Del Mar College
Corpus Christi, TX

Cherie R. Rebar, PhD, MBA, RN, COI
Vice President for Communication
    and Marketing
Connect: RN2ED
Beavercreek, OH
Professor of Nursing
Wittenberg University
Springfield, OH
Adjunct Faculty
Mercy College of Ohio
Toledo, OH

Jeffrey W. Schultz, MS, APRN, ACNP-BC, CCNS,
    RN-BC, CCRN, CEN, NE-BC, NR-P
Senior Advanced Practice Provider
Cardiovascular Intensive Care Unit
North Florida Regional Medical Center
Flight Nurse
ShandsCair Critical Care Transport Program
University of Florida Health
Gainesville, FL

Nathan Shiflett, DO
Psychiatry Residency Program Director
Chillicothe VA Medical Center
Chillicothe, OH

Tracy Taylor, DNP, RN
Instructor of Clinical Practice
College of Nursing
The Ohio State University
Columbus, OH

John L. Weimer, Jr., MS, RN, AEMT, CEN,
    NEA-BC, FACHE
Vice President of Emergency and
    Trauma Services
Department of Administration
Kettering Health Network
Kettering Medical Center
Kettering, OH

Previous contributors

Julie Briggs, RN, BSN, MHA

Laura M. Criddle, PhD, RN, CEN, CFRN, FAEN

Laurie Donaghy, BSN, RN, CEN

Mary Jones, DNP, CNM, ENP-BC, FNP-BC

Sharon L. Lee, APRN, MSN, FNP-C

Lisa Matamoros, RN-BC, DNP, CEN, CPEN

Donna M. Roe, DNP, APRN, BC, CEN

Jane Von Dohre, MSN, RN, CEN

Melissa S. Wafer, RN, MSN, CEN

Robin Walsh, RN, BSN

Preface

The need for emergency nursing to remain incredibly easy continues as we look with confidence and anticipation into the future of health care. Each year adds to the list of new health care challenges and opportunities.

With 136.9 million visits annually to emergency departments per the Centers for Disease Control and Prevention, it is no surprise that knowledgeable emergency nurses are relied on to provide the quickest and best possible care.

One key role of the emergency nurse is to quickly assess the patient's chief concern and act if necessary. *Emergency Nursing Made Incredibly Easy! Third Edition* will help the nurse hone these vital skills. This book covers the evidence-based triage process and holistic care issues such as culture and pain considerations. Subsequent chapters focus on physiologic systems, covering neurologic, cardiac, respiratory, gastrointestinal, and musculoskeletal emergencies. It also discusses wound care management, genitourinary and gynecologic emergencies, obstetric emergencies, maxillofacial and ocular emergencies, psychiatric emergencies, environmental emergencies, mass casualty events and disaster response, and shock and multisystem trauma.

The clear language and illustrations will help readers anticipate and assess certain conditions and prevent predictable complications. Recurring topics for each section include how to assess the patient, diagnostic tests that may be done, and treatment options to anticipate. A *Quick quiz* at the end of each chapter tests the reader's knowledge on the information presented.

In addition, icons draw your attention to important issues:

Ages and stages—highlights age-related changes and how they affect your patient's health

Stay on the ball—focuses on critical areas involving possible dangers, risks, complications, or contraindications

Education edge—offers patient-teaching tips

This book can help practicing emergency nurses learn more about their current position. It can also help student nurses, and nurses from other specialties, build confidence in knowing how to respond in emergent situations. We are proud to be able to introduce you to the newest edition of *Emergency Nursing Made Incredibly Easy!*—a wonderful tool that will help you navigate the challenging and rewarding world of emergency nursing.

Enjoy!

Nicole M. Heimgartner, DNP, RN, COI

Cherie R. Rebar, PhD, MBA, RN, COI

Carolyn J. Gersch, PhD, RN, CNE

Educational Strategists
Connect: RN2ED

Contents

Chapter 1

Emergency department basics

Just the facts

In this chapter, you'll learn:

♦ roles and responsibilities of an emergency nurse
♦ credentials for emergency nurses
♦ ways to work with a interprofessional team
♦ ways to incorporate clinical tools and best practices into your care.

What is emergency nursing?

Emergency nursing is the delivery of specialized care to a variety of ill or injured patients. Such patients may be unstable, have complex needs, and require intensive and vigilant nursing care. Others may have minor problems. No matter the reason for coming to the emergency department (ED), all patients feel that their problems are emergencies.

Common illnesses and injuries seen in patients in EDs include:

- orthopedic injuries, including fractures, strains, and sprains
- traumatic injuries from such events as car collisions, falls, mass casualties, and natural and man-made disaster
- cardiovascular disorders, such as heart failure and acute coronary syndromes (unstable angina and myocardial infarction [MI])
- respiratory disorders, such as acute respiratory failure, pulmonary embolism, and asthma
- gastrointestinal (GI) and hepatic disorders, such as acute pancreatitis, GI bleeding, acute liver failure, acute cholecystitis, and bowel obstructions
- renal disorders, such as acute and chronic renal failure, kidney stones, and urinary tract infections
- shock due to hypovolemia, sepsis, cardiac dysfunction, acute spinal cord injury, and anaphylaxis
- metabolic disorders, such as diabetic ketoacidosis
- pediatric ailments, such as gastroenteritis, bronchiolitis, febrile seizures, and appendicitis
- drug/alcohol overdoses
- integumentary issues, including lacerations and abrasions
- gynecologic and obstetric problems

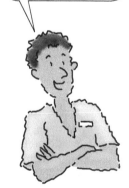

Emergencies come in all makes and models. This chapter tunes up your ED expertise!

- neurologic disorders such as strokes and head injuries
- psychiatric emergencies
- injuries resulting from violence and abuse, including knife- and gun-related trauma.

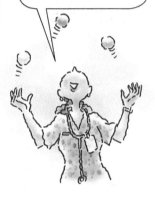

Juggling the variety of patient needs in the ED can be tough, but we'll make sure you're prepared!

Meet the emergency nurse

An emergency nurse is responsible for making sure that all patients and members of their families receive close attention and the best care possible.

What do you do?

As an emergency nurse, you may fill many roles in the emergency setting, such as staff nurse, nurse educator, nurse manager, clinical nurse specialist (CNS), nurse practitioner, flight nurse, sexual assault nurse examiner, trauma care specialist, or nurse researcher. (See *Role call*.)

Where do you work?

As an emergency nurse, you may work in various settings, including:
- hospital EDs
- triage centers
- urgent care centers
- trauma centers
- care flight programs
- emergency response units
- poison control centers
- prehospital care environments
- rural clinics.

What makes you special?

A nurse who specializes in emergencies accepts a wide range of responsibilities, including:
- being an advocate
- using sound clinical judgment
- demonstrating caring practices
- collaborating with a interprofessional team
- demonstrating an understanding of cultural diversity
- providing patient and family teaching.

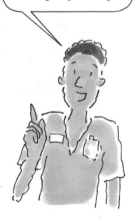

Patient advocacy is one of the most important aspects of emergency nursing.

Advocacy

An advocate is a person who works on another person's behalf. As a patient advocate, you should also address the concerns of family members and the community whenever possible (Gurney et al., 2017).

Role call

By filling various nursing and management roles, an emergency nurse helps promote optimum health, prevent illness, and aid coping with illness or death. Here are various capacities in which an emergency nurse may function.

Staff nurse
- Makes independent assessments
- Plans and implements patient care
- Provides direct nursing care
- Makes clinical observations and executes interventions
- Administers medications and treatments
- Promotes activities of daily living
- Coordinates care of patients

Nurse educator
- Assesses patients' and families' learning needs; plans and implements teaching strategies to meet those needs
- Evaluates effectiveness of teaching
- Educates peers and colleagues
- Uses excellent interpersonal skills to ensure optimal performance and outcomes

Nurse manager
- Acts as an administrative representative of the unit
- Ensures that effective and quality nursing care is provided in a timely and fiscally sound environment

Clinical nurse specialist
- Participates in education and direct patient care
- Consults with patients and family members
- Collaborates with other nurses and health care team members to deliver high-quality care

Nurse practitioner
- Provides primary health care to patients and families; can function independently
- May obtain histories and conduct physical examinations
- Orders laboratory and diagnostic tests and interprets results
- Diagnoses disorders
- Treats patients
- Counsels and educates patients and families

Nurse researcher
- Reads current nursing literature
- Applies information in practice
- Collects data
- Conducts research studies
- Serves as a consultant during research study implementation

Flight nurse
- Performs advanced procedures in the field, such as intubation, central line placement, and chest tube placement

Sexual assault nurse examiner
- Examines patients and collects evidence in cases of known or suspected sexual assault
- May testify at trials regarding their findings

Trauma care specialist
- May function in trauma centers as staff nurse or trauma coordinator
- Maintains records related to an emergency department's trauma level designation

---

As an advocate, especially for a patient who may not be able to advocate for himself or herself in an emergency setting, you're also responsible for (Rainer, 2015):
- protecting the patient's rights
- assisting the patient and the family in the decision-making process by providing education and support
- negotiating with other members of the health care team on behalf of the patient and family
- keeping the patient and family informed about the care plan
- advocating for flexible visitation in the ED
- respecting and supporting the decisions of the patient and family

- serving as a liaison between the patient and family and other members of the health care team
- respecting the patient's values and cultures
- acting in the patient's best interest
- preventing injuries in the community by educating families about poison safety, use of car restraints, and safe sleeping tips for infants to prevent sudden infant death syndrome.

Stuck in the middle

Being a patient advocate can sometimes cause conflict between you and family members. For example, a patient may have an advance directive requesting no resuscitation but the family may not approve.

It may also cause conflict between your professional duty and the patient's personal values. For example, the patient may be a Jehovah's Witness and refuse a blood transfusion (Malkin et al., 2016). In this case, you should consult your facility's ethics committee as well as its policies and procedures.

I realize we have different ideas about emergency care, but let's do what's best for the patient.

Clinical judgment

An emergency nurse needs to exercise clinical judgment in a fast-paced and stressful environment. To develop sound clinical judgment, you need critical thinking skills. Critical thinking is a complex mixture of knowledge, intuition, logic, common sense, and experience (Emergency Nurses Association, 2012).

Why be critical?

Critical thinking fosters understanding of issues and enables you to quickly find answers to difficult questions. It isn't a trial-and-error method, yet it isn't strictly a scientific problem-solving method either.

Critical thinking enhances your ability to identify a patient's needs. It also enables you to use sound clinical decision making and to determine which nursing actions/interventions best meet a patient's needs.

Developing critical thinking skills

Critical thinking skills improve with increasing clinical and scientific experience. The best way for you to develop critical thinking skills is by asking questions and learning. You should never be afraid to ask a question even if you are an experienced nurse.

Always asking questions

The first question you should find the answer to is "What are the patient's symptoms or diagnosis?" If it's a diagnosis with which you aren't familiar, look it up and read about it. Find the answers to questions like these:

- What are the signs and symptoms?
- What's the usual cause?
- What complications can occur?

In addition to the answers to diagnosis-related questions, also be sure to find out:

- What are the patient's physical examination findings?
- Which laboratory and diagnostic tests are necessary?
- Does the patient have risk factors? If so, are they significant? What interventions would minimize those risk factors?
- What are the patient's cultural beliefs? How can you best address the patient's cultural concerns?
- What are the possible complications? What type of monitoring is needed to watch for complications?
- What are the usual medications and treatments for the patient's condition? (If you aren't familiar with the medications or treatments, look them up in a reliable source or consult a colleague.)

Critical thinking and the nursing process

Critical thinking skills are necessary when applying the nursing process—assessment, planning, implementation, and evaluation—and making patient care decisions.

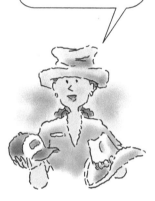

No matter what it looks like, be sure to put on your critical thinking cap for the next steps.

Caring practice

Caring practice is the use of a therapeutic and compassionate environment to focus on the patient's needs. Although care is based on standards and protocols, it must also be individualized to each patient.

Caring practice also involves:

- maintaining a safe environment
- interacting with the patient and the family members in a compassionate and respectful manner throughout the ED stay
- supporting the family when a patient dies unexpectedly.

Collaboration

Collaboration allows a health care team to use all available resources for the patient. An emergency nurse is part of a interprofessional team in which each person contributes expertise. The collaborative goal is to optimize patient outcomes. As a nurse, you may often serve as the coordinator of such collaborative teams.

Cultural diversity

Culture is defined as the way people live and how they behave in a social group. This behavior is learned and passed on from generation to generation. Acknowledging and respecting patients' diverse cultural beliefs is a necessary part of high-quality care.

Keep an open mind

An emergency nurse is expected to demonstrate awareness and sensitivity toward a patient's religion, lifestyle, family makeup, socioeconomic status, age, gender, and values. Be sure to assess cultural factors and concerns and integrate them into the care plan.

Education

As an educator, an emergency nurse is the facilitator of patient, family, and staff education. Patient education involves teaching patients and their families about:
- the patient's illness
- the importance of managing comorbid disorders (such as diabetes, arthritis, and hypertension)
- diagnostic and laboratory testing
- planned surgical procedures, including preoperative and postoperative expectations
- instructions on specific patient care, such as wound care and range-of-motion exercises
- medications that are prescribed
- illness and injury prevention
- home care instructions and follow-up appointments.

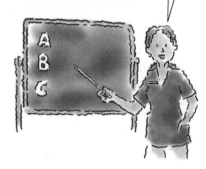

Patients, families, and staff members—everyone needs some education from an emergency nurse.

Staff as students

Emergency nurses also commonly serve as staff educators. Examples of staff teaching topics you may need to address include:
- how to use new equipment
- how to interpret diagnostic test results
- how to administer a new medication.

Becoming an emergency nurse

Most nursing students are only briefly exposed to emergency nursing. Much of the training required to become an emergency nurse is learned on the job.

Learning by doing

On-the-job training is central to gaining the extensive skills required of an emergency nurse. Your facility may provide a competency-based orientation program for new emergency nurses. In such a program, you gain knowledge and experience while working in the ED and a preceptor (a staff nurse or CNS with specialized training in emergency nursing) provides guidance.

An orientation period allows a nurse time to acquire the knowledge and technical skills needed to work in the emergency environment. Such technical skills include working with cardiac monitoring systems, mechanical ventilators, hemodynamic monitoring devices, autotransfusers, and intracranial pressure (ICP) monitoring devices. In addition, it is very important for the ED nurse to develop time management and prioritization skills and have an assertive attitude to advocate for the patient. These skills and attitudes are important to being successful in achieving optimum outcomes.

Gaining credentials

The Emergency Nurses Association (ENA) is one of the world's largest specialty nursing organizations, with more than 42,000 members. The strategic goals of ENA are to promote excellence in emergency nursing through community, knowledge, quality and safety, and advocacy (ENA, 2018).

Through ENA, you can become certified as an emergency nurse or emergency flight nurse. Certification, demonstrated through earning your certified emergency nurse (CEN) or certified emergency flight nurse credentials, states you're a professional, with proficiency and skill in a highly specialized area of nursing. Emergency nurses can obtain certification through the Board of Certification for Emergency Nursing.

CEN certification requires renewal after 4 years. Nurses can recertify by taking the examination again or by demonstrating continuing education in emergency nursing.

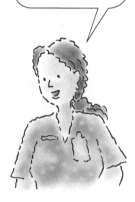

There's lots of incentive to freshen up your CEN certification over time.

Help wanted

Certification isn't mandatory to work as an emergency nurse, but it's certainly encouraged. Many units prefer to hire nurses with certification because it means that they have demonstrated expertise and commitment to emergency nursing.

Safety first

The goal of any nursing certification program is to promote safe nursing care. CEN certification is evidence that a nurse has demonstrated clinical excellence and recognizes the importance of patient safety. Certification validates the nurse's qualifications and specialized clinical knowledge.

What's in it for me?

For most nurses, the main reason for seeking CEN certification is personal fulfillment, but there are other rewards as well. Many institutions reimburse nurses for taking the examination, and others offer monetary incentives to nurses with CEN certification.

Nursing responsibilities

As an emergency nurse, you're responsible for all parts of the nursing process: assessing, planning, implementing, and evaluating care of all patients in your care. Remember that each of these steps gives you an opportunity to exercise your critical thinking skills.

Assessment

Emergency nursing requires that you continuously assess the patient for subtle changes in condition and monitor all equipment being used. Caring for emergency patients always involves patient assessment, which includes physical and psychological statuses. As part of the patient assessment, the emergency nurse may use highly specialized equipment such as cardiac monitors, hemodynamic monitoring devices, and ICP monitoring devices. The nurse will also be required to incorporate laboratory and diagnostic study findings when assessing a patient.

Planning

Planning requires you to consider the patient's psychological and physiologic needs and set realistic patient goals. The result is an individualized care plan for your patient. To ensure safe passage through the emergency environment, you must also anticipate changes in the patient's condition. For example, for a patient admitted with a diagnosis of MI, you should monitor cardiac rhythm and anticipate rhythm changes. If an arrhythmia such as complete heart block develops, you may need to change the treatment plan and establish new goals.

What's the problem?

In planning, be sure to address present and potential problems, such as:
- pain
- anxiety and fear
- cardiac arrhythmias
- respiratory distress
- mental status changes
- altered hemodynamic states

- impaired physical mobility
- impaired skin integrity
- fluid volume deficit.

Implementation

As a nurse, you must implement specific interventions to address existing and potential patient problems.

A call to intervene

Examples of interventions include:
- monitoring and treating cardiac arrhythmias
- managing pain
- offering emotional support
- monitoring responses to therapy.

Evaluation

It's necessary for you to continually evaluate a patient's response to interventions. Use such evaluations to change the care plan as needed to make sure that your patient continues to work toward achieving optimum outcome goals.

Emergency essentials

What comes to mind when you hear the word *emergency*? Do you think of a motor vehicle collision, a drowning, or a patient with cardiac arrest coming through the doors of the ED? Or do you visualize a postoperative patient experiencing respiratory distress or a patient falling while trying to walk to the bathroom? Emergencies occur everywhere. No matter what your area of expertise is, you'll encounter emergencies in your nursing career. This section gives an overview of emergency situations and your role in responding to patients who need your help.

It's quite a laundry list, but the answers to these questions provide valuable patient information.

Information station

When a patient arrives in the ED by ambulance, it's important to get as much information as you can from the prehospital care providers. For instance, if the patient was involved in an accident, you'll want to know certain information.

Danger details

- How did the accident occur?
- What type of accident was it?
- If it was a motor vehicle collision, did the vehicle sustain exterior/interior or front/rear end damage?

Patient particulars

- Was the patient restrained?
- Did the patient have to be extricated from the vehicle?
- Was the patient ambulatory at the scene?
- If the patient sustained a burn injury, was the patient found in an enclosed space?
- If the burn resulted from a fire, was the fire accompanied by an explosion?

Injuries sustained

- What injuries have the prehospital care providers identified or suspected?
- What are the patient's chief concerns?

Vital vitals

- What vital signs have care providers obtained before arriving in the ED?
- What treatment has the patient received and what was the patient's response?

Systematic systems

All patients with traumatic injuries should be assessed rapidly with a systematic method used consistently for all patients. The ENA has developed the Trauma Nursing Core Course to teach nurses such a method for assessing trauma patients. The ENA method uses primary and secondary surveys to rapidly identify life-threatening emergencies and prioritize care.

Primary survey

The primary survey begins with an assessment of airway, breathing, and circulation—the ABCs learned in nursing school. The ENA recommends additional assessment parameters: neurologic status—designated as *disability* (*D*)—and exposure and environment—designated as *E* (ENA, 2019). (See *Primary assessment of the trauma patient.*) The ABCDE primary survey consists of—you guessed it—five steps.

A is for airway

Before you assess a trauma patient's airway, immobilize the cervical spine through initial stabilization and by applying a cervical collar.

Primary assessment of the trauma patient

The chart that follows outlines the parameters for assessing the trauma patient along with their associated assessment steps and appropriate interventions.

Parameter	Assessment	Interventions
A = Airway	• Airway patency	• Institute cervical spine immobilization until X-rays determine whether the patient has a cervical spine injury. • Position the patient. • To open the airway, make sure that the neck is midline and stabilized; next, perform the jaw-thrust maneuver.
B = Breathing	• Respirations (rate, depth, effort) • Breath sounds • Chest wall movement and chest injury • Position of trachea (midline or deviation)	• Administer 100% oxygen with a bag valve mask. • Use airway adjuncts, such as an oropharyngeal or a nasopharyngeal airway, an endotracheal tube, an esophageal–tracheal combitube, or cricothyrotomy, as indicated. • Suction the patient as needed. • Remove foreign bodies that may obstruct breathing. • Treat life-threatening conditions, such as pneumothorax or tension pneumothorax.
C = Circulation	• Pulse and blood pressure • Bleeding or hemorrhage • Capillary refill and color of skin and mucous membranes • Cardiac rhythm	• Start cardiopulmonary resuscitation, medications, and defibrillation or synchronized cardioversion. • Control hemorrhaging with direct pressure or pneumatic devices. • Establish intravenous access and fluid therapy (isotonic fluids and blood). • Treat life-threatening conditions such as cardiac tamponade.
D = Disability	• Neurologic assessment, including level of consciousness, pupils, and motor and sensory function	• Institute cervical spine immobilization until X-rays confirm the absence of cervical spine injury.
E = Exposure and environment	• Expose for injuries and maintain a warm environment once exposed.	• Examine the patient to determine the extent of injuries. • Provide warm blankets and warmed fluids or use overhead warmer. If an environmental exposure is determined, the use of institute-appropriate therapy (warming therapy for hypothermia or cooling therapy for hyperthermia) may be indicated.

Until proven otherwise, assume that the patient who has sustained a major trauma has a cervical spine injury.

When continuing your assessment, note whether the patient can speak; if the patient is able to speak, the airway is patent. Open the airway of an unresponsive patient with the head-tilt, chin-lift method or with modified jaw thrust in the trauma patient. Check for obstructions to the airway, such as the tongue (the most common obstruction), blood, loose teeth, or vomitus. Clear airway obstructions immediately using the jaw-thrust or chin-lift technique to maintain cervical spine immobilization. You may need to use suction if blood or vomitus is present.

Insert a nasopharyngeal or oropharyngeal airway if necessary; however, remember that an oropharyngeal airway can only be used on an unconscious patient. An oropharyngeal airway stimulates the gag reflex in a conscious or semiconscious patient. If a nasopharyngeal or oropharyngeal airway fails to provide a patent airway, the patient may require intubation.

B is for breathing

Assess the patient for spontaneous respirations, noting their rate, depth, and symmetry. Obtain oxygen saturation with pulse oximetry. Is the patient using accessory muscles to breathe? Do you hear breath sounds bilaterally? Do you detect tracheal deviation or jugular vein distention? Does the patient have an open chest wound? All major trauma patients require high-flow oxygen. If the patient doesn't have spontaneous respirations or if breathing is ineffective, ventilate the patient by using a bag valve mask device until intubation can be achieved.

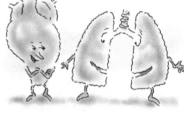

All right, just because the primary survey puts airway and breathing before circulation doesn't mean you can gloat.

C is for circulation

Check for the presence of peripheral pulses. Determine the patient's blood pressure. What's the patient's skin color? Does the patient exhibit pallor, flushing, or some other discoloration? What's the patient's skin temperature? Is it warm, cool, or clammy to the touch? Is the patient diaphoretic? Is there obvious bleeding? All major trauma patients need at least two large-bore intravenous (IV) lines because they may require large amounts of fluids and blood. A fluid warmer should be used if possible. If the patient exhibits external bleeding, apply direct pressure over the site. If the patient has no pulse, initiate cardiopulmonary resuscitation immediately.

D is for disability

Perform a neurologic assessment. Use the Glasgow Coma Scale to assess the patient's baseline status. Maintain cervical spine immobilization until X-rays confirm that there's no cervical injury. If the patient isn't alert and oriented, conduct further assessments using the secondary survey.

E is for exposure and environment

Expose the patient to perform a thorough assessment. Remove all clothing to assess injuries. Remember that if the patient has bullet holes or knife tears through clothing, don't cut through these areas. Law enforcement will count on you to preserve evidence as necessary. Environmental control means keeping the patient warm. If you have removed the patient's clothes, cover the patient with warm blankets. You may need to use an overhead warmer, especially with an infant or a small child. Use fluid warmers when administering large amounts of IV fluids. A cold patient has numerous problems with healing.

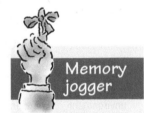

Memory jogger

You may also assess a patient using this mnemonic: A Very Practical Use (AVPU).

A = Alert, oriented patient

V = responds to Voice

P = responds to Pain

U = Unresponsive patient

Remember that the primary ABCDE survey is a rapid assessment intended to identify life-threatening emergencies that must be treated before the assessment continues.

Secondary survey

After the primary survey is completed, perform a more detailed secondary survey, which includes a head-to-toe assessment. The ENA (2017) recommends additional assessment data such as vital signs, family presence, and focused adjuncts designated as F; give comfort measures designated as G; history and head-to-toe assessment designated as H; and inspect posterior surfaces designated as I. This part of the examination identifies all injuries sustained by the patient. At this time, a care plan is developed and diagnostic tests are ordered.

F is for family matters/full set of vital signs/focused adjuncts

Obtain a full set of vital signs initially, including respirations, pulse, blood pressure, and temperature. If you suspect chest trauma, get blood pressures in both arms.

Next, perform these five interventions:

1. Initiate cardiac monitoring.
2. Obtain continuous pulse oximetry readings. Be aware, however, that readings may be inaccurate if the patient is cold or in shock.
3. Insert a urinary catheter to monitor accurate intake and output measurements. Many urinary catheters also record core body temperatures. Don't insert a urinary catheter if there's blood at the urinary meatus.
4. Insert a nasogastric (NG) tube for stomach decompression. Injuries such as a facial fracture contraindicate the use of an NG tube; if a facial fracture is suspected, insert the tube orally instead. Depending on your facility's policy and procedures, the healthcare provider may insert the NG tube when a facial fracture is suspected.
5. Obtain laboratory studies as ordered, such as type and cross-matching for blood; a complete blood count or hematocrit and hemoglobin level; toxicology and alcohol screens, if indicated; a pregnancy test, if necessary; and serum electrolyte levels. Obtain radiologic studies as ordered such as computed tomography scans and X-rays. You may be asked to assist the physician with a focused assessment with sonography for trauma (FAST exam) for patients to determine if there is presence of free air in the peritoneum.

Facilitate the presence of the patient's family. Several organizations, including the ENA and the American Heart Association, endorse the practice of allowing the patient's family to be present during resuscitation (ENA, 2017). It's important, however, to assess the family's needs before offering permission to be present. Family members may need emotional

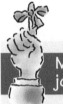

Memory jogger

The acronym SAMPLE is a mnemonic that will help you remember the types of information you'll need to obtain for the patient's history.

Subjective: What does the patient say? How did the accident occur? Does the patient remember? What symptoms does the patient report?

Allergies: Does the patient have allergies, and if so, what allergies? Is the patient wearing a medical identification bracelet?

Medications: Does the patient take medications on a regular basis, and if so, what medications? What medications has the patient taken in the past 24 hours?

Past medical history: Has the patient been treated for medical conditions, and if so, which ones? Has the patient had surgery, and if so, what type of surgery?

Last meal eaten, Last tetanus shot, Last menses: When was the last time the patient had anything to eat or drink? When was the patient's most recent tetanus shot? (If unknown, administer one in the emergency department.) If the patient is a female of childbearing age, when was her last menses? Could she be pregnant?

Events/Environment leading to injury: How did the accident occur? Inquire about precipitating factors, if any. For instance, the patient being seen for injuries sustained in a motor vehicle accident may have had the accident because of a myocardial infarction while driving. Likewise, the patient who sustained a fall might have fallen due to dizziness or tripping over an object.

and spiritual support from you or from a member of the clergy. If a family member wishes to be present during resuscitation, assign a health care professional to explain procedures as they're performed.

G for give comfort measures

During a tense trauma situation, the urgency of the assessment and treatment processes may cause you to overlook the patient's fears. Remember to talk to the patient and explain the examination and interventions being administered. An encouraging word and tone can go a long way to comfort and calm a frightened patient. Comfort measures also include the administration of pain medication and sedation as needed.

H is for history and head–to–toe assessment

Obtain the patient's history, remembering to obtain as much information as possible to determine the presence of coexisting conditions, or alcohol or drug use, that could affect care or factors that might have precipitated the trauma. The mnemonic SAMPLE will help you remember the information needed. SAMPLE stands for Subjective data, Allergies, Medications, Past medical history, Last meal eaten, and Events/Environment leading to the injury.

Next, perform a head-to-toe assessment, starting at the patient's head and working your way down to the feet. Don't forget to check all posterior surfaces. Logroll the patient (with assistance, if necessary) to assess for injuries to the back. Address life-threatening injuries immediately.

Triage

Triage is a method of prioritizing patient care according to the type of illness or injury and the urgency of the patient's condition. It's used to ensure appropriate care is provided in a timely manner to meet the patient's needs (Falconer et al., 2018).

Many people with nonurgent conditions come to the ED because it's their only source of medical care; this increase in nonurgent cases has necessitated a means of quickly identifying and treating those patients with more serious conditions. The triage nurse must be able to rapidly assess the nature and urgency of problems for many patients and prioritize their care based on that assessment.

Guidelines for triage-based care is based on a five-tier system:

1. *Level I: resuscitation*—This level includes patients who need immediate nursing and medical attention, such as those with cardiopulmonary arrest, major trauma, severe respiratory distress, and seizures.
2. *Level II: emergent*—These patients need immediate nursing assessment and rapid treatment. Patients who may be assessed as level II include those with head injuries, chest pain, stroke, asthma, and sexual assault injuries.
3. *Level III: urgent*—These patients need quick attention but can wait as long as 30 minutes for an assessment and treatment. Such patients might report to the ED with signs of infection, mild respiratory distress, or moderate pain.
4. *Level IV: less urgent*—Patients in this triage category can wait up to 1 hour for an assessment and treatment; they may include those with an earache, chronic back pain, upper respiratory symptoms, and a mild headache.
5. *Level V: nonurgent*—These patients can wait up to 2 hours (possibly longer) for an assessment and treatment; those with sore throat, menstrual cramps, and other minor symptoms are typically assigned to level V.

If you can't decide which triage level is best for a patient, assign the patient to the higher level.

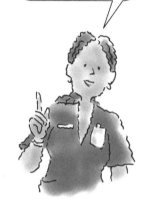

The triage method prioritizes ailments so that all patients receive appropriate care.

Once divided

Carefully document the patient's chief concern and vital signs, the triage assessment, and the triage category to which you've assigned the patient. It's also important to document pertinent negatives. For example, if the patient is experiencing chest pain without cardiac symptoms, be sure to note "Patient reports nonradiating left chest pain; denies shortness of breath, diaphoresis, or nausea. Pain increases with movement and deep inspiration." Quote the patient when appropriate.

As you perform triage, tell the patients you interview that you're the triage nurse and that you'll be performing a screening assessment. Be attentive to what's occurring beyond your current assessment because it may be necessary to leave the patient if a patient with a more critical situation arrives in the ED.

Stay in touch

Maintain communication with patients waiting to be summoned to a treatment room because a patient's status may change—improving or worsening—during an extended period in the waiting room. Patients appreciate information on the reasons for waiting room delays.

Interprofessional teamwork

Nurses working with emergency patients commonly collaborate with a interprofessional team of health care professionals. The team approach helps caregivers to meet the diverse needs of individual patients.

The whole goal

The goal of collaboration is to provide effective and comprehensive (holistic) care. Holistic care addresses the biologic, psychological, social, and spiritual dimensions of a person.

Team huddle

An interprofessional team providing direct patient care may consist of many professionals, including:
- registered nurses (RNs)
- doctors
- advanced practice nurses (such as CNSs and nurse practitioners)
- licensed practical nurses (LPNs)
- respiratory therapists, paramedics, ED health care providers, and others. (See *Meet the team.*)

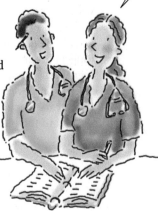

When we coordinate efforts, ED professionals make beautiful working relationships together.

Working with registered nurses

Teamwork is essential in the stressful environment of the ED. The emergency nurse should be able to work well with all members of the team.

Meet the team

Various members of the interprofessional team have collaborative relationships with emergency nurses. Here are some examples.

Patient care technician
- Responsible for providing direct patient care to critically ill patients
- Bathes patients
- Obtains vital signs
- Assists with transportation of patients for testing

Pastoral caregiver
- Also known as a *chaplain*
- Meets patient's and family's spiritual and religious needs
- Provides support and empathy to the patient and the family
- Delivers patient's last rites if requested

Stroke team
- Assesses persons coming to the emergency department with symptoms of an acute stroke
- Assesses patients for appropriateness of thrombolytic therapy and other needed treatments
- Commonly includes a nurse, a neurologist, and a radiologist
- Can participate in hospital and community education related to stroke prevention, early signs and symptoms, and treatments

Social services
- Assist patients and families with such problems as difficulty paying for medications, follow-up physician visits, and other health-related issues
- Assist patients with travel and housing if needed

Child protective services
- Designed to protect children from abusive situations
- Preserve the family unit, if possible, while ensuring the safety of children

The buddy system

It's important to have a colleague to look to for moral support, physical assistance with a patient, and problem solving. No one person has all the answers, but together, nurses have a better chance of solving problems.

Working with doctors

Patients in the ED are usually seen by an ED doctor who will probably have no prior knowledge of the patient. Consults made to the patient's primary care doctor can help fill in the blanks, as can assessments from specialists within your facility. Specialists commonly called to the ED to assess and treat patients include:

- cardiologists
- neurologists
- orthopedists
- gynecologists
- psychiatrists
- pediatricians.

In addition, if you work in a teaching institution, you may also interact on a regular basis with medical students, interns, and residents who are under the direction of the attending doctor.

Working with advanced practice nurses

Advanced practice nurses—CNSs and acute care nurse practitioners (ACNPs)—are increasingly employed in EDs. An advanced practice nurse may be employed by a hospital and assigned to a specific unit or may be employed by a doctor to assist in caring for and monitoring patients. The advanced practice nurse assists staff nurses in clinical decision making and enhances the quality of patient care, which improves patient care outcomes.

The roles of a lifetime

The traditional roles of a CNS are:
- clinician
- educator
- researcher
- consultant
- manager.

The CNS offers support and guidance to staff nurses as they care for patients. The CNS assists with problem solving when complex care is necessary for patients and their families. In addition, the CNS may develop research projects dealing with problems identified on the unit.

On a role

An ACNP has the responsibilities traditionally held by a nurse practitioner. These responsibilities may include:
- conducting comprehensive health assessments
- diagnosing
- prescribing pharmacologic and nonpharmacologic treatments. An ACNP may also conduct research and manage care.

Working with licensed practical nurses

In some EDs, LPNs are members of the health care team. Generally, an LPN collaborates with an RN to deliver patient care. The RN is responsible for and delegates specific tasks to the LPN, whose duties may include caring directly for patients and collecting data. The LPN may also administer approved medications, assist with procedures, and record vital signs.

Working with respiratory therapists

An emergency nurse also commonly collaborates with respiratory therapists in caring for emergency patients.

Respiration-related roles

The role of a respiratory therapist is to monitor and manage the respiratory status of patients. To do this, the respiratory therapist may:

- administer breathing treatments
- suction patients
- collect specimens
- obtain arterial blood gas values
- manage ventilator changes.

Clinical tools

The interprofessional team uses various tools to promote safe and comprehensive holistic care. These tools include clinical pathways, practice guidelines, and protocols.

Clinical pathways

Clinical pathways (also known as *critical pathways*) are care management plans for patients with a given diagnosis or condition.

Follow the path

Clinical pathways are typically generated and used by departments that deliver care for similar conditions to many patients. An interprofessional committee of clinicians at the facility usually develops clinical pathways. The overall goals are to:

- establish a standard approach to care for all providers in the department
- establish roles for various members of the health care team
- provide a framework for collecting data on patient outcomes.

Tried and true

Pathways are based on evidence from research and clinical practice. The committee gathers and uses information from peer-reviewed literature and experts outside the facility.

Outlines and timelines

Clinical pathways usually outline the duties of all professionals involved with patient care. They follow specific timelines for indicated actions. They also specify expected patient outcomes, which serve as checkpoints for the patient's progress and caregiver's performance.

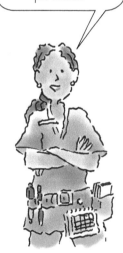

The tools of your trade? Clinical pathways, practice guidelines, and protocols.

Practice guidelines

Practice guidelines specify courses of action to be taken in response to a diagnosis or condition. Practice guidelines aid decision making by health care providers and patients. They're interprofessional in nature and can be used to coordinate care by multiple providers.

Let an expert be your guide

Expert health care providers usually write practice guidelines. They condense large amounts of information into easily usable formats, combining clinical expertise with the best available clinical evidence. Practice guidelines are used to:

- streamline care
- control variations in practice patterns
- distribute health care resources more effectively.

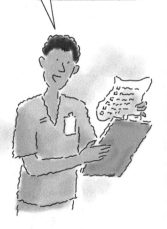

Always check where practice guidelines come from before you apply them to your patient.

The evidence is in

Practice guidelines are valuable sources of information. They indicate which tests and treatments are appropriate and provide a framework for building a standard of care (a statement describing an expected level of care or performance).

Consider the source

Like research-based information, clinical guidelines should be evaluated for the quality of their sources. It's a good idea to read the developers' policy statement about how evidence was selected and what values were applied in making recommendations for care (Carman et al., 2013).

Protocols

Protocols are facility-established sets of procedures for a given circumstance. Their purpose is to outline actions that are most likely to produce optimal patient outcomes.

First things first

Protocols describe a sequence of actions a health care provider should take to establish a diagnosis or begin a treatment regimen. For example, a chest pain protocol outlines a bedside strategy for managing patients with chest pain.

Protocols facilitate the delivery of consistent, cost-effective care. They're also educational resources for clinicians who strive to keep abreast of current best practices (Castner et al., 2013). Protocols may be either highly directive or flexible, allowing health care provider to use clinical judgment.

Input from experts

Nursing or medical experts write protocols, commonly with input from other health care providers. Protocols may be approved by legislative bodies, such as boards of nursing or medical boards. Hospital committees may approve other types of protocols for various facilities.

Transport

Patients who are hospitalized rarely stay in their room for their entire visit; they're transported for diagnostic tests, procedures, and surgery. The ED patient is no different. Trauma patients can experience either an interfacility or intrafacility transport journey.

Not so simple

Moving a patient from one place to another sounds simple. However, it isn't quite so easy when a patient is hemodynamically unstable; has airway or respiratory compromise; requires continuous cardiac monitoring, continuous infusion of IV fluids, or medications; or has an artificial airway or mechanical ventilation. In these instances, patients must be accompanied by an RN who's trained and prepared to handle any emergency situation that can happen.

Before any transport, the patient's condition must be evaluated to ensure safety.

Interfacility transport

An *interfacility transport* is one that moves the patient from the ED to another health care facility. Interfacility transport happens on the ground with a paramedic ambulance or critical care transport or by air (usually by helicopter, but fixed- and rotary-wing planes may also be used).

ED on wheels (or wings)

Interfacility transport vehicles are like EDs on wheels. They can safely handle the transport of critically ill patients and are staffed with critical care transport teams that include specially trained paramedics, specially trained RNs, and emergency flight nurses. The staff is trained to handle intra-aortic balloon pumps and invasive pressure and end-tidal carbon dioxide monitoring.

Sure it's costly, but you can't beat air transport for a dramatic entrance!

Movin' out

Trauma patients are moved from their original facility to another for several reasons. The patient may be moved due to a need for higher level of medical care or special services not offered at the original facility. Alternatively, the patient may be moved to another hospital due to family and patient convenience or where the patient's healthcare provider is located.

Cha-ching

Interfacility transport doesn't come without a price. Air transport can be very costly in more ways than one; it's expensive, and airplanes can only land at approved airports. This mode of travel also requires that the patient be transported via ambulance to the airplane and then from the airplane to the facility. This loading and unloading can cause the patient unneeded stress.

Helicopter transport is expensive and can cost up to four times the cost of an ambulance. Its advantage is the ability to land at the scene of an accident and at hospitals equipped with heliport pads. This advantage decreases the amount of transport time needed to get the patient to a qualified facility. This advantage is weather dependent and may not be optimal in every situation.

Intrafacility transport

An *intrafacility transport* involves transporting the patient from the ED to another area of the receiving hospital such as an inpatient unit, the X-ray or imaging department, or the operating room.

Movin' in

Stable ED patients may be transported to another area of the hospital by ancillary support staff provided that they don't require continuous monitoring. Examples of stable patients may include pregnant patients without abdominal trauma, persistent uterine contractions, or signs of imminent birth and patients with:
- closed head injuries
- abdominal pain but who have stable vital signs
- closed head injuries without altered level of consciousness, neurologic impairment, or severe agitation
- mild injuries or illnesses that carry minimal risk of becoming unstable.

Communication

Regardless of which type of transport the patient requires, communication is vital to the patient's survival in coming to your facility, going to another facility, or just moving within your facility. Complete documentation of the patient's condition, procedures, laboratory test results, monitoring parameters, and medications is paramount.

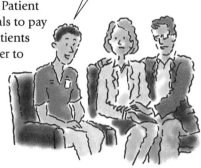

Communication is key during patient transport.

All in the know

In 2015, The Joint Commission established certain National Patient Safety Goals to urge nurses and other health care professionals to pay stronger attention to the accuracy of medications given to patients as they transition from one care setting or health care provider to another. Medication reconciliation should occur whenever a patient moves from one location to another location in a health care facility, from one health care facility to another, or when there is a change in the caregivers responsible for the patient.

When giving report about a patient, be sure to include:
- the patient's name, age, allergies, weight, medical history, and daily medications
- when the current symptoms first occurred
- when the patient first arrived in the ED
- critical laboratory values
- diagnostic and interventional procedures that the patient received
- IV sites and size of catheters as well as fluids infusing, rate of infusion, and dose of any added medications
- medications given to the patient and their response
- endotracheal tube size (if the patient is intubated); depth of insertion and ventilator settings
- the patient's vital signs.

Family matters

Make sure that the patient's family is kept informed of plans to transport the patient. A traumatic event is stressful enough for the family, and being kept abreast of the patient's condition as well as plans for transporting the patient may help allay fears.

Best practices

As new procedures and medicines become available, nurses committed to excellence regularly update and adapt their practices. An approach known as *best practices* is an important tool for providing high-quality care.

Best for all concerned

The term *best practices* refers to clinical practices, treatments, and interventions that result in the best possible outcomes for the patient and your facility.

The best practice approach is generally a team effort that draws on various types of information. Common sources of information used to identify best practices are research data, personal experience, and expert opinion.

Emergency research

The goal of emergency nursing research is to improve the delivery of care and thereby improve patient outcomes. Nursing care is commonly based on evidence that's derived from research. Evidence can be used to support current practices or to change practices. (See *Research and nursing*.)

The best way to get involved in research is to be a good consumer of nursing research. You can do so by reading nursing journals and being aware of the quality of research and reported results. The ENA publishes the *Journal of Emergency Nursing*, which has many pertinent research articles.

Share and share alike

Don't be afraid to share research findings with colleagues. Sharing promotes sound clinical care, and all involved may learn about easier and more efficient ways to care for patients.

Research and nursing

All scientific research is based on the same basic process, which consists of these steps:

1. **Identify a problem.** Identifying problems in the emergency environment isn't difficult. An example of such a problem is maintaining body temperature in a trauma patient.

2. **Conduct a literature review.** The goal of this step is to see what has been published about the identified problem.

3. **Formulate a research question or hypothesis.** In the case of body temperature, one question is "Which method of warming is most effective in a trauma patient?"

4. **Design a study.** The study may be experimental or nonexperimental. The nurse must decide what data should be collected and how to collect that data.

5. **Obtain consent.** The nurse must obtain consent to conduct research from the study participants. Most facilities have an internal review board that must approve such permission for studies.

6. **Collect data.** After the study is approved, the nurse can begin conducting the study and collecting the data.

7. **Analyze the data.** The nurse analyzes the data and states the conclusions derived from the analysis.

8. **Share the information.** Lastly, the researcher shares the collected information with other nurses through publications and presentations.

Evidence-based care

Evidence-based care isn't based on tradition, custom, or intuition. It's derived from various concrete sources, such as:
- formal nursing research
- clinical knowledge
- scientific knowledge.

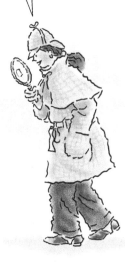

Hmmm... the evidence points to an alternate treatment.

An evidence-based example

Research results may provide insight into the treatment of a patient who, for example, doesn't respond to a medication or treatment that seemed effective for other patients.

In this example, you may believe that a certain drug should be effective for pain relief based on previous experience with that drug. The trouble with such an approach is that other factors can contribute to pain relief such as the route of administration, the dosage, and concurrent treatments.

First, last, and always

Regardless of the value of evidence-based care, you should always use professional clinical judgment when dealing with emergency patients and their families. Remember that each patient's condition ultimately dictates treatment.

Quick quiz

1.   Which essential qualification does the nurse need to work in an emergency department?
    A.   Have a baccalaureate degree
    B.   Have certification in emergency nursing
    C.   Be able to diagnose patient's medical problems
    D.   Use the nursing process in delivering nursing care

Answer: D. The professional nurse uses the nursing process (assessment, planning, implementation, and evaluation) to care for emergency patients.

2.   The nurse who has completed professional certification in emergency nursing can assuredly:
    A.   obtain a pay raise.
    B.   obtain an administrative position.
    C.   function as an advanced practice nurse.
    D.   validate knowledge and skills in emergency nursing.

Answer: D. The purpose of professional certification is to validate knowledge and skill in a particular area. Certification is a demonstration of excellence and commitment to the nurse's chosen specialty area.

3.   How does the nurse describe the purpose of the interprofessional team in delivery of patient care in the emergency setting?
   A.   Decreases filings of lawsuits
   B.   Assists the nurse in performing patient care
   C.   Provides holistic, comprehensive care to patients
   D.   Replaces the need for primary care in the emergent setting

Answer: C. The purpose of the interprofessional team is to provide comprehensive care to the emergency patient.

4.   How does the emergency nurse effectively participate in the research process?
   A.   Analyzes studies
   B.   Conducts research
   C.   Consumes published research
   D.   Participates in facility internal review board

Answer: C. The emergency nurse reads research articles and determines whether they are applicable to practice. Research findings are not useful unless they are incorporated into practice when indicated.

5.   How does the emergency nurse articulate the purpose of evidence-based care?
   A.   It improves patient outcomes
   B.   It refutes traditional nursing practices.
   C.   It validates traditional nursing practices.
   D.   It establishes a body of knowledge unique to nursing.

Answer: A. Although evidence-based practices may validate or refute traditional practice, its purpose is to improve patient outcomes.

Scoring

☆☆☆   If you answered all five questions correctly, take a bow! You're basically a whiz when it comes to emergency nursing basics.

☆☆   If you answered three or four questions correctly, there's no room for criticism! Your critical thinking skills are basically intact.

☆   If you answered fewer than three questions correctly, the situation is emergent! Review the chapter and you'll be on the right pathway.

Selected references

Carman, M., Wolf, L., Baker, K., et al. (2013). Translating research to practice: Bringing emergency nursing research full circle to the bedside. *Journal of Emergency Nursing, 39*(6), 657–659. doi:10.1016/j.jen.2013.09.004

Castner, J., Grinslade, S., Guay, J., et al. (2013). Registered nurse scope of practice and ED complaint-specific protocols. *Journal of Emergency Nursing, 39*(5), 467.e3–473.e3. doi:10.1016/j.jen.2013.02.009

Emergency Nurses Association. (2012). *Sheehy's manual of emergency care* (7th ed.). St. Louis, MO: Elsevier.

Emergency Nurses Association. (2017). *Clinical practice guideline: Family presence during invasive procedures and resuscitation. Does family presence have a positive or negative influence on the patient, family, and staff during invasive procedures and resuscitation?* Retrieved from https://www.ena.org/practice-research/research /CPG/Documents/FamilyPresenceCPG.pdf

Emergency Nurses Association. (2018). *ENA has 2020 vision: Five year strategic plan.* Retrieved from https://www.ena.org/docs/default-source/default-document-library/enastrategicplan.pdf?sfvrsn=5c367de2_2

Emergency Nurses Association. (2019). *Trauma nursing core course: Provider manual* (8th ed.). Des Plaines, IL: Author.

Falconer, S., Karuppan, C., Kiehne, E., et al. (2018). ED triage process improvement: Timely vital signs for less acute patients. *Journal of Emergency Nursing, 44*(6), 589–597. doi:10.1016/j.jen.2018.05.006

Gurney, D., Gillespie, G. L., McMahon, M., et al. (2017). Nursing code of ethics: Provisions and interpretative statements for emergency nurses. *Journal of Emergency Nursing, 43*(6), 497–503. doi: 10.1016/j/jen.2017.09.011

Malkin, M., Lenart, J., Walsh, C. A., et al. (2016). Transfusion ethics in a pediatric Jehovah's Witness trauma patient: Simulation case. *MedEdPORTAL, 12.* doi:10.15766/mep_2374-8265.10450

Rainer, J. (2015). Speaking up: Factors and issues in nurses advocating for patients when patients are in jeopardy. *Journal of Nursing Care Quality, 30*(1), 53–62.

The Joint Commission. (2015). *National patient safety goals effective January 1, 2015.* Retrieved from http://www.jointcommission.org/assets/1/6/2015_npsg _hap.pdf

Chapter 2

Holistic care

Just the facts

In this chapter, you'll learn:

- ◆ family dynamics to consider when you provide care
- ◆ issues that affect emergency patients and their families
- ◆ ways to assess and manage pain in emergency patients
- ◆ principles of ethical decision making
- ◆ concepts related to end-of-life decisions and how they're important to your care.

What is holistic health care?

Holistic health care revolves around a notion of totality. The goal of holistic care is to meet not only the patient's physical needs but also social, spiritual, and emotional needs.

A new dimension

Holistic care addresses all dimensions of a person, including:

- physical
- emotional
- social
- spiritual.

Only by considering these dimensions can the health care team provide high-quality holistic care. You should strive to provide holistic care to all emergency patients, even if their physical needs seem more pressing than other needs.

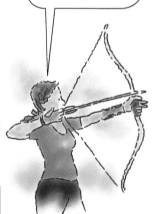

Holistic care aims to treat the entire patient from the inside out.

Holistic care issues

The road to delivering the best holistic care is strewn with various issues, including:

- patient and family issues
- cognitive issues
- ethics issues.

Patient and family issues

A family is defined as a group of two or more persons who possibly live together in the same household, perform certain interrelated social tasks, and share an emotional bond. Families can profoundly influence the individuals within them.

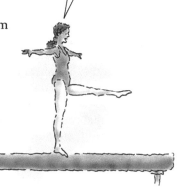

Keep in mind that the stress from a medical emergency can really throw a family off-balance.

Family ties

A family is a dynamic system. During stress-free times, this system tends to maintain homeostasis, meaning that it exists in a stable state of harmony and balance. However, when a crisis sends one family member into the emergency department (ED), the rest may feel a tremendous strain and family homeostasis is thrown off. The major effects of such imbalances are:

- increased stress levels
- reorganization of family roles.

Slipping on emotional turmoil

The emergency patient's condition may change rapidly (within minutes or hours); the result of such physiologic instability is emotional turmoil and psychological stress for the family. Family members may use whatever coping mechanisms they have, such as seeking support from friends or clergy. The longer the patient remains in the ED, however, the more stress and psychological distress increases for the patient and his or her family.

Circle out of round

When sudden critical illness or injury disrupts the family circle, a patient can no longer fulfill certain role responsibilities. Such roles are typically:

- financial (if the patient is a major contributor to the family's monetary stability)
- social (if the patient fills such roles as spouse, parent, mediator, or disciplinarian).

Unprepared for the worst

Family members may also worry about the possible death of the patient. The suddenness of the illness or injury may overwhelm the family and put it into a crisis state. The ramifications of the patient's illness or injury may cause other family members to feel hopeless and helpless.

Nursing responsibilities

The patient's family members need guidance and support during the stay in the ED and beyond. An emergency nurse's responsibility to family is to provide information about:
- nursing care of the patient
- the patient's prognosis and expected treatments.

Lend a hand

Because you're regularly exposed to members of the patient's family, you can help them during their time of crisis. For example, you can observe the family's anxiety level and, if necessary, refer them to another member of the multidisciplinary team, such as a social worker or chaplain.

You can also help the family solve problems by helping them:
- verbalize the immediate problem
- identify support systems
- recall how they handled stress in the past.

Such assistance helps the family focus on the present issue. It also allows them to solve problems and regain some sense of control over their lives.

Lend an ear, too

You can also help the family cope with their feelings during this stressful time. Two ways to do this are by encouraging expression of feelings (such as by crying or discussing the issue) and providing empathy.

Because you asked

During a patient's stay in the ED, families come to rely on the opinions of professionals and commonly ask for their input. They need honest information given to them in terms they can understand. In many cases, you're the health care team member who provides this information.

Living with the decision

A nurse can use phrases such as "I know that you would like me to decide what's best for your loved one, but I can't make that decision because you're the ones who will have to live with the outcome." The emergency nurse then needs to reinforce and acknowledge the family's decision and accept their feelings.

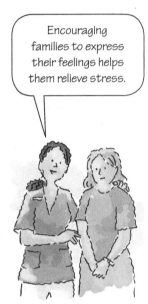

Encouraging families to express their feelings helps them relieve stress.

Cultural considerations

Cultural influences can affect how a family copes with the hospitalization of a loved one. A patient's cultural background can also affect many aspects of care, such as:

- patient and family roles during illness
- communication between health care providers and the patient and family
- feelings of the patient and family regarding end-of-life issues
- family views regarding health care practices
- pain management
- nutrition
- spiritual support.

Consider culture

To provide effective holistic care, you must honor the patient's cultural beliefs and values. Because culture can impact care, you should perform a cultural assessment. (See *Assessing cultural considerations*, page 32.)

Conducting a cultural assessment enables you to:

- recognize a patient's cultural responses to illness and hospitalization
- determine how the patient and the family define health and illness
- determine the family's beliefs about the cause of the illness.

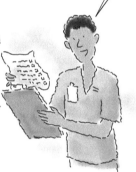

Culture affects many aspects of patient care, including pain management.

Cognitive issues

A patient in an ED may feel overwhelmed by technology. Although this equipment is essential for patient care, it can create an environment that's foreign to the patient, which can result in disturbed cognition (thought-related function) and anxiety. In addition, the disease process can affect cognitive function in an emergency patient. For example, a patient with metabolic disturbances or hypoxia can experience confusion and changes in sensorium (mental clarity).

Fair to compare

When assessing cognitive function, the first question you should ask is "What was your previous level of functioning?" If the patient can't answer this question, ask a family member.

It's a factor

Many factors impact a patient's cognitive function while in the ED, including:

- invasion of personal space
- medications
- pain
- sensory input.

Assessing cultural considerations

A cultural assessment yields the information you need to administer high-quality nursing care to members of various cultural populations. The goal of the cultural assessment quest is to gain awareness and understanding of cultural variations and their effects on the care you provide. For each patient, you and other members of the multidisciplinary team use the findings of a cultural assessment to develop an individualized care plan.

When performing a cultural assessment, be sure to ask questions that yield certain information about the patient and his or her family, including questions about:

- cultural health beliefs
- communication methods
- cultural restrictions
- social networks
- nutritional status
- religion
- values and beliefs.

Here are examples of the types of questions you should consider for each patient.

Cultural health beliefs

- What does the patient believe caused the illness? A patient may believe that the illness is the result of an imbalance in yin and yang, punishment for a past transgression, or the result of divine wrath.
- How does the patient typically express pain?
- What does the patient believe promotes health? Beliefs can range from eating certain foods to wearing amulets for good luck.
- In what types of healing practices (such as herbal remedies and healing rituals) does the patient engage?

Communication differences

- What language does the patient speak?
- Does the patient require an interpreter?
- How does the patient want to be addressed?
- What are the styles of nonverbal communication (e.g., eye contact or touching)?

Cultural expressions

- How does the patient's cultural group express emotion?
- How are feelings about death, dying, and grief expressed?
- How is modesty expressed or protected?
- Does the patient have restrictions related to exposure of parts of the body?

Social networks

- What are the roles of each family member during health and illness?
- Who makes the legal and health care decisions for the patient?

Nutrition

- What's the meaning of food and eating to the patient?
- What types of food does the patient eat? Foods to be avoided?
- Does the patient's food need to be prepared a certain way?

Religion

- What's the role of religious beliefs and practices during illness?
- Does the patient believe that special rites or blessings need to be performed?
- Are there healing rituals or practices that must be followed?

Invasion of personal space

Personal space is the unmarked boundary or territory around a person. Several factors—such as cultural background and social situation—influence a patient's interpretation of personal space. A patient's personal space is limited in many ways by the emergency environment—for example, due to the confines of bed rest, lack of privacy, and use of invasive equipment.

You can try to increase your patient's sense of personal space—even within the emergency environment—by simply remembering to show common courtesy, such as:

- asking permission to perform a procedure or look at a wound or dressing
- pulling the curtain or closing the door
- knocking before you enter the patient's room.

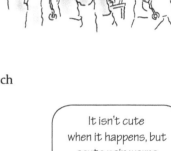

If you think finding personal space in the ED is hard, imagine what it's like for a patient!

Medications

Many medications can cause adverse central nervous system reactions and affect cognitive function. A few examples include:

- inotropics—such as digoxin (Lanoxin), which can cause agitation, hallucinations, malaise, dizziness, vertigo, and paresthesias
- corticosteroids—such as prednisone, which can cause euphoria, psychotic behavior, insomnia, vertigo, headache, paresthesias, and seizures
- benzodiazepines—such as lorazepam (Ativan), which can cause drowsiness, sedation, disorientation, amnesia, unsteadiness, and agitation
- opioid analgesics—such as hydromorphone (Dilaudid), which can cause sedation, clouded sensorium, euphoria, dizziness, light-headedness, and somnolence.

Pain control issues

Because fear of pain is a major concern for many emergency patients, pain management is an important part of your care. Emergency patients are exposed to many types of procedures—such as intravenous (IV) procedures, cardiac monitoring, and intubation—that cause discomfort and pain. Pain is classified as acute or chronic.

Acute pain

Acute pain is caused by tissue damage due to injury or disease. It varies in intensity from mild to severe and lasts briefly. Acute pain is considered a protective mechanism because it warns of present or potential tissue damage or organ disease. It may result from a traumatic injury, surgical or diagnostic procedure, or medical disorder.

Examples include:

- pain experienced after a traumatic injury
- pain experienced during invasive procedures
- pain of acute myocardial infarction.

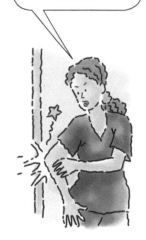

It isn't cute when it happens, but acute pain warns of potential tissue damage or organ disease.

Help is at hand

Acute pain can be managed effectively with analgesics, such as opioids and nonsteroidal anti-inflammatory drugs (NSAIDs). It generally subsides when the underlying problem is resolved.

Chronic pain

Chronic pain is ongoing pain that lasts 6 months or longer. It may be as intense as acute pain but isn't a warning of tissue damage. Some patients in the ED may experience chronic pain as well as acute pain.

Examples of chronic pain include:
- arthritis pain
- chronic back pain
- chronic pain from cancer.

Don't be fooled

The nervous system adapts to chronic pain. This adaptation means that many typical manifestations of pain—such as abnormal vital signs and facial grimacing—cease to exist. Therefore, chronic pain should be assessed as often as acute pain (generally, at least every 2 hours or more often, depending on the patient's condition). Assess chronic pain by questioning the patient.

Pain assessment

When it comes to pain assessment for emergency patients, it's especially important for the nurse to have good assessment skills. The most valid pain assessment comes from the patient's own reports.

A pain assessment includes questions about:
- *location.* Ask the patient to tell you where the pain is; there may be more than one area of pain.
- *intensity.* Ask the patient to rate the pain using a pain scale.
- *quality.* Ask how the pain feels: sharp, dull, aching, or burning.
- *onset, duration, and frequency.* Ask when the pain started, how long it lasts, and how often it occurs.
- *alleviating and aggravating factors.* Ask what makes the pain feel better and what makes it worse.
- *associated factors.* Ask whether other problems are associated with the pain, such as nausea and vomiting.
- *effects on lifestyle.* Ask whether appetite, sleep, relationships, emotions, and work are affected.

Choose a tool

Many pain assessment tools are available. Whichever you choose, make sure it's used consistently so that everyone on the health care team is speaking the same language when addressing the patient's pain.

Common pain-rating scales

These common pain-rating scales are examples of the rating systems you can use to help a patient quantify pain levels.

Visual analog scale

To use the visual analog scale, ask the patient to place a line across the scale to indicate the current level of pain. The scale is a 10-cm line with "No pain" at one end and "Pain as bad as it can be" at the other end. The pain rating is determined by using a ruler to measure the distance, in millimeters, from "No pain" to the patient's mark.

No pain _____ **Pain as bad as it can be**

Numeric rating scale

To use the numeric rating scale, ask the patient to choose a number from 0 (indicating no pain) to 10 (indicating the worst pain imaginable) to indicate his or her current pain level. The patient may circle the number on the scale or verbally state the number that best describes the pain.

No pain | 0 1 2 3 4 5 6 7 8 9 10 11 12 | **Pain as bad as it can be**

Wong-Baker FACES® scale

A patient age 3 or older or an adult patient with language difficulty may not be able to describe the current pain level using the visual analog scale or the numeric rating scale. In that case, use a faces scale like the one that follows. Ask your patient to choose the face on a scale from 0 to 10 that best represents the severity of current pain.

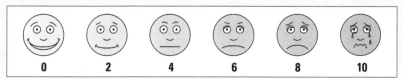

| 0 | 2 | 4 | 6 | 8 | 10 |

©2015 Wong-Baker FACE® Foundation. Used with permission.

The three most common pain assessment tools used by clinicians are the visual analog scale, numeric rating scale, and faces scale. (See *Common pain-rating scales*.)

Silent suffering

Many patients can't verbally express feelings of pain. For example, a patient may be unable to speak due to intubation or have an altered level of consciousness ranging from confusion to unresponsiveness. In such cases, it's up to the nurse to ascertain the patient's pain level.

Body and mind

There are many physiologic and psychological responses to pain that a nurse should watch for during a pain assessment. Nurses in the ED must remember that some patients are not familiar with many of the terms used in the medical environment and lack health literacy. Health literacy deficits have been linked with increased mortality, lower patient satisfaction with health care, and overuse of ED for health care needs (Nierengarten, 2018).

Some examples of physiologic responses to pain are:
- tachycardia
- tachypnea
- dilated pupils
- increased or decreased blood pressure
- pallor
- nausea and vomiting
- loss of appetite
- agitation.

Psychological responses to pain may manifest as:
- fear
- anxiety
- confusion
- depression
- sleep deprivation.

Pain particulars

When communicating aspects of a patient's pain to the health care provider, make sure you:
- describe the pain by location, intensity, and duration
- indicate possible causes of the pain if known
- describe how the patient is responding to the pain or any treatment interventions.

Pain management

Achieving adequate pain control in the ED depends on effective pain assessment and the use of pharmacologic and nonpharmacologic treatments.

To provide the best holistic care possible, work with the primary health care provider and other members of the health care team to develop an individualized pain management program for each patient.

Pharmacologic pain management

Pharmacologic pain management is common in EDs. Three classes of medications commonly used by the emergency nurse are:
- nonopioids
- opioids
- adjuvant medications.

A trio of opioids

Opioids block the release of neurotransmitters that send pain signals to the brain. The three categories of opioids are opioid agonists (opioid analgesics), opioid antagonists (opioid reversal agents), and mixed opioid agonist–antagonists.

Opioid agonists

Opioid agonists relieve pain by binding to pain receptors, which, in effect, produce pain relief. Examples of opioid agonists are:

• morphine (Duramorph)
• fentanyl (Duragesic)
• hydromorphone (Dilaudid)
• codeine
• oxycodone.

Opioid antagonists

Opioid antagonists attach to opiate receptors without producing agonistic effects. They work by displacing the opioid at the receptor site and reversing the analgesic and respiratory depressant effects of the opioid. Examples of opioid antagonists are:

• naloxone (Narcan)
• naltrexone.

Mixed opioid agonist–antagonists

Mixed opioid agonist–antagonists relieve pain by binding to opiate receptors to effect varying degrees of agonistic and antagonistic activity. They carry a lower risk of toxic effects and drug dependency than opioid agonists and opioid antagonists. However, they are not commonly used for pain control. Examples of mixed opioid agonist–antagonists are:

• buprenorphine
• butorphanol.

Nonopioids are number 1

Nonopioids are the first choice for managing mild pain. They decrease pain by inhibiting inflammation at the injury site. Examples of nonopioids are:

- acetaminophen (Tylenol)
- NSAIDs, such as ibuprofen (Advil) and naproxen (Naprosyn)
- salicylates such as aspirin.

    NSAIDs should be avoided for patients at risk for bleeding or those with severe liver disease.

Opioid option

Opioids are narcotics that contain a derivative of the opium (poppy) plant and other synthetic drugs that imitate natural opioids. Opioids work by blocking the release of neurotransmitters involved in transmitting pain signals to the brain. There are three categories of opioids. (See *A trio of opioids*.)

Adjuvants are all right

Adjuvant analgesics are drugs that have other primary indications but are used as analgesics in some circumstances. Adjuvants may be given in combination with opioids or alone to treat patients with chronic pain. Drugs used as adjuvant analgesics include:

- anticonvulsants, such as carbamazepine (Carbatrol), clonazepam (Klonopin), and gabapentin (Neurontin)
- tricyclic antidepressants, such as nortriptyline (Pamelor)
- benzodiazepines, such as alprazolam (Xanax), diazepam (Valium), and lorazepam (Ativan)
- corticosteroids, such as dexamethasone and methylprednisolone (Medrol).

> Adjuvant analgesics work alone or with a partner to help alleviate chronic pain.

Drug administration

A common route of pain medication administration in the ED is IV bolus on an as-needed basis. It's the preferred route for opioid therapy, especially when short-term pain relief is needed—for example, during procedures such as wound care. The benefit of this method is rapid pain control. On the downside, with IV bolus administration, the patient experiences alternating periods of pain control and pain.

Nonpharmacologic pain management

Pain control isn't achieved solely with medications. Nonpharmacologic means are useful adjuncts in managing pain. Some common nonpharmacologic pain control methods are:

- distraction—such as television viewing and reading
- music therapy—a form of sound therapy using rhythmic sound to communicate, relax, and encourage healing (effective for brief periods of time)
- hypnosis—used to achieve *symptom suppression*, to block awareness of pain, or *symptom substitution*, which allows a positive interpretation of pain
- guided imagery—in which the patient visualizes a soothing image while the nurse describes pleasant sensations (For example, the patient may picture himself or herself at the beach while you describe the sounds of the waves and birds and the feel of the warm sun and a breeze on the patient's skin.)
- relaxation therapy—a form of meditation used to focus attention on a single sound or image or on the rhythm of breathing
- heat application (thermotherapy)—application of dry or moist heat to decrease pain (Heat enhances blood flow, increases tissue metabolism, and decreases vasomotor tone; it also may relieve pain due to muscle aches or spasms, itching, or joint pain.)
- cold application (cryotherapy)—constricts blood vessels at the injury site, reducing blood flow to the site (Cold slows edema development, prevents further tissue damage, and minimizes bruising; it may be more effective than heat in relieving such pain as muscle aches or spasms, itching, incision pain, headaches, and joint pain.)

> Imagery gives me a vacation away from pain.

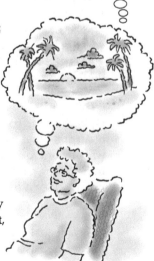

- transcutaneous electrical nerve stimulation—in which electrodes transmit mild electrical impulses to the brain to block pain impulses
- massage therapy—manipulation of soft tissue to enhance healing that can reduce anxiety, muscle tension, and pain (McMillan et al., 2018).

Sensory input

Sensory stimulation in any environment may be perceived as pleasant or unpleasant and comfortable or painful. The emergency environment tends to stimulate all five senses:

1. auditory
2. visual
3. gustatory
4. olfactory
5. tactile.

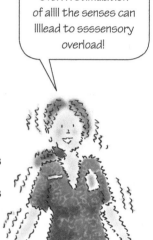

Overrrrstimulation of allll the senses can lllead to ssssensory overload!

Too much or too little

Patients in the ED don't have control over the environmental stimulation around them. They may experience sensory deprivation, sensory overload, or both. *Sensory deprivation* can result from a reduction in the quantity and quality of normal and familiar sensory input, such as the normal sights and sounds encountered at home. *Sensory overload* results from an increase in the amount of unfamiliar sounds and sights in the emergency environment, such as beeping cardiac monitors, ringing telephones, overhead paging systems, and voices.

When environmental stimuli exceed the patient's ability to cope with the stimulation, the patient may experience anxiety, confusion, and panic as well as delusions.

Ethical issues

Nurses who work in EDs routinely deal with ethical dilemmas. You'll recognize a situation as an ethical dilemma in these circumstances:

- More than one solution exists; that is, there's no clear "right" or "wrong" way to handle a situation.
- Each solution carries equal weight.
- Each solution is ethically defensible.

The value of values

Ethical dilemmas in EDs commonly revolve around quality-of-life issues for the patient, especially as they relate to end-of-life decisions—such as do-not-resuscitate orders, life support, and patients' requests for no heroic measures. When considering quality of life, make sure others don't impose their own value system on the patient. Each person has a set of personal values that are influenced by environment and culture. Nurses also have a set of professional values.

Code of ethics

The American Nurses Association (ANA) and Emergency Nurses Association (ENA) have established a code of ethics (ANA, 2015; Gurney et al., 2017). The ANA code of ethics for nurses provides information that's necessary for a practicing nurse to use professional skills in providing the most effective holistic care possible, such as serving as a patient advocate and striving to protect the health, safety, and rights of each patient (ANA, 2015). The current ANA code of ethics may be reviewed online to enhance the nurse's understanding regarding a variety of topics including holistic patient care: https://www.nursingworld.org/coe-view-only.

End-of-life decisions

The threat of death is common in EDs. Perhaps at no other time is the holistic care of patients and their families as important as it is during this time. End-of-life decisions are almost always difficult for patients, families, and health care professionals to make. Nurses are in a unique position as advocates to assist patients and their families through this process. Nurses have an obligation to educate patients and their families regarding their legal right to self-determination and end-of-life decisions.

Unsolvable mysteries

Your primary role as a patient advocate is to promote the patient's wishes. In many instances, however, a patient's wishes aren't known. That's when ethical decision making takes priority. Decisions aren't always easy to make and the answers aren't always clear cut. At times, such ethical dilemmas may seem unsolvable.

A question of quality

It's sometimes difficult to determine what can be done to achieve good quality of life and what can simply be achieved, technologically speaking. Technologic advances sometimes seem to exceed our ability to analyze the ethical dilemmas associated with them.

Years ago, death was considered a natural part of life and most people died at home, surrounded by their families. Today, most people die in hospitals, and death is commonly regarded as a medical failure rather than a natural event. Sometimes, it's hard for you to know whether you're assisting in extending the patient's life or delaying the patient's death.

Consulting the committee

Most hospitals have ethics committees that review ethical dilemmas. The nurse may consider consulting the ethics committee if:
- the health care provider disagrees with the patient or family regarding treatment of the patient
- health care providers disagree among themselves about treatment options
- family members disagree about what should be done.

Determining medical futility

Medical futility refers to treatment that's hopeless or interventions that aren't likely to benefit the patient even though they may appear to be effective. For example, a patient with a terminal illness who's expected to die experiences cardiac arrest. Cardiopulmonary resuscitation may be effective in restoring a heartbeat but may still be deemed futile because it doesn't change the patient's outcome.

Dealing with cardiac arrest

In case of cardiac arrest (sudden stoppage of the heart), an emergency patient may be described by a code status. This code status describes the orders written by the health care provider describing what resuscitation measures should be carried out by the nurse and should be based on the patient's wishes regarding resuscitation measures. When cardiac arrest occurs, you must ensure that resuscitative efforts are initiated or that unwanted resuscitation doesn't take place.

Who decides?

The wishes of a competent, informed patient should always be honored. However, when a patient can't make decisions, the health care team—consisting of the patient's family, nursing staff, and physicians—may have to make end-of-life decisions for the patient.

Advance directives

Most people prefer to make their own decisions regarding end-of-life care. It's important that patients discuss their wishes with their loved ones; however, many don't. Instead, total strangers may be asked to make important health care decisions when patients can't do so. That's why it's important for people to make choices ahead of time and to make these choices known by developing advance directives.

The Patient Self-Determination Act requires hospitals and other institutions to make information available to patients on advance directives. However, it isn't mandatory for patients to have advance directives. Although ED nurses should understand the advance directive process, it should be understood that during a stressful ED visit is not the time for patients and family members to make these difficult decisions. Advance directives are best determined after a diagnosis and prior to any ED or hospital visit (Miller, 2017).

Where there's a will, there's a law

There are two types of advance directives:

- *living will*
- *durable power of attorney for health care.*

A living will states what treatments a patient will accept and what treatments the patient will refuse in case terminal illness renders the patient unable to make those decisions at the time. For example, a patient may be willing to accept artificial nutrition but not hemodialysis.

Durable power of attorney is the appointment of a person—chosen by the patient—to make decisions on the patient's behalf if the patient can no longer do so. Durable power of attorney for health care doesn't give the chosen individual authority to access business accounts; the power is strictly related to health care decisions (Ignatavicius et al., 2018).

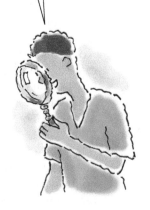

Although they aren't mandatory, advance directives can take a lot of the mystery out of end-of-life care decisions.

It takes two

After an advance directive is written, two witnesses must sign it. This document can be altered or canceled at any time. For more information, check the laws regarding advance directives for the state in which you practice.

Organ donation

When asked, most people say that they support organ donation. However, only a small percentage of qualified organs are ever donated. Tens of thousands of names are on waiting lists for organs in the United States alone. Organ transplantation is successful for many patients, giving them additional, high-quality years of life.

The Uniform Anatomical Gift Act governs the donation of organs and tissues. In addition, most states have legislation governing the procurement of organs and tissues. Some require medical staff to ask about organ donation on every death. Other states require staff to notify a regional organ procurement agency that then approaches the family. Become familiar with the laws of your state and the policies of the facility in which you practice.

Standards deviation

Medical criteria for organ donation vary from state to state. Many organ procurement agencies want to be notified of all deaths and imminent deaths so that they, not the medical staff, can determine if the patient is a potential candidate for organ donation.

Donations accepted

Any patient who donates organs must first be declared brain dead. Death used to be defined as the cessation of respiratory and cardiac function. However, developments in technology have made this definition obsolete. We now rely on brain death criteria to determine an individual's death.

Quick quiz

1.   Which statement regarding culture and health does the nurse recognize as accurate?
   A.   Cultural impacts will have a positive effect on patient's outcomes.
   B.   Culture doesn't affect the patient's hospitalization.
   C.   Cultural factors can affect patient and family roles during illness.
   D.   Culture rarely impacts decisions about health.

Answer: C. Cultural factors can have a major impact on patient and family roles during illness. Culture affects the patient's and family members' feelings about illness, pain, and end-of-life issues, among other things. Cultural beliefs do not always coincide with positive patient outcomes. Due to some cultural beliefs, the nurse may not be able to complete lifesaving interventions.

2.   The ED nurse is caring for a patient whose cognitive function seems slightly impaired. Which factor does the nurse assess to determine the cause? Select all that apply.
   A.   Pain presence
   B.   Anxiety or fear
   C.   Current health status
   D.   Medication being taken
   E.   Invasion of personal space

Answer: A, B, C, D, and E. All of these factors can impact the patient's cognitive function while in the ED.

3.   The nurse is caring for a patient who experienced a mild ankle sprain. Which treatment order would the nurse question?
   A.   Naproxen
   B.   Ibuprofen
   C.   Oxycodone
   D.   Acetaminophen

Answer: C. Nonopioids are the first choice for managing mild pain. Oxycodone is an opioid which is used for severe pain; therefore, the nurse will question this treatment order.

Scoring

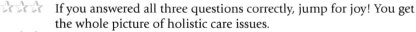

★★★   If you answered all three questions correctly, jump for joy! You get the whole picture of holistic care issues.

★★   If you answered two questions correctly, we won't issue a complaint! You're ready to join the team.

★   If you answered fewer than two questions correctly, don't worry; it isn't an ethical dilemma! Just review the chapter and try again.

Selected references

American Nurses Association. (2015). *Code of ethics for nurses with interpretive statements.* Retrieved from https://www.nursingworld.org/coe-view-only

Gurney, D., Gillespie, G. L., McMahon, M. P., et al. (2017). Nursing code of ethics: Provisions and interpretative statements for emergency nurses. *Journal of Emergency Nursing, 43*(6), 497–503. Retrieved from https://www.ena.org/docs/default-source/resource-library/practice-resources/ethics/ethics.pdf?sfvrsn=cb143931_8

Ignatavicius, D., Workman, L., & Rebar, C. (2018). *Medical-surgical nursing: Concepts for interprofessional collaborative care* (9th ed.). St. Louis, MO: Elsevier.

McMillan, K., Glaser, D., & Radovich, P. (2018). The effect of massage on pain and anxiety in hospital patients: An observational study. *MedSurg Nursing, 27*(1), 14–18.

Miller, B. (2017). Nurses in the know: The history and future of advance directives. *Online Journal of Issues in Nursing, 22*(3). doi:10.3912/OJIN.Vol22No03PPT57

Nierengarten, M. (2018). Improving health literacy. *Contemporary OB/GYN, 63*(6), 42–45.

Chapter 3

Neurologic emergencies

Just the facts

In this chapter, you'll learn:

◆ key areas to assess when dealing with neurologic emergencies

◆ important diagnostic tests and procedures used for neurologic emergencies

◆ common neurologic emergencies and their treatments.

Understanding neurologic emergencies

The neurologic system is a highly complex system that plays a major role in regulating many body functions. Emergencies that affect the neurologic system can be life-threatening. In the event of an emergency involving the neurologic system, you, the nurse, must thoroughly assess the patient and be astute to subtle changes, which may indicate potential deterioration in condition. The nurse formulates a plan for interventions based on the focused assessment findings. These interventions must be implemented quickly to minimize the risks to the patient.

Assessment

A complete and thorough assessment of the nervous system is vital. Damage to the nervous system can cause problems in daily function (Johns Hopkins Medicine, n.d.). Because the nervous system is complex, assessment of subtle and elusive changes can be difficult. A thorough health history and investigation of physical signs of impairment are necessary data to collect when you assess a patient for possible neurologic impairment.

I know this is difficult, but a detailed history is the basis of neurologic emergency assessment. Now, tell me more about your childhood brain injury.

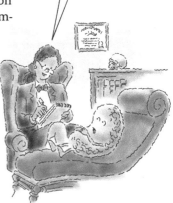

Check the records

In the event a patient cannot be interviewed because of the condition or impairment, evaluation of the patient's electronic medical record could provide you information about the patient's history. Other important sources of information may be provided by family members and the emergency medical response team that may have provided transportation of the patient to the emergency department (ED).

History

To collect a focused health history, gather details about the patient's current state of health, previous health status, lifestyle, environment, and family health (Lewis et al., 2017).

Friends and family fill in

A patient with a neurologic emergency may have trouble remembering or relating information. When gathering information about the health history, you should first allow the patient to answer questions. If the patient's family or close friends are available, they may be able to assist in validating or correcting details of the patient's health history.

Current health

Discover the patient's chief concern by asking such questions as "Can you tell me why you came to the hospital?" or "Can you describe what has been concerning you lately?" When documenting subjective reports, use the patient's own words.

Common concerns

If your patient is suffering from a neurologic emergency, symptoms may include headaches, visual disturbances, motor disturbances (such as weakness, tremors, paresthesia, paresis, and paralysis), seizures, sensory deviations, and an altered level of consciousness (LOC) (Johns Hopkins Medicine, n.d.).

Details, please

Encourage the patient to describe details of the current condition by asking such questions as:
- Can you describe your headache?
- When did you start feeling dizzy?
- What were you doing when the numbness started?
- Have you ever had seizures or tremors?
- Have you ever had weakness or paralysis in your arms or legs?
- Do you have trouble urinating, walking, speaking, understanding others, reading, or writing?
- How is your memory and ability to concentrate (Lewis et al., 2017)?

Previous health

Many chronic diseases affect the neurologic system, so ask questions about the patient's past health and use of medications. Specifically, ask whether the patient has had any:

- major illnesses
- recurrent minor illnesses
- injuries
- surgical procedures
- allergies.

Lifestyle

Ask questions about the patient's cultural and social background as well as the living environment because these affect care decisions. Note the patient's education level, occupation, and hobbies. Asking about family or support the patient may have is also important. As you gather this information, assess the patient's self-image. Also ask about smoking, alcohol consumption, and recreational drug use.

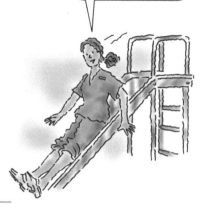

A patient's hobbies can really "play" into the neurologic assessment. Be sure to ask about them!

Physical examination

A complete neurologic examination is long and detailed. When performing a neurologic assessment, the nurse must first identify if an emergency exists. Decreasing level of LOC during assessment is an abnormal assessment finding, which should prompt the nurse to a potential emergency (Lewis et al., 2017). Depending on the nature of the patient's condition, limit your examination to specific problem areas or stop your examination entirely to intervene if the patient exhibits signs and symptoms of deterioration. If your initial screening indicates a neurologic problem, you will need to conduct a more detailed assessment (Lewis et al., 2017).

Top-to-bottom examination

Examine the patient's neurologic system in an orderly way. Beginning with the highest levels of neurologic function and working down to the lowest, assess these five areas:

1. mental status
2. cranial nerve function
3. sensory function
4. motor function
5. reflexes.

Quick check of mental status

To quickly screen your patient for disordered thought processes, ask the questions below. An incorrect answer to any question may indicate the need for a more detailed mental status examination. Make sure that you know the correct answers before asking the questions.

Question	Function screened
What is your name?	Orientation to person
What is your mother's name?	Orientation to other people
What year is it?	Orientation to time
Can you tell me where you are?	Orientation to place
How old are you?	Memory
Where were you born?	Remote memory
What did you have for breakfast?	Recent memory
Who is the president of the United States?	General knowledge
Can you count backward from 20 to 1?	Attention span and calculation skills

Mental status

Mental status assessment begins when you observe and talk to the patient. Components of the mental status assessment include general appearance, cognition, mood, and affect (Lewis et al., 2017). Responses to your questions reveal clues about the patient's orientation and memory. Use these clues as a guide during the physical assessment.

No easy answers

Be sure to ask questions that require more than yes-or-no answers. Otherwise, confusion or disorientation might not be revealed. If you have doubts about a patient's mental status, perform a screening examination. (See *Quick check of mental status.*)

Three-part exam

Use the mental status examination to check these three parameters:
1. LOC
2. speech
3. cognitive function.

Level of consciousness

Watch for any change in the patient's LOC. Changes in LOC are the earliest and most sensitive indicator of changes in neurologic status. Changes can indicate worsening or improvement in neurologic status.

Descriptions and definitions

Many terms are used to describe LOC, and definitions differ widely among health care providers. To avoid confusion, clearly describe the patient's response to various stimuli and avoid using words such as:

- lethargic
- stuporous
- comatose.

The Glasgow Coma Scale offers an objective way to assess the patient's LOC (Glasgow Coma Scale, n.d.). (See *Using the Glasgow Coma Scale*, page 50.)

Looking at LOC

Start by quietly observing the patient's behavior. If the patient appears to be sleeping or unconscious, try to rouse the patient by providing an appropriate stimulus in this order:

1. auditory
2. tactile
3. painful (Baird, 2016).

Speech

Listen to how well the patient expresses thoughts (Baird, 2016). Are the words spoken appropriate, does the patient seem to have problems finding or articulating words, or is the speech slurred?

It's hard to say

To assess for dysarthria (difficulty forming words), ask the patient to repeat the phrase "No ifs, ands, or buts." Assess speech comprehension by determining the patient's ability to follow instructions and cooperate with your examination.

Language changes

Keep in mind that language performance tends to fluctuate with the time of day and changes in physical condition. A healthy person may have language difficulty when ill or fatigued. However, increasing speech difficulties may indicate deteriorating neurologic status, which warrants further evaluation. Also consider the patient's level of language proficiency based on age, culture, and baseline deficits.

When, then who

To quickly test your patient's orientation, memory, and attention span, use the mental status screening questions. Orientation to time is usually disrupted first; orientation to person, last. Always consider the

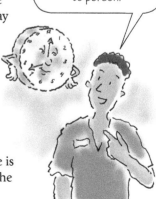

A patient's orientation to time is usually disrupted before the orientation to person.

Using the Glasgow Coma Scale

The Glasgow Coma Scale is used to convey the level of consciousness of a patient. The findings describe the patient's baseline mental status and may be used to monitor trends in responsiveness (Glasgow Coma Scale, n.d.).

The scale is used to test the patient's ability to respond to verbal, motor, and sensory stimulation; the results are then scored. A patient who is alert; can follow simple commands; and is oriented to time, place, and person receives a score of 15 points. A lower score in one or more categories may signal an impending neurologic crisis. A total score of 8 or less indicates severe neurologic damage (Glasgow Coma Scale, n.d.). Of the three components, motor response is the least affected by confounding variables and most predictive of neurologic outcome.

Test	Score	Patient's response
Eye-opening response		
Spontaneously	4	Opens eyes spontaneously
To speech	3	Opens eyes in response to verbal stimulus
To pain	2	Opens eyes only on painful stimulus
None	1	Doesn't open eyes in response to stimulus
Verbal response		
Oriented	5	Is oriented to person, place, and time
Confused	4	Tells incorrect year
Inappropriate words	3	Replies randomly with words
Incomprehensible	2	Moans or screams
None	1	Doesn't respond
Motor response		
Obeys commands	6	Responds to simple commands
Localizes pain	5	Reaches toward painful stimulus and tries to remove it
Withdraws from pain	4	Moves away from painful stimulus
Abnormal flexion	3	Assumes a decorticate posture (shown below)
Abnormal extension	2	Assumes a decerebrate posture (shown below)
None	1	Doesn't respond; just lies flaccid
Total score		

patient's environment and physical condition when assessing orientation. Environmental stimuli can alter the patient's orientation to time. For example, a patient admitted to the ED may not be oriented to date because of the events, the activity, bright lights, and noise in the department itself, but the patient may still remember the year.

Thought content

Disordered thought patterns may indicate delirium or psychosis. Assess thought pattern by evaluating the clarity and cohesiveness of the patient's ideas. Does the patient converse smoothly with logical transitions between ideas? Does the patient have hallucinations (sensory perceptions that lack appropriate stimuli) or delusions (beliefs not supported by reality) (Halter, 2018)?

Insight on insight

Test your patient's insight by finding out whether the patient:
- has a realistic view of self
- is aware of illness and circumstances.
  For example, you might ask "What do you think caused your back pain?" Expect different patients to have different degrees of insight. For instance, a patient may attribute chest discomfort to indigestion rather than acknowledge having had a heart attack.

Lost in emotion

Throughout the interview, assess your patient's emotional status. Note the patient's mood, emotional lability or stability, and the appropriateness of emotional responses. You may assess the patient's mood by asking the patient to express feelings about the future. Keep in mind that signs and symptoms of depression in an older adult patient may differ from those of children and young adults (Halter, 2018). (See *Depression and older adult patients.*)

Cranial nerve function

Cranial nerve assessment reveals valuable information about the condition of the central nervous system (CNS), especially the brainstem. The 12 cranial nerves form the juncture between the brain (the CNS) and the head and neck (the peripheral nervous system) (Johns Hopkins Medicine, n.d.). (See *Identifying cranial nerves*, page 52.)

Under pressure

Because of their location, some cranial nerves are more vulnerable to the effects of increasing intracranial pressure (ICP). Therefore, a neurologic screening assessment of the CNS focuses on these key nerves:
- oculomotor (CN III)
- abducens (CN VI) (Lewis et al., 2017).

Remember that even healthy patients have different levels of inSIGHT.

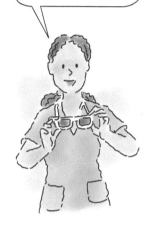

Ages and stages

Depression and older adult patients

Symptoms of depression in older adults may be different from those found in other patients. For example, rather than the usual sad affect seen in patients with depression, older adult patients may exhibit atypical signs such as decreased function, disturbed sleeping with early morning wakening, increased agitation, indecisiveness, and a sense of hopelessness (Lewis et al., 2017).

Identifying cranial nerves

Each cranial nerve is identified with the letters *CN*, and a Roman numeral, such as: *CN I, CN II, CN III*, and so on. The locations of the cranial nerves as well as their functions are shown below.

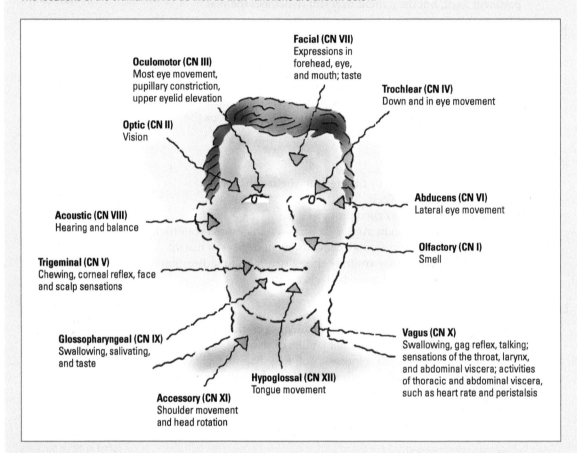

Facial (CN VII)
Expressions in forehead, eye, and mouth; taste

Oculomotor (CN III)
Most eye movement, pupillary constriction, upper eyelid elevation

Trochlear (CN IV)
Down and in eye movement

Optic (CN II)
Vision

Abducens (CN VI)
Lateral eye movement

Acoustic (CN VIII)
Hearing and balance

Olfactory (CN I)
Smell

Trigeminal (CN V)
Chewing, corneal reflex, face and scalp sensations

Glossopharyngeal (CN IX)
Swallowing, salivating, and taste

Vagus (CN X)
Swallowing, gag reflex, talking; sensations of the throat, larynx, and abdominal viscera; activities of thoracic and abdominal viscera, such as heart rate and peristalsis

Hypoglossal (CN XII)
Tongue movement

Accessory (CN XI)
Shoulder movement and head rotation

Get on some other nerves

Evaluate all cranial nerves if the patient's history or symptoms indicate a potential CNS emergency or when performing a complete nervous system assessment.

See about sight

Next, assess the optic (CN II) and oculomotor (CN III) nerves:
- To assess the optic nerve, check visual acuity and visual fields. Do this by using a Snellen eye chart, starting with large print and moving to small print.

- To assess the oculomotor nerve, check pupil size, pupil shape, direct and consensual response to light, and directions of gaze. When assessing pupil size, look for trends such as a gradual change in the size of one pupil or appearance of unequal pupils (Baird, 2016; Lewis et al., 2017). (See *Recognizing pupillary changes*, page 54.)

Funny face

To test the motor portion of the facial nerve (CN VII) to assess for possible stroke or Bell palsy, ask the patient to:
- wrinkle the forehead
- raise and lower the eyebrows
- smile to show teeth
- puff out the cheeks (Johns Hopkins Medicine, n.d.).

Also, with the patient's eyes tightly closed, attempt to open the eyelids. As you conduct each part of this test, look for symmetry.

Bouncing and spinning

To test the vestibular portion of the acoustic nerve, observe the patient for nystagmus (abnormal eye movement) (Lewis et al., 2017) and disturbed balance, such as in a cerebellar stroke or Ménière disease. Note reports of the room spinning or dizziness.

Check the pipes

Test the glossopharyngeal (CN IX) and vagus nerves (CN X) together because their innervation overlaps in the pharynx:
- The glossopharyngeal nerve is responsible for swallowing, salivating, and taste perception on the posterior one-third of the tongue.
- The vagus nerve controls swallowing and is responsible for voice quality (Johns Hopkins Medicine, n.d.).

First, assess these nerves by listening to the patient's vocal quality. Then check the gag reflex by touching the tip of a tongue blade against the posterior pharynx and asking the patient to open wide and say "ah." Watch for the symmetrical upward movement of the soft palate and uvula and the midline position of the uvula. Abnormal findings may indicate stroke, expanding hematoma of the neck, palate infection, neuromuscular disease, or airway foreign body.

Shrug it off

To assess for possible stroke or upper spinal cord injury, assess the spinal accessory nerve (CN XI), which controls the sternocleidomastoid muscles and the upper portion of the trapezius muscles. Press down on the patient's shoulders while he or she attempts to shrug against this resistance. Note shoulder strength and symmetry while inspecting and palpating the trapezius muscles.

Recognizing pupillary changes

Use this table as a guide to recognize pupillary changes and identify possible causes.

Pupillary change	Possible causes
Unilateral, dilated (≥4 mm), and nonreactive 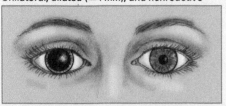	• Uncal herniation with oculomotor nerve compression • Brainstem compression • Cranial nerve (CN) III compression or injury • Increased intracranial pressure • Head trauma with subdural or epidural hematoma, or orbital injury (Good & Kirkwood, 2018)
Bilateral, dilated (≥4 mm), and nonreactive 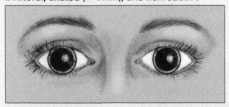	• Severe brain damage • Sympathomimetic intoxication (e.g., cocaine, methamphetamine) • Anticholinergic poisoning (e.g., atropine) • Severe brain anoxia and ischemia (Good & Kirkwood, 2018)
Bilateral, midsize, and nonreactive 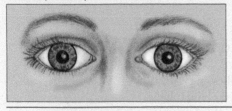	• Midbrain involvement caused by edema, hemorrhage, infarction, laceration, or contusion
Bilateral, small, equal, reactive 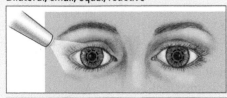	• Bilateral diencephalic damage originating from the hypothalamus • Metabolic dysfunction (Good & Kirkwood, 2018)
Bilateral, pinpoint (≤1 mm), and usually nonreactive 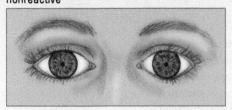	• Lesions of the pons, usually associated with hemorrhage (Good & Kirkwood, 2018)

Recognizing pupillary changes *(continued)*

Pupillary change	Possible causes
Unilateral, small (1.5 mm), and nonreactive 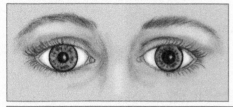	• Disruption of sympathetic nerve supply to the head caused by spinal cord lesion above the first thoracic vertebra
Nonreactive, mispositioned 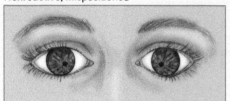	• Midbrain damage

To further test the trapezius muscles, apply resistance from one side while the patient tries to return the head to midline position (Johns Hopkins Medicine, n.d.).

Test tongue toughness

To assess the hypoglossal nerve (CN XII), follow these steps:
- Ask the patient to stick out the tongue. Look for any deviation from the midline, atrophy, or fasciculations.
- Test tongue strength by asking the patient to push the tongue against the cheek as you apply resistance. Repeat on the opposite side. Observe the tongue for symmetry.
- Test speech by asking the patient to repeat the sentence "Round the rugged rock that ragged rascal ran."

Sensory function

Assess the sensory system to evaluate the ability of the:
- sensory receptors to detect stimulus
- afferent nerves to carry sensory nerve impulses to the spinal cord
- sensory tracts in the spinal cord to carry sensory messages to the brain (VanMeter & Hubert, 2014).

This might hurt

To test for pain sensation, instruct the patient to close both eyes and then touch above the area of sensory loss to find the line of demarcation, first with the sharp end of a safety pin and then with the dull end.

Motor function

Assess motor function to aid evaluation of these structures and functions:

- cerebral cortex and initiation of motor activity by way of the pyramidal pathways
- corticospinal tract's ability to carry motor messages down the spinal cord
- lower motor neurons' capacity to carry efferent impulses to the muscles
- muscles' capability to carry out motor commands
- cerebellum and basal ganglia's ability to coordinate and fine-tune movement (VanMeter & Hubert, 2014).

Acts of strength

To assess arm muscle strength, ask the patient to push you away as you apply resistance. Then ask the patient to extend both arms, palms up. When evaluating strength, assess bilaterally. Note any muscle weakness or hypertrophy (Baird, 2016). Have the patient close both eyes and maintain this position for 20 to 30 seconds. Observe the arm for downward drifting and pronation (Baird, 2016).

To gauge leg strengths, ask the patient to lift each leg off the bed while in a supine position.

Grace and gait

Assess the patient's coordination and balance. Note whether the patient can sit and stand without support. If appropriate, observe as the patient walks.

While evaluating the patient, note imbalances and abnormalities. When cerebellar dysfunction is present, the patient has a wide-based, unsteady gait. Deviation to one side may indicate a cerebellar lesion on that side (Baird, 2016).

> A wide, unsteady gait might help me here, but in a patient with a neurologic emergency, it signals cerebellar dysfunction.

Extreme coordination

Test the extremities for coordination by having the patient touch his or her nose and then your outstretched finger as you move your finger. Repeat this action faster and faster. The patient's movements should be accurate and smooth.

Test cerebellar function further by assessing rapid alternating movements. Tell the patient to use the thumb of one hand to touch each finger of the same hand in rapid sequence. Repeat with the other hand.

Abnormalities can indicate cerebellar disease, stroke, ethanol toxicity, or a cerebellar infarct (Baird, 2016).

Present and absent actions

Motor responses in an unconscious patient may be appropriate, inappropriate, or absent. Appropriate responses, such as localization or withdrawal, mean that the sensory and corticospinal (motor) pathways are functioning. Inappropriate responses, such as decorticate (abnormal flexion) or decerebrate posturing (abnormal extension), indicate dysfunction (Baird, 2016).

Motor responses will be limited in a patient who cannot follow commands or is unresponsive. When assessing, be sure to note whether any stimulus produces a response and describe that response.

Superficially speaking

You can elicit superficial reflexes using light and tactile stimulation such as stroking or scratching the skin.

Because these reflexes are cutaneous, the more you try to elicit them in succession, the less response you'll get. Therefore, observe carefully the first time you stimulate these reflexes.

Superficial reflexes include the plantar, pharyngeal, and abdominal reflexes. How to test these reflexes:

- To test the *plantar reflex*, use an applicator stick, tongue blade, reflex hammer handle, or key and slowly stroke the lateral side of the patient's sole from the heel to the great toe. The normal response in an adult is plantar (downward) flexion of the toes. Upward movement of the great toe and fanning of the other toes—called *Babinski reflex*—is abnormal (Baird, 2016; McKinney et al., 2018). (See *Babinski reflex in infants.*)
- To test the *pharyngeal reflex* of CN IX and CN X, instruct the patient to widely open the mouth. Then, touch the back of the pharynx with a tongue blade. Normally, doing so causes the patient to gag.
- To test the *abdominal reflex* and intactness of thoracic spinal segments T8, T9, and T10, use the tip of the handle on the reflex hammer to stroke one side and then the opposite side of the patient's abdomen above the umbilicus. Repeat on the lower abdomen. Normally, the abdominal muscles contract and the umbilicus deviates toward the stimulated side.

Write it down

After you examine the patient, document your findings using a grading scale to rate each reflex. Document the rating for each reflex at the appropriate site on a stick figure.

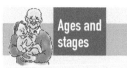

Ages and stages

Babinski reflex in infants

Babinski reflex can be elicited in some normal infants—sometimes until age 2 years. However, plantar flexion of the toes is seen in more than 90% of normal infants.

Diagnostic tests

Diagnostic testing to evaluate the nervous system typically includes imaging studies. Other tests such as lumbar puncture may also be used (Baird, 2016).

Diagnostic testing may be routine for you, but it can be frightening for the patient. Try to prepare the patient and the family for each test and follow-up monitoring procedure. Some tests can be performed at the patient's bedside, but many require transportation to the imaging department.

Imaging studies

The most common imaging studies used to detect neurologic disorders include angiography, computed tomography (CT) scan, magnetic resonance imaging (MRI), and spinal X-rays.

Angiography

Angiographic studies of the brain include CT angiography (most common) and traditional digital subtraction angiography (DSA). During CT angiography, the technician injects a radiopaque contrast medium into a vessel. This procedure highlights cerebral vessels, making it easier to:

- detect stenosis or occlusion associated with thrombus or spasm
- identify aneurysms and arteriovenous malformations (AVMs)
- locate vessel displacement associated with tumors, abscesses, cerebral edema, hematomas, or herniation
- assess collateral circulation (Baird, 2016).

Nursing considerations

- Explain the procedure to the patient and answer all questions.
- Confirm the patient is not allergic to iodine or shellfish because a person with such allergies may have an adverse reaction to the contrast medium. If the patient has a confirmed allergy, communicate this with the health care provider. The patient may need to be medicated prior to the procedure.
- Ensure any preprocedure tests have been completed and results are reviewed and available on the patient's chart; this includes evaluation of renal function (serum creatinine and blood urea nitrogen [BUN] levels) and coagulation studies (prothrombin time [PT], partial thromboplastin time [PTT], and platelet count) (Baird, 2016). Notify the health care provider of abnormal results prior to the procedure.

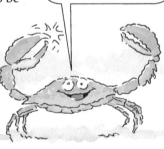

Not to sound crabby, but if your patient is allergic to me or iodine, he or she might have an adverse reaction to the contrast medium.

- Explain to the patient he or she may feel a flushed sensation in the face as the dye is injected.
- Ensure the patient maintains bed rest as prescribed and monitor the patient's vital signs.
- Monitor the catheter insertion site for signs of bleeding.
- If an arterial injection site was used, the patient may need a pressure device such as a FemoStop over the catheter site; monitor the patient's peripheral pulse in the extremity used for catheter insertion.
- Unless contraindicated, encourage the patient to drink more fluids and increase the intravenous (IV) flow rate as ordered; the increase in fluid intake will help flush the dye from the body.
- Monitor the patient for neurologic changes and such complications as hemiparesis, hemiplegia, aphasia, and impaired LOC.
- Monitor for adverse reactions to the contrast medium, which may include restlessness, tachypnea, respiratory distress, tachycardia, facial flushing, urticaria, nausea, and vomiting (Baird, 2016).

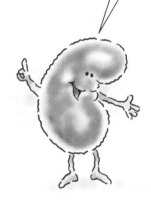

Don't forget me! Check evaluation of renal function before the procedure and report anything abnormal.

Steady, Freddie

- Instruct the patient to remain still during the angiogram.
- Explain that he or she may feel flushed or have a metallic taste in the mouth as the contrast medium is injected.
- Tell the patient to alert care providers immediately if he or she feel discomfort or shortness of breath.
- Unless contraindicated, encourage the patient to drink more fluids for the rest of the day to flush the contrast medium from the body (Baird, 2016).

Computed tomography spine scanning

CT scanning of the spine is used to assess such disorders as herniated disk, spinal cord tumors, spinal stenosis, fractures, subluxations, and distraction injuries.

Computed tomography brain scanning

CT scanning of the brain is used to detect brain contusions, calcifications, cerebral atrophy, hydrocephalus, inflammation, space-occupying lesions (tumors, hematomas, and abscesses), vascular anomalies (AVM, aneurysms, infarctions, and blood clots), foreign bodies, and bony displacement.

Nursing considerations

- Confirm that the patient is not allergic to iodine or shellfish to avoid an adverse reaction to the contrast medium, if contrast is being used.
- If the test calls for a contrast medium, inform the patient that contrast is injected intravenously.

- Ensure preprocedure tests, including evaluation of renal function (serum creatinine and BUN levels), are available on the patient's chart and have been reviewed; keep in mind the contrast medium is excreted through the kidneys and can cause acute renal failure.
- Teach the patient that he or she may feel flushed or notice a metallic taste in the mouth when the contrast medium is injected.
- Explain to the patient what to expect during the procedure. Depending on the procedure and type of equipment, the CT scanner may circle around the patient. Explain to the patient he or she will need to lie still during the test.
- Inform the patient and family that the contrast medium may discolor the patient's urine for 24 hours.
- Expect the health care provider to prescribe an increase in IV flow rate after the test if the patient's oral intake is being restricted or oral intake is contraindicated; otherwise, suggest that the patient drink more fluids to flush the medium out of the body (Baird, 2016).

Magnetic resonance imaging

MRI generates detailed pictures of soft tissue structures. The test may involve the use of a contrast medium such as gadolinium (Pagana et al., 2017).

Sharper images

Compared with conventional radiographs and CT scans, MRI provides superior visualization of soft tissues, sharply differentiating healthy, benign, cancerous, injured, edematous, and atrophied tissue and clearly revealing blood vessels. In addition, MRI permits imaging in multiple planes, including sagittal and coronal views in regions where bones normally hamper visualization. Angiograms can also be performed in conjunction with MRI (Baird, 2016).

MRI is especially useful for studying the CNS because it can reveal structural abnormalities associated with such conditions as transient ischemic attack (TIA), tumors, multiple sclerosis, cerebral edema, and hydrocephalus (Baird, 2016).

Nursing considerations

- Confirm that the patient isn't allergic to the contrast medium (usually gadolinium).
- If the test calls for a contrast medium, tell the patient that the medium is injected intravenously into an existing IV line or that a new line may be inserted.
- Explain that the procedure can take up to 90 minutes; tell the patient that he or she must remain still for intervals of 5 to 20 minutes.

- Ensure that all metallic items such as hair clips, bobby pins, jewelry (including body piercing jewelry), watches, eyeglasses, hearing aids, and dentures are removed from the patient's body.
- Carefully screen the patient for contraindications to MRI.
- Explain that the test is painless but that the machinery may seem loud and frightening and the tunnel confining. According to facility policy, you may be able to offer the patient earplugs or headphones to listen to music to reduce the noise.
- Provide sedation as ordered to promote relaxation during the test.
- After the procedure, increase the IV flow rate as ordered or encourage the patient to increase oral fluid intake to flush the contrast medium from the body (Baird, 2016).

Spinal radiographs

The health care provider may order anteroposterior and lateral spinal X-rays when spinal disease is suspected or when injury to the cervical, thoracic, lumbar, or sacral vertebral segments exists.

Depending on the patient's condition, other X-ray images may be taken from special angles, such as the open-mouth view (to identify possible odontoid fracture).

Spinal X-rays are used to detect spinal fracture; displacement and subluxation; and destructive lesions, such as primary and metastatic bone tumors. Once common, in many cases, CT scanning is now substituted for standard radiographs.

Nursing considerations

- Reassure the patient that X-rays are painless.
- As prescribed, administer an analgesic before the procedure if the patient has existing pain; this will help make the patient more comfortable.
- Remove the patient's cervical collar as soon as cervical X-rays reveal no injury and a written removal order has been obtained.

Other tests

In addition to imaging studies, lumbar puncture is another neurologic test.

Lumbar puncture

During lumbar puncture, a sterile needle is inserted into the subarachnoid space of the spinal canal, usually between the third and fourth lumbar vertebrae. A health care provider does the lumbar puncture. The procedure requires sterile technique and careful patient positioning (Baird, 2016).

Why do it?

Lumbar puncture is used to:
- detect blood and bacteria in cerebrospinal fluid (CSF)
- obtain CSF specimens for laboratory analysis
- measure intraspinal pressure
- relieve increased ICP by removing CSF.

Contraindications and cautions

Lumbar puncture is contraindicated in patients with lumbar deformity or infection at the puncture site. This procedure is performed cautiously in patients with increased ICP because the rapid decrease of pressure that follows withdrawal of CSF can cause tonsillar herniation and medullary compression.

Nursing considerations

- Describe the procedure to the patient and family, explaining that the procedure may cause some discomfort.
- Assist in positioning the patient and provide support (Lewis et al., 2017).
- Reassure the patient that a local anesthetic is administered before the test. Tell the patient to report any tingling or sharp pain as the anesthetic is injected.
- According to facility policy, monitor the patient for bleeding; signs of neurologic deficits; and complications, such as headache, fever, back spasms, or seizures (Lewis et al., 2017).

Treatments

For many of your patients with neurologic emergencies, medication or drug therapy is essential.
- Fibrinolytics are used to treat patients with acute ischemic stroke.
- Anticonvulsants are used to control seizures.
- Corticosteroids are used to reduce inflammation (Good & Kirkwood, 2018).

Other types of drugs commonly used to treat patients with neurologic emergencies include:
- analgesics
- anticoagulants and antiplatelets
- anticonvulsants
- benzodiazepines
- calcium channel blockers
- corticosteroids
- diuretics
- thrombolytics

- antipsychotics
- antibiotics
- antiparkinson agents (Good & Kirkwood, 2018).

Heads up!

When caring for a patient undergoing medication therapy, stay alert for severe adverse reactions and interactions with other drugs (Lewis et al., 2017; U.S. Food and Drug Administration, 2018). (See *Selected drugs used in neurologic emergencies*, pages 64 and 65.)

Surgery

Life-threatening neurologic disorders occasionally call for emergency surgery. Surgery commonly involves craniotomy, a procedure to open the skull and expose the brain.

Be ready before and after

You may only be responsible for the patient's care before surgery. After surgery the patient is typically admitted to an intensive care unit (ICU) or neurologic ICU for close monitoring.

Craniotomy

During craniotomy, a surgical opening into the skull exposes the brain. This procedure allows various treatments, such as ventricular shunting, excision of a tumor or abscess, repair of ruptured aneurysm, aneurysm clipping (destroys the aneurysm by placing one or more surgical clips on the neck of an aneurysm), removal of bone fragment or foreign objects, and decompress the brain (Swearingen, 2016).

Condition and complexity count

The degree of risk depends on your patient's condition and the complexity of the surgery. Craniotomy raises the risk of having various complications, such as:
- infection
- hemorrhage
- respiratory compromise
- increased ICP.

Nursing considerations
- Encourage the patient and family to ask questions about the procedure. Provide clear answers to reduce confusion and anxiety and enhance effective coping (Swearingen, 2016).
- Explain that some or all of the patient's head will likely be shaved before surgery.

Selected drugs used in neurologic emergencies

Use this table to find out about common neurologic drugs and their indications and adverse effects.

Drug	Indications	Adverse effects
Opioid analgesics		
Morphine (Duramorph)	• Severe pain	• Respiratory depression, apnea, bradycardia, seizures, sedation
Oxycodone	• Mild to moderate pain	• Respiratory depression, bradycardia, sedation, constipation
Anticonvulsants		
Fosphenytoin (Cerebyx)	• Status epilepticus, seizures during neurosurgery	• Increased intracranial pressure, cerebral edema, somnolence, bradycardia, QT prolongation, heart block
Phenytoin (Dilantin)	• Generalized tonic–clonic seizures, status epilepticus, nonepileptic seizures after head trauma	• Stevens–Johnson syndrome, arrhythmias
Anticoagulants		
Heparin (standard or low molecular weight)	• Embolism prophylaxis after cerebral thrombosis in evolving stroke	• Hemorrhage, thrombocytopenia
Antiplatelets		
Aspirin	• Transient ischemic attacks, thromboembolic disorders	• Gastrointestinal bleeding, acute renal insufficiency, thrombocytopenia, hepatic dysfunction
Ticlopidine	• Thrombotic stroke prophylaxis	• Thrombocytopenia, agranulocytosis
Barbiturates		
Phenobarbital	• All types of seizures except absence seizures and febrile seizures in children; also used for status epilepticus, sedation, and drug withdrawal	• Respiratory depression, apnea, bradycardia, angioedema, Stevens–Johnson syndrome
Benzodiazepines		
Diazepam (Valium)	• Status epilepticus, anxiety, acute alcohol withdrawal, muscle spasm	• Respiratory depression, bradycardia, cardiovascular collapse, drowsiness, acute withdrawal syndrome
Lorazepam (Ativan)	• Status epilepticus, anxiety, agitation	• Drowsiness, acute withdrawal syndrome
Calcium channel blockers		
Nimodipine	• Neurologic deficits caused by cerebral vasospasm after aneurysm rupture	• Decreased blood pressure, tachycardia, edema

Selected drugs used in neurologic emergencies *(continued)*

Drug	Indications	Adverse effects
Corticosteroids		
Dexamethasone, methylprednisolone (Solu-Medrol)	• Cerebral edema or severe inflammation in brain tumor patients	• Heart failure, cardiac arrhythmias, edema, circulatory collapse, thromboembolism, pancreatitis, peptic ulceration
Diuretics		
Furosemide (Lasix)	• Edema, hypertension	• Renal failure, thrombocytopenia, agranulocytosis, volume depletion, dehydration
Mannitol (Osmitrol)	• Cerebral edema, increased intracranial pressure	• Heart failure, seizures, fluid and electrolyte imbalance
Hypertonic saline	• Cerebral edema, increased intracranial pressure	• Fluid and electrolyte imbalance
Fibrinolytics		
Alteplase (recombinant tissue plasminogen activator) (Activase)	• Acute ischemic stroke	• Cerebral hemorrhage, spontaneous bleeding, allergic reaction
Serotonin inhibitors		
Sumatriptan (Imitrex)	• Acute migraine or cluster-type headache	• Blood pressure alterations

Adapted from Lewis, S., Bucher, L., Heitkemper, M., et al. (2017). Problems related to movement and coordination. In J. Kwong & D. Roberts (Eds.), *Medical-surgical nursing: Assessment and management of clinical problems* (10th ed., pp. 1293–1445). St. Louis, MO: Elsevier; and U.S. Food and Drug Administration. (2018). *Drugs@FDA: FDA approved drug products.* Retrieved from https://www.accessdata.fda.gov/scripts/cder/daf/index.cfm

- Explain that postoperatively the patient will likely be in the ICU initially for close monitoring. Explain that a large head dressing and possibly drains will be in place, and the patient cannot pull or tug on these (Swearingen, 2016).
- Teach the patient to report a sweet or salty taste because this may be a sign of CSF leak (Swearingen, 2016).
- Provide emotional support to the patient and family as they cope with the concept of surgery and allow them to discuss fears and anxiety (Swearingen, 2016).

Cerebral aneurysm repair

Surgical or endovascular interventions are the only sure ways to prevent rupture or rebleeding of a cerebral aneurysm. Alternatively, coils may be inserted (percutaneously through the femoral artery) to occlude the aneurysm. This approach avoids craniotomy and associated complications (Good & Kirkwood, 2018).

Nursing considerations

- Tell the patient and family that, after the procedure, the patient will likely be transferred to the ICU for close monitoring. Explain that several IV lines, an endotracheal tube (ET), and mechanical ventilation may be needed.
- Give emotional support to the patient and family to help them cope with the upcoming surgery.

Common disorders

In the ED, you're likely to encounter patients with common neurologic emergencies, especially head trauma, increased ICP, seizures, spinal cord injury, stroke, subarachnoid hemorrhage (SAH), meningitis, and subdural hematoma. Regardless of the disorder, your priority is always to ensure vital functioning—that is, airway, breathing, and circulation.

Traumatic brain injury

Traumatic brain injury (TBI) results from any impact or injury to the brain; the traumatic insult to the brain causes physical, intellectual, emotional, social, or vocational deviations (Good & Kirkwood, 2018). Children ages 0 to 4 years, young adults ages 15 to 24, and older adults ages 75 years or older are at highest risk for TBI (Good & Kirkwood, 2018).

To put it bluntly

TBI is generally defined as a blow to the head (sometimes referred to as *blunt trauma*) or a penetrating injury that impacts normal brain function (American Association of Neurological Surgeons, 2018).

Open and exposed

In penetrating trauma, as the name suggests, a foreign object in the scalp, skull, meninges, or brain tissue exposes the cranial contents to the environment. The risk of infection is high. Possible complications of both blunt and penetrating trauma include:

- increased ICP due to edema or hematoma formation
- infection (in open wounds)
- respiratory depression and failure
- brain herniation.

Mortality and prevention

TBIs contribute to 30% of all injury-related deaths in the United States. In 2010, approximately 2.5 million people sustained a TBI (Centers for Disease Control and Prevention [CDC], 2019a). Preventative measures for TBI include:

- wearing seat belts and using age-appropriate car seats
- wearing helmets during activities such as when playing baseball or contact sports, riding a bicycle or motorcycle, or skiing
- making living areas safer for seniors by removing tripping hazards and installing handrails on stairways
- making living areas safer for children by using safety devices such as gates for stairways and window guards for open windows (CDC, 2019a).

What causes it

Leading causes of TBI:

- motor vehicle crashes
- falls
- sports-related injuries
- recreational injuries
- war-related injuries
- interpersonal violence (CDC, 2019a; Lewis et al., 2017).

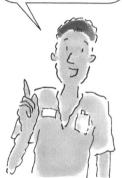

The cranial vault protects the brain from physical blows.

How it happens

The brain is shielded by the cranial vault (composed of skin, bone, meninges, and CSF), which intercepts the force of a physical blow. Below a certain level of force, the cranial vault prevents energy from damaging the brain.

The degree of traumatic head injury is proportional to the amount of force reaching the intracranial tissues. In addition, until ruled out, you must presume that cervical spine injuries are present in patients with blunt traumatic head injuries.

Case closed

Blunt trauma is typically a sudden acceleration or deceleration (or both) injury. In the patient who sustains a coup–contrecoup injury, the head hits an object injuring cranial tissues near the point of impact (coup); the force then pushes the brain against the opposite side of the skull, causing a second (contrecoup) impact (Lewis et al., 2017).

Contusions and lacerations occur as the brain's soft tissues slide over the rough bones of the skull, including the skull base. The brain may also endure rotational shearing forces, which are particularly damaging to the cerebrum (Lewis et al., 2017).

What to look for

Types of head trauma include:

- concussion
- contusion
- laceration
- epidural hematoma
- intraparenchymal hematoma
- skull fractures
- generalized edema
- subdural hematoma (Lewis et al., 2017).

    Each type is associated with specific signs and symptoms (Lewis et al., 2017). (See *Hidden hematoma* and *Types of head injury*, pages 70 to 73.)

What tests tell you

These diagnostic tests are used for head injury:

- A head CT scan will show cranial fractures; ischemic or necrotic tissue; cerebral edema; a shift in brain tissue; herniation; traumatic hydrocephalus; and subdural, epidural, and intracerebral hematomas from ruptured blood vessels.
- Cerebral angiography (usually performed with CT) shows the location of vascular disruption or reduced blood flow.
- MRI can assess diffuse axonal injuries but is NOT indicated emergently.

How it's treated

Treatment may be surgical or supportive.

May be surgical

Surgical treatment includes:

- craniotomy and decompression craniectomy
- evacuation of a hematoma
- ventricular drain insertion.

    Early surgical intervention can remove embedded foreign bodies and skull fragments, evacuate hematomas, and control bleeding. Such measures reduce the risk of infection and further brain damage.

The supportive nurse

Provide supportive treatment as prescribed, which may include:

- close observation to detect changes in neurologic status suggesting deterioration
- cleaning, debridement, and repair of any wounds associated with skull fractures
- diuretics, such as mannitol or hypertonic saline, to reduce cerebral edema
- analgesics to relieve reports of headache and reduce metabolic demands

Ages and stages

Hidden hematoma

An older person with cerebral atrophy has a larger subdural space. After a seemingly minor head injury, bleeding may occur without symptoms. Chronic alcoholics are also at risk for cerebral atrophy. Diagnosis of the subdural hematoma in these patients is delayed because symptoms are similar to other health problems.

- anticonvulsants such as phenytoin to prevent seizures
- respiratory support, including mechanical ventilation and ET tube intubation, for any patient with a Glasgow Coma Scale score of 8 or less.

What to do

- Institute cardiac monitoring and be alert for rate changes or arrhythmias.
- Maintain a patent airway. Monitor ventilatory status with end-tidal CO_2 measurement, pulse oximetry, or arterial blood gas (ABG) analysis.
- Any patient with a Glasgow Coma Scale score of less than or equal to 8 should have an ET tube and mechanical ventilation in place, unless altered LOC is likely to be of short duration (e.g., the post-ictal patient, the intoxicated patient, the concussed patient with an improving LOC).
- In a patient with a moderate or severe brain injury, insert an oral gastric tube to decompress the stomach. Avoid using a nasogastric tube in any patient with potential midface trauma.
- Monitor vital signs often. Initially, monitor vital signs continuously and examine the patient for additional injuries; continue to check vital signs and neurologic status, including LOC and pupil size, every 15 minutes.
- Maintain spinal immobilization until the spine has been cleared; once cleared, remove the spine board as soon as possible.
- Assess hemodynamic parameters to help evaluate cerebral perfusion pressure (CPP). CPP should be maintained at less than or equal to 70 mm Hg at all times.

Metabolic medicine

- Administer medications as ordered to reduce brain stimuli. If necessary, use continuous infusions of such agents as midazolam, fentanyl (Sublimaze), or morphine to reduce metabolic demand and ICP.
- Observe the patient closely for signs of hypoxia, hypotension, or increased ICP, such as headache, dizziness, irritability, anxiety, and such changes in behavior as agitation.
- Carefully monitor the patient for CSF leakage from the ears or nose.
- Elevate the head of the bed 30 degrees. Keep the nose and the navel in alignment.
- Position the patient to promote secretion drainage. If you detect CSF leakage from the nose, place a gauze pad under the nostrils. Do not suction through the nose, instead, use the mouth. CSF leakage from the ear indicates the patient has a skull fracture and ruptured tympanic membrane.

> After head trauma, a halo signals CSF leakage.

(Text continues on page 72.)

Types of head injury

Here's a summary of the signs and symptoms and diagnostic test findings for different types of head injury.

Type	Description
Concussion (minor traumatic brain injury)	• A blow to the head hard enough to move the brain within the skull; this causes temporary neural dysfunction. • Glasgow Coma Scale score is usually normal within 24 to 48 hours, but symptoms can persist for months. • Repeated injuries have a cumulative effect on the brain and may cause death or severe disability due to second impact syndrome.
Contusion (bruising of brain tissue; more serious than concussion)	• Acceleration–deceleration (including coup–contrecoup) injuries disrupt normal nerve function in the bruised area. Patients frequently experience concussion as well. • Injury can be directly beneath the site of impact or opposite the impact. • Brain may strike bony prominences inside the skull (especially the sphenoidal ridges), causing contusions to the frontal and temporal lobes. • Often at a site of fracture
Diffuse axonal injury (DAI)	• This condition involves a high-energy mechanism of injury, with extensive damage to the brain structures, primarily the white matter of the brain. • The axons in the cerebral hemispheres, corpus callosum, and brainstem are sheared, most commonly at the gray–white matter interface disconnecting the axons and "unwiring" the brain. • DAI is commonly accompanied by damage to blood vessels and other brain tissues.
Subdural hematoma (SDH)	• Accumulation of blood in the subdural space (between the dura and arachnoid mater) • This condition may be acute, subacute, or chronic and is almost always unilateral because SDH expansion is limited by the falx cerebri. • SDH is usually associated with torn bridging veins that connect the cerebral cortex to the underside of the dura. Occasionally, this is the result of parenchymal or venous sinus tears. • Acute hematomas are a surgical emergency. Subacute and chronic SDHs can be managed urgently.
Intracerebral hematoma	• Traumatic or spontaneous disruption of cerebral vessels in the brain parenchyma causing neurologic deficits (usually occurs within the frontal and temporal lobes) • Shear forces from brain movement cause vessel laceration and hemorrhage into the parenchyma. • Patients with severe head injuries—particularly penetrating injuries—almost always have intraparenchymal bleeding.

Signs and symptoms	Diagnostic test findings
• Short-term disruption of the reticular activating system that may or may not be associated with loss of consciousness • Vomiting from localized injury and brainstem dysfunction • Anterograde and retrograde amnesia (in which the patient can't recall events immediately after the injury or events that led up to the traumatic incident) correlating with severity of injury; all related to disruption of reticular activating system • Irritability or lethargy • Behavior out of character • Reports dizziness, nausea, or severe headache	• The diagnosis of concussion is based on history and clinical findings. Computed tomography (CT) scans will be negative and should be avoided unless additional injuries are considered likely.
• Scalp wounds from direct injury may or may not be present. • Labored respiration and loss of consciousness secondary to increased pressure from bruising • As the bruise evolves, symptoms progress. Findings reflect a slow but progressive deterioration in mental status: Drowsiness, confusion, disorientation, agitation, and violence are signs of increased intracranial pressure (ICP) associated or focal cerebral deficits. • Other findings, such as hemiparesis, pupillary changes, and posturing, are related to the location, number, and size of the contusions.	• CT scan may show changes in tissue density; possible displacement of the surrounding structures; and evidence of ischemic tissue, hematomas, and fractures. However, because bruises develop over time, initial CT findings may be minimal. Repeat CT in 12 to 24 hours will better reflect the extent of injury.
• Immediate and profound loss of consciousness for a minimum of 6 hours with possible decerebrate or decorticate posture; the effects of injury may be profound and are associated with residual neurologic dysfunction.	• Because the changes of DAI are microscopic, the initial CT scan appears normal. Within 6 hours, changes may be visible on magnetic resonance imaging. At 12 to 72 hours, CT reveals widespread cerebral edema.
• Worsening headache from enlarging hematoma • Unilateral (ipsilateral) pupil enlargement from increased ICP • Gradual or rapidly deteriorating level of consciousness	• CT scan reveals a hematoma that oozes across the brain surface but stops at the midline. • CT evidence of subdural mass and brain tissue shifting • In the patient with a chronic SDH, the cerebrospinal fluid (CSF) is yellow (indicating old blood) and has a relatively low protein level.
• Findings depend entirely on the site and amount of bleeding and accompanying injuries. Patients may be unresponsive immediately or may deteriorate gradually due to increasing ICP and mass effect from the hemorrhage. • Common findings include motor and sensory deficits as well as decorticate or decerebrate responses from compression of corticospinal tracts and brainstem.	• CT scan identifies the bleeding site(s).

(continued)

Types of head injury *(continued)*

Type	Description
Skull fracture	• Types of skull fractures include linear and depressed. • Fractures of the anterior and middle fossae of the skull base are more common and less lethal than posterior fossa fractures. • A blow to the head causes one or more fracture types. Skull fractures may not be problematic unless the brain is exposed, bone fragments are driven into neural tissue, a major vessel is damaged, or the dura is torn.

Adapted from Good, V. S., & Kirkwood, P. L. (2018). *Advanced critical care nursing* (2nd ed.). St. Louis, MO: Elsevier; and Lewis, S., Bucher, L., Heitkemper, M., et al. (2017). Problems related to movement and coordination. In J. Kwong & D. Roberts (Eds.), *Medical-surgical nursing: Assessment and management of clinical problems* (10th ed., pp. 1293–1445). St. Louis, MO: Elsevier.

Seizure watch

- Posttraumatic seizures greatly increase the brain's metabolic demands and must be prevented in any patient with a moderate or severe brain injury. Institute seizure prophylaxis as necessary to ensure patient safety.
- Depending on the underlying injury, you may need to prepare the patient for immediate imaging and surgical intervention as indicated.
- After the patient is stabilized, clean and dress superficial scalp wounds.
- Explain all procedures and treatments to the patient and family.
- Provide instructions for follow-up care for the patient with a concussion who will be discharged. (See *After a concussion*, page 74.)

Increased intracranial pressure

ICP refers to the pressure produced by the contents within the skull. The skull is normally a rigid structure, which contains three components:
1. blood
2. CSF
3. brain tissue.

Signs and symptoms	Diagnostic test findings
• May be asymptomatic, findings largely depend on the extent of underlying brain trauma • Discontinuity and displacement of bone structures occur with severe fractures, but most skull fractures are nondisplaced. • Motor, sensory, and cranial nerve dysfunction is associated with skull fractures. • Persons with anterior fossa skull fractures may have periorbital ecchymosis (raccoon eyes), anosmia (loss of smell due to first cranial nerve involvement), and pupil abnormalities (second and third cranial nerve involvement). • CSF rhinorrhea (leakage through the nose), CSF otorrhea (leakage from the ear), hemotympanum (blood accumulation at the tympanic membrane), ecchymosis over the mastoid bone (Battle sign), and facial paralysis (seventh cranial nerve injury) accompany middle fossa skull fractures. • Signs of medullary dysfunction, such as cardiovascular and respiratory failure, accompany posterior fossa skull fracture.	• CT scan reveals scalp swelling, fractures, and intracranial damage.

Tip the scales

Normally, the body maintains a balance of intracranial volume. However, any condition that increases intracranial contents will cause ICP to rise. Significant or rapid ICP elevations are poorly tolerated by the brain and may result in herniation.

What causes it

Increased ICP can be caused by any condition that increases any of the three components of the intracranial vault. Causes include:
- hemorrhage
- edema
- hydrocephalus
- space-occupying lesions (tumors, abscesses, cysts, foreign bodies, and AVMs)
- infection (e.g., meningitis, encephalitis)
- metabolic disorders (e.g., hepatic encephalopathy).

How it happens

Under normal circumstances, a change in the volume of one of the intracranial contents triggers a reciprocal change in one or more of the components to maintain a consistent pressure. When this balance

After a concussion

The patient with a concussion (mild traumatic brain injury) may be discharged from the emergency department (ED). In such cases, the patient and family need instructions on how to monitor the patient at home and when the patient should seek medical care. Include the following in your discharge teaching:

• Ensure that a responsible person, such as a family member, will be with the patient at home for the next 24 hours.

• Provide brain rest. Encourage the patient to sleep and avoid all stimulation and vigorous or potentially dangerous activity.

• Teach the family member how to check the patient's neurologic status every 1 to 2 hours. Observe for confusion, difficulty walking, changes in level of consciousness, projectile vomiting, unequal pupils, lethargy, irritability, difficulty arousing, failure to eat, or continuous crying.

• Advise the family member to immediately notify 911 or bring the patient to an ED if any of these findings occur (Hartjes, 2018).

becomes altered, ICP increases. Initially, the body compensates by regulating the volume of the three substances via:

• displacing CSF into the spinal canal
• increasing absorption or decreasing production of CSF
• limiting blood flow to the head
• forcing brain tissue out of the skull (herniation).

When these compensatory mechanisms become overtaxed, small changes in volume lead to big changes in pressure.

What to look for

Initial signs and symptoms of increased ICP are subtle. Findings include changes in the patient's LOC, pupils, motor responses, and vital signs.

Early symptoms

• Headache
• Increased blood pressure (intermittently)
• Nausea and vomiting
• Muscle weakness or motor changes on the side opposite the lesion and positive pronator drift
• Varied LOC (initially) (The patient may become restless, anxious, or quiet, or you may note a need for increased stimulation to be aroused.)

Further compromise
- Hemiparesis
- Hemiplegia
- Abnormal respirations
- Cannot be aroused (as ICP continues to increase)
- Pupillary changes (may reveal dilation, constriction of one pupil and not the other, a sluggish reaction by both pupils, pupillary changes only on one side, or unequal pupils)
- Seizures

Severe increased ICP
- Absent doll's eye reflex
- Bradycardia
- Systolic hypertension
- Widened pulse pressure
- Hyperthermia
- Pupils fixed and dilated

What tests tell you

The patient with increased ICP typically undergoes diagnostic testing to determine the underlying cause of the problem. Such tests may include:
- cerebral angiography to evaluate cerebral blood flow and evidence of vascular disruption
- CT imaging to evaluate for hematomas, other lesions, ischemic tissue, CSF accumulation, or fractures.

How it's treated

Treatment focuses on correcting the underlying problem and controlling ICP and may include:
- osmotic diuresis with mannitol or hypertonic saline.

What to do

- Institute cardiac monitoring and be alert for cardiac changes or arrhythmias.
- Closely monitor vital signs and neurologic status, including LOC and pupil size.
- Maintain a patent airway. Monitor oxygenation and ventilation status using pulse oximetry, end-tidal CO_2 measurement, and ABG analysis as ordered.
- Administer medications as ordered. If necessary, use continuous infusions of such agents as midazolam, fentanyl, morphine, or propofol to reduce cerebral metabolic demand.
- If an ICP monitoring system is inserted, continuously monitor ICP waveform and pressure.

Hypertonic IV saline solutions can help knock out increased ICP.

- Elevate the head of the bed 30 degrees (appropriate for most patients).
- Institute seizure precautions as necessary to minimize the risk of injury.
- Explain all procedures and treatments to the patient's family.
- Prepare to transfer the patient to an ICU when indicated.

What to avoid

- Avoid extreme hip, knee, and neck flexion because these actions increase ICP.
- Minimize procedures that might increase ICP, such as suctioning.

Seizures

Seizures are paroxysmal events associated with the abnormal electrical discharge of neurons in the brain. Seizures are an indication of an underlying problem rather than a primary disease state. A patient with a seizure disorder experiences recurrent seizures. However, many seizures aren't a part of a seizure disorder. Rather, the seizures result from isolated events such as fever, toxin exposure, alcohol withdrawal, or brain injury.

Primary and secondary

A primary seizure disorder (epilepsy) is idiopathic, occurring without any apparent structural changes in the brain. Secondary seizure disorder is characterized by structural changes or metabolic alterations of the neuronal membranes, causing increased automaticity.

Who's affected . . .

Epilepsy affects 1% to 2% of the population; approximately 3.4 million people live with epilepsy (CDC, 2019b). The incidence is highest in children and older adults. Seizure control can generally be achieved if the patient adheres strictly to prescribed therapy.

. . . and how

Complications of seizures include hypoxia or anoxia, traumatic injury, aspiration, neuronal damage, depression, and anxiety.

What causes it

For many of the seizures, the etiology is unknown (epilepsy). Some possible causes of secondary seizure disorder include:

- anoxia
- birth trauma (such as inadequate oxygen supply to the brain, blood incompatibility, or intracranial hemorrhage)

- infectious diseases (meningitis, encephalitis, or brain abscess)
- head injury or trauma
- perinatal infection.

How it happens

In the patient with a seizure disorder, certain neurons in the brain depolarize easily or become hyperexcitable, firing more readily than normal when stimulated. Once an impulse is generated, the electrical current spreads to surrounding cells, which fire in turn. The impulse potentially cascades to:

- cortical, subcortical, and brainstem areas
- a single area of the brain (a partial seizure)
- both sides of the brain (a generalized seizure).

Increase O$_2$ or else

The brain's metabolic demand for oxygen increases dramatically during a generalized seizure. If this demand isn't met, hypoxia and brain damage result. Glucose demands are elevated as well.

Firing of inhibitory neurons causes the excited neurons to slow and eventually stop. When this inhibitory action fails, the result is status epilepticus (continuous seizures or seizures occurring one right after another). Without treatment, the resulting anoxia is fatal.

What to look for

The hallmark of a seizure disorder is recurring seizures, which can be classified as partial or generalized. Some patients are affected by more than one type. (See *Identifying types of seizures*, page 78.)

What tests tell you

Here are possible primary diagnostic results of tests for seizure disorders:

- A CT scan may indicate abnormalities in internal brain structures such as a tumor or cyst, but most seizure patients will have a normal brain CT.
- MRI may indicate abnormalities in internal brain structures but is not indicated in emergent situation.
- Electroencephalography is used to confirm the presence of seizure activity and can be useful to determine the classification of the disorder (Lewis et al., 2017).

How it's treated

First-line treatment consists of drug therapy specific to the seizure type. The goal of therapy is to reduce seizures using the fewest drugs possible.

Identifying types of seizures

Use these definitions to understand different seizure types. Keep in mind that some patients may be affected by more than one type.

Partial seizures

Arising from a localized (or "focal") area of the brain, they may remain focal or can spread to the entire brain, evolving into a generalized seizure. The two types of partial seizures are simple partial seizures and complex partial seizures.

Simple partial seizures

These seizures originate in one area of the brain and do NOT alter consciousness. The patient is awake, appropriate, and aware of the symptoms. Clinical findings depend on brain location. Simple partial seizures occurring on the motor strip will cause motor findings such as repetitive jerking or stiffening in an extremity, accompanied by tingling sensation in the same area (Lewis et al., 2017). Seizures in the occipital lobe can cause hallucinations or flashing lights, whereas those in memory regions can produce déjà vu. The patient remains alert at all times and fully aware of the seizure event.

Complex partial seizures

Like the patient with a simple partial seizure, the complex partial seizure patient exhibits focal findings, which reflect the area of brain involvement. However, the person experiencing a complex partial seizure is conscious but is significantly altered. Findings vary but typically include purposeless behaviors, such as a glassy stare, picking at clothing, aimless wandering, lip-smacking or chewing motions, or unintelligible speech.

Complex partial seizures usually last a few seconds or minutes. Afterward, mental confusion may be present. The patient has no memory of actions during a complex partial seizure (Lewis et al., 2017).

Generalized seizures

Generalized seizures involve a loss of consciousness, but there are several types. Types include *absence, myoclonic, clonic, tonic, generalized tonic–clonic*, and *atonic*.

Absence seizures

Absence seizures (formerly referred to as *petit mal seizures*) are most common in children. The seizure usually begins with a brief change in the level of consciousness,

signaled by blinking or rolling of the eyes, a blank stare, and slight mouth movements. The patient maintains posture but is unconscious.

Such seizures last 1 to 10 seconds. Uncontrolled, seizures can recur up to 100 times per day and can progress to a generalized tonic–clonic seizure (Lewis et al., 2017).

Myoclonic seizures

This rare form of seizures is marked by brief, involuntary muscle jerks of the body or extremities, which may occur in a rhythmic manner (Lewis et al., 2017).

Clonic seizures

Clonic seizures are characterized by bilateral rhythmic, jerking movements.

Tonic seizures

Tonic seizures are characterized by a sudden increase in bilateral muscle tone, usually of the arms, but may also include the legs.

Tonic–clonic seizures

This is the classic, most readily recognized seizure pattern. Tonic–clonic seizures often begin with a loud cry caused by air rushing from the lungs and through the vocal cords. The patient loses consciousness and falls to the ground. The body stiffens (the tonic phase) and then alternates between episodes of muscle spasm and relaxation (the clonic phase). Tongue biting, incontinence, labored breathing, apnea, and cyanosis are frequent accompaniments.

The seizure usually stops in 2 to 5 minutes. Afterward, the patient will regain consciousness but remains somewhat confused (referred to as the *postictal phase*). He or she may have difficulty talking and may experience drowsiness, fatigue, headache, muscle soreness, and extremity weakness and may fall into a deep sleep.

Atonic seizures

An atonic seizure is characterized by a general loss of postural tone and temporary loss of consciousness. It occurs most commonly in children and is sometimes called a *drop attack* because the child falls (Lewis et al., 2017).

For tonic–clonic seizures

Commonly prescribed drugs for the control of generalized tonic–clonic seizures (alternating episodes of muscle spasm and relaxation) include phenytoin (Dilantin), carbamazepine (Tegretol), phenobarbital, and primidone (Mysoline) (Lewis et al., 2017).

When medications don't work . . .

If multidrug therapy fails, treatment of chronic seizures may include surgical removal of a focal lesion or ablation of a neural pathway to attain long-term seizure reduction. Vagal nerve stimulation is also becoming a popular option for the long-term management of patients with certain seizure disorders.

Continuous

In some cases, a patient may experience continuous seizures or recurrent seizures lasting at least 20 to 30 minutes. In these patients, immediate intervention is necessary. (See *Status epilepticus*, page 80.)

What to do for the patient with a generalized tonic–clonic seizure

- Ensure patient safety.
- Protect the patient's airway by positioning. Never place anything in the patient's mouth.
- Administer supplemental oxygen as needed.
- Obtain a blood glucose level as indicated.
- Initiate IV or intraosseous (IO) access.
- Administer naloxone if opioid toxicity is suspected (this is a very rare cause of tonic–clonic seizures).
- Administer diazepam (Valium) or lorazepam (Ativan) IV, IO, or rectally as prescribed to control seizures.
- Institute cardiac monitoring and be alert for cardiac changes or arrhythmias.
- Monitor a patient receiving anticonvulsants for signs of toxicity, such as nystagmus, ataxia, lethargy, dizziness, drowsiness, slurred speech, irritability, nausea, and vomiting.
- When administering fosphenytoin (Cerebyx) IV, use a large vein and administer the drug according to the guidelines. Monitor vital signs continuously during the infusion and for 10 to 20 minutes after the infusion is complete. Be alert for signs of hypotension.
- If the patient has a history of anticonvulsant medication use, draw a drug level and send the specimen to the laboratory.

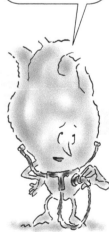

Be alert for cardiac changes after seizures.

Stay on the ball

Status epilepticus

Status epilepticus is a continuous seizure state that must be interrupted by emergency measures. It can occur during all types of seizures. Status epilepticus is easy to recognize in the patient with a tonic–clonic event but may be very difficult to recognize in a patient with a sensory focal seizure or an atonic seizure. In these cases, patients may appear to have psychiatric or other medical problems.

Always an emergency

Status epilepticus can result from withdrawal from antiepileptic medications; hypoxic or metabolic encephalopathy; acute head trauma; or septicemia secondary to encephalitis, meningitis, toxins, or hypothermia. The cause may also be idiopathic.

Act fast

Emergency treatment for all types of status epilepticus consists of benzodiazepine administration such as lorazepam (Ativan) or diazepam (Valium). High doses may be necessary. Intravenous (IV) dextrose 50% is given when seizures are secondary to hypoglycemia, and IV thiamine is administered to seizing patients with chronic alcohol use disorder and those experiencing withdrawal. After the seizure has stopped, administer a longer acting antiepileptic agent such as fosphenytoin (Cerebyx) or phenytoin (Dilantin) as prescribed (Lewis et al., 2017).

Tonic–clonic seizure interventions

If the patient has a tonic–clonic seizure, follow these steps:
- Do not restrain the patient during a seizure.
- Place the patient in a lying position; loosen any tight clothing; and put something soft, such as a pillow, under the head.
- Clear the area of hard objects.
- Don't force anything into the patient's mouth.
- Turn the patient or the patient's head to the side to allow secretions to drain.
- After the seizure, reassure the patient, orient to time and place, and inform the patient that he or she experienced a seizure.

Spinal cord injury

Spinal injuries include fractures, subluxations, and dislocations of the vertebral column. They usually result from trauma to the head, neck, or back. Injuries to the 5th, 6th, or 7th cervical; 12th thoracic; and 1st, 4th, and 5th lumbar vertebrae are most common. Thoracic spine fractures (in otherwise healthy adults) are unusual and suggest the application of significant force.

Dangerous damage

The real danger with spinal injury is spinal cord damage due to cutting, pulling, edema, twisting, contusion, and compression. Spinal cord injury can occur at any level, and the damage it causes may be partial or can involve the entire cord diameter. Complications of spinal cord injury include neurogenic shock and spinal shock.

What causes it

The most serious spinal cord injuries are the result of motor vehicle collisions, falls, and sports injuries; diving into shallow water; and gunshot or stab wounds. Less serious injuries commonly occur from lifting heavy objects and minor falls. Spinal cord dysfunction can also result from many different medical disorders.

How it happens

Spinal cord trauma results from deforming forces. Types of trauma include:
- hyperextension
- hyperflexion
- rotational twisting
- vertebral compression (axial loading)
- distraction (pulling apart).

During spinal cord trauma
- An injury may cause microscopic damage in the gray matter or white matter or macroscopic damage (tearing, compression, and disruption) to the spinal cord tissue, blood vessels, or meningeal layers.
- Areas of hemorrhage within the cord can gradually increase in size until the entire cord is filled with blood, which causes cord necrosis.
- Edema, with or without hemorrhage, causes compression and decreases the blood supply. The spinal cord loses perfusion and becomes ischemic. Edema and hemorrhage are usually greatest in the two segments above and below the injury.
- Edema contributes to the patient's dysfunction by increasing pressure and compressing the nerves. For example, edema near the third to fifth cervical vertebrae may interfere with respiration.

What to look for

In your assessment, look for:
- history of trauma, a neoplastic lesion, a CSF collection, or an infection that could produce a spinal abscess
- muscle spasms and back or neck pain that worsens with movement
- point tenderness (pain) on spinal palpation
- pain that radiates to other areas, such as the arms or legs

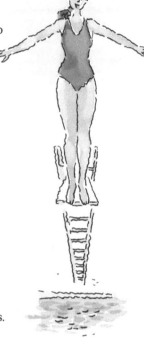

Look out below! Diving into shallow water is a leading cause of serious spinal cord trauma.

- sensory loss ranging from mild paresthesia to complete anesthesia; in milder injury, symptoms may be delayed several days or weeks
- ecchymosis, pain, edema, guarding, tenderness, and bony crepitus over the spine and paraspinal area
- loss of the bulbocavernous reflex. Test by assessing for the presence of anal sphincter squeeze when the clitoris or glans is pinched (or when an indwelling urinary catheter is tugged).
- loss of rectal tone
- neck pain induced by coughing
- a sensation of hot water or an electric shock running down the patient's back
- diaphragmatic breathing.

Specifically speaking

Specific signs and symptoms depend on the type and degree of injury. (See *Types of spinal cord injury.*)

What tests tell you

Diagnosis of acute spinal cord injuries are based on the results of these diagnostic tests:
- Spinal radiographs are used much less frequently than in the past because they do not adequately image the cord.
- CT scans visualize bony stability and alignment.
- MRI scans are indicated whenever cord injury is suggested by CT or clinical exam.
- Neurologic evaluation is used to locate the level of injury and assess cord damage.

How it's treated

The primary treatment after spinal injury is immediate immobilization to stabilize the spine and prevent further cord damage. Other treatment is supportive.

Spinal immobilization limits further neurologic injury. Immobilization devices include head supports, cervical collars, gentle skeletal traction, halo device placement, or surgical fixation.

What to do

- Immediately stabilize the patient's spine. As with all spinal injuries, suspect cord damage until proven otherwise. Initially, use a rigid cervical collar, lateral head immobilizer, and backboard. However, it is crucial to get an order to remove these devices as soon as possible to minimize their complications.
- If the patient has a helmet in place, remove it if possible, according to facility policy. Ensure that at least two people are participating in the removal process.
- Check the patient's airway and respiratory rate and effectiveness.

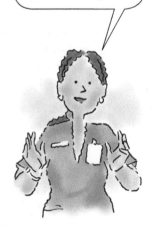

Immediate immobilization after the injury may help prevent further spinal cord damage.

Types of spinal cord injury

Spinal cord injury may be classified as complete or incomplete. An incomplete injury may be an anterior cord syndrome, central cord syndrome, or Brown–Séquard syndrome, depending on the area of cord affected.

Type	Description	Signs and symptoms
Complete injury	• All tracts of the spinal cord are completely disrupted. • All functions involving the spinal cord below the level of injury are completely and permanently lost.	• Loss of motor function (quadriplegia or tetraplegia) with cervical cord transection; paraplegia with thoracic cord disruption • Muscle flaccidity • Loss of all reflexes and sensory function below the level of injury • Bladder and bowel atony • Paralytic ileus • Loss of vasomotor tone below the level of injury • Unstable blood pressure • Loss of perspiration below the level of injury • Dry, pale, or flushed skin • Respiratory impairment
Incomplete injury: central cord syndrome	• The central position of the cord is affected. • Typically from a cervical hyperextension injury	• Motor deficits greater in the upper extremities and torso than in lower extremities • Variable degree of bladder dysfunction depending on the level of the lesion
Incomplete injury: anterior cord syndrome	• Typically from a cervical hyperflexion injury • Cord injury results from bone fragments or occlusion of the anterior spinal artery.	• Loss of motor function below the level of injury • Loss of pain and temperature sensations below the level of injury • Intact deep touch, pressure, proprioception (position), and vibration senses
Incomplete injury: Brown–Séquard syndrome	• Hemisection of the cord (damage to cord on only one side) • Most common in stabbing and gunshot wounds	• Ipsilateral paralysis or paresis below the level of injury • Ipsilateral loss of touch, pressure, vibration, and position sense below the level of injury • Contralateral loss of pain and temperature sensations below the level of injury

- Evaluate the patient's LOC.
- Perform a neurologic assessment to establish baseline motor and sensory status and frequently reassess neurologic status for changes.
- Assess respiratory status closely at least every hour initially. Obtain baseline, oxygen saturation, and end-tidal CO_2 and negative inspiratory force measurements and reassess frequently. Auscultate breath sounds and check the patient's ability to manage secretions as necessary.
- Administer supplemental oxygen as indicated.

- Begin cardiac monitoring and assess cardiac status frequently, at least every hour initially. Monitor blood pressure and hemodynamic status frequently.
- If the patient becomes hypotensive, prepare to administer fluids and vasopressors.
- Anticipate gastric tube insertion and low intermittent suctioning. Assess the abdomen for distention.

Distention prevention

- Insert an indwelling urinary catheter as prescribed to prevent bladder distention. Monitor intake and output.
- Institute measures to prevent hypothermia, such as applying a forced air warmer. Keep the patient covered when possible and administer warmed IV fluids as prescribed.
- Begin measures to prevent skin breakdown due to immobilization.
- Monitor laboratory test results including electrolytes, BUN and creatinine levels, complete blood count (CBC), and urinalysis.
- Assess for signs of neurogenic shock, such as bradycardia (pink, warm skin below the injury and cool, pale skin above it).
- Assess for signs of spinal shock, such as flaccid paralysis and loss of deep tendon and perianal reflexes.
- Prepare the patient for surgical stabilization if necessary.
- Provide emotional support to the patient and family (Kumar et al., 2018; Swearingen, 2016; VanMeter & Hubert, 2014).

Stroke

Stroke, sometimes known as a *brain attack*, is a sudden impairment of cerebral circulation in one or more blood vessels. Stroke interrupts or diminishes blood supply to the brain and causes serious damage to brain tissues.

The sooner the better

The sooner circulation returns to normal after a stroke, the better your patient's chances are for a good neurologic recovery. However, about one-half of patients who survive a stroke remain permanently disabled, and many experience stroke recurrence within weeks, months, or years.

Number three

Stroke is the third most common cause of death in the United States and the most common cause of neurologic disability. Stroke affects more than 750,000 people each year and is fatal in about one-half of cases (Lewis et al., 2017).

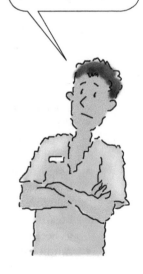

It's sad but true; one-half of all stroke survivors remain permanently disabled.

What causes it

Stroke typically results from one of three causes:

1. thrombosis of an intracranial vessel, occluding an artery that supplies the brain
2. embolism from a thrombus generated outside the brain, such as in the heart, aorta, or common carotid artery
3. hemorrhage from an intracranial artery or vein, such as from hypertension, ruptured aneurysm, AVM, trauma, or hemorrhagic disorder.

Risk factor facts

Risk factors that predispose a patient to stroke include:

- cardiac disease, including dysrhythmias, coronary artery disease, myocardial infarction, dilated cardiomyopathy, and valvular disease
- cigarette smoking
- diabetes mellitus
- familial hyperlipidemia
- family history of stroke
- history of TIA (See *TIA and older adults*.)
- hypertension
- increased alcohol intake
- obesity and a sedentary lifestyle
- use of hormonal contraceptives (Mayo Clinic, 2019b).

How it happens

Regardless of the cause, the underlying event leading to stroke is oxygen and nutrient deprivation in the brain cells. Here's what happens:

- In the event of a stroke, arterial flow is interrupted and autoregulatory mechanisms maintain cerebral circulation until collateral circulation develops to deliver blood to the affected area.
- If the compensatory mechanisms become overworked or cerebral blood flow remains impaired for more than a few minutes, oxygen deprivation leads to infarction of brain tissue.
- The brain cells rapidly cease to function because they cannot engage in anaerobic metabolism or store glucose or glycogen for later use.

Ischemic stroke

When a thrombotic or embolic stroke causes ischemia:

- Some of the neurons served by the occluded vessel die from lack of oxygen and nutrients.
- Cerebral infarction then occurs in which tissue injury triggers an inflammatory response that in turn increases ICP.
- Injury to the surrounding cells disrupts metabolism and leads to changes in ionic transport, localized acidosis, and free radical formation.

Ages and stages

TIA and older adults

To assess for a history of transient ischemic attack (TIA), ask an older adult patient about recent falls—especially frequent falls. Doing so is important because an older patient is less likely to forget about or minimize frequent falls than he or she is to report other TIA symptoms.

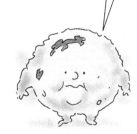

Cellular swelling is one consequence of ischemic stroke.

- Calcium, sodium, and water accumulate in the injured cells, and excitatory neurotransmitters are released.
- Continued cellular injury and edema set up a cycle of further neuronal damage.

Hemorrhagic stroke

Here's what happens when a hemorrhage causes a stroke:

- Vessel rupture impairs cerebral perfusion, which causes infarction. The free blood acts as a space-occupying mass, exerting pressure on nearby brain tissues.
- The brain's regulatory mechanisms attempt to maintain equilibrium by increasing blood pressure to maintain CPP. The increased ICP displaces CSF from the skull, thus restoring intracranial equilibrium.
- If the area of hemorrhage is small or located in noneloquent tissue, the patient may have minimal neurologic deficits. If the bleeding is heavy, ICP increases rapidly and perfusion to surrounding tissues stops. Even if the pressure returns to normal, it may be too late to save brain cells.
- Initially, ruptured cerebral blood vessels constrict to limit blood loss. This vasospasm further compromises blood flow, leading to more ischemia and cellular damage.
- If a clot forms in the vessel, decreased blood flow through the vessel also promotes ischemia.
- If the blood enters the subarachnoid space, meningeal irritation occurs.
- Blood cells in the CSF circulation occlude the arachnoid villi, causing communicating hydrocephalus.

What to look for

Clinical features of stroke vary, depending on the artery affected (and, consequently, the portion of the brain it supplies), the severity of the damage, and the extent of collateral circulation that develops to help the brain compensate for decreased blood supply (Lewis et al., 2017). (See *Stroke signs and symptoms*.)

Left is right and right is left

A stroke in the left cerebral hemisphere produces symptoms on the right side of the body; in the right hemisphere, symptoms appear on the left side. Common signs and symptoms of stroke include sudden onset of:

- hemiparesis on the side opposite the affected portion of the brain (commonly more severe in the face and arm than in the leg because the middle cerebral artery is more often affected than is the anterior cerebral artery)
- unilateral sensory deficits (such as numbness or tingling) on the same side as the hemiparesis

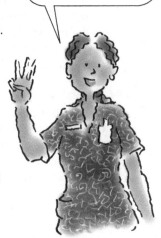

Blurred vision, slurred speech, and hemiparesis are just three stroke symptoms.

Stroke signs and symptoms

With stroke, functional loss reflects damage to the area of the brain that's normally perfused by the occluded or rup-tured artery. Although one patient may experience only mild hand weakness, another may develop unilateral paralysis.

Local hypoxia and ischemia can produce edema that affects distal parts of the brain, causing further neurologic deficits. Here are the signs and symptoms that accompany stroke at different sites.

Site	Signs and symptoms	
Middle cerebral artery	• Aphasia • Dysphasia • Dyslexia (reading problems) • Dysgraphia (difficulty writing)	• Visual field cuts • Hemiparesis on the affected side, which is more severe in the face and arm than in the leg
Internal carotid artery	• Headaches • Weakness • Paralysis • Numbness • Sensory changes • Vision disturbances such as blurring on the affected side	• Altered level of consciousness • Bruits over the carotid artery • Aphasia • Dysphagia • Ptosis
Anterior cerebral artery	• Confusion • Weakness • Numbness on the affected side (especially in the arm) • Paralysis of the contralateral foot and leg • Incontinence	• Intellectual and memory impairment • Poor coordination • Impaired motor and sensory functions • Personality changes, such as flat affect and distractibility
Vertebral or basilar artery	• Mouth and lip numbness • Dizziness • Weakness on the affected side • Vision deficits, such as color blindness, lack of depth perception, and diplopia	• Poor coordination • Dysphagia • Slurred speech • Amnesia • Ataxia
Posterior cerebral artery	• Visual field cuts • Sensory impairment • Dyslexia	• Coma • Blindness from ischemia in the occipital area

- slurred or indistinct speech or the inability to understand speech (aphasia)
- blurred or indistinct vision, double vision, or vision loss in one eye (usually described as a curtain coming down or "grayout" of vision)
- mental status changes or loss of consciousness (particularly when associated with one of the above symptoms)
- very severe headache with hemorrhagic stroke (SAH stroke).

What tests tell you

Test findings that help diagnose a stroke:

- CT scanning discloses structural abnormalities, edema, and lesions, such as nonhemorrhagic infarction and aneurysms. Results are used to differentiate a stroke from other disorders, such as a tumor or hematoma. Patients with TIA generally have a normal CT scan. CT scanning shows evidence of hemorrhagic stroke immediately and of ischemic (thrombotic or embolic) stroke within 72 hours after the onset of symptoms. CT scans should be obtained within 25 minutes of patient arrival in the ED, and results should be available within 45 minutes of arrival to determine whether hemorrhage is present. (If hemorrhagic stroke is present, fibrinolytic therapy is contraindicated.)
- Cerebral angiography shows details of disruption or displacement of the cerebral circulation by occlusion or hemorrhage.
- DSA is used to evaluate patency of the cerebral vessels and shows evidence of occlusion of the cerebral vessels, a lesion, or vascular abnormalities.
- A carotid duplex scan is a high-frequency ultrasound that shows blood flow through the carotid arteries and reveals stenosis due to atherosclerotic plaques or blood clots.

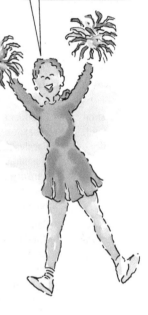

Give me a CT scan and a DSA! These two tests can help you identify a stroke today!

Go with the flow

- Brain CT scans show ischemic areas, but findings may not be conclusive for up to 2 weeks after stroke.
- No laboratory tests confirm the diagnosis of stroke, but some tests aid diagnosis and some are used to establish a baseline for fibrinolytic therapy. A blood glucose test shows whether the patient's symptoms are related to hypoglycemia. Hemoglobin level and hematocrit may be elevated in the patient with severe occlusion. Baseline values to be obtained before fibrinolytic therapy begins include CBC, platelet count, PTT, PT-international normalized ratio (INR), fibrinogen level, and a serum chemistry panel.

How it's treated

The goal in the ischemic stroke patient who meets inclusion criteria is to begin fibrinolytic therapy within 60 minutes of ED arrival. (See *Suspected stroke procedures*.)

Drugs of choice

Fibrinolytic agents (formerly called *thrombolytics*) are the drugs of choice in treating an ischemic stroke patient. However, the patient must first meet strict criteria to be considered for this intervention. (See *Who's suited for thrombolytic therapy?* page 90.)

Suspected stroke procedures

• Recognize signs and symptoms of stroke and initiate emergency medical services.
• Transfer to hospital and initiate interventions (within 10 minutes of arrival).
• Neurologic examination, evaluation by the stroke team, and head computed tomography (CT) scan complete (within 25 minutes of arrival)
• Head CT scan interpreted (within 45 minutes)
  – No head bleed
• Ischemic stroke is possible; investigate fibrinolytic therapy options/exclusions.
  – Qualifies for fibrinolytic therapy
• Give tissue plasminogen activator within 60 minutes.

Drugs for acute stroke management

Drug therapy for the management of acute stroke includes:
- fibrinolytics for emergency reversal of vessel occlusion in the ischemic stroke patient
- aspirin or ticlopidine as an antiplatelet agent to prevent recurrent ischemic stroke
- benzodiazepines to treat patients with seizure activity (usually seizures only occur with hemorrhagic strokes)
- anticonvulsants to treat patients with seizures or to prevent them after the patient's condition has stabilized
- antihypertensive and antiarrhythmic agents to treat patients with cardiovascular risk factors for recurrent stroke
- analgesics to relieve the headaches that may follow a hemorrhagic stroke.

Under the knife

Depending on the type, etiology, and extent of the stroke, the patient may undergo:
- craniotomy to remove a hematoma
- aneurysm clipping or coiling
- carotid endarterectomy or stent placement to restore carotid perfusion
- extracranial bypass to circumvent an artery that's blocked by occlusion or stenosis
- percutaneous intra-arterial interventions to remove the clot or reopen the vessel with a clot extractor, stent, or direct fibrinolytic administration.

What to do

Your facility may have a stroke protocol and stroke team composed of specially trained health care providers who respond to potential stroke

Stay on the ball

Who's suited for thrombolytic therapy?

Not every stroke patient is a candidate for intravenous (IV) fibrinolytic therapy. Each patient must be evaluated to see whether established criteria are met.

Criteria that must be present for a patient to be considered for fibrinolytic therapy include:

• age 18 years or older
• acute ischemic stroke associated with significant neurologic deficits
• onset of symptoms less than 4.5 hours before treatment begins (Mayo Clinic, 2019a).

Criteria that must *not* be present
In addition to meeting the previous criteria, the patient must not:

• exhibit evidence of subarachnoid hemorrhage during pretreatment evaluation
• have a history of recent (within 3 months) serious head trauma or stroke
• have uncontrolled hypertension at the time of treatment (blood pressure greater than 185 mm Hg systolic or 110 mm Hg diastolic)
• have active bleeding on examination
• have known bleeding diathesis involving but not limited to:
  – heparin administration within 48 hours of stroke onset and an upper limit normal partial thromboplastin time
  – platelet count less than 100,000/mL
• have a brain computed tomography scan showing a multilobar infarction
• have experienced arterial puncture at a noncompressible site within the last 7 days
• have blood glucose less than 50 mg/dL.

The patient may be considered for fibrinolytic therapy after careful consideration and examination of the risk, these criteria that may be present include:

• seizure at onset of stroke
• major surgery or serious trauma within past 14 days
• recent gastrointestinal or urinary tract hemorrhage within past 21 days
• recent myocardial infarction within past 3 months.

patients. When a patient shows signs and symptoms of a stroke, first evaluate the patient with a stroke screening tool such as the National Institutes of Health Stroke Scale (National Institutes of Health, n.d.).

After your initial assessment, call the stroke team if your facility has one. They will evaluate the patient, complete a neurologic assessment, report findings, and facilitate rapid and appropriate care of the patient. Such care includes emergency interventions, diagnostic tests, and transfer to the ICU. During this time, do the following:

• Secure and maintain the patient's airway and anticipate the potential need for ET intubation and mechanical ventilation.

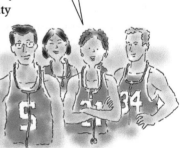

Once you've assessed, call for the best—the stroke team! They'll be able to provide further evaluation.

Multiple monitors

- Monitor oxygen saturation levels via pulse oximetry and ABG results as ordered. Administer supplemental oxygen as ordered to maintain oxygen saturation greater than 90%.
- Place the patient on a cardiac monitor and observe for cardiac arrhythmias.
- Assess the patient's neurologic status frequently, at least every 15 to 30 minutes initially and then hourly as indicated. Observe for signs of deterioration.
- Obtain laboratory studies as ordered, such as CBC, PT, INR, and PTT.
- Prepare to administer labetalol as prescribed to keep the patient's blood pressure less than 185 mm Hg systolic and less than 110 mm Hg diastolic.
- Assess hemodynamic status frequently. Give fluids as ordered and monitor IV infusions to avoid overhydration, which may increase ICP.
- Assess the patient receiving fibrinolytic therapy for signs and symptoms of bleeding every 15 to 30 minutes and institute bleeding precautions. Monitor results of coagulation studies.

Anticonvulsant, antiplatelet, anticoagulation

- Monitor the patient for seizures and administer anticonvulsants as prescribed. Institute safety precautions to prevent injury.
- If the patient had a TIA, administer an antiplatelet agent as prescribed. Administer anticoagulants such as heparin if the patient shows signs of stroke progression or evidence of embolic stroke. Monitor coagulation studies closely.
- If the patient is not a candidate for thrombolytic therapy, prepare to administer heparin anticoagulation as prescribed.
- Initiate steps to prevent skin breakdown.
- Provide meticulous eye and mouth care.
- Maintain communication with the patient. If the patient is aphasic, set up a simple method of communicating.
- Provide psychological support.
- Anticipate transfer to the ICU or interventional radiology as appropriate.

Subarachnoid hemorrhage

SAH refers to bleeding that occurs into the subarachnoid space. CSF normally occupies this space. Serious SAHs are associated with aneurysm rupture.

An aneurysm is a weakness in the wall of an artery that causes that area of the artery to dilate or bulge. These vascular defects can occur in any portion of the brain but are most common in the cerebrum. The most frequent form of brain aneurysm is a congenital *berry aneurysm*, a saclike outpouching of an artery. Aneurysms usually arise at an arterial junction in the circle of Willis, the circular anastomosis forming the major cerebral arteries at the base of the brain.

> Did you say subarachnid? I'm scared of spiders!

> No, I said subarachnoid, as in hemorrhage, which might be scarier!

Women are more prone

The incidence of cerebral aneurysm rupture is slightly higher in women than in men, especially those in their late 40s or early to mid-50s, but—because they are usually congenital—a cerebral aneurysm rupture can occur at any age in either gender.

What causes it

The primary cause of serious SAH is rupture of an aneurysm. Besides berry aneurysms, subarachnoid bleeding may result from an AVM, from a degenerative process, or from both. The most common cause of SAH is trauma, but in most cases, the bleeding is minor.

How it happens

Aneurysmal SAH occurs when blood flow exerts pressure against a weakened arterial wall. The pressure causes the wall to stretch and become overblown like a balloon resulting in rupture. Rupture is followed by hemorrhage in which blood spills into the subarachnoid space normally occupied by CSF. Sometimes, blood also spills into brain tissue, where the subsequent clot can cause potentially fatal increased ICP and brain tissue damage.

What to look for

The patient with SAH will experience symptoms of blood in the subarachnoid space. Findings, which may have persisted for days, include:
- headache
- intermittent nausea and vomiting
- nuchal rigidity
- photophobia
- back and leg stiffness.

Without warning

Aneurysm rupture usually occurs abruptly and without warning, causing:
- sudden, severe headache from increased pressure due to bleeding into a closed space
- nausea and projectile vomiting related to increased ICP

Grading of cerebral aneurysm rupture

Subarachnoid hemorrhage (SAH) severity varies from patient to patient, depending on the site and amount of bleeding. Five grades characterize SAH severity:

• *Grade I: minimal bleeding*—The patient is alert, with no neurologic deficit; may have a slight headache and nuchal rigidity.

• *Grade II: mild bleeding*—The patient is alert, with a mild to severe headache and nuchal rigidity; may have third nerve palsy.

• *Grade III: moderate bleeding*—The patient is confused or drowsy, with nuchal rigidity and, possibly, a mild focal deficit.

• *Grade IV: severe bleeding*—The patient is unconscious, with nuchal rigidity and, possibly, mild to severe hemiparesis.

• *Grade V: moribund (usually fatal)*—If the rupture is nonfatal, the patient is in a deep coma or decerebrate.

- altered LOC (possibly including deep coma, depending on the severity and location of bleeding) due to increased pressure caused by increased cerebral blood volume
- meningeal irritation due to bleeding into the meninges and resulting in nuchal rigidity, back and leg pain, fever, restlessness, irritability, occasional seizures, photophobia, and blurred vision
- hemiparesis, hemisensory defects, dysphagia, and vision defects due to bleeding into the brain tissues
- diplopia, ptosis, dilated pupil, and inability to rotate the eye caused by compression on the oculomotor nerve if the aneurysm is near the internal carotid artery.

Making the grade

Typically, the ruptured intracranial aneurysm is graded according to the patient's signs and symptoms. (See *Grading of cerebral aneurysm rupture*.)

What tests tell you

The following tests aid SAH diagnosis:
- Cerebral angiography identifies the site of bleeding and reveals altered cerebral blood flow, vessel lumen diameter, and differences in arterial filling.
- CT scan reveals evidence of hemorrhage and may identify an aneurysm.
- Lumbar puncture and analysis of CSF will reveal blood in the CSF.
- Transcranial Doppler studies are used to detect vasospasm.

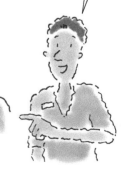

Older adult patients, or ones with serious diseases, may opt for conservative treatment instead of surgery.

How it's treated

Emergency treatment begins with oxygenation and ventilation. Then, to reduce the risk of rebleeding, the neurosurgeon or neuroradiologist may attempt to repair the aneurysm. Repair options include clipping, coiling, or even wrapping the aneurysm (in the case of giant aneurysms).

Today, endovascularly inserted detachable (Guglielmi) metal coils are routinely used to occlude aneurysms.

The coils protect against further hemorrhage by reducing blood pulsations in the vessel and sealing the hole or weak area of the wall. Eventually, clots form, and the aneurysm is separated from the parent vessel by the formation of new connective tissue.

What to do

- Establish and maintain a patent airway and anticipate the need for supplementary oxygen or mechanical ventilatory support. Monitor ABG levels.
- Initiate cardiac monitoring and be alert for cardiac changes and arrhythmias.
- Position the patient to promote pulmonary drainage and prevent aspiration and upper airway obstruction.
- Limit stimulation (such as bed rest, limited visitors, and avoidance of coffee and physical activity) to minimize the risk of rebleeding and avoid increased ICP until the aneurysm has been secured.
- Monitor LOC and vital signs frequently. Avoid rectal temperature measurement.
- Accurately record intake and output.

Watch out

- Be alert for findings that may indicate an enlarging aneurysm, rebleeding, intracranial clot, increased ICP, or vasospasm. Signs and symptoms include decreased LOC, unilateral enlarged pupil, onset or worsening of hemiparesis or motor deficit, increased blood pressure, slowed pulse rate, worsening of headache or sudden onset of a headache, renewed or worsened nuchal rigidity, seizures, and renewed or persistent vomiting.
- If the patient develops vasospasm—evidenced by focal motor deficits, increasing confusion, and worsening headache—initiate therapy as ordered. The calcium channel blocker nimodipine may reduce smooth muscle spasm and maximize perfusion during spasm. During therapy, assess the patient for fluid overload.
- Turn the patient often and institute measures to reduce the risks associated with bed rest.

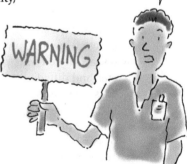

These danger signs may indicate an enlarging aneurysm or other problems.

WARNING

Rebound effects

- Inform the patient and family about the condition, planned treatments, and possible complications.
- Prepare the patient for surgery or transfer to the ICU as appropriate; provide preoperative teaching if the patient's condition permits (Baxter, 2018; Hartjes, 2018; Pagana et al., 2017).

Quick quiz

1. After falling from a tall ladder, a patient is transported to the ED. What is the priority nursing intervention?
    A. Assess full range of motion to determine extent of injury.
    B. Call for an immediate chest X-ray.
    C. Immobilize the patient's head and neck.
    D. Open the airway with a head-tilt, chin-lift maneuver.

Answer: C. All patients with suspected head injury or potential injury to the spinal column need to be stabilized to prevent any further damage to the spinal cord. The nurse's first intervention should be to immobilize the head and neck. Spinal immobilization limits further neurologic injury. Immobilization devices may include head supports and cervical collars.

2. A patient is admitted with thrombotic stroke. In the first 24 hours after admission, what is the priority nursing assessment?
    A. Pupil size and pupillary response
    B. Bowel sounds
    C. Cholesterol levels
    D. Echocardiogram

Answer: A. Pupil size and pupillary response must be assessed as changes would indicate possible involvement of the cranial nerves. Bowel sounds should be assessed but is not the priority. Cholesterol levels are important to consider for long-term wellness, and echocardiogram is associated with cardiac system not related to the patient with a thrombotic stroke.

3. Which statement best describes a lucid interval?
    A. An interval when the patient has garbled speech
    B. An interval when the patient is oriented and then becomes somnolent
    C. An interval when the patient is alert but cannot recall recent events
    D. An interval when the patient has warning symptoms, such as auras

Answer: B. A lucid interval is described as a brief period of unconsciousness followed by alertness and then again loses consciousness.

Dysarthria describes garbled speech. An interval when the patient is alert but cannot recall events is known as amnesia. Visual disturbances (auras) and other warning symptoms typically occur before seizures.

4.   A patient is at risk for increased ICP. Which would be priority for the nurse to monitor?
   A.   Tachycardia
   B.   Decreased systolic blood pressure
   C.   Unequal pupil size
   D.   Decreasing body temperature

Answer: C. Increasing ICP causes unequal pupils as a result of the pressure on CN III. Increasing ICP causes increased systolic blood pressure, bradycardia, and increase in body temperature.

Scoring

☆☆☆   If you answered all four questions correctly, pat yourself on the back! You're a neurologic emergency know-it-all.

☆☆   If you answered three questions correctly, stand tall! You're emerging as an emergency expert.

☆   If you answered fewer than three questions correctly, don't worry! Just "head" back to the beginning of the chapter and try again.

Selected references

American Association of Neurological Surgeons. (2018). *Traumatic brain injury.* Retrieved from https://www.aans.org/en/Patients/Neurosurgical-Conditions-and-Treatments/Traumatic-Brain-Injury

Baird, M. S. (2016). *Manual of critical care nursing: Nursing interventions and collaborative management* (7th ed.). St. Louis, MO: Elsevier.

Baxter, C. A. (2018). Neurological emergencies. In V. Sweet (Ed.), *Emergency nursing core curriculum* (7th ed., pp. 349–364). St. Louis, MO: Elsevier.

Centers for Disease Control and Prevention. (2019a). *Basic information about traumatic brain injury.* Retrieved from https://www.cdc.gov/traumaticbraininjury/basics.html

Centers for Disease Control and Prevention. (2019b). *Epilepsy data and statistics.* Retrieved from https://www.cdc.gov/epilepsy/data/index.html

Glasgow Coma Scale. (n.d.). *What is GCS?* Retrieved from http://www.glasgowcomascale.org/what-is-gcs/

Good, V. S., & Kirkwood, P. L. (2018). *Advanced critical care nursing* (2nd ed.). St. Louis, MO: Elsevier.

Halter, M. (2018). *Varcarolis' foundations of psychiatric mental health nursing: A clinical approach* (8th ed.). St. Louis, MO: Elsevier.

Hartjes, T. M. (2018). *AACN core curriculum for high acuity, progressive, and critical care nursing* (7th ed.). St. Louis, MO: Elsevier.

Johns Hopkins Medicine. (n.d.). *Neurological exam*. Retrieved from https://www.hopkins medicine.org/healthlibrary/conditions/adult/nervous_system_disorders /neurological_exam_85,P00780

Kumar, V., Abbas, A. K., & Aster, J. C. (2018). *Robbins basic pathology* (10th ed.). Philadelphia, PA: Elsevier.

Lewis, S., Bucher, L., Heitkemper, M., et al. (2017). Problems related to movement and coordination. In J. Kwong & D. Roberts (Eds.), *Medical-surgical nursing: Assessment and management of clinical problems* (10th ed., pp. 1293–1445). St. Louis, MO: Elsevier.

Mayo Clinic. (2019a). *Stroke: Diagnosis & treatment*. Retrieved from https://mayoclinic .org/disease-conditions/stroke/diagnosis-treatment/drc-20350119

Mayo Clinic. (2019b). *Stroke: Symptoms & causes*. Retrieved from https://www.mayo clinic.org/diseases-conditions/stroke/symptoms-causes/syc-20350113

McKinney, E. S., James, S. R., Murray, S. S., et al. (2018). *Maternal-child nursing* (5th ed.). St. Louis, MO: Elsevier.

National Institutes of Health. (n.d.). *NIH Stroke Scale*. Retrieved from https://www .stroke.nih.gov/documents/NIH_Stroke_Scale.pdf

Pagana, K. D., Pagana, T. J., & Pagana, T. N. (2017). *Mosby's diagnostics & laboratory test reference* (13th ed.). St. Louis, MO: Elsevier.

Swearingen, P. (2016). *All-in-one nursing care planning resource: Medical-surgical, pediatric, maternity, and psychiatric* (4th ed.). St. Louis, MO: Elsevier.

U.S. Food and Drug Administration. (2018). *Drugs@FDA: FDA approved drug products*. Retrieved from https://www.accessdata.fda.gov/scripts/cder/daf/index.cfm

VanMeter, K. C., & Hubert, R. J. (Eds.). (2014). Nervous system disorders. In *Gould's Pathophysiology for the health professions* (5th ed., pp. 325–385). St. Louis, MO: Elsevier.

Chapter 4

Cardiac emergencies

Just the facts

In this chapter, you'll learn:

◆ emergency assessment of the cardiovascular system

◆ diagnostic tests and procedures for cardiovascular emergencies

◆ cardiovascular disorders in the emergency department and their treatments.

Understanding cardiac emergencies

The cardiovascular system is a major control system in the body, playing a key role in cellular nutrition and circulation. It's responsible for carrying life-sustaining oxygen and nutrients via the blood to all cells of the body. When faced with an emergency involving the cardiovascular system, you must assess the patient thoroughly, always being alert for subtle changes that might indicate a potential deterioration in the patient's condition. A thorough nursing assessment forms the basis for your interventions, which must be instituted quickly to minimize potentially life-threatening risks to the patient.

Assessment

Assessment of a patient's cardiovascular system includes a health history and physical examination. If you can't interview the patient because of the condition, you may gather history information from the patient's family members, the patient's primary nurse or other health care providers, or the emergency medical response team.

Health history

To obtain the health history of a patient's cardiovascular system, begin by introducing yourself and then obtain information on the patient's chief concern, personal and family health, and chest pain or pressure or other adverse symptoms, if any.

Chief concern

Use the seven attributes of a symptom, listed below, to obtain details about the patient's chief concern:

1. location (Where is it? Does it radiate?)
2. quality (What's it like?)
3. quantity or severity (How bad is it on a 1 to 10 scale?)
4. timing (When does/did it start? How long does it last? How often does it occur?)
5. setting or environmental factors (including personal activities and contributing factors, such as climbing stairs or exercising)
6. factors that make it better or worse
7. associated manifestations.

Personal and family health

Ask the patient for details about family history and past medical history. Also ask about:

- current health habits, such as smoking, alcohol intake, caffeine intake, exercise, and dietary intake of fat and sodium
- stressors in the patient's life and coping strategies used to deal with them
- environmental or occupational factors
- activities of daily living
- drugs the patient is taking, including prescription medications, over-the-counter or herbal preparations, or illicit drugs
- menopause (if applicable)
- previous surgeries.

Reports of chest pain or pressure

Many patients with cardiovascular problems report chest pain or pressure. Use the seven attributes of a symptom to get a complete picture of the patient's discomfort.

Where, what, and why?

If the patient isn't in distress, ask open-ended questions that require more than yes-or-no responses (i.e., "Tell me about your pain." vs. "Are you in pain?"). Use familiar expressions rather than medical terms whenever possible. (See *Cardiac questions*, page 100.)

In their own words

It is important to let the patients describe their condition using their own words. Ask for a description about the location, radiation, intensity, and duration of pain and precipitating, exacerbating, or relieving factors to obtain an accurate description of chest pain (Ignatavicius et al., 2018). (See *Differentiating chest pain*, page 101.)

Cardiac questions

To thoroughly assess your patient's cardiac function, be sure to ask these questions:

- Are you in pain?
- Where's the pain located?
- Does the pain feel like a burning, tight, squeezing, or pressure sensation?
- Does the pain radiate to your arm, neck, back, or jaw?
- When did the pain begin?
- What relieves or aggravates it?
- Are you experiencing nausea, dizziness, or sweating?

- Do you feel short of breath? Has trouble with breathing ever awakened you from sleep?
- Does your heart ever pound or skip a beat? When?
- Do you ever get dizzy, feel faint, or have you ever fainted? When?
- Do you experience swelling in your ankles or feet? When? Does anything relieve the swelling?
- Have you had to limit your activities?

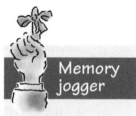

Memory jogger

To remember the order in which you should perform assessment of the cardiovascular system, just think, "I'll **P**roperly **P**erform **A**ssessment."

I—Inspection

P—Palpation

P—Percussion

A—Auscultation

Physical examination

Cardiac emergencies affect people of all ages, ethnicities, and cultures and can take many forms. To best identify abnormalities, use a consistent, methodical approach to the physical examination. Because of the emergency nature of the patient's condition, remember you may need to limit the examination to specific problem areas or stop the examination entirely to intervene if the patient exhibits signs or symptoms of a deteriorating condition. If your initial screening indicates a cardiac problem, you will need to conduct a more detailed assessment.

The heart of it

When performing an assessment of a patient's heart health, proceed in this order:

1. inspection
2. palpation
3. percussion
4. auscultation (Jarvis, 2016).

Inspection
First, take a moment to assess the patient's general appearance.

First impressions

Is the patient alert? Does the patient appear anxious? Is the patient excessively thin or obese? Note the patient's skin color. Are the fingers clubbed? (Clubbing is a sign of chronic hypoxia caused by a lengthy cardiovascular or respiratory disorder.) If the patient is dark skinned, inspect mucous membranes for pallor.

Stay on the ball

Differentiating chest pain

Use this table to help you more accurately assess chest pain/pressure.

What it feels like	Where it's located	What makes it worse	What causes it	What makes it better
Aching, squeezing, pressure, heaviness, burning pain; usually subsides within 10 minutes	Substernal; may radiate to jaw, neck, arms, and back	Eating, physical effort, smoking, cold weather, stress, anger, hunger, lying down	Angina pectoris	Rest, nitroglycerin (*Note*: Unstable angina appears even at rest.)
Tightness or pressure; burning, aching pain, possibly accompanied by shortness of breath, diaphoresis, weakness, anxiety, or nausea; sudden onset; lasts ½ hour to 2 hours	Typically across chest but may radiate to jaw, neck, arms, or back	Exertion, anxiety	Acute myocardial infarction	Nitroglycerin and opioid analgesics such as morphine, oxygen, cardiac medications
Sharp and continuous; may be accompanied by friction rub; sudden onset	Substernal; may radiate to neck or left arm	Deep breathing, supine position	Pericarditis	Sitting up, leaning forward, anti-inflammatory drugs
Excruciating, tearing pain; may be accompanied by blood pressure difference between right and left arm; sudden onset	Retrosternal, upper abdominal, or epigastric; may radiate to back, neck, or shoulders	Not applicable	Dissecting aortic aneurysm	Emergency intervention with percutaneous endovascular graft procedure or aneurysmectomy surgery; intravenous morphine for pain control and beta blocker for blood pressure control
Sudden, stabbing pain; may be accompanied by cyanosis, dyspnea, or cough with hemoptysis	Over lung area	Inspiration	Pulmonary embolus	Oxygen, place patient in high Fowler position, administer anticoagulants or fibrinolytics as prescribed; antianxiety medications
Sudden, severe pain; sometimes accompanied by dyspnea, increased pulse rate, decreased breath sounds, or deviated trachea	Lateral thorax	Normal respiration	Pneumothorax	Analgesics, chest tube insertion

From Ignatavicius, D. D., Workman, L., & Rebar, C. (2018). *Medical-surgical nursing: Concepts for interprofessional collaborative care* (9th ed.). St. Louis, MO: Elsevier.

Check the chest

Next, inspect the chest. Note landmarks you can use to describe your findings as well as structures underlying the chest wall. Look for pulsations, symmetry of movement, retractions, or heaves (strong outward thrusts of the chest wall that display during systole).

Arms and legs, too

Inspect the patient's arms or legs, noting color; hair distribution; and lesions, ulcers, or edema.

Light the way

Position a *light source, such as a penlight, so that it casts a shadow on the patient's chest.* Note the location of the apical impulse. This location is also usually the point of maximal impulse (PMI) and should be located in the fifth intercostal space medial to the left midclavicular line.

The apical impulse indicates how well the left ventricle is working because it corresponds to the apex of the heart. To find the apical impulse in a woman with large breasts, displace the breasts during the examination.

Neck next

Continue inspection by observing the vessels in the neck. Note the carotid artery pulsations, which should be brisk and localized and don't decrease when the patient is upright, during inhalation or exhalation, or when palpated. Also inspect the jugular veins. The internal jugular vein has a softer, undulating pulsation, which changes in response to position, breathing, and palpation.

Then go for the jugular

Check the jugular venous pulse by positioning the patient supine with the head of the bed elevated 30 to 45 degrees. Turn the patient's head slightly away from you. Normally, the highest pulsation takes place no more than 1½" (3.8 cm) above the sternal notch. If pulsations appear higher, it indicates elevation in central venous pressure (CVP) and jugular vein distention.

Abnormal findings

Here are some of the abnormal findings you may note on inspection and what such findings indicate:

- Cyanosis, pallor, or cool or cold skin may indicate poor cardiac output and tissue perfusion.
- Skin may be flushed if the patient has a fever.
- Absence of body hair on the arms or legs may indicate diminished arterial blood flow to those areas.

> Lack of arm or leg hair can be a sign of decreased arterial blood flow.

Palpating the apical impulse

The apical impulse is associated with the first heart sound and carotid pulsation. To ensure that you're feeling the apical impulse and not a muscle spasm or some other pulsation, use one hand to palpate the patient's carotid artery and the other to palpate the apical impulse. Then compare the timing and regularity of the impulses. The apical impulse should roughly coincide with the carotid pulsation.

Note the amplitude, size, intensity, location, and duration of the apical impulse. You should feel a gentle pulsation in an area about ½" to ¾" (1.5 to 2 cm) in diameter.

Elusive impulse

The apical impulse may be difficult to palpate in patients who are obese or pregnant and in patients with thick chest walls. If it's difficult to palpate with the patient lying supine, have the patient lie on the left side or sit upright.

- Swelling or *edema* may indicate heart failure or venous insufficiency. It may also be caused by varicosities or thrombophlebitis.
- Chronic right-sided heart failure may cause ascites and generalized edema.
- Inspection may reveal barrel chest (rounded thoracic cage caused by chronic obstructive pulmonary disease), scoliosis (lateral curvature of the spine), or kyphosis (convex curvature of the thoracic spine). If severe enough, these conditions can impair cardiac output by preventing chest expansion and inhibiting heart muscle movement.
- Retractions (visible indentations of the soft tissue covering the chest wall) or the use of accessory muscles to breathe typically result from a respiratory disorder, but a congenital heart defect or heart failure may also cause them.

Palpation

Note skin temperature, turgor, and texture. Using the ball of your hand and then your fingertips, gently palpate over the precordium to find the apical impulse. Note heaves or thrills (fine vibrations that feel like the purring of a cat). (See *Palpating the apical impulse.*)

Palpate the potentials

Also palpate the sternoclavicular, aortic, pulmonic, tricuspid, and epigastric areas for abnormal pulsations. Pulsations aren't usually felt in these areas. However, an aortic arch pulsation in the sternoclavicular area or an abdominal aorta pulsation in the epigastric area may be a normal finding in a thin patient.

Refill, please

Check capillary refill and time by assessing the nail beds on the fingers and toes. Refill time should be less than 3 seconds. If you are unable to obtain capillary refill and time because of patient injuries or disease, firmly press in the sternal area and assess for blanching in 3 seconds.

And compare

Palpate for the pulse on each side of the neck, comparing pulse volume and symmetry. Don't palpate both carotid arteries at the same time or press too firmly. If you do, the patient may faint or become bradycardic.

Regular and equal

All pulses should be regular in rhythm and equal in strength.
Pulses are graded on a scale from 0 to 4+:
- 4+ is bounding.
- 3+ is increased.
- 2+ is normal.
- 1+ is weak.
- 0 is absent.

Abnormal findings

Abnormal findings on palpation may reveal:
- weak pulse, indicating low cardiac output or increased peripheral vascular resistance such as in arterial atherosclerotic disease (Note that older adult patients commonly have weak pedal pulses.)
- strong bounding pulse, commonly found in hypertension and in high cardiac output states, such as exercise, pregnancy, anemia, and thyrotoxicosis
- apical impulse that exerts unusual force and lasts longer than one-third of the cardiac cycle—a possible indication of increased cardiac output
- displaced or diffuse impulse, possibly indicating left ventricular hypertrophy
- pulsation in the aortic, pulmonic, or right ventricular area, which is a sign of chamber enlargement or valvular disease
- pulsation in the sternoclavicular or epigastric area, which is a sign of an aortic aneurysm

What a thrill!

- palpable thrill, which is an indication of blood flow turbulence and is usually related to valvular dysfunction (Determine how far the thrill radiates and make a mental note to listen for a murmur at this site during auscultation.)
- heave along the left sternal border, which is an indication of right ventricular hypertrophy

- heave over the left ventricular area, which is a sign of a ventricular aneurysm (A thin patient may experience a heave with exercise, fever, or anxiety because of increased cardiac output and more forceful contraction.)
- displaced PMI, which is a possible indication of left ventricular hypertrophy caused by volume overload from mitral or aortic stenosis, septal defect, acute myocardial infarction (MI), or another disorder.

Percussion

Percussion is less useful than other assessment methods, but it may help you locate the cardiac borders.

Border patrol

Begin percussing at the anterior axillary line and continue toward the sternum along the fifth intercostal space. The sound changes from resonance to dullness over the left border of the heart, normally at the midclavicular line. The right border of the heart is usually aligned with the sternum and can't be percussed.

Auscultation

You can learn a great deal about the heart by auscultating for heart sounds. Cardiac auscultation requires a methodical approach.

Erb and friends

First, identify the auscultation sites, including the sites over the four cardiac valves, at Erb point, and at the third intercostal space at the left sternal border. Use the bell to hear low-pitched sounds and the diaphragm to hear high-pitched sounds. (See *Heart sound sites*, page 106.)

Auscultate for heart sounds with the patient in three positions:
1. lying on the back with the head of the bed raised 30 to 45 degrees
2. sitting up
3. lying on the left side.

Upward, downward, zigward, zagward

Use a zigzag pattern over the precordium. Start at the apex and work upward or at the base and work downward. Whichever approach you use, be consistent. Use the diaphragm to listen as you go in one direction; use the bell as you come back in the other direction. Be sure to listen over the entire precordium, not just over the valves. Note the patient's heart rate and rhythm.

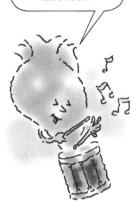

Percussion isn't the best way to assess, but it's definitely the catchiest!

Heart sound sites

When auscultating for heart sounds, place the stethoscope over the four traditional sites where movement of blood through valves and valve closure are best heard, as illustrated here. Erb point is also pictured and is where you may hear S_2 better.

Auscultation sites are identified by the names of heart valves but aren't located directly over the valves. Rather, these sites are located along the pathway blood takes as it flows through the heart's chambers and valves.

1. Aortic area: second intercostal space, right of sternal border
2. Pulmonic area: second intercostal space, left of sternal border
3. Tricuspid area: left lower sternal border
4. Mitral valve area: fifth intercostal space, midclavicular line
5. Erb point: third intercostal space, left of sternal border

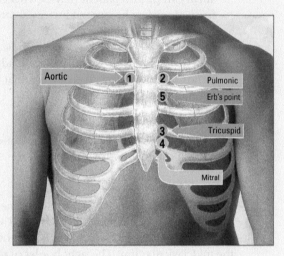

1, 2, 3, 4, and more

Systole is the period of ventricular contraction:
- As pressure in the ventricles increases, the mitral and tricuspid valves snap closed. The closure produces the first heart sound, S_1.
- At the end of ventricular contraction, the aortic and pulmonic valves snap shut. The snap produces the second heart sound, S_2.
- Always identify S_1 and S_2 and then listen for adventitious sounds, such as a third or fourth heart sound (S_3 and S_4).
- Also listen for murmurs (vibrating, blowing, or rumbling sounds) and rubs (harsh, scratchy, scraping, or squeaking sounds).

Listen for the "dub"

Start auscultating at the aortic area where the S_2 is loudest. An S_2 is best heard at the base of the heart at the end of ventricular systole. It occurs when the pulmonic and aortic valves close and is generally described as sounding like "dub." Its sound is shorter, higher pitched, and louder than S_1. When the pulmonic valve closes later than the aortic valve during inspiration, you hear a split S_2.

Rub-a-"dub"-"lub"! The S_2 sound is high-pitched and loud, whereas the S_1 sound is low-pitched and dull.

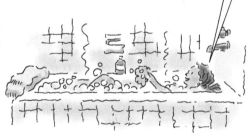

Listen for the "lub"

From the base of the heart, move to the pulmonic area and then down to the tricuspid area. Then move to the mitral area, where S_1 is the loudest.

An S_1 is best heard at the apex of the heart. It results from closure of the mitral and tricuspid valves and is generally described as sounding like "lub." It's low-pitched and dull. An S_1 occurs at the beginning of ventricular systole. It may be split if the mitral valve closes just before the tricuspid valve.

Auscultation awareness!

Also auscultate the major arteries, such as the carotid, femoral, and popliteal arteries, using the bell of the stethoscope to assess for bruits.

Abnormal findings

On auscultation, you may detect S_1 and S_2 heart sounds that are accentuated, diminished, or inaudible. Other abnormal heart sounds—such as S_3, S_4, and murmurs—may result from pressure changes, valvular dysfunctions, and conduction defects (Ignatavicius et al., 2018). (See *Interpreting abnormal heart sounds.*)

Third heart sound

The third heart sound—known as S_3 or *ventricular gallop*—is a low-pitched noise best heard by placing the bell of the stethoscope at the apex of the heart.

Kentucky galloper

Its rhythm resembles a horse galloping, and its cadence resembles the word "Ken-tuc-ky" (lub-dub-by). Listen for S_3 with the patient in a supine or left lateral decubitus position.

An S_3 usually sounds during early diastole to middiastole, at the end of the passive filling phase of either ventricle. Listen for this sound immediately after S_2. It may signify that the ventricle isn't compliant enough to accept the filling volume without additional force.

Fourth heart sound

The fourth heart sound, or S_4, is abnormal and occurs late in diastole, just before the pulse upstroke. It immediately precedes the S_1 of the next cycle. Known as the *atrial* or *presystolic gallop*, it occurs during atrial contraction.

Tennessee walker

An S_4 shares the same cadence as the word "Ten-nes-see" (le-lub-dub). It's heard best with the bell of the stethoscope and with the patient in the supine position.

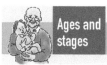

Ages and stages

Interpreting abnormal heart sounds

An S_3 may occur normally in a child or young adult less than 35 years old. In a patient older than age 35, however, it can indicate a disorder, such as:
- right-sided heart failure
- left-sided heart failure
- pulmonary congestion
- intracardiac blood shunting
- myocardial infarction
- anemia
- thyrotoxicosis.

Common S_4
S_4 may appear in older adult patients with stiffened ventricles.

Identifying heart murmurs

To identify a heart murmur, first listen closely to determine its timing in the cardiac cycle. Then determine its other characteristics, including quality, pitch, and location as well as possible causes.

Timing	Quality and pitch	Location	Possible causes
Midsystolic (systolic ejection)	Harsh and rough with medium to high pitch	Pulmonic	Pulmonic stenosis
	Harsh and rough with medium to high pitch	Aortic and suprasternal notch	Aortic stenosis
Holosystolic (pansystolic)	Harsh with high pitch	Tricuspid	Ventricular septal defect
	Blowing with high pitch	Mitral, lower left sternal border	Mitral insufficiency
	Blowing with high pitch	Tricuspid	Tricuspid insufficiency
Early diastolic	Blowing with high pitch	Mid-left sternal edge (not aortic area)	Aortic insufficiency
	Blowing with high pitch	Pulmonic	Pulmonic insufficiency
Middiastolic to late diastolic	Rumbling with low pitch	Apex	Mitral stenosis
	Rumbling with low pitch	Tricuspid, lower right sternal border	Tricuspid stenosis

What S_4 says

An S_4 may indicate cardiovascular disease, such as:

- acute MI
- hypertension
- anemia
- aortic stenosis
- cardiomyopathy
- coronary artery disease (CAD)
- elevated left ventricular pressure
- pulmonary stenosis
- pulmonary emboli (Ignatavicius et al., 2018).

If the S_4 sound persists, it may indicate impaired ventricular compliance or volume overload.

Murmurs

A murmur, which is longer than a heart sound, makes a vibrating, blowing, or rumbling noise. Just as turbulent water in a stream babbles as it passes through a narrow point, turbulent blood flow produces a murmur.

If you detect a murmur, identify where it's loudest; pinpoint when it sounds during the cardiac cycle; and describe its pitch, pattern, quality, and intensity. (See *Identifying heart murmurs*.)

Location, location, and . . . timing

Murmurs can start in any cardiac auscultatory site and may radiate from one site to another. To identify the radiation area, auscultate from the site where the murmur seems loudest to the farthest site where it's still heard. Note the anatomic landmark of the farthest site.

Pinpoint its presence

Determine whether the murmur happens during systole (between S_1 and S_2) or diastole (between S_2 and the next S_1). Then pinpoint when in the cardiac cycle the murmur takes place—for example, during middiastole or late systole. A murmur heard throughout systole is called a *holosystolic* (or *pansystolic*) *murmur*, and a murmur heard throughout diastole is called a *pandiastolic murmur*. Occasionally, murmurs run through both portions of the cycle (continuous murmur).

Pitch

Depending on the rate and pressure of blood flow, pitch may be high, medium, or low. You can best hear a low-pitched murmur with the bell of the stethoscope, a high-pitched murmur with the diaphragm, and a medium-pitched murmur with both.

Pattern

Crescendo is produced when the velocity of blood flow increases and the murmur becomes louder. Decrescendo is produced when velocity decreases and the murmur becomes quieter. A crescendo–decrescendo pattern describes a murmur with increasing loudness followed by increasing softness.

Quality

The volume of blood flow, the force of the contraction, and the degree of valve compromise all contribute to murmur quality. Terms used to describe quality include *musical, blowing, harsh, rasping, rumbling,* or *machinelike.*

Intensity

Use a standard, six-level grading scale to describe the intensity of the murmur:
1. grade I—extremely faint; barely audible even to the trained ear
2. grade II—soft and low; easily audible to the trained ear
3. grade III—moderately loud; about equal to the intensity of normal heart sounds
4. grade IV—loud with a palpable thrill at the murmur site

5. grade V—very loud with a palpable thrill; audible with the stethoscope in partial contact with the chest
6. grade VI—extremely loud, with a palpable thrill; audible with the stethoscope over, but not in contact with, the chest (Ignatavicius et al., 2018).

Rubs

To detect a pericardial friction rub, use the diaphragm of the stethoscope to auscultate in the third left intercostal space along the lower left sternal border.

Rubbed the wrong way

Listen for a harsh, scratchy, scraping, or squeaking sound throughout systole, diastole, or both. To enhance the sound, have the patient sit upright and lean forward or exhale. A rub usually indicates pericarditis.

Bruits

Sounds aren't normally heard over the carotid arteries. A bruit, which sounds like buzzing or blowing, could indicate arteriosclerotic plaque formation. When you auscultate for the femoral and popliteal pulses, check for a bruit or other abnormal sounds. A bruit over the femoral or popliteal artery usually indicates narrowed vessels.

Bothersome bruits

During auscultation of the central and peripheral arteries, you may notice a continuous bruit caused by turbulent blood flow. A bruit over the abdominal aorta usually indicates an aneurysm (weakness in the arterial wall that allows a sac to form) or a dissection (a tear in the layers of the arterial wall).

Diagnostic tests

Advances in diagnostic testing allow for earlier and easier diagnosis and treatment of cardiac emergencies. For example, in some patients, echocardiography—a noninvasive, risk-free test—can provide as much diagnostic information on valvular heart disease as cardiac catheterization, an invasive, high-risk test.

Cardiac monitoring

Cardiac monitoring is a form of electrocardiography (ECG) that enables continuous observation of the heart's electrical activity. It's an essential assessment tool in the emergency department (ED) and is used to continually monitor the patient's cardiac status to enable rapid identification and treatment of abnormalities in rate, rhythm, or conduction.

A test with 12 views

The 12-lead ECG measures the heart's electrical activity and records it as waveforms. It's one of the most valuable and commonly used diagnostic tools; however, it isn't 100% diagnostic and is used in conjunction with other tests. The standard 12-lead ECG uses a series of electrodes placed on the patient's extremities and chest wall to assess the heart from 12 different views (leads). The 12 leads include three bipolar limb leads (I, II, and III), three unipolar augmented limb leads (aV_R, aV_L, and aV_F), and six unipolar precordial limb leads (V_1 to V_6). The limb leads and augmented leads show the heart from the frontal plane. The precordial leads show the heart from the horizontal plane. (See *Precordial lead placement*, page 112.)

> Cardiac monitoring lets you assess the heart from the vantage of 12 different views.

Up, down, and across . . .

Scanning up, down, and across the heart, each lead transmits information about a different area. The waveforms obtained from each lead vary depending on the location of the lead in relation to the wave of electrical stimulus, or *depolarization*, passing through the myocardium.

. . . from top to bottom . . .

The six limb leads record electrical activity in the heart's frontal plane. This plane is a view through the middle of the heart from top to bottom. Electrical activity is recorded from the anterior to the posterior axis.

. . . and, finally, horizontal

The six precordial leads provide information on electrical activity in the heart's horizontal plane, a transverse view through the middle of the heart, dividing it into upper and lower portions. Electrical activity is recorded from a superior or an inferior approach.

Practice pointers

- Use a systematic approach to interpret the ECG recording. Compare the patient's previous ECG with the current one, if available, to help identify changes.
- Determine the heart rate: A normal heart rate is between 60 and 100 beats per minute. Less than 60 beats per minute is bradycardia, and greater than 100 beats per minute is tachycardia.
- P waves should be smooth, rounded, and upright in most leads, and there should be a P wave for every QRS complex.
- PR intervals should always be constant and measure between 0.12 and 0.20 second.
- QRS complex should always be constant and normally measures between 0.04 and 0.10 second.

Precordial lead placement

To record a 12-lead electrocardiography (ECG), place electrodes on the patient's arms and left leg and place a ground lead on the patient's right leg. The three standard limb leads (I, II, and III) and the three augmented leads (aV_R, aV_L, and aV_F) are recorded using these electrodes. Then, to record the precordial chest leads, place electrodes as follows:

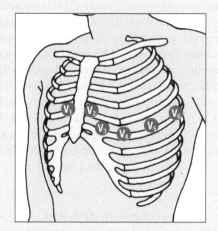

- V_1—fourth intercostal space (ICS), right sternal border
- V_2—fourth ICS, left sternal border
- V_3—midway between V_2 and V_4
- V_4—fifth ICS, left midclavicular line
- V_5—fifth ICS, left anterior axillary line
- V_6—fifth ICS, left midaxillary line.

In order to obtain additional information for more accurate diagnosis of a posterior wall or right ventricular myocardial infarction, a 15- or 18-lead ECG may be used, which will give a more direct view of the walls involved (Baird, 2016).

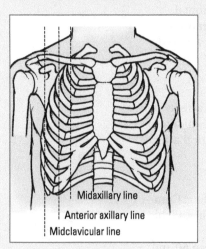

Midaxillary line
Anterior axillary line
Midclavicular line

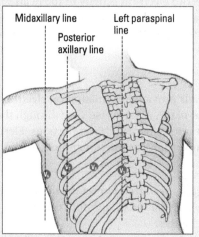

Midaxillary line

Posterior axillary line

Left paraspinal line

- ST segments should be relatively isoelectric with minimal deviation. ST segment elevation greater than 1 mm above the baseline and ST segment depression greater than 0.5 mm below the baseline are considered abnormal. Abnormal ST segment can indicate myocardial ischemia, infarction, pericarditis, ventricular hypertrophy, or abnormal potassium levels.

- T waves normally deflect upward in leads I, II, and V_3 to V_6. Excessively tall, flat, or inverted T waves accompanying such symptoms as chest pain may indicate ischemia.
- QT interval should be equal to or less than half of the previous R-R interval. Lengthening of the QT interval can occur with some medications and can lead to lethal dysrhythmias.
- A normal Q wave generally has a duration of less than 0.04 second. An abnormal Q wave has a duration of 0.04 second or more, a depth greater than 4 mm, or a height one-fourth of the R wave. Abnormal Q waves indicate myocardial necrosis, developing when depolarization can't follow its normal path because of damaged tissue in the area (Ignatavicius et al., 2018).

Cardiac marker studies

Analysis of cardiac markers (proteins) aids diagnosis of acute MI.

Release those enzymes!

After infarction, damaged cardiac tissue releases significant amounts of enzymes into the blood. Serial measurement of enzyme levels reveals the extent of damage and helps monitor the progress of healing.

Heart enzymes

Cardiac troponin I and T are preferred biomarker tests for MI because they are sensitive and specific to cardiac injury, and results can be obtained and evaluated quickly. Troponin levels begin to rise within 2 hours of symptom onset. (See *Release of cardiac enzymes and proteins*, page 114.) Serial troponin values should be assessed, and a predictable rise and fall of troponin value will occur with MI (Reeder & Kennedy, 2018).

Prior to the development of highly specific troponin testing, use of the isoenzyme CK-MB found specifically in heart muscle was commonly used as an indicator of cardiac injury. Use of CK-MB has declined as troponin is preferred for diagnosis and assessment of infarction in most settings (Jaffe & Morrow, 2018).

Brain natriuretic peptide (BNP) is an amino acid secreted by the ventricles in response to the heart muscle stretching. An increase in serum BNP level can indicate heart failure (Huether & McCance, 2016; Ignatavicius et al., 2018).

Practice pointers

- After any cardiac enzyme test, handle the collection tube gently to prevent hemolysis and send the sample to the laboratory immediately. A delay can affect test results.

Release of cardiac enzymes and proteins

Because they're released by damaged tissue, serum proteins and isoenzymes (catalytic proteins that vary in concentration in specific organs) can help identify the compromised organ and assess the extent of damage. After an acute myocardial infarction, cardiac enzymes and proteins rise and fall in characteristic patterns, as shown in the graph.

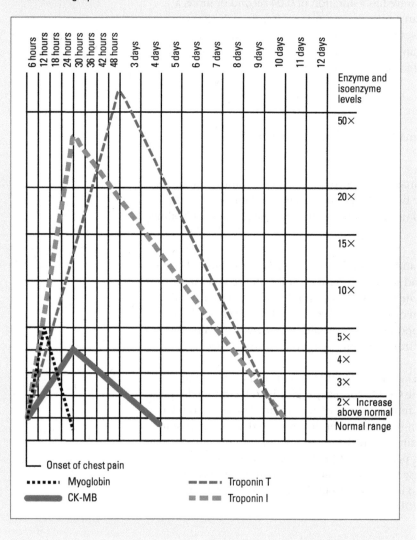

Echocardiography

Echocardiography is used to examine the size, shape, and motion of cardiac structures. It's done using a transducer placed at an acoustic window (an area where bone and lung tissue are absent) on the patient's chest. The transducer directs sound waves toward cardiac structures, which reflect these waves.

Echocardiography aka Echo

The transducer picks up the echoes, converts them to electrical impulses, and relays them to an echocardiography machine for display on a screen and for recording on a strip chart or videotape. The most commonly used echocardiography techniques are motion mode (M-mode) and two-dimensional.

Motion mode

In *M-mode echocardiography*, a single, pencil like ultrasound beam strikes the heart, producing an "ice pick," or vertical, view of cardiac structures. This mode is especially useful for precisely viewing cardiac structures.

Echo in 2-D

In *two-dimensional echocardiography*, the ultrasound beam rapidly sweeps through an arc, producing a cross-sectional, or fan-shaped, view of cardiac structures. This technique is useful for recording lateral motion and providing the correct spatial relationship between cardiac structures. In many cases, both techniques are performed to complement each other. Patients who come to the ED with atrial fibrillation who require an echocardiogram may have mildly distorted images because of the rapid motion of the heart.

TEE combination

In *transesophageal echocardiography* (*TEE*), ultrasonography is combined with endoscopy to provide a better view of the heart's structures. (See *A closer look at TEE*.)

Echo abnormalities

The echocardiogram may detect mitral stenosis, mitral valve prolapse, aortic insufficiency, wall motion abnormalities, and pericardial effusion (excess pericardial fluid).

A closer look at TEE

In transesophageal echocardiography (TEE), a small transducer is attached to the end of a gastroscope and inserted into the esophagus so that images of the heart's structure can be taken from the posterior of the heart. This test causes less tissue penetration and interference from chest wall structures and produces high-quality images of the thoracic aorta (except for the superior ascending aorta, which is shadowed by the trachea).

TEE is used to diagnose or evaluate:
• congenital heart disease
• endocarditis
• intracardiac thrombi
• thoracic and aortic disorders
• tumors
• valvular disease or repairs.

Practice pointers

- Explain the procedure and instruct the patient to remain still during the test because movement can distort results.
- Tell the patient that conductive gel is applied to the chest and that a quarter-sized transducer is placed directly over it. Because pressure is exerted to keep the transducer in contact with the skin, warn the patient that minor discomfort may be experienced.
- After the procedure, remove the conductive gel from the skin with a tissue or cloth.

Hemodynamic monitoring

Hemodynamic monitoring is an invasive procedure used to assess cardiac function and determine the effectiveness of therapy by measuring:

- blood pressure
- cardiac output
- intracardiac pressures
- mixed oxygen saturation (Baird, 2016; Ignatavicius et al., 2018; Pagana & Pagana, 2018; Urden et al., 2018). (See *Putting hemodynamic monitoring to use.*)

Getting involved

Hemodynamic monitoring involves insertion of a catheter into the vascular system. The types of hemodynamic monitoring include:

- arterial blood pressure monitoring
- pulmonary artery pressure (PAP) monitoring using the internal and external jugular and subclavian veins. (Femoral and antecubital veins may be used but aren't the sites of choice.)

Arterial blood pressure monitoring

In arterial blood pressure monitoring, the health care provider inserts a catheter into the radial or femoral artery to measure blood pressure or obtain samples of arterial blood for diagnostic tests such as arterial blood gas (ABG) studies. A transducer transforms the flow of blood during systole and diastole into a waveform, which appears on an oscilloscope.

Pulmonary artery pressure monitoring

Continuous PAP and intermittent pulmonary artery occlusion pressure (PAOP) measurements provide important information about left ventricular function and preload. Use this information for monitoring, aiding diagnosis, refining assessment, guiding interventions, and projecting patient outcomes; however, this monitoring requires

Putting hemodynamic monitoring to use

Hemodynamic monitoring provides information on intracardiac pressures, arterial pressure, and cardiac output. To understand intracardiac pressures, picture the heart and vascular system as a continuous loop with constantly changing pressure gradients that keep the blood moving. Hemodynamic monitoring records the gradients within the vessels and heart chambers. Cardiac output indicates the amount of blood ejected by the heart each minute.

Pressure and description	Normal values	Causes of increased pressure	Causes of decreased pressure
Central venous pressure or right atrial pressure			
The central venous pressure or right atrial pressure shows right ventricular function and end-diastolic pressure.	Normal mean pressure ranges from 2 to 5 mm Hg (3 to 8 cm H_2O) (Urden et al., 2018).	• Right-sided heart failure • Volume overload • Tricuspid valve stenosis or insufficiency • Constrictive pericarditis • Pulmonary hypertension • Cardiac tamponade • Right ventricular infarction	• Reduced circulating blood volume
Right ventricular pressure			
Typically, the health care provider measures right ventricular pressure only when initially inserting a pulmonary artery catheter. Right ventricular systolic pressure normally equals pulmonary artery systolic pressure; right ventricular end-diastolic pressure, which reflects right ventricular function, equals right atrial pressure.	Normal systolic pressure ranges from 20 to 30 mm Hg and normal diastolic pressure, from 0 to 5 mm Hg (Urden et al., 2018).	• Mitral stenosis or insufficiency • Pulmonary disease • Hypoxemia • Constrictive pericarditis • Chronic heart failure • Atrial and ventricular septal defects • Patent ductus arteriosus	• Reduced circulating blood volume
Pulmonary artery pressure			
Pulmonary artery systolic pressure shows right ventricular function and pulmonary circulation pressures. Pulmonary artery diastolic pressure reflects left ventricular pressures, specifically left ventricular end-diastolic pressure, in a patient without significant pulmonary disease.	Systolic pressure normally ranges from 15 to 28 mm Hg. The mean pressure usually ranges from 5 to 16 mm Hg (Pagana & Pagana, 2018).	• Left-sided heart failure • Increased pulmonary blood flow (left or right shunting, as in atrial or ventricular septal defects) • Any condition causing increased pulmonary arteriolar resistance (such as pulmonary hypertension, volume overload, mitral stenosis, or hypoxia)	• Reduced circulating blood volume
Pulmonary artery occlusion pressure (wedge)			
Pulmonary artery occlusion pressure (PAOP) reflects left atrial and left ventricular pressures, unless the patient has mitral stenosis. Changes in PAOP reflect changes in left ventricular filling pressure.	The mean pressure normally ranges from 5 to 12 mm Hg (Urden et al., 2018).	• Left-sided heart failure • Mitral stenosis or insufficiency • Hypervolemia • Pericardial tamponade	• Reduced circulating blood volume

special training. If PAP is implemented, the patient will be transferred to a critical care area as soon as possible for continued care.

PAP purposes

PAP monitoring is indicated for patients who:
- are hemodynamically unstable
- need fluid management or continuous cardiopulmonary assessment
- are receiving multiple or frequently administered cardioactive drugs
- are experiencing shock, trauma, pulmonary or cardiac disease, or multiple organ dysfunction syndrome.

PAP's parts

A pulmonary artery (PA) catheter has up to six lumens that gather hemodynamic information. In addition to distal and proximal lumens used to measure pressures, a PA catheter has a balloon inflation lumen that inflates the balloon for PAOP measurement and a thermistor connector lumen that allows cardiac output measurement. Some catheters also have a pacemaker wire lumen that provides a port for pacemaker electrodes and measures continuous mixed venous oxygen saturation.

PAP and PAOP procedures

In PAP or PAOP measurement, the health care provider inserts the balloon-tipped, multilumen catheter into the patient's internal jugular or subclavian vein. When the catheter reaches the right atrium, the balloon is inflated to float the catheter through the right ventricle into the PA. When the catheter is in the PA, PAOP measurement is possible through an opening at the catheter's tip. The catheter is then deflated and rests in the PA, allowing diastolic and systolic PAP readings.

The balloon should be totally deflated except when taking a PAOP reading because prolonged wedging can cause pulmonary infarction.

Practice pointers

Nursing considerations depend on the type of hemodynamic monitoring conducted.

Arterial blood pressure monitoring
- Explain the procedure to the patient and family, if possible.
- After catheter insertion, observe the pressure waveform to assess arterial pressure.

> Careful... overinflating a PA catheter balloon can distend the PA and rupture vessels.

- Assess the insertion site for signs of infection, such as redness and swelling. Notify the health care provider immediately if you note such signs.
- Document the date and time of catheter insertion, catheter insertion site, type of flush solution used, type of dressing applied, and patient's tolerance of the procedure.

PAP monitoring

- After catheter insertion, a specially trained registered nurse (RN) will inflate the balloon with a syringe to take PAOP readings. Care must be maintained not to inflate the balloon with too much air. Overinflation could distend the PA, causing vessel rupture. The balloon should not be wedged for a prolonged period because prolonged wedging could lead to a pulmonary infarction.
- After each PAOP reading, the line is flushed per facility policy. If the specially trained RN encounters difficulty, the health care provider should be notified.
- Make sure that stopcocks are properly positioned and connections are secure. Loose connections may introduce air into the system or cause blood backup, leakage of deoxygenated blood, or inaccurate pressure readings. Also make sure the lumen hubs are properly identified to serve the appropriate catheter ports.

Irritation prevention

- Because the catheter can slip back into the right ventricle and irritate it, check the monitor for a right ventricular waveform to detect the problem promptly.
- To minimize valvular trauma, make sure the balloon is deflated whenever the catheter is withdrawn from the PA to the right ventricle or from the right ventricle to the right atrium.
- Document the date and time of catheter insertion, the health care provider who performed the procedure, the catheter insertion site, pressure waveforms and values for the various heart chambers, the balloon inflation volume required to obtain a wedge tracing, arrhythmias that took place during or after the procedure, the type of flush solution used and its heparin concentration (if any), the type of dressing applied, and the patient's tolerance of the procedure.

Cardiac output monitoring

Cardiac output—the amount of blood ejected by the heart in 1 minute—is monitored to evaluate cardiac function. The normal range for cardiac output is 4 to 8 L per minute. The most widely used method for monitoring cardiac output is the bolus thermodilution technique through the PA catheter.

On the rocks or room temperature

To measure cardiac output, a solution is injected into the right atrium through a port on a PA catheter. Room temperature injectant (usually 10 mL of saline solution) may be used depending on the facility policy and the patient status (Urden et al., 2018).

This indicator solution mixes with the blood as it travels through the right ventricle into the PA, and a thermistor on the catheter registers the change in temperature of the flowing blood. A computer then plots the temperature change over time as a curve and calculates flow based on the area under the curve.

To be continued

Some PA catheters contain a filament that permits continuous cardiac output monitoring. Using such a device, an average cardiac output value is determined over a 3-minute span; the value is updated every 30 to 60 seconds. This type of monitoring allows close scrutiny of the patient's hemodynamic status and prompt intervention in case problems arise.

Better assessor

Cardiac output is better assessed by calculating cardiac index, which takes body size into account. To calculate the patient's cardiac index, divide cardiac output by body surface area, a function of height and weight. The normal cardiac index ranges from 2.5 to 4.2 L/minute/m^2 for adults or 3.5 to 6.5 L/minute/m^2 for pregnant women.

Physiologic changes can affect the cardiac output and the cardiac index; they include:
- decreased preload
- increased preload
- vasoconstriction (changes in afterload)
- vasodilation (changes in afterload)
- hypothermia.

Practice pointers
- Make sure your patient doesn't move during the procedure because movement can cause an error in measurement.
- Perform cardiac output measurements and monitoring at least every 2 to 4 hours, especially if the patient is receiving vasoactive or inotropic agents or if fluids are being added or restricted.

- Discontinue cardiac output measurements when the patient is hemodynamically stable and weaned from vasoactive and inotropic medications.
- Monitor the patient for signs and symptoms of inadequate perfusion, including restlessness, fatigue, changes in level of consciousness (LOC); decreased capillary refill time; diminished peripheral pulses; oliguria; and pale, cool skin.
- Add the fluid volume injected for cardiac output determinations to the patient's total intake.
- Record the patient's cardiac output, cardiac index, and other hemodynamic values and vital signs at the time of measurement. Note the patient's position during measurement (Baird, 2016; Urden et al., 2018).

Treatments

Many treatments are available for patients with cardiac emergencies. Commonly used treatment measures include drug therapy; surgery; balloon catheter treatments; and other treatments, such as defibrillation, synchronized cardioversion, and pacemaker insertion.

Drug therapy

Types of drugs used to improve cardiovascular function include oxygen, adrenergics, adrenergic blockers, antianginals, antiarrhythmics, anticoagulants, antiplatelets, antihypertensives, cardiac glycosides and phosphodiesterase inhibitors (PDIs), beta-adrenergic blockers, angiotensin-converting enzyme (ACE) inhibitors, diuretics, and thrombolytics.

Adrenergics

Adrenergic drugs are also called *sympathomimetics* because they produce effects similar to those produced by the sympathetic nervous system.

Classified by chemical

Adrenergic drugs are classified in two groups based on their chemical structure—catecholamines (naturally occurring and synthetic) and noncatecholamines. (See *Understanding adrenergics*, page 122.)

Understanding adrenergics

Adrenergic drugs produce effects similar to those produced by the sympathetic nervous system. They can affect alpha-adrenergic receptors, beta-adrenergic receptors, or dopamine receptors. However, most of the drugs stimulate the alpha and beta receptors, mimicking the effects of norepinephrine and epinephrine. Dopaminergic drugs act on receptors typically stimulated by dopamine. Use this table to learn about the indications and adverse reactions associated with these drugs.

Drugs	Indications	Adverse reactions
Catecholamines		
Dobutamine	• Increases cardiac output in short-term treatment of cardiac decompensation from depressed contractility	• Headache • Tachycardia • Cardiac arrhythmias (premature ventricular contractions) • Hypertension
Dopamine	• Adjunct in shock to increase cardiac output, blood pressure, and urine flow	• Dyspnea • Bradycardia • Palpitations • Tachycardia • Cardiac arrhythmias (ventricular) • Hypotension • Widened QRS • Angina • Necrosis at intravenous (IV) site with infiltration
Epinephrine	• Anaphylaxis • Bronchospasm • Hypersensitivity reactions • Restoration of cardiac rhythm in cardiac arrest	• Restlessness • Anxiety • Headache • Tachycardia • Palpitations • Cardiac arrhythmias (ventricular fibrillation) • Precordial pain (in patients with ischemic heart disease) • Necrosis at IV site with infiltration
Norepinephrine (Levophed)	• Gastrointestinal bleeding • Maintains blood pressure in acute hypotensive states	• Headache • Bradycardia • Hypertension • Necrosis at IV site with infiltration
Noncatecholamines		
Ephedrine	• Maintains blood pressure in acute hypotensive states, especially with spinal anesthesia • Treatment of orthostatic hypotension and bronchospasm	• Restlessness • Anxiety • Dizziness • Headache • Cardiac arrhythmias (ventricular fibrillation) • Nausea

Adapted from American Heart Association. (2016). *Advanced cardiovascular life support provider manual* (16th ed.). Dallas, TX: Author; Burchum, J. R., & Rosenthal, L. D. (2018). *Lehne's pharmacology for nursing care* (10th ed.). St. Louis, MO: Elsevier; Kee, J. L., Hayes, E. R., & McCuistion, L. E. (2015). *Pharmacology: A patient-centered nursing process approach* (8th ed.). St. Louis, MO: Elsevier; and U.S. Food and Drug Administration. (2018). *Drugs@FDA: FDA approved drug products*. Retrieved from https://www.accessdata.fda.gov/scripts/cder/daf/index.cfm

Which receptor

Therapeutic use of adrenergic drugs depends on which receptors they stimulate and to what degree. Adrenergic drugs can affect:
- alpha-adrenergic receptors
- beta-adrenergic receptors
- dopamine receptors.

Mimicking norepinephrine and epinephrine

Most of the adrenergic drugs produce their effects by stimulating alpha- and beta-adrenergic receptors. These drugs mimic the action of norepinephrine or epinephrine.

Doing it like dopamine

Dopaminergic drugs act primarily on receptors in the sympathetic nervous system that are stimulated by dopamine.

Catecholamines

Because of their common basic chemical structure, catecholamines share certain properties. They stimulate the nervous system, constrict peripheral blood vessels, increase heart rate, and dilate the bronchi (Kee et al., 2015). They can be manufactured in the body or in a laboratory.

Excitatory or inhibitory

Catecholamines primarily act directly. When catecholamines combine with alpha or beta receptors, they cause an excitatory or inhibitory effect. Typically, activation of alpha receptors generates an excitatory response except for intestinal relaxation. Activation of the beta receptors mostly produces an inhibitory response except in the cells of the heart, where norepinephrine produces excitatory effects.

How heartening

The clinical effects of catecholamines depend on the dosage and the route of administration. Catecholamines are potent inotropes, meaning they make the heart contract more forcefully. As a result, the ventricles empty more completely with each heartbeat, increasing the workload of the heart and the amount of oxygen it needs to do this harder work.

Rapid rates

Catecholamines also produce a positive chronotropic effect, which means they cause the heart to beat faster. The heart beats faster because catecholamines increase the depolarization rate of pacemaker cells in the sinoatrial (SA) node of the heart. As catecholamines cause blood vessels to constrict and blood pressure to increase, the heart rate decreases as the body tries to prevent an excessive increase in blood pressure.

Fascinating rhythm

Catecholamines can cause the Purkinje fibers (an intricate web of fibers that carry electrical impulses into the ventricles of the heart) to fire spontaneously, possibly producing abnormal heart rhythms, such as premature ventricular contractions and fibrillation. Epinephrine is likelier than norepinephrine to produce this spontaneous firing.

Noncatecholamines

Noncatecholamine adrenergic drugs have a variety of therapeutic uses because of the many effects these drugs can have on the body, such as the local or systemic constriction of blood vessels. Noncatecholamines can directly act to stimulate alpha activity or selectively exert beta activity. Ephedrine is a direct-acting noncatecholamine that combines both actions (Burchum & Rosenthal, 2018).

Adrenergic blockers

Adrenergic blocking drugs, also called *sympatholytic drugs,* are used to disrupt sympathetic nervous system function. (See *Understanding adrenergic blockers.*)

Impending impulses

Adrenergic blockers work by blocking impulse transmission (and thus sympathetic nervous system stimulation) at adrenergic neurons or adrenergic receptor sites. The action of the drugs at these sites can be exerted by:
- interrupting the action of sympathomimetic (adrenergic) drugs
- reducing available norepinephrine
- preventing the action of cholinergic drugs.

Classified information

Adrenergic blockers are classified according to their site of action as alpha-adrenergic blockers or beta-adrenergic blockers.

Alpha-adrenergic blockers

Alpha-adrenergic blockers work by interrupting the actions of sympathomimetic drugs at alpha-adrenergic receptors. The interruption results in:
- relaxation of the smooth muscle in the blood vessels
- increased dilation of blood vessels
- decreased blood pressure.

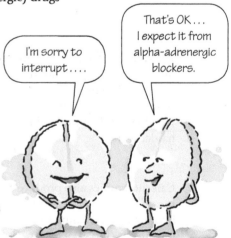

Understanding adrenergic blockers

Adrenergic blockers block impulse transmission at adrenergic receptor sites by interrupting the action of adrenergic drugs, reducing the amount of norepinephrine available, and blocking the action of cholinergics.

Drugs	Indications	Adverse reactions
Alpha-adrenergic blockers		
Prazosin (Minipress)	• Hypertension	• Orthostatic hypotension • Reflex tachycardia • Nasal congestion (Burchum & Rosenthal, 2018)
Beta-adrenergic blockers		
Nonselective Nadolol (Corgard), propranolol (Inderal), sotalol (Betapace)	• Prevention of complications after myocardial infarction, angina, hypertension, supraventricular arrhythmias, situational anxiety, heart failure	• Hypotension • Bradycardia • Peripheral vascular insufficiency • Heart failure • Bronchoconstriction • Sore throat • Atrioventricular block
Selective Acebutolol, atenolol (Tenormin), bisoprolol, esmolol (Brevibloc), and metoprolol (Lopressor)	• Hypertension, angina, cardiac dysrhythmias	• Heart failure (decreased cardiac output) • Bradycardia • Heart block

Adapted from Burchum, J. R., & Rosenthal, L. D. (2018). *Lehne's pharmacology for nursing care* (10th ed.). St. Louis, MO: Elsevier; Kee, J. L., Hayes, E. R., & McCuistion, L. E. (2015). *Pharmacology: A patient-centered nursing process approach* (8th ed.). St. Louis, MO: Elsevier; and U.S. Food and Drug Administration. (2018). *Drugs@FDA: FDA approved drug products*. Retrieved from https://www.accessdata.fda.gov/scripts/cder/daf/index.cfm

Alpha-adrenergic blockers work in one of two ways:

1. They interfere with or block the synthesis, storage, release, and reuptake of norepinephrine by neurons.
2. They antagonize epinephrine, norepinephrine, or adrenergic (sympathomimetic) drugs at alpha receptor sites.

Not very discriminating

Alpha receptor sites are either alpha$_1$ or alpha$_2$ receptors. Alpha-adrenergic blockers include drugs that block stimulation of alpha$_1$ receptors and that may block alpha$_2$ stimulation.

Reducing resistance

Alpha-adrenergic blockers occupy alpha receptor sites on the smooth muscle of blood vessels, which prevents catecholamines from occupying and stimulating the receptor sites. As a result, blood vessels dilate, increasing local blood flow to the skin and other organs. The decreased peripheral vascular resistance (resistance to blood flow) helps to decrease blood pressure.

Beta-adrenergic blockers

Beta-adrenergic blockers, the most widely used adrenergic blockers, prevent stimulation of the sympathetic nervous system by inhibiting the action of catecholamines and other sympathomimetic drugs at beta-adrenergic receptors.

Selective (or not)

Beta-adrenergic drugs are selective or nonselective. Nonselective beta-adrenergic drugs affect:
- $beta_1$ receptor sites (located mainly in the heart)
- $beta_2$ receptor sites (located in the bronchi, blood vessels, and uterus).

Highly discriminating

Selective beta-adrenergic drugs primarily affect the $beta_1$-adrenergic sites. They include atenolol, esmolol, acebutolol, and metoprolol.

Intrinsically sympathetic

Some beta-adrenergic blockers, such as pindolol and acebutolol, have intrinsic sympathetic activity. The sympathetic activity means that, instead of attaching to beta receptors and blocking them, these beta-adrenergic blockers attach to beta receptors and stimulate them. These drugs are sometimes classified as *partial agonists*.

Widely effective

Beta-adrenergic blockers have widespread effects in the body because they produce their blocking action not only at the adrenergic nerve endings but also in the adrenal medulla. Effects on the heart include:
- increased peripheral vascular resistance
- decreased blood pressure
- decreased force of contractions of the heart
- decreased oxygen consumption by the heart
- slowed conduction of impulses between the atria and ventricles
- decreased cardiac output (Ignatavicius et al., 2018; Kee et al., 2015).

Selective or nonselective

Some of the effects of beta-adrenergic blocking drugs depend on whether the drug is classified as selective or nonselective. Selective beta-adrenergic blockers, which preferentially block $beta_1$ receptor sites, reduce stimulation of the heart. They're commonly called *cardioselective beta-adrenergic blockers*.

Nonselective beta-adrenergic blockers, which block beta$_1$ and beta$_2$ receptor sites, reduce stimulation of the heart and cause the bronchioles of the lungs to constrict. The constriction causes bronchospasm in patients with chronic obstructive lung disorders (Ignatavicius et al., 2018; Kee et al., 2015).

Antianginals

When the oxygen demands of the heart exceed the amount of oxygen being supplied, areas of heart muscle become ischemic (not receiving enough oxygen). When the heart muscle is ischemic, a person experiences chest pain. The condition is known as *angina* or *angina pectoris*.

Reduce demand, increase supply

Although angina's cardinal symptom is chest pain, the drugs used to treat angina aren't typically analgesics. Instead, antianginal drugs correct angina by reducing myocardial oxygen demand (the amount of oxygen the heart needs to do its work), increasing the supply of oxygen to the heart, or both.

The top three

The three classes of commonly used antianginal drugs include:
1. nitrates (for acute angina)
2. beta-adrenergic blockers (for long-term prevention of angina)
3. calcium channel blockers (used when other drugs fail to prevent angina). (See *Understanding antianginal drugs*, page 128.)

Nitrates

Nitrates are the drug of choice for relieving acute angina.

Antiangina effect

Nitrates cause the smooth muscle of the veins and, to a lesser extent, the arteries to relax and dilate. Here's what happens:
- When the veins dilate, less blood returns to the heart.
- Decreased blood return reduces the amount of blood in the ventricles at the end of diastole, when the ventricles are full. (The blood volume in the ventricles just before contraction is called *preload*.)
- By reducing preload, nitrates reduce ventricular size and ventricular wall tension so the left ventricle doesn't have to stretch as much to pump blood. The reduction in size and tension in turn reduces the oxygen requirements of the heart.
- As the coronary arteries dilate, more blood is delivered to the myocardium, improving oxygenation of the ischemic tissue (Ignatavicius et al., 2018; Kee et al., 2015).

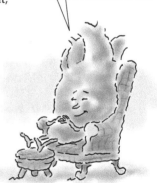

Nitrates help the smooth muscles of my veins relax, kick back, and forget all about angina.

Understanding antianginal drugs

Antianginal drugs are effective in treating patients with angina because they reduce myocardial oxygen demand, increase the supply of oxygen to the heart, or both. Use the table to learn about the indications and adverse reactions associated with these drugs.

Drugs	Indications	Adverse reactions
Nitrates		
Isosorbide dinitrate, isosorbide mononitrate, and nitroglycerin	• Relief and prevention of angina	• Dizziness • Headache • Hypotension • Increased heart rate
Beta-adrenergic blockers		
Atenolol (Tenormin), metoprolol (Lopressor), nadolol (Corgard), and propranolol (Inderal)	• First-line therapy for hypertension • Long-term prevention of angina	• Angina • Arrhythmias • Bradycardia • Bronchial constriction • Diarrhea • Fainting • Fluid retention • Heart failure • Nausea • Shock • Vomiting
Calcium channel blockers		
Amlodipine (Norvasc), diltiazem (Cardizem), nicardipine, nifedipine (Procardia), and verapamil (Calan)	• Long-term prevention of angina	• Arrhythmias • Dizziness • Flushing • Headache • Heart failure • Hypotension • Orthostatic hypotension • Persistent peripheral edema • Weakness

Adapted from Ignatavicius, D. D., Workman, L., & Rebar, C. (2018). *Medical-surgical nursing: Concepts for interprofessional collaborative care* (9th ed.). St. Louis, MO: Elsevier; Kee, J. L., Hayes, E. R., & McCuistion, L. E. (2015). *Pharmacology: A patient-centered nursing process approach* (8th ed.). St. Louis, MO: Elsevier; and U.S. Food and Drug Administration. (2018). *Drugs@FDA: FDA approved drug products.* Retrieved from https://www.accessdata.fda.gov/scripts/cder/daf/index.cfm

Reducing resistance

The arterioles provide the most resistance to the blood pumped by the left ventricle (called *peripheral vascular resistance*). Nitrates decrease afterload by dilating the arterioles, reducing resistance, easing the heart's workload, and easing oxygen demand.

Beta-adrenergic blockers

Beta-adrenergic blockers are used for long-term prevention of angina and are one of the main types of drugs used to treat hypertension.

Down with everything

Beta-adrenergic blockers decrease blood pressure and block beta-adrenergic receptor sites in the heart muscle and conduction system. These actions decrease the heart rate and reduce the force of the heart's contractions, resulting in lower demand for oxygen.

Calcium channel blockers

Calcium channel blockers are commonly used to prevent angina that doesn't respond to nitrates or beta-adrenergic blockers. Some calcium channel blockers are also used as antiarrhythmics.

Preventing passage

Calcium channel blockers are indicated for use with chronic stable angina, variant angina, or patients with hypertension who continue to have angina while treated with beta blockers. Calcium channel blockers are not indicated with acute MI (Ignatavicius et al., 2018; Reeder & Kennedy, 2018). Calcium channel blockers prevent the passage of calcium ions across the myocardial cell membrane and vascular smooth muscle cells, causing dilation of the coronary and peripheral arteries. The dilation in turn decreases the force of the heart's contractions and reduces the workload of the heart.

Rate reduction

By preventing arterioles from constricting, calcium channel blockers also reduce afterload. In addition, decreasing afterload decreases oxygen demands of the heart.

Conduction reduction

Calcium channel blockers also reduce the heart rate by slowing conduction through the SA and atrioventricular (AV) nodes. A slower heart rate reduces the heart's need for oxygen.

Antiarrhythmics

Antiarrhythmics are used to treat arrhythmias, which are disturbances of the normal heart rhythm. (See *Understanding antiarrhythmics,* pages 130 and 131.)

Understanding antiarrhythmics

Antiarrhythmics are used to restore normal heart rhythm in patients with arrhythmias. The table provides examples of drugs within these classes and associated indications and adverse reactions.

Drugs	Indications	Adverse reactions
Class IA antiarrhythmics		
Disopyramide (Norpace), procainamide	• Atrial fibrillation • Atrial flutter • Paroxysmal atrial tachycardia • Ventricular tachycardia	• Abdominal cramping • Anorexia • Bitter taste • Diarrhea • Nausea and vomiting • Ringing in ears
Class IB antiarrhythmics		
Lidocaine (Xylocaine)	• Alternative to amiodarone in cardiac arrest from ventricular fibrillation or pulseless ventricular tachycardia	• Bradycardia • Drowsiness • Hypotension • Confusion • Paresthesia
Class IC antiarrhythmics		
Flecainide, propafenone (Rythmol SR)	• Ventricular tachycardia, ventricular fibrillation, supraventricular arrhythmias	• Propafenone: bronchospasm, gastrointestinal symptoms • New arrhythmias
Class II antiarrhythmics		
Acebutolol, esmolol (Brevibloc), and propranolol (Inderal)	• Atrial flutter, atrial fibrillation, paroxysmal atrial tachycardia, ventricular arrhythmias	• Arrhythmias • Bradycardia • Bronchoconstriction • Diarrhea • Heart failure • Hypotension • Nausea and vomiting
Class III antiarrhythmics		
Amiodarone	• Life-threatening ventricular dysrhythmias, atrial fibrillation	• Anorexia • Hypotension • Severe pulmonary toxicity • Thyroid toxicity • Liver toxicity • Corneal microdeposits • Photosensitivity

Understanding antiarrhythmics *(continued)*

Drugs	Indications	Adverse reactions
Class III antiarrhythmics (continued)		
Dofetilide (Tikosyn)	• Atrial fibrillation and atrial flutter	• QT prolongation • Torsades de pointes • Ventricular arrhythmias • Headache • Chest pain • Dizziness
Dronedarone (Multaq)	• Atrial fibrillation and atrial flutter	• Weakness • Diarrhea • Bradycardia • Heart failure exacerbation or new onset • QT prolongation • Liver toxicity • May cause worsening renal failure
Class IV antiarrhythmics		
Diltiazem (Cardizem) and verapamil (Calan)	• Supraventricular arrhythmias	• Atrioventricular block • Bradycardia • Dizziness • Flushing (with diltiazem) • Hypotension • Peripheral edema • Heart failure
Miscellaneous antiarrhythmics		
Adenosine	• Paroxysmal supraventricular tachycardia	• Chest discomfort • Hypotension • Dyspnea • Facial flushing • Shortness of breath

Adapted from American Heart Association. (2016). *Advanced cardiovascular life support provider manual* (16th ed.). Dallas, TX: Author; Burchum, J. R., & Rosenthal, L. D. (2018). *Lehne's pharmacology for nursing care* (10th ed.). St. Louis, MO: Elsevier; and U.S. Food and Drug Administration. (2018). *Drugs@FDA: FDA approved drug products*. Retrieved from https://www.accessdata.fda.gov /scripts/cder/daf/index.cfm

Benefits vs. risks

Unfortunately, many antiarrhythmic drugs can worsen or cause arrhythmias, too. Thus, the benefits of antiarrhythmic therapy must be weighed against the associated risks.

Four classes plus . . .

Antiarrhythmics are categorized into four major classes: I (which includes IA, IB, and IC), II, III, and IV. The mechanisms of action of antiarrhythmic drugs vary widely, and a few drugs exhibit properties common to more than one class. One drug, adenosine, doesn't fall into any of these classes.

Class I antiarrhythmics

Class I antiarrhythmics are sodium channel blockers. This group is the largest group of antiarrhythmic drugs. Class I agents are commonly subdivided into classes IA, IB, and IC.

Class IA antiarrhythmics

Class IA antiarrhythmics control arrhythmias by altering the myocardial cell membrane and interfering with autonomic nervous system control of pacemaker cells.

No (para)sympathy

Class IA antiarrhythmics also block parasympathetic stimulation of the SA and AV nodes. Because stimulation of the parasympathetic nervous system causes the heart rate to slow down, drugs that block the parasympathetic nervous system increase the conduction rate of the AV node.

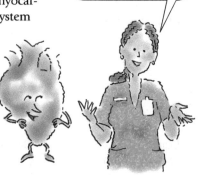

Talk about overbearing! Class IA antiarrhythmics interfere with myocardial cell membrane, parasympathetic stimulation of SA nodes, and more!

Rhythmic risks

The increase in the conduction rate can produce dangerous increases in the ventricular heart rate if rapid atrial activity is present, as in a patient with atrial fibrillation. In turn, the increased ventricular heart rate can offset the ability of the antiarrhythmics to convert atrial arrhythmias to a regular rhythm.

Class IB antiarrhythmics

Lidocaine, a class IB antiarrhythmic, is one of the antiarrhythmics commonly used in treating patients with acute ventricular arrhythmias.

Class IB drugs work by blocking the rapid influx of sodium ions during the depolarization phase of the heart's depolarization–repolarization cycle. The blocking action results in a decreased refractory period, which reduces the risk of arrhythmia.

Make a IB line for the ventricle

Because class IB antiarrhythmics especially affect the Purkinje fibers and myocardial cells in the ventricles, they're used only in treating patients with ventricular arrhythmias.

Class IC antiarrhythmics

Class IC antiarrhythmics are used to treat patients with certain severe, refractory (resistant) ventricular arrhythmias. Class IC antiarrhythmics include flecainide and propafenone.

Slowing the seeds of conduction

Class IC antiarrhythmics primarily slow conduction along the heart's conduction system. Moricizine decreases the fast inward current of sodium ions of the action potential. The decrease depresses the depolarization rate and effective refractory period.

Class II antiarrhythmics

Class II antiarrhythmics include the beta-adrenergic antagonists, also known as *beta-adrenergic blockers*.

Receptor blockers

Class II antiarrhythmics block beta-adrenergic receptor sites in the conduction system of the heart. As a result, the ability of the SA node to fire spontaneously (automaticity) is slowed. The ability of the AV node and other cells to receive and conduct an electrical impulse to nearby cells (conductivity) is also reduced.

Strength reducers

Class II antiarrhythmics also reduce the strength of the heart's contractions. When the heart beats less forcefully, it doesn't require as much oxygen to do its work.

Class III antiarrhythmics

Class III antiarrhythmics are used to treat patients with ventricular arrhythmias and atrial fibrillation and flutter. Amiodarone is the most widely used class III antiarrhythmic. Dofetilide (Tikosyn) and dronedarone (Multaq) are also class III antiarrhythmics used for atrial fibrillation and atrial flutter.

One way to two way

Although the exact mechanism of action isn't known, class III antiarrhythmics are thought to suppress arrhythmias by converting a unidirectional block to a bidirectional block. They have little or no effect on depolarization.

Miscellaneous antiarrhythmics

The class IV antiarrhythmics include calcium channel blockers. These drugs block the movement of calcium during phase 2 of the action potential and slow conduction and the refractory period of calcium-dependent tissues, including the AV node. The calcium channel blockers used to treat patients with arrhythmias are verapamil and diltiazem. Miscellaneous antiarrhythmics also include adenosine.

Adenosine

Adenosine is an injectable antiarrhythmic drug indicated for acute treatment of paroxysmal supraventricular tachycardia.

Depressing the pacemaker

Adenosine depresses the pacemaker activity of the SA node, reducing the heart rate and the ability of the AV node to conduct impulses from the atria to the ventricles.

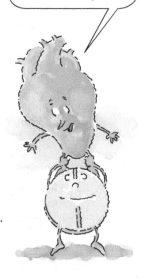

A little aspirin a day keeps the blood clots away!

Anticoagulants

Anticoagulants are used to reduce the ability of the blood to clot (Burchum & Rosenthal, 2018; FDA, 2018). (See *Understanding anticoagulants*.) Major categories of anticoagulants include antiplatelet drugs, heparin, and oral anticoagulants.

Antiplatelet drugs are used to prevent arterial thromboembolism, especially in patients at risk for MI, stroke, and arteriosclerosis (hardening of the arteries). They interfere with platelet activity in different drug-specific and dose-related ways.

Low is good

Low dosages of aspirin suppress platelet aggregation by inhibiting the enzyme that is required to break down thromboxane A_2 (TXA$_2$). TXA$_2$ can promote platelet aggregation.

Anticlumping

Clopidogrel inhibits platelet aggregation by blocking adenosine di-phosphate receptors on platelets, thereby preventing the clumping of platelets.

Heparin

Heparin is used to prevent clot formation. Low-molecular-weight heparin (LMWH), such as dalteparin and enoxaparin, prevents deep vein thrombosis (a blood clot in the deep veins, usually of the legs) in surgical patients. Heparin is unable to cross membranes, including those in the gastrointestinal tract; therefore, heparin is administered intravenously and LMWH therapy is administered subcutaneously. Be aware, however, that a patient placed on any form of heparin is at risk for developing heparin-induced thrombocytopenia. Although the risk of severe adverse effects is low, you must monitor the patient's platelet count. A decrease in platelet count is cause for alarm and should be addressed and closely monitored. All patients on any type of anticoagulants should be monitored for bleeding (Burchum & Rosenthal, 2018).

Understanding anticoagulants

Anticoagulants reduce the blood's ability to clot and are included in the treatment plans for many patients with cardio-vascular disorders. The table includes common examples of drugs in this category as well as associated indications and adverse reactions.

Drugs	Indications	Adverse reactions
Heparins		
Heparin and low-molecular-weight heparins, such as dalteparin (Fragmin) and enoxaparin (Lovenox)	• Deep vein thrombosis • Embolism prophylaxis • Prevention of complications after myocardial infarction (MI) • Pulmonary embolism	• Bleeding • Heparin-induced thrombocytopenia
Oral anticoagulants		
Warfarin (Coumadin)	• Atrial arrhythmias • Deep vein thrombosis prophylaxis • Used to prevent thrombosis in veins and within the atria of the heart	• Bleeding • Numerous drugs interact adversely with warfarin
Direct oral anticoagulants		
Fondaparinux (Arixtra), rivaroxaban (Xarelto), apixaban (Eliquis), edoxaban (Savaysa), betrixaban (Bevyxxa), dabigatran (Pradaxa)	• Deep vein thrombosis • Acute pulmonary embolus • Stroke prevention • Used to prevent thrombosis in veins and within the atria of the heart	• Bleeding • Anemia
Antiplatelet drugs		
Aspirin, ticlopidine, clopidogrel (Plavix), prasugrel (Effient), ticagrelor (Brilinta), vorapaxar (Zontivity)	• Decreases the risk of death after MI • Used to prevent thrombosis in arteries • Prevents complications of prosthetic heart valves • Chronic stable angina	• Bleeding • Gastrointestinal distress • Headache

Adapted from Burchum, J. R., & Rosenthal, L. D. (2018). *Lehne's pharmacology for nursing care* (10th ed.). St. Louis, MO: Elsevier; and U.S. Food and Drug Administration. (2018). *Drugs@FDA: FDA approved drug products.* Retrieved from https://www.accessdata.fda.gov/scripts/cder/daf/index.cfm

No new clots

Because it doesn't affect the synthesis of clotting factors, heparin can't dissolve already formed clots. It does prevent the formation of new thrombi. Here's how it works:

- Heparin inhibits the formation of thrombin and fibrin by activating antithrombin III.
- Antithrombin III then inactivates factors IXa, Xa, XIa, and XIIa in the intrinsic and common pathways. The end result is prevention of a stable fibrin clot.

- In low doses, heparin increases the activity of antithrombin III against factor Xa and thrombin and inhibits clot formation. Much larger doses are necessary to inhibit fibrin formation after a clot has formed. The relationship between dose and effect is the rationale for using low-dose heparin to prevent clotting.
- Whole blood clotting time, prothrombin time (PT) and partial thromboplastin time (PTT) are prolonged during heparin therapy. However, these times may be only slightly prolonged with low or ultra-low preventive doses. Protamine sulfate is the antidote for heparin overdose (Burchum & Rosenthal, 2018; Kee et al., 2015).

Circulate freely

Heparin can be used to prevent clotting when a patient's blood must circulate outside the body through a machine, such as a cardiopulmonary bypass or hemodialysis.

Oral anticoagulants

Oral anticoagulants alter the ability of the liver to synthesize vitamin K–dependent clotting factors, including prothrombin and factors VII, IX, and X (Lilley et al., 2017). Clotting factors already in the bloodstream continue to coagulate blood until they become depleted, so anticoagulation doesn't begin immediately.

A long history

Warfarin (Coumadin) is the oldest oral anticoagulant and works by suppressing four specific clotting factors (VII, IX, X, and prothrombin). The factors are dependent on an active form of vitamin K and inhibit the enzyme that creates an active form of vitamin K. In the past, warfarin was the major oral anticoagulant available in the United States. Effective treatment with warfarin requires regular monitoring of coagulation time, specifically the PT and the international normalized ratio. Bleeding is a significant risk with warfarin, and patients should be monitored closely and instructed on signs of bleeding. The antidote for warfarin is vitamin K (phytonadione). Although warfarin is still used, direct oral anticoagulants (DOACs) have presented a new option for oral anticoagulation therapy that presents a lower risk of bleeding and require less monitoring of coagulation times (Burchum & Rosenthal, 2018).

Direct oral anticoagulants

DOACs, also called *novel oral anticoagulants*, were developed as an oral anticoagulant with fewer drug interactions and a fixed dosing schedule. These drugs inhibit a specific enzyme in the coagulation cascade (Garcia & Crowther, 2019). Drugs in this class do not require frequent blood monitoring to tailor and determine dosing, have a lower risk of bleeding, and have a quick onset. One of the more common drugs in this class is dabigatran due to ease of use as well as an available reversal agent (idarucizumab) that can be used for life-threatening bleeding or if emergent surgical intervention is required (Garcia & Crowther, 2019).

Antihypertensives

Antihypertensive drugs act to reduce blood pressure. They're used to treat patients with hypertension, a disorder characterized by high systolic blood pressure, high diastolic blood pressure, or both.

Know the program

Although treatment for hypertension begins with beta-adrenergic blockers and diuretics, antihypertensives are used if those drugs aren't effective. Antihypertensive therapy includes the use of sympatholytics (other than beta-adrenergic blockers), vasodilators, ACE inhibitors, and angiotensin receptor blockers alone or in combination (Burchum & Rosenthal, 2018; Lilley et al., 2017; FDA, 2018). (See *Understanding antihypertensives*, pages 138 and 139.)

Sympatholytics

Sympatholytic drugs include several different types of drugs. However, all of these drugs work by inhibiting or blocking the sympathetic nervous system, which causes dilation of the peripheral blood vessels or decreases cardiac output, thereby reducing blood pressure.

Where and how

Sympatholytic drugs are classified by their site or mechanism of action and include:
- centrally acting sympathetic nervous system inhibitors, such as clonidine
- alpha blockers, such as doxazosin and prazosin
- mixed alpha- and beta-adrenergic blockers such as carvedilol.

Vasodilators

The two types of vasodilating drugs include calcium channel blockers and direct vasodilators. These drugs decrease systolic and diastolic blood pressure.

Calcium stoppers

Calcium channel blockers produce arteriolar relaxation by preventing the entry of calcium into the cells. This relaxation prevents the contraction of vascular smooth muscle.

Understanding antihypertensives

Antihypertensives are prescribed to reduce blood pressure in patients with hypertension.

The table includes common examples of drugs in this category as well as associated indications and adverse reactions.

Drugs	Indications	Adverse reactions
Sympatholytic drugs		
Central-acting sympathetic nervous system inhibitors Clonidine (Catapres), guanfacine, and methyldopa	• Hypertension	• Drowsiness • Hypotension (alpha blockers) • Dry mouth • Bradycardia
Alpha blockers Doxazosin (Cardura), prazosin (Minipress)	• Hypertension	• Orthostatic hypotension • Headache • Dizziness • Gastrointestinal upset
Mixed alpha- and beta-adrenergic blockers Labetalol	• Hypertension • Hypertensive emergency	• Orthostatic hypotension • Palpitations • Syncope
Vasodilators		
Hydralazine and nitroprusside (Nitropress)	• Used in combination with other drugs to treat moderate to severe hypertension • Nitroprusside: hypertensive emergency	Hydralazine • Myocardial infarction, hypotension, headache, tachycardia, edema, nausea, vomiting, diarrhea, systemic lupus erythematosus, rash, angina, blood dyscrasias Nitroprusside • Hypotension • Hypothyroidism • Bradycardia • Decreased platelet aggregation • Methemoglobinemia • Rarely: cyanide toxicity
Angiotensin-converting enzyme inhibitors		
Benazepril (Lotensin), captopril, enalapril (Vasotec), fosinopril, lisinopril (Zestril), quinapril (Accupril), ramipril (Altace)	• Heart failure • Hypertension	• Angioedema • Hypotension • Fatigue • Headache • Increased serum potassium concentrations • Persistent cough • Dizziness • Nausea • Diarrhea or constipation

Understanding antihypertensives *(continued)*

Drugs	Indications	Adverse reactions
Calcium channel blocker		
Amlodipine (Norvasc)	• Hypertension	• Peripheral edema • Flushing • Headache • Dizziness • Bradycardia • Atrioventricular block
Angiotensin II receptor blockers		
Losartan, eprosartan, valsartan, irbesartan, and olmesartan	• Hypertension • Heart failure	• Chest pain • Fatigue • Hypoglycemia • Diarrhea • Urinary tract infection • Anemia • Weakness
Alpha₁ and beta receptor blockers		
Carvedilol (Coreg)	• Hypertension • Heart failure	• Bradycardia

Adapted from Burchum, J. R., & Rosenthal, L. D. (2018). *Lehne's pharmacology for nursing care* (10th ed.). St. Louis, MO: Elsevier; Lilley, L. L., Collins, S. R., & Snyder, J. S. (2017). *Pharmacology and the nursing process* (8th ed.). St. Louis, MO: Elsevier; and U.S. Food and Drug Administration. (2018). *Drugs@FDA: FDA approved drug products.* Retrieved from https://www.accessdata.fda.gov/scripts/cder/daf/index.cfm

Direct dial

Direct vasodilators act on arteries, veins, or both. They work by relaxing peripheral vascular smooth muscles, causing the blood vessels to dilate. The dilation decreases blood pressure by increasing the diameter of the blood vessels, reducing total peripheral resistance.

Hydralazine is usually used to treat patients with resistant or refractory hypertension. Nitroprusside is reserved for use in hypertensive crisis.

ACE inhibitors

ACE inhibitors reduce blood pressure by interrupting the renin–angiotensin–aldosterone system.

Without ACE inhibition

Here's how the renin–angiotensin–aldosterone system works:
- Normally, the kidneys maintain blood pressure by releasing the hormone renin.
- Renin acts on the plasma protein angiotensinogen to form angiotensin I.

- Angiotensin I is then converted to angiotensin II.
- Angiotensin II, a potent vasoconstrictor, increases peripheral resistance and promotes the excretion of aldosterone.
- Aldosterone, in turn, promotes the retention of sodium and water, increasing the volume of blood the heart needs to pump.

With ACE inhibition

ACE inhibitors work by preventing the conversion of angiotensin I to angiotensin II. As angiotensin II is reduced, arterioles dilate, reducing peripheral vascular resistance.

Less water, less work

By reducing aldosterone secretion, ACE inhibitors promote the excretion of sodium and water. Less sodium and water reduces the amount of blood the heart needs to pump, resulting in lower blood pressure.

Angiotensin II receptor antagonists

Unlike ACE inhibitors, which prevent production of angiotensin, angiotensin II receptor antagonists block the action of angiotensin II, a major culprit in the development of hypertension, by attaching to tissue-binding receptor sites.

Calcium channel blockers

Calcium channel blockers block the binding of calcium to receptors, which causes smooth muscle relaxation that decreases blood pressure (Lilley et al., 2017).

Cardiac glycosides and phosphodiesterase inhibitors

Cardiac glycosides and PDIs increase the force of the heart's contractions. Increasing the force of contractions is known as a *positive inotropic effect*, so these drugs are also called *inotropic agents* (affecting the force or energy of muscular contractions). (See *Understanding cardiac glycosides and PDIs*.)

Slower rate

Cardiac glycosides, such as digoxin, also slow the heart rate (called a *negative chronotropic effect*) and slow electrical impulse conduction through the AV node (called a *negative dromotropic effect*).

The short and long of it

PDIs, such as milrinone, are typically used for short-term management of heart failure or long-term management in patients awaiting heart transplant surgery.

Boosting output

PDIs improve cardiac output by strengthening contractions. These drugs are thought to help move calcium into the cardiac cell or to

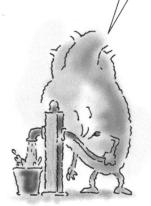

The more water and sodium excreted thanks to ACE inhibitors, the less blood I need to pump. Thank goodness—my arm is killing me!

Understanding cardiac glycosides and PDIs

Cardiac glycosides and phosphodiesterase inhibitors have a positive inotropic effect on the heart, meaning they increase the force of contraction.

The table includes common examples of drugs in this category as well as associated indications and adverse reactions.

Drugs	Indications	Adverse reactions
Cardiac glycoside		
Digoxin (Lanoxin)	• Heart failure • Atrial fibrillation	• Digoxin toxicity (abdominal pain, arrhythmias, depression, headache, insomnia, irritability, nausea, vision disturbances) • Bradycardia or tachycardia • Hypotension • Fatigue • Confusion • Convulsions • Colored vision • Gastrointestinal disturbances (anorexia, nausea, vomiting, diarrhea)
Phosphodiesterase inhibitors		
Milrinone	• Heart failure refractory to digoxin, diuretics, and vasodilators	• Arrhythmias • Chest pain • Hypotension

From Burchum, J. R., & Rosenthal, L. D. (2018). *Lehne's pharmacology for nursing care* (10th ed.). St. Louis, MO: Elsevier; Lilley, L. L., Collins, S. R., & Snyder, J. S. (2017). *Pharmacology and the nursing process* (8th ed.). St. Louis, MO: Elsevier; and U.S. Food and Drug Administration. (2018). *Drugs@FDA: FDA approved drug products.* Retrieved from https://www.accessdata.fda.gov/scripts/cder/daf/index.cfm

increase calcium storage in the sarcoplasmic reticulum. By directly relaxing vascular smooth muscle, they also decrease peripheral vascular resistance (afterload) and the amount of blood returning to the heart (preload).

Diuretics

Diuretics are used to promote the excretion of water and electrolytes by the kidneys. By doing so, diuretics play a major role in treating hypertension and other cardiovascular conditions. (See *Understanding diuretics*, page 142.)

The major diuretics used as cardiovascular drugs include:
- loop diuretics
- potassium-sparing diuretics
- thiazide and related diuretics.

Loop diuretics

Loop (high-ceiling) diuretics are highly potent drugs.

Understanding diuretics

Diuretics are used to treat patients with various cardiovascular conditions. They work by promoting the excretion of water and electrolytes by the kidneys. The table includes common examples of drugs in this category as well as associated indications and adverse reactions.

Drugs	Indications	Adverse reactions
Thiazide and related diuretics		
Hydrochlorothiazide, chlorthalidone, metolazone (Zaroxolyn)	• Hypertension • Heart failure	• Hypokalemia • Hyperglycemia • Hyperlipidemia • Hyperuricemia • Orthostatic hypotension • Dehydration • Gastrointestinal (GI) disturbances
Loop diuretics		
Bumetanide (Bumex), ethacrynic acid (Edecrin), furosemide (Lasix), and torsemide (Demadex)	• Edema • Heart failure • Hypertension	• Hypokalemia • Dehydration • Hyperuricemia • Hypocalcemia • Hyperglycemia • Hyponatremia • Orthostatic hypotension • Hearing loss
Potassium-sparing diuretics		
Amiloride (Midamor), spironolactone (Aldactone), and triamterene (Dyrenium)	• Hypertension • Diuretic-induced hypokalemia in patients with heart failure • Heart failure	• Hyperkalemia • Dizziness • Headache • GI upset

Adapted from Burchum, J. R., & Rosenthal, L. D. (2018). *Lehne's pharmacology for nursing care* (10th ed.). St. Louis, MO: Elsevier; Lilley, L. L., Collins, S. R., & Snyder, J. S. (2017). *Pharmacology and the nursing process* (8th ed.). St. Louis, MO: Elsevier; and U.S. Food and Drug Administration. (2018). *Drugs@FDA: FDA approved drug products.* Retrieved from https://www.accessdata.fda.gov/scripts/cder/daf/index.cfm

High potency, big risk

Loop diuretics are the most potent diuretics available, producing the greatest volume of diuresis (urine production). They also carry a high potential for causing severe adverse reactions.

In the loop

Loop diuretics receive their name because they act primarily on the thick ascending loop of Henle (the part of the nephron responsible for concentrating urine) to increase the secretion of sodium, chloride, and water. These drugs may also inhibit sodium, chloride, and water reabsorption.

Potassium-sparing diuretics

Potassium-sparing diuretics have weaker diuretic and antihypertensive effects than other diuretics, but they have the advantage of conserving potassium.

Potassium-sparing effects

The direct action of the potassium-sparing diuretics on the distal tubule of the kidneys produces:
- increased urinary excretion of sodium and water
- increased excretion of chloride and calcium ions
- decreased excretion of potassium and hydrogen ions.
    These effects lead to reduced blood pressure and increased serum potassium levels.

Thiazide and related diuretics

Thiazide and related diuretics are considered the first-line drugs for hypertension. They work by reducing volume and arterial resistance.

Sodium stoppers

Thiazide and related diuretics work by preventing sodium from being reabsorbed in the kidney. As sodium is excreted, it pulls water along with it. Thiazide and related diuretics also increase the excretion of chloride, potassium, and bicarbonate, which can result in electrolyte imbalances.

Stability with time

Initially, these drugs decrease circulating blood volume, leading to a reduced cardiac output. However, if therapy is maintained, cardiac output stabilizes but plasma fluid volume decreases.

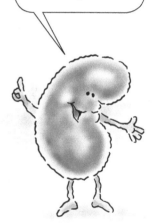

Sodium once, shame on you; sodium twice, shame on me! Thiazide diuretics prevent me from reabsorbing the stuff.

Thrombolytics

Thrombolytic drugs are used to dissolve a preexisting clot or thrombus and are commonly used in an acute or emergency situation. They work by converting plasminogen to plasmin, which lyses (dissolves) thrombi, fibrinogen, and other plasma proteins (Burchum & Rosenthal, 2018; Lilley et al., 2017). (See *Understanding thrombolytics*, page 144.)

    Some commonly used thrombolytic drugs include:
- reteplase
- alteplase
- tenecteplase.

Understanding thrombolytics

Thrombolytic (or fibrinolytic) drugs are prescribed to dissolve a preexisting clot or thrombus. These drugs are typically used in acute or emergency situations. The table includes common examples of drugs in this category as well as associated indications and adverse reactions.

Drugs	Indications	Adverse reactions
Alteplase (tissue plasminogen activator), reteplase, tenecteplase	• Acute ischemic stroke • Acute myocardial infarction • Arterial thrombosis • Pulmonary embolus	• Bleeding • Intracranial hemorrhage

Adapted from U.S. Food and Drug Administration. (2018). *Drugs@FDA: FDA approved drug products.* Retrieved from https://www .accessdata.fda.gov/scripts/cder/daf/index.cfm

Surgery

Types of surgery used to treat cardiovascular system disorders include coronary artery bypass graft (CABG), vascular repair, and insertion of a ventricular assist device (VAD).

Coronary artery bypass graft

CABG circumvents an occluded coronary artery with an autogenous graft (usually a segment of the saphenous vein from the leg or internal mammary artery), thereby restoring blood flow to the myocardium. CABG is one of the most commonly performed cardiac surgeries used to restore blood flow from occluded vessels that cannot be opened using percutaneous coronary intervention (PCI) (Ignatavicius et al., 2018). The need for CABG is determined by the results of cardiac catheterization and patient symptoms.

Why bypass?

If successful, CABG can relieve anginal pain, improve cardiac function, and possibly enhance the patient's quality of life.

CABG varieties

CABG techniques vary according to the patient's condition and the number of arteries being bypassed. Newer surgical techniques, such as the mini-CABG and direct coronary artery bypass, can reduce the risk of cerebral complications and accelerate recovery for patients requiring grafts of only one or two arteries. In some patients, it's possible to perform the CABG procedure without using a heart–lung bypass machine.

Nursing considerations

When caring for a patient who is undergoing CABG, your major roles include patient teaching and caring for the patient's changing cardiovascular needs:

- Check and record vital signs and hemodynamic parameters frequently, possibly every 5 to 15 minutes depending on the patient's condition and facility protocol.
- Administer medications and titrate according to the patient's response as prescribed.
- Monitor ECGs continuously for disturbances in heart rate and rhythm.
- Reinforce the health care provider's explanation of the surgery.
- Explain the complex equipment and procedures used in the critical care unit (CCU) or postanesthesia care unit (PACU).
- Explain to the patient upon awakening from surgery, an endotracheal (ET) tube may be in place and connected to a mechanical ventilator. Additionally, the patient will have continuous cardiac monitoring, a chest tube, an indwelling urinary catheter, arterial lines, epicardial pacing wires, and, possibly, a PA catheter. Inform the patient that the equipment will be removed as soon as possible.
- Make sure that the patient or a responsible family member has signed a consent form.

I think if I take the coronary artery bypass instead of the freeway, I can avoid anginal pain AND make good time.

Vascular repair

Vascular repair may be needed to treat patients with:

- vessels damaged by arteriosclerotic or thromboembolic disorders, trauma, infections, or congenital defects
- vascular obstructions that severely compromise circulation
- vascular disease that doesn't respond to drug therapy or nonsurgical treatments such as balloon catheterization
- life-threatening dissecting or ruptured aortic aneurysms
- limb-threatening acute arterial occlusion.

Repair review

Vascular repair methods include aneurysm resection, grafting, embolectomy, vena caval filtering, and endarterectomy. The surgery used depends on the type, location, and extent of vascular occlusion or damage.

Nursing considerations

- Make sure the patient and family understand the health care provider's explanation of the surgery and possible complications.

- Inform the patient that a general anesthetic will be used for the procedure and the patient will awaken from the anesthetic in the CCU or PACU. Explain that an intravenous (IV) line will be placed, ECG electrodes will be on the patient's chest for continuous cardiac monitoring, and, possibly, an arterial line or a PA catheter will be inserted to provide continuous pressure monitoring. A urinary catheter may be used to allow accurate output measurement. If necessary, the patient will be intubated and placed on mechanical ventilation.
- Before surgery, perform a complete vascular assessment. Take vital signs to provide a baseline. Evaluate the strength and sound of the blood flow and the symmetry of the pulses and note bruits. Record the temperature of the extremities; any sensitivity to motor and sensory stimuli; and pallor, cyanosis, or redness. Rate peripheral pulse volume and strength on a scale of 0 (pulse absent) to 4 (bounding and strong pulse). Check capillary refill time by blanching the fingernails or toenails. Normal refill time is less than 3 seconds.
- Auscultate heart, breath, and bowel sounds and report abnormal findings. Monitor the ECG for abnormalities in heart rate or rhythm. Also monitor other pressure readings and carefully record intake and output.
- Withhold food according to the surgeon's orders and facility policy.
- If the patient is awaiting surgery for aortic aneurysm repair, be on guard for signs and symptoms of acute dissection or rupture. Notify the health care provider immediately if the patient experiences sudden severe pain in the chest, abdomen, or lower back; severe weakness; diaphoresis; tachycardia; or a precipitous drop in blood pressure.

Percutaneous coronary intervention

PCI is a nonsurgical way to open coronary vessels narrowed by arteriosclerosis. It's usually used with cardiac catheterization to assess the stenosis and efficacy of angioplasty.

In PCI, a balloon-tipped catheter is inserted into a narrowed coronary artery. The procedure, performed in the cardiac catheterization laboratory under local anesthesia, relieves pain caused by angina and myocardial ischemia. A stent may be placed during the PCI procedure to help prevent vasospasms and repeated occlusion.

Plaque, meet Balloon

When the guide catheter's position at the occlusion site is confirmed by angiography, the physician carefully introduces a double-lumen balloon into the catheter and through the lesion, where a marked increase in the pressure gradient is obvious. The physician alternately inflates and deflates the balloon until arteriography verifies successful arterial dilation and a decrease in the pressure gradient. With balloon inflation, the plaque is compressed against the vessel wall, allowing coronary blood to flow more freely.

Nursing considerations
- Describe the procedure to the patient and family and tell them the procedure takes 1 to 3 hours to complete.
- Explain that a catheter will be inserted into an artery or a vein in the patient's wrist or groin and that pressure may be felt as the catheter moves along the vessel.
- Reassure the patient that although awake during the procedure, the patient will be given a sedative. Instruct the patient to report angina during the procedure.
- Explain that the physician injects a contrast medium to outline the location of the lesion. Warn the patient that a hot, flushing sensation or transient nausea may occur during the injection.
- Check the patient's history for allergies; if the patient has had allergic reactions to shellfish, iodine, or contrast media, notify the health care provider.

Take two aspirins and call me . . .
- If prescribed by the health care provider, administer a dose of aspirin before the procedure to prevent platelet aggregation.
- Make sure the patient signs an informed consent form.
- Restrict food and fluids before the procedure.
- Make sure that the results of coagulation studies, complete blood count (CBC), serum electrolyte studies, blood typing and cross-matching, blood urea nitrogen (BUN), and serum creatinine are available.
- Obtain baseline vital signs and assess peripheral pulses; continue to assess the patient's vital signs and oxygen saturation frequently.
- Apply ECG electrodes and insert an IV line if not already in place. Monitor IV infusions as indicated.
- Administer oxygen through a nasal cannula.
- If prescribed by the health care provider, administer a sedative to decrease patient anxiety.

Other treatments

Other treatments for cardiovascular disorders include synchronized cardioversion, defibrillation, and pacemaker insertion.

Synchronized cardioversion

Synchronized cardioversion is an elective or emergency procedure used to treat unstable tachyarrhythmias (such as atrial flutter, atrial fibrillation, and supraventricular tachycardia and ventricular tachycardia). It's also the treatment of choice for patients with arrhythmias that don't respond to drug therapy.

Electrifying experience

In synchronized cardioversion, an electric current is delivered to the heart to correct an arrhythmia. Compared with defibrillation, it uses much lower energy levels and is synchronized to deliver an electric charge to the myocardium at the peak R wave.

The procedure causes immediate depolarization, interrupting reentry circuits (abnormal impulse conduction resulting when cardiac tissue is activated two or more times, causing reentry arrhythmias) and allowing the SA node to resume control.

Synchronizing the electrical charge with the R wave ensures that the current won't be delivered on the vulnerable T wave and disrupt repolarization. Thus, it reduces the risk that the current will strike during the relative refractory period of a cardiac cycle and induce ventricular fibrillation (AHA, 2016; Ignatavicius et al., 2018).

Nursing considerations
- Describe the elective procedure to the patient and make sure an informed consent is obtained.
- Obtain a baseline 12-lead ECG.
- If prescribed, administer a sedative.
- Apply conductive gel to the paddles or attach "hands-free" defibrillation pads to the chest wall; position the pads so that one pad is to the right of the sternum, just below the clavicle, and the other is at the fifth or sixth intercostal space in the left anterior axillary line.
- Turn on the defibrillator and select the ordered energy level as suggested by the advanced cardiac life support (ACLS) guidelines, usually between 50 and 100 joules.
- Activate the synchronized mode by depressing the synchronizer switch.
- Check that the machine is sensing the R wave correctly.
- Place the paddles on the chest and apply firm pressure OR if using "hands-free" defibrillation pads, attach them to the chest wall.
- Charge the paddles or defibrillation pads.
- Instruct other personnel to stand clear of the patient and the bed to avoid the risk of an electric shock by stating "all clear."

- Discharge the current by pushing both paddles' DISCHARGE buttons simultaneously or, if using the defibrillation pads, pressing the discharge button on the machine.

Repeat, repeat, and repeat again

- If cardioversion is unsuccessful, repeat the procedure two or three times as ordered, gradually increasing the energy with each additional countershock.
- If normal rhythm is restored, continue to monitor the patient and provide supplemental ventilation as long as needed.
- If the patient's cardiac rhythm changes to ventricular fibrillation, switch the mode from SYNCHRONIZED to DEFIBRILLATE and defibrillate the patient immediately after charging the machine.
- When using handheld paddles, continue to hold the paddles on the patient's chest until the energy is delivered.

In sync

- Remember to reset the SYNC MODE on the defibrillator after each synchronized cardioversion. Resetting the switch is necessary because most defibrillators automatically reset to an unsynchronized mode.
- Document the use of synchronized cardioversion, the rhythm before and after cardioversion, the amperage used, and how the patient tolerated the procedure.

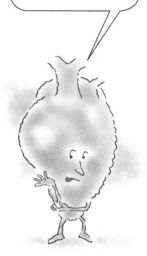

Resetting the SYNC MODE defibrillator switch after each cardioversion ensures that the machine stays synchronized.

Defibrillation

In defibrillation, electrode paddles or self-adhesive pads are used to direct an electric current through the patient's heart. The current causes the myocardium to depolarize, which in turn encourages the SA node to resume control of the heart's electrical activity.

The electrode paddles or self-adhesive pads delivering the current may be placed on the patient's chest. Electrical current may be applied directly to the myocardium during cardiac surgery. Most defibrillators are biphasic.

Positively speaking

A *biphasic defibrillator* delivers the electrical current in a positive direction for a specified duration and then reverses and flows in a negative direction for the remaining time of the electrical discharge. The biphasic defibrillator delivers two currents of electricity and lowers the defibrillation threshold of the heart muscle, making it possible to successfully defibrillate ventricular fibrillation with smaller amounts of energy.

Adjustable

Additionally, the biphasic defibrillator is able to adjust for differences in impedance or the resistance of the current through the chest, thereby reducing the number of shocks needed to terminate ventricular fibrillation. Also, damage to the myocardial muscle is reduced because of the lower energy levels used and fewer shocks needed.

Act early and quickly

Because some arrhythmias, such as ventricular fibrillation, can cause death if not corrected, the success of defibrillation depends on early recognition and quick treatment. In addition to treating ventricular fibrillation, defibrillation may also be used to treat ventricular tachycardia that doesn't produce a pulse.

Nursing considerations
- Assess the patient to determine if a pulse is present. If no pulse is present, call for help and perform cardiopulmonary resuscitation (CPR) until the defibrillator and other emergency equipment arrive.
- Connect the monitoring leads of the defibrillator to the patient and assess cardiac rhythm in two leads.
- Expose the patient's chest and apply hands-free pads appropriately. (See *Defibrillator paddle placement.*)
- Turn on the defibrillator and set energy level following ACLS guidelines.

Charge!! And discharge!

- Charge the paddles by pressing the CHARGE button, which is located on the machine.
- Clear the patient (ensure no staff or oxygen is touching the bed or patient). Once clear, administer the shock. The appropriate energy used to shock the patient depends on the type of defibrillator used—monophasic or biphasic. For defibrillation, if the machine is biphasic, the initial dose is 120 to 200 joules. Further shocks with equivalent or higher doses of energy may be considered. If the defibrillator is monophasic, the machine should be set at 360 joules for an adult patient (AHA, 2016).
- Reassess the patient's pulse and give 2 minutes of CPR. Reassess cardiac rhythm.
- If necessary, prepare to defibrillate a second time at the appropriate setting, according to the defibrillator recommendations. Announce that you're preparing to defibrillate and follow the procedure described previously.
- Reassess the patient and continue CPR.

Defibrillator paddle placement

Here's a guide to correct paddle placement for defibrillation.

Anterolateral placement

For anterolateral placement, place one paddle to the right of the upper sternum, just below the right clavicle. Place the other over the fifth or sixth intercostal space at the left anterior axillary line.

Anteroposterior placement

For anteroposterior placement, place the anterior paddle directly over the heart at the precordium, to the left of the lower sternal border. Place the flat posterior paddle under the patient's body beneath the heart and immediately below the scapula (but not under the vertebral column).

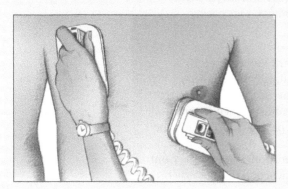

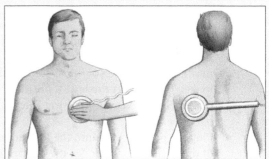

- If the patient still has no pulse after the first two cycles of defibrillation and CPR, begin administering appropriate medications such as epinephrine per ACLS guidelines. Also, consider possible causes for failure of the patient's rhythm to convert, such as acidosis and hypoxia.

Rhythm restoration

- If defibrillation restores a normal rhythm, assess the patient. Obtain baseline ABG levels and a 12-lead ECG. Provide supplemental oxygen, ventilation, and medications as needed. Prepare the defibrillator for immediate reuse.
- Document the procedure, including the patient's ECG rhythms before and after defibrillation; the number of times defibrillation was performed; the voltage used during each attempt; whether a pulse returned; the dosage, route, and time of drugs administered; whether CPR was used; how the airway was maintained; and the patient's outcome.
- Prepare the patient for possible insertion of an implantable cardioverter–defibrillator (ICD).

Transcutaneous pacemaker

A transcutaneous pacemaker, also referred to as *external* or *noninvasive pacing*, is a temporary pacemaker that's used in an emergency. The device consists of an external, battery-powered pulse generator and a lead or electrode system.

Dire straits

In a life-threatening situation, a transcutaneous pacemaker works by sending an electrical impulse from the pulse generator to the patient's heart by way of two large electrodes that are placed on the front and back of the patient's chest.

Transcutaneous pacing is quick and effective, but it's used only until the health care provider can institute transvenous pacing.

Nursing considerations

- Attach monitoring electrodes to the patient in the lead I, II, or III position. Do so even if the patient is already on telemetry monitoring because you must connect the electrodes to the pacemaker. If you select the lead II position, adjust the left leg electrode placement to accommodate the anterior pacing electrode and the patient's anatomy.
- Plug the patient cable into the ECG input connection on the front of the pacing generator. Set the selector switch to the MONITOR ON position.
- You should see the ECG waveform on the monitor. Adjust the R wave beeper volume to a suitable level and activate the alarm by pressing the ALARM ON button. Set the alarm for 10 to 20 beats lower and 20 to 30 beats higher than the intrinsic rate.
- Press the START/STOP button for a printout of the waveform.
- Now you're ready to apply the two pacing electrodes.

Proper placement

- First, make sure the patient's skin is clean and dry to ensure good skin contact.
- Pull off the protective strip from the posterior electrode (marked BACK) and apply the electrode on the left side of the back, just below the scapula and to the left of the spine.
- The anterior pacing electrode (marked FRONT) has two protective strips—one covering the jellied area and one covering the outer ring. Expose the jellied area and apply it to the skin in the anterior position—to the left of the precordium in the usual V_2 to V_5 position. Move the electrode around to get the best waveform. Then expose the electrode's outer rim and firmly press it to the skin. (See *Proper electrode placement.*)

Proper electrode placement

Place the two pacing electrodes for a transcutaneous pacemaker at heart level on the patient's chest and back (as shown). The placement ensures that the electrical stimulus must travel only a short distance to the heart.

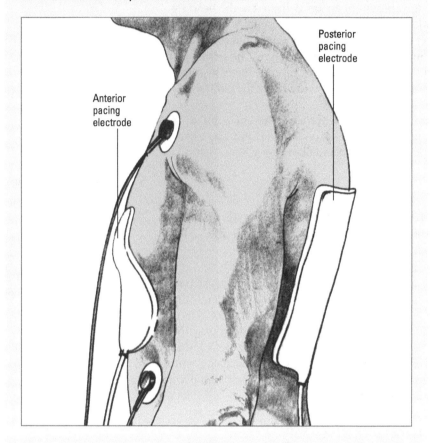

Posterior pacing electrode

Anterior pacing electrode

Now to pacing

- After making sure the energy output in milliamperes (mA) is on, connect the electrode cable to the monitor output cable.
- Check the waveform, looking for a tall QRS complex in lead II.
- Next, turn the selector switch to PACER ON. Tell the patient a thumping or twitching sensation may be felt with pacing. Reassure the patient that you will administer a medication as prescribed to help decrease the discomfort associated with transcutaneous pacing.

Set the beat

- Now set the rate dial to 10 to 20 beats higher than the patient's intrinsic rate. Look for pacer artifact or spikes, which will appear as you increase the rate. If the patient doesn't have an intrinsic rhythm, set the rate at 60.
- Slowly increase the amount of energy delivered to the heart by adjusting the OUTPUT MA dial. Do so until capture is achieved; you'll see a pacer spike followed by a widened QRS complex that resembles a permanent ventricular contraction. The setting is the pacing threshold. To ensure consistent capture, increase output by 10%. Don't go higher because you could cause the patient needless discomfort.
- With full capture, the patient's heart rate should be approximately the same as the pacemaker rate set on the machine. The usual pacing threshold is between 40 and 60 mA.

Them bones, them bones

- Don't place the electrodes over a bony area because bone conducts current poorly. For female patients, place the anterior electrode under the patient's breast but not over her diaphragm.

Check back with the vitals

- After placement of a transcutaneous pacemaker, assess the patient's vital signs, skin color, LOC, and peripheral pulses to determine the effectiveness of the paced rhythm. Perform a 12-lead ECG to serve as a baseline and then perform additional ECGs daily or with clinical changes. If possible, also obtain a rhythm strip before, during, and after pacemaker placement; any time that pacemaker settings are changed; and whenever the patient receives treatment because of a complication due to the pacemaker.
- Continuously monitor the ECG reading, noting capture, sensing, rate, intrinsic beats, and competition of paced and intrinsic rhythms. If the pacemaker is sensing correctly, the sense indicator on the pulse generator should flash with each beat.

Common disorders

In the ED, you're likely to encounter patients with common cardiac emergencies, especially acute coronary syndrome, aortic aneurysm, cardiac arrest, cardiac arrhythmias, cardiac contusion, cardiac tamponade, heart failure, and hypertensive crisis. Regardless of the disorder, the priorities are always to ensure vital functioning—that is, airway, breathing, and circulation.

Acute coronary syndrome

Patients with acute coronary syndrome have some degree of coronary artery occlusion. The degree of occlusion defines whether the acute coronary syndrome is:

- unstable angina
- non–ST segment elevation MI (non-STEMI)
- ST segment elevation MI (STEMI).

Plaque's place

The development of acute coronary syndrome begins with a rupture or erosion of plaque, an unstable and lipid-rich substance. The rupture results in platelet adhesions, fibrin clot formation, and thrombin activation.

What causes it

Patients with certain risk factors appear to face a greater likelihood of developing acute coronary syndrome. These factors include:

- diabetes
- family history of heart disease
- hypertension
- obesity
- high-fat, high-carbohydrate diet
- sedentary lifestyle
- menopause
- hyperlipoproteinemia
- smoking
- stress.

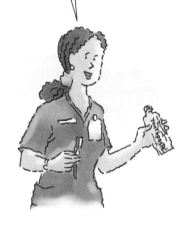

Plaque erosion on the teeth may be welcome but not around the heart.

How it happens

Acute coronary syndrome most commonly results when a thrombus progresses and occludes blood flow. (An early thrombus doesn't necessarily block blood flow.) The effect is an imbalance in myocardial oxygen supply and demand.

Degree and duration

The degree and duration of blockage dictate the type of infarct:

- If the patient has *unstable angina,* a thrombus partially occludes a coronary vessel. The thrombus is full of platelets. The partially occluded vessel may have distal microthrombi that cause necrosis in some myocytes.
- If smaller vessels infarct, the patient is at higher risk for MI, which may progress to a *non-STEMI.* Only the innermost layer of the heart is damaged.

Identifying symptoms of MI

The cardinal symptom of a myocardial infarction (MI) is persistent, intense substernal pain that may radiate to the left arm, jaw, neck, or shoulder blades. The pain is unrelieved by rest or nitroglycerin and may last several hours. Some patients with an MI, such as older adult patients and those with diabetes, may not experience pain at all. Other patients experience only mild pain; for example, female patients who experience atypical chest pain with an MI may present with reports of indigestion and fatigue. Any patient may experience atypical chest pain, but it's more common in women.

- *STEMI* results when reduced blood flow through one of the coronary arteries causes myocardial ischemia, injury, and necrosis. The damage extends through all myocardial layers.

What to look for

A patient with angina typically experiences:
- burning
- squeezing
- crushing tightness in the substernal or precordial chest that may radiate to the left arm, neck, jaw, or shoulder blade. (See *Identifying symptoms of MI*.)

It hurts when I do this

Angina may most commonly follow physical exertion but may also follow emotional excitement, cold exposure, or a large meal. Angina is commonly relieved by nitroglycerin and rest. It's less severe and shorter lived than the pain of acute MI.

Angina has different forms:
1. *stable*—predictable pain, in frequency and duration, which can be relieved with nitrates and rest
2. *unstable*—increased pain, which can occur with exertion or at rest; can be easily induced; increases in number of attacks or intensity
3. *Prinzmetal or a variant*—pain from unpredictable coronary artery spasm
4. *preinfarction angina*—angina that occurs in the days or weeks before a patient experiences an MI (Ignatavicius et al., 2018).

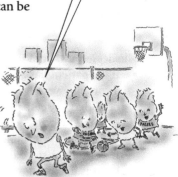

Patients with angina often experience a burning or squeezing sensation after physical exertion. I think I'll sit this one out!

Pinpointing infarction

The site of myocardial infarction (MI) depends on the vessels involved:
• Occlusion of the circumflex branch of the left coronary artery causes a lateral wall infarction.
• Occlusion of the anterior descending branch of the left coronary artery leads to an anterior wall infarction.
• True posterior or inferior wall infarctions generally result from occlusion of the right coronary artery or one of its branches.
• Right ventricular infarctions can also result from right coronary artery occlusion, can accompany inferior infarctions, and may cause right-sided heart failure.
• In an ST segment elevation MI, tissue damage extends through all myocardial layers; in a non–ST segment elevation MI, damage occurs only in the innermost layer.

My, my, MI pain

A patient with MI experiences severe, persistent chest pain that isn't relieved by rest or nitroglycerin. The pain may be described as crushing or squeezing. The pain is usually substernal but may radiate to the left arm, jaw, neck, or shoulder blades.

And many more

Other signs and symptoms of MI include:
• anxiety
• feeling of impending doom
• nausea and vomiting
• perspiration
• shortness of breath
• cool extremities
• fatigue
• hypotension or hypertension
• muffled heart sounds
• palpable precordial pulse
• dysrhythmias.

What tests tell you

These tests are used to diagnose CAD:
• ECG during an anginal episode shows ischemia. Serial 12-lead ECGs may be normal or inconclusive during the first few hours after an MI. Abnormalities include non-STEMI and STEMI. (See *Pinpointing infarction*.)
• Coronary angiography reveals coronary artery stenosis or obstruction and collateral circulation and shows the condition of the arteries beyond the narrowing.

- Myocardial perfusion imaging during treadmill exercise discloses ischemic areas of the myocardium, visualized as "cold spots."
- With MI, serial cardiac enzymes troponin T and I values will elevate.

How it's treated

For patients with angina, the goal of treatment is to reduce myocardial oxygen demand or increase oxygen supply. These treatments are used to manage angina:

- Nitrates reduce myocardial oxygen consumption and increase collateral blood flow to the myocardium by dilating the coronary arteries (Ignatavicius et al., 2018).
- Beta-adrenergic blockers may be administered to reduce the workload and oxygen demands of the heart.
- If angina is caused by coronary artery spasm, calcium channel blockers may be given.
- Antiplatelet drugs minimize platelet aggregation and the danger of coronary occlusion.
- Antilipemic drugs can reduce elevated serum cholesterol or triglyceride levels.
- Obstructive lesions may necessitate CABG or PCI. Other alternatives include laser angioplasty, minimally invasive surgery, rotational atherectomy, or stent placement.

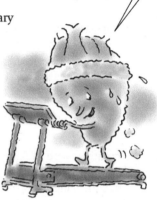

Myocardial perfusion imaging during treadmill exercise reveals the myocardium's ischemic areas.

MI relief

The goals of treatment for MI are to relieve pain, stabilize heart rhythm, revascularize the coronary artery, preserve myocardial tissue, and reduce cardiac workload. Here are some guidelines for treatment:

- Thrombolytic therapy should be started within 2 to 4 hours of the onset of symptoms (unless contraindications exist). Thrombolytic therapy involves administration of alteplase, tenecteplase, or reteplase.
- PCI (via cardiac catheterization) is the preferred option for restoring blood flow due to MI. Many facilities have a "door to balloon time" policy as time is of the essence when blood flow to the myocardium is compromised (Gibson et al., 2018). Review your facility policy.
- Oxygen is administered to increase oxygenation of the blood.
- Nitroglycerin is administered as prescribed to relieve chest pain. With an MI, nitroglycerin is administered sublingually or intravenously.
- Morphine is administered as analgesia because pain stimulates the sympathetic nervous system, leading to an increase in heart rate and vasoconstriction.
- Aspirin is administered to inhibit platelet aggregation.

Patency protection

- All patients who receive fibrinolytic therapy should be prescribed anticoagulation (IV heparin, enoxaparin) as well as antiplatelet drugs such as clopidogrel to increase the chances of patency in the affected coronary artery (Burchum & Rosenthal, 2018).
- Amiodarone, lidocaine, transcutaneous pacing patches (or a transvenous pacemaker), defibrillation, or epinephrine may be used if arrhythmias are present.
- Physical activity is limited initially to reduce cardiac workload, thereby limiting the area of necrosis.
- IV nitroglycerin is administered in patients without hypotension, bradycardia, or excessive tachycardia to reduce afterload and preload and to relieve chest pain.
- Glycoprotein IIb/IIIa inhibitors (such as abciximab [ReoPro]) are administered to patients with continued unstable angina and non-STEMI, with acute chest pain, or following invasive cardiac procedures to reduce platelet aggregation.
- IV beta-adrenergic blocker is administered early to patients with evolving acute MI; it's followed by oral therapy to reduce heart rate and to reduce myocardial oxygen requirements. Beta blockers have been shown to decrease morbidity and mortality in patients with MIs (Ignatavicius et al., 2018).
- ACE inhibitors are administered to those with evolving MI with ST segment elevation or left bundle branch block to reduce afterload and preload and to prevent remodeling.
- Laser angioplasty, atherectomy, stent placement, or transmyocardial revascularization may be initiated.
- Lipid-lowering drugs are administered to patients with elevated low-density lipoprotein and cholesterol levels.

What to do

- On admission, monitor and record the patient's ECG, blood pressure, temperature, and heart and breath sounds. Also, assess and record the severity, location, type, and duration of pain.
- Obtain a 12-lead ECG and assess heart rate and blood pressure when the patient experiences acute chest pain.
- Monitor the patient's hemodynamic status closely. Be alert for indicators suggesting decreased cardiac output, such as decreased blood pressure, increased heart rate, increased PAP, increased PAOP, decreased cardiac output measurements, and decreased right atrial pressure.
- Assess urine output hourly.
- Monitor the patient's oxygen saturation levels and notify the health care provider if oxygen saturation falls below 90%.

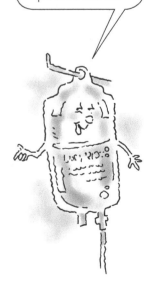

IV heparin, nitroglycerin, and beta-adrenergic blocker can help patients with MI.

- Monitor the patient's blood pressure after giving nitroglycerin, especially the first dose.
- During episodes of chest pain, monitor ECG, blood pressure, and PA catheter readings (if applicable) to determine changes.
- Frequently monitor ECG rhythm strips to detect heart rate changes and arrhythmias.
- Obtain serial measurements of cardiac enzyme levels as prescribed.
- Watch for crackles in the lungs, cough, tachypnea, and edema, which may indicate impending left-sided heart failure. Carefully monitor weight, intake and output, respiratory rate, serum enzyme levels, ECG waveforms, and blood pressure. Auscultate for S_3 or S_4 heart sounds.
- Prepare the patient for cardiac catheterization or reperfusion therapy as indicated. (The use of fibrinolytic should only be considered if PCI is delayed greater than 120 minutes.)
- Administer and titrate medications as prescribed (primary measures include morphine, oxygen, nitroglycerin, aspirin). Avoid intramuscular injections; IV administration provides more rapid symptom relief.
- Organize patient care and activities to allow rest periods. If the patient is immobilized, assist with repositioning often and use intermittent compression devices. Gradually increase the patient's activity level as tolerated.

Treating the heart

ACLS certification is highly important training for every ED nurse. The AHA provides guidelines for treating life-threatening perfusion issues of the brain and heart. Facilities usually require nurses working in critical areas to obtain ACLS certification. These guidelines are updated every few years based on research and are considered the standard of care. Whether it is acute coronary syndrome, electrolyte imbalance, or hypovolemia leading to a cardiac perfusion issue requiring advanced intervention, the ACLS-certified nurse needs to be aware and implement the current guidelines and standards of care set forth by the AHA for ACLS.

Aortic aneurysm

An aortic aneurysm is a localized outpouching or an abnormal dilation in a weakened arterial wall. Aortic aneurysm is typically found in the aorta between the renal arteries and the iliac branches, but the abdominal, thoracic, or ascending arch of the aorta may be affected.

What causes it

The exact cause of an aortic aneurysm is unclear, but several factors place a person at risk, including:

- family history
- atherosclerosis
- hypertension
- hyperlipidemia
- tobacco use
- advanced age
- pregnancy
- Marfan syndrome
- syphilis
- preexisting aneurysm (in advanced age)
- trauma.

How it happens

Aneurysms arise from a defect in the middle layer of the arterial wall (*tunica media* or medial layer). When the elastic fibers and collagen in the middle layer are damaged, stretching and segmental dilation occur. As a result, the medial layer loses some of its elasticity, and it fragments. Smooth muscle cells are lost and the wall thins.

Thin and thinner

The thinned wall may contain calcium deposits and atherosclerotic plaque, making the wall brittle. As a person ages, the elastin in the wall decreases, further weakening the vessel. If hypertension is present, blood flow slows, resulting in ischemia and additional weakening (Ignatavicius et al., 2018).

Wide vessel, slow flow

When an aneurysm begins to develop, lateral pressure increases, causing the vessel lumen to widen and blood flow to slow. Over time, mechanical stressors contribute to elongation of the aneurysm.

Blood forces

Hemodynamic forces may also play a role, causing pulsatile stresses on the weakened wall and pressing on the small vessels that supply nutrients to the arterial wall. In aortic aneurysms, the stress and pressure cause the aorta to become bowed and tortuous.

What to look for

Most patients with aortic aneurysms are asymptomatic until the aneurysms enlarge and compress surrounding tissue. A large aneurysm may produce signs and symptoms that mimic an MI, renal calculi, lumbar disk disease, or duodenal compression.

When symptoms arise

Usually, the patient exhibits symptoms if rupture, expansion, embolization, thrombosis, or pressure from the mass on surrounding structures exists. Rupture is more common if the patient also has hypertension or if the aneurysm is larger than 6 cm. If the patient has a suspected thoracic aortic aneurysm, assess for:

- difficulty breathing
- reports of sudden, excruciating, tearing pain that moves from the anterior to the posterior
- hoarseness or coughing
- nausea and vomiting
- diaphoresis
- hematemesis
- dysphagia
- aortic insufficiency murmur
- hemoptysis
- palpable pulsations at the left sternoclavicular joint
- tachycardia
- unequal blood pressure and pulse when measured in both arms.

Acute expansion

When there's an acute expansion of a thoracic aortic aneurysm, assess for:

- severe hypertension
- neurologic changes
- jugular vein distention
- new murmur of aortic sufficiency
- right sternoclavicular lift
- tracheal deviation
- hypovolemic shock.

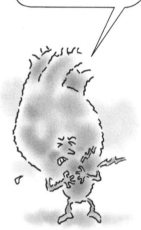

A sudden, tearing pain that moves from the anterior to the posterior is a sure sign of aortic aneurysm.

What tests tell you

No specific laboratory test diagnoses an aortic aneurysm; however, several other tests may be helpful:

- If blood is leaking from the aneurysm, leukocytosis and a decrease in hemoglobin and hematocrit may be noted.
- Computed tomography (CT) scanning with contrast is used for assessing the size and location of an aneurysm (Ignatavicius et al., 2018).
- TEE allows visualization of the thoracic aorta. It's commonly combined with Doppler flow studies to provide information about blood flow.
- Abdominal ultrasonography or echocardiography can be used to determine the size, shape, length, and location of the aneurysm.

- Anteroposterior and lateral X-rays of the chest or abdomen can be used to detect aortic calcification and widened areas of the aorta.
- Magnetic resonance imaging (MRI) can disclose the aneurysm's size and effect on nearby organs.
- Serial ultrasonography at 6-month interval reveals growth of small aneurysms.
- Aortography is used to determine the aneurysm's approximate size and the patency of visceral vessels.

How it's treated

Aneurysm treatment may involve surgery and appropriate drug therapy. Aortic aneurysms usually require resection and replacement of the aortic section using a vascular or Dacron graft. However, keep these points in mind:

- If the aneurysm is small and produces no symptoms, surgery may be delayed, with regular physical examination and ultrasonography or CT scans performed to monitor progression.
- Large or symptomatic aneurysms are at risk for rupture and need immediate repair.
- Endovascular grafting may be an option for a patient with an abdominal aortic aneurysm. The procedure, which can be done using local or regional anesthesia, is a minimally invasive procedure whereby the walls of the aorta are reinforced to prevent expansion and rupture of the aneurysm.
- Medications to control blood pressure, relieve anxiety, and control pain are also prescribed.

Emergency measures

Rupture of an aortic aneurysm is a medical emergency requiring immediate treatment, including:

- resuscitation with fluid and blood replacement
- IV propranolol to reduce myocardial contractility
- IV nitroprusside to reduce blood pressure and maintain it at 90 to 100 mm Hg systolic
- IV morphine to relieve pain
- arterial line and indwelling urinary catheter to monitor the patient's condition preoperatively.

What to do

- A patient with an actual or suspected aortic aneurysm rupture presents a medical emergency. Place the patient on continuous monitoring. Monitor blood pressure and pulse in extremities and compare findings bilaterally. If the difference in systolic blood pressure exceeds 10 mm Hg, notify the health care provider immediately.

- Assess cardiovascular status frequently, including heart rate, rhythm, ECG, and cardiac enzyme levels. MI can develop if an aneurysm ruptures along the coronary arteries.
- Obtain blood samples to evaluate kidney function by assessing BUN, creatinine, and electrolyte levels. Measure intake and output, hourly if necessary, depending on the patient's condition.
- Monitor CBC for evidence of blood loss, including decreased hemoglobin, hematocrit, and red blood cell (RBC) count.

ABGs and arterial lines

- Obtain an arterial sample for ABG analysis, as prescribed, and monitor cardiac rhythm. Assist with arterial line insertion to allow for continuous blood pressure monitoring. Assist with insertion of a PA catheter to assess hemodynamic balance.
- Administer beta blockers to decrease blood pressure, heart rate, and left ventricular contractility.
- Administer IV morphine as prescribed, to relieve pain if present.
- Administer nitroprusside sodium (Nitropress) IV only after beta blockers have been initiated because the heart rate can increase and potentially extend the dissection.
- Observe the patient for signs of rupture, which may be immediately fatal. Watch closely for signs of acute blood loss, such as decreasing blood pressure; increasing pulse and respiratory rates; restlessness; decreased LOC; and cool, clammy skin.

Rupture response

- Prepare the patient for emergency surgery.
- If rupture does take place, insert a large-bore IV catheter, begin fluid resuscitation, and administer nitroprusside sodium IV, as prescribed, usually to maintain a mean arterial pressure (MAP) of 70 to 80 mm Hg. Also administer propranolol IV (to reduce left ventricular ejection velocity), as prescribed, until the heart rate ranges from 60 to 80 beats per minute. Expect to administer additional doses every 4 to 6 hours until oral medications can be used.
- If the patient is experiencing acute pain, administer morphine IV as prescribed.
- Inform the patient and family of transfer to the CCU after surgery.

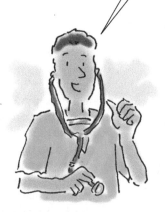

Pay close attention to blood pressure in an aortic aneurysm patient. Check it every 2 to 4 hours or more.

Cardiac arrest

Cardiac arrest is the absence of mechanical functioning of the heart muscle. The heart stops beating or beats abnormally and doesn't pump effectively. If blood circulation isn't restored within minutes, cardiac arrest can lead to the loss of arterial blood pressure, brain damage, and death.

What causes it

Cardiac arrest can be caused by a wide variety of conditions, including acute MI, ventricular fibrillation, ventricular tachycardia, severe trauma, hypovolemia, metabolic disorders, brain injury, respiratory arrest, drowning, or drug overdose.

How it happens

In cardiac arrest, myocardial contractility stops, resulting in a lack of cardiac output. An imbalance in myocardial oxygen supply and demand follows, leading to myocardial ischemia, tissue necrosis, and death.

What to look for

The patient experiencing a cardiac arrest suddenly loses consciousness. Spontaneous respirations are absent, and the patient has no palpable pulse.

What tests tell you

No specific diagnostic tests are used to confirm a cardiac arrest. However, cardiac monitoring or ECG may reveal an underlying cardiac arrhythmia, such as ventricular fibrillation or asystole.

How it's treated

Treatment of cardiac arrest involves basic and ACLS measures in conjunction with treating the underlying cause of the arrest. The ultimate goal of treatment is to restore the patient's cardiac rhythm and function.

What to do

- Determine responsiveness and notify the health care provider and rapid response team.
- Initiate CPR. (See *Adult BLS cardiac arrest algorithm*, page 166.)
- Monitor cardiac rhythm.
- Assist with ET intubation and mechanical ventilation.
- Follow ACLS protocols; administer medications as prescribed. (See *ACLS adult cardiac arrest algorithm*, page 167.)
- Assist with defibrillation for ventricular fibrillation or pulseless ventricular tachycardia.

(Text continues on page 168.)

Adult BLS cardiac arrest algorithm

The algorithm shows the basic life support (BLS) steps to follow when you suspect cardiac arrest in an adult patient.

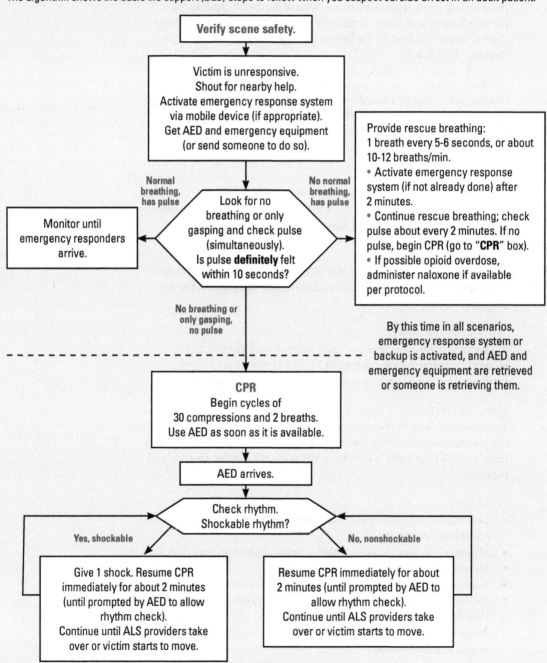

Verify scene safety.

Victim is unresponsive.
Shout for nearby help.
Activate emergency response system
via mobile device (if appropriate).
Get AED and emergency equipment
(or send someone to do so).

Provide rescue breathing:
1 breath every 5-6 seconds, or about
10-12 breaths/min.
• Activate emergency response
system (if not already done) after
2 minutes.
• Continue rescue breathing; check
pulse about every 2 minutes. If no
pulse, begin CPR (go to "**CPR**" box).
• If possible opioid overdose,
administer naloxone if available
per protocol.

Normal
breathing,
has pulse

No normal
breathing,
has pulse

Look for no
breathing or only
gasping and check pulse
(simultaneously).
Is pulse **definitely** felt
within 10 seconds?

Monitor until
emergency responders
arrive.

No breathing or
only gasping,
no pulse

By this time in all scenarios,
emergency response system or
backup is activated, and AED and
emergency equipment are retrieved
or someone is retrieving them.

CPR
Begin cycles of
30 compressions and 2 breaths.
Use AED as soon as it is available.

AED arrives.

Check rhythm.
Shockable rhythm?

Yes, shockable

No, nonshockable

Give 1 shock. Resume CPR
immediately for about 2 minutes
(until prompted by AED to allow
rhythm check).
Continue until ALS providers take
over or victim starts to move.

Resume CPR immediately for about
2 minutes (until prompted by AED to
allow rhythm check).
Continue until ALS providers take
over or victim starts to move.

ACLS adult cardiac arrest algorithm

The algorithm shows the American Heart Association's guidelines for treating a patient in cardiac arrest.

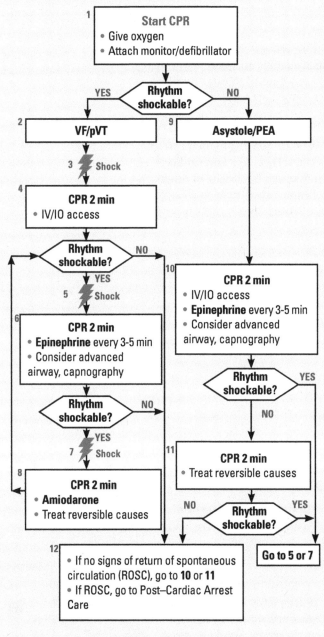

CPR Quality

- Push hard (at least 2 inches [5 cm]) and fast (100-120/min) and allow complete chest recoil.
- Minimize interruptions in compressions.
- Avoid excessive ventilation.
- Rotate compressor every 2 minutes, or sooner if fatigued.
- If no advanced airway, 30:2 compression-ventilation ratio.
- Quantitative waveform capnography.
  - If P_{ETCO_2} <10 mm Hg, attempt to improve CPR quality.
- Intra-arterial pressure
  - If relaxation phase (diastolic) pressure <20 mm Hg, attempt to improve CPR quality.

Shock Energy for Defibrillation

- **Biphasic:** Manufacturer recommendation (e.g., initial dose of 120-200 J); if unknown, use maximum available. Second and subsequent doses should be equivalent, and higher doses may be considered.
- **Monophasic:** 360 J

Drug Therapy

- **Epinephrine IV/IO dose:** 1 mg every 3-5 minutes
- **Amiodarone IV/IO dose:** First dose: 300 mg bolus. Second dose: 150 mg.

Advanced Airway

- Endotracheal intubation or supraglottic advanced airway
- Waveform capnography or capnometry to confirm and monitor ET tube placement
- Once advanced airway in place, give 1 breath every 6 seconds (10 breaths/min) with continuous chest compressions

Return of Spontaneous Circulation (ROSC)

- Pulse and blood pressure
- Abrupt sustained increase in P_{ETCO_2} (typically ≥40 mm Hg)
- Spontaneous arterial pressure waves with intra-arterial monitoring

Reversible Causes

- **H**ypovolemia
- **H**ypoxia
- **H**ydrogen ion (acidosis)
- **H**ypo-/hyperkalemia
- **H**ypothermia
- **T**ension pneumothorax
- **T**amponade, cardiac
- **T**oxins
- **T**hrombosis, pulmonary
- **T**hrombosis, coronary

Cardiac arrhythmias

In cardiac arrhythmia, abnormal electrical conduction or automaticity changes heart rate and rhythm.

Asymptomatic to catastrophic

Cardiac arrhythmias vary in severity, from those that are mild, asymptomatic, and require no treatment (such as sinus arrhythmia in which heart rate increases and decreases with respiration) to catastrophic ventricular fibrillation, which requires immediate resuscitation.

Organized by origin and effects

Cardiac arrhythmias are generally classified according to their origin (atrial, ventricular, or supraventricular). Their effect on cardiac output and blood pressure, partially influenced by the site of origin, determines their clinical significance. Lethal arrhythmias, such as ventricular tachycardia and ventricular fibrillation, are a major cause of sudden cardiac death.

What causes it

Common causes of cardiac arrhythmias include:
- drug toxicity
- congenital defects
- acid–base imbalances
- electrolyte imbalances
- cellular hypoxia
- connective tissue disorders
- degeneration of the conductive tissue
- hypertrophy of the heart muscle
- myocardial ischemia or infarction
- organic heart disease.

How it happens

Cardiac arrhythmias may result from:
- abnormal electrical conduction
- escape beats (additional abnormal heart beats resulting from a very slow heart rate)
- enhanced automaticity
- reentry.

What to look for

When a patient presents with a history of symptoms suggesting cardiac arrhythmias or has been treated for a cardiac arrhythmia, be alert for:
- reports of precipitating factors, such as exercise, smoking, sleep patterns, emotional stress, exposure to heat or cold, caffeine intake, position changes, or recent illnesses

Look out! Escape beats are a major cause of arrhythmias!

- attempts to alleviate the symptoms, such as coughing, rest, medications, or deep breathing
- reports of sensing the heart's rhythm, such as palpitations, irregular beating, skipped beats, or rapid or slow heart rate.

A matter of degree

Physical examination findings vary depending on the arrhythmia and the degree of hemodynamic compromise. Circulatory failure, along with an absence of pulse and respirations, is found with asystole, ventricular fibrillation, and, sometimes, ventricular tachycardia.

That's not all

Additional findings may include:
- dizziness
- weakness
- chest pains
- cold and clammy extremities
- hypotension
- dyspnea
- pallor
- reduced urine output
- syncope (with severely impaired cerebral circulation).

What tests tell you
- A 12-lead ECG is the standard test for identifying cardiac arrhythmias. A 15-lead ECG (in which additional leads are applied to the right side of the chest) or an 18-lead ECG (in which additional leads are also added to the posterior scapular area) may be done to provide more definitive information about the patient's right ventricle and posterior wall of the left ventricle (AHA, 2016; Ignatavicius et al., 2018; Urden et al., 2018). (See *Understanding cardiac arrhythmias,* pages 170 to 177.)
- Laboratory testing may reveal electrolyte abnormalities, hypoxemia or acid–base abnormalities (with ABG analysis), or drug toxicities as the cause of arrhythmias.
- Electrophysiologic testing may be used to identify the mechanism of an arrhythmia and location of accessory pathways and to assess the effectiveness of antiarrhythmic drugs.

How it's treated
The goals of treatment for cardiac arrhythmias are to return pacer function to the sinus node, increase or decrease ventricular rate to

(Text continues on page 178.)

Understanding cardiac arrhythmias

Here's an outline of many common cardiac arrhythmias and their features, causes, and treatments. Use a normal electrocardiogram strip, if available, to compare normal cardiac rhythm configurations with the rhythm strips shown here. Characteristics of normal sinus rhythm include:

- ventricular and atrial rates of 60 to 100 beats per minute
- regular and uniform QRS complexes and P waves
- PR interval of 0.12 to 0.20 second
- QRS duration <0.12 second
- identical atrial and ventricular rates, with constant PR intervals.

Arrhythmia and features

Sinus tachycardia

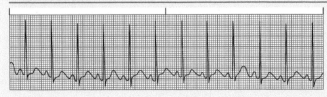

- Atrial and ventricular intervals regular
- Rate >100 beats per minute; rarely >150 beats per minute
- Normal P waves preceding each QRS complex

Sinus bradycardia

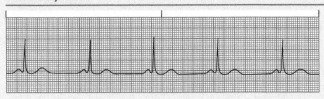

- Atrial and ventricular intervals regular
- Rate <60 beats per minute
- Normal P waves preceding each QRS complex

Paroxysmal supraventricular tachycardia

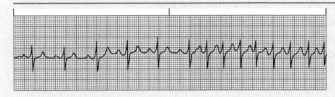

- Atrial and ventricular intervals regular
- Heart rate >160 beats per minute; rarely exceeds 250 beats per minute
- P waves regular but aberrant; difficult to differentiate from preceding T waves
- P waves preceding each QRS complex
- Sudden onset and termination of arrhythmia

Causes	Treatment
• Normal physiologic response to fever, exercise, anxiety, pain, dehydration • May also accompany shock, left-sided heart failure, cardiac tamponade, hyperthyroidism, anemia, hypovolemia, pulmonary embolism (PE), and anterior wall myocardial infarction (MI) • Can occur with use of some drugs such as atropine, epinephrine, isoproterenol, quinidine, caffeine, alcohol, cocaine, amphetamines, and nicotine	• Treatment of underlying cause • Oxygen if hypoxemic • Beta-adrenergic blockers or calcium channel blocker as prescribed
• Normal in a well-conditioned heart, as in an athlete • Increased intracranial pressure; increased vagal tone due to straining during defecation, vomiting, intubation, or mechanical ventilation; sick sinus syndrome (SSS); hypothyroidism; and inferior wall MI • May also occur with anticholinesterase, beta-adrenergic blocker, digoxin, and morphine use	• No treatment is necessary unless patient is symptomatic. • Treatment of underlying cause • Atropine per advanced cardiac life support (ACLS) protocol if persistent bradycardia causes hypotension, an altered mental status, signs of shock, ischemic chest pain, or acute heart failure
• Intrinsic abnormality of atrioventricular (AV) conduction system • Physical or psychological stress, hypoxia, hypokalemia, cardiomyopathy, congenital heart disease, MI, valvular disease, Wolff-Parkinson-White syndrome, cor pulmonale, hyperthyroidism, and systemic hypertension • Digoxin toxicity; use of caffeine, marijuana, or central nervous system stimulants	• If QRS complex is narrow and regular and patient is stable, perform vagal maneuvers; carotid massage by physician only • Intravenous (IV) administration of adenosine as prescribed • If patient is unstable, immediate synchronized cardioversion • If QRS complex is narrow and irregular, the health care provider can control the rate using calcium channel blockers or beta-adrenergic blockers. • If QRS complex is wide and irregular, antiarrhythmics such as amiodarone may be prescribed; if ineffective, then magnesium may be prescribed.

(continued)

Understanding cardiac arrhythmias *(continued)*

Arrhythmia and features

Atrial flutter and fibrillation

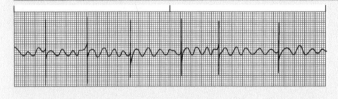

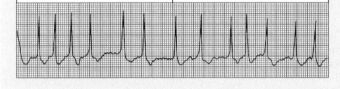

Atrial flutter
- Atrial rhythm regular; rate 250 to 400 beats per minute
- Ventricular rate variable, depending on degree of AV block (usually 60 to 100 beats per minute)
- No P waves; atrial activity appears as flutter waves (F waves); sawtooth configuration common in lead II
- QRS complexes are uniform in shape but commonly irregular in rhythm.

Atrial fibrillation
- Atrial rhythm grossly irregular
- Ventricular rhythm grossly irregular, may be normal rate or rapid ventricular response
- QRS complexes of uniform configuration and duration
- PR interval indiscernible
- No P waves; atrial activity appears as erratic, irregular, baseline fibrillatory waves (F waves).

Junctional rhythm

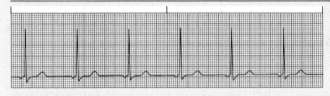

- Atrial and ventricular rhythms regular; atrial rate 40 to 60 beats per minute; ventricular rate usually 40 to 60 beats per minute (60 to 100 beats per minute is accelerated junctional rhythm)
- P waves preceding, hidden within (absent), or after QRS complex; usually inverted if visible
- PR interval (when present) <0.12 second
- QRS complex configuration and duration normal, except in aberrant conduction

First-degree AV block

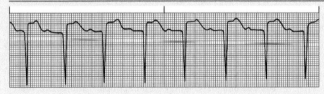

- Atrial and ventricular intervals regular
- PR interval >0.20 second
- P wave precedes QRS complex.
- QRS complex normal

Causes	Treatment
• Atrial fibrosis • Loss of muscle mass • Heart failure, chronic obstructive pulmonary disease, thyrotoxicosis, constrictive pericarditis, ischemic heart disease, sepsis, PE, rheumatic heart disease, hypertension, mitral stenosis, atrial irritation, or complication of coronary bypass or valve replacement surgery, diabetes mellitus, obesity, advanced age, excessive alcohol intake, "holiday heart syndrome" • Nifedipine and digoxin use	• If patient is unstable with a ventricular rate >150 beats per minute, immediate cardioversion following trans-esophageal echocardiograph verifying the absence of clot formation in heart chambers • If patient is stable, follow ACLS protocol and drug therapy as prescribed, which may include calcium channel blockers such as diltiazem (Cardizem), beta-adrenergic blockers such as metoprolol (Lopressor), antiarrhythmics such as amiodarone (Cordarone) or dronedarone (Multaq), or digoxin (Lanoxin). • Anticoagulation therapy may be prescribed. • In some patients with refractory atrial fibrillation uncontrolled by drugs, electrophysiologic studies and radiofrequency catheter ablation may be performed (Ignatavicius et al., 2018).
• Inferior wall MI or ischemia, hypoxia, vagal stimulation, and SSS • Acute rheumatic fever • Valve surgery • Digoxin toxicity	• Treatment of underlying cause • Atropine for symptomatic slow rate • Pacemaker insertion if patient doesn't respond to drugs • Discontinuation of digoxin, if prescribed • If accelerated junctional, beta blockers and calcium channel blockers may be prescribed.
• Possible in healthy persons • Inferior wall MI or ischemia, hypothyroidism, hypokalemia, and hyperkalemia • Digoxin toxicity; use of, beta-adrenergic blockers, calcium channel blockers, flecainide	• Usually, patients are asymptomatic and require no treatment. • If symptomatic, treat underlying cause. • Atropine may be prescribed if severe symptomatic bradycardia develops. • Use caution with administration of digoxin, calcium channel blockers, and beta-adrenergic blockers (Sauer, 2019a).

(continued)

Understanding cardiac arrhythmias *(continued)*

Arrhythmia and features

Second-degree AV block Mobitz I (Wenckebach)

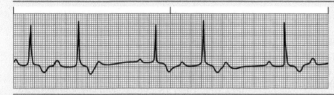

- Atrial rhythm regular
- Ventricular rhythm irregular
- Atrial rate exceeds ventricular rate.
- PR interval progressively longer with each cycle until QRS complex disappears (dropped beat); PR interval shorter after dropped beat

Second-degree AV block Mobitz II

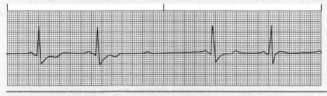

- Atrial rhythm regular
- Ventricular rhythm regular or irregular, with varying degree of block
- PR interval constant for conducted beats
- P waves normal size and shape, but some aren't followed by a QRS complex

Third-degree AV block (complete heart block)

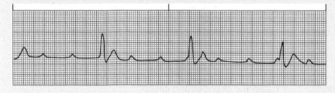

- Atrial rhythm regular
- Ventricular rhythm regular and rate slower than atrial rate
- No relation between P waves and QRS complexes
- No constant PR interval
- QRS duration normal (junctional pacemaker) or wide and bizarre (ventricular pacemaker)

Premature ventricular contraction

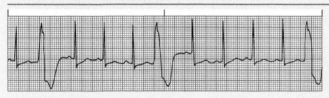

- Atrial rhythm regular
- Ventricular rhythm irregular
- QRS complex premature, usually followed by a complete compensatory pause
- QRS complex wide and distorted, usually >0.12 second
- Premature QRS complexes occurring alone or in pairs, alternating with normal beats; focus from one or more sites
- Ominous when clustered, multifocal, with R-wave-on-T pattern

Causes	Treatment
• Inferior wall MI, cardiac surgery, acute rheumatic fever, and vagal stimulation • Digoxin toxicity; use of beta blockers	• Treatment of underlying cause • Atropine or transcutaneous pacemaker may be prescribed for symptomatic bradycardia. • Discontinuation of digoxin, if prescribed
• Coronary artery disease (CAD), MI, cardiomyopathy • Digoxin toxicity	• Temporary or permanent pacemaker • Atropine, dopamine, or epinephrine for symptomatic hypotension, angina, or bradycardia • Discontinuation of digoxin, if prescribed • May progress to third-degree (complete) heart block (Sauer, 2019b)
• MI, congenital abnormality, rheumatic fever, myocarditis, amyloidosis, cardiomyopathy • Digoxin toxicity • Beta blockers, calcium channel blockers	• Atropine or dopamine, for symptomatic bradycardia • Transcutaneous or permanent pacemaker (Sauer, 2019c)
• Heart failure; chronic or acute MI or ischemia; myocardial irritation by ventricular catheter or a pacemaker; mitral valve prolapse, hypercapnia; hypoxia, hypokalemia; hypocalcemia; hypomagnesemia; acidosis • Drug toxicity • Caffeine, tobacco, or alcohol use • Psychological stress, anxiety, fever, pain, or exercise	• If warranted, procainamide or amiodarone may be prescribed. • Treatment of underlying cause • Discontinuation of drug causing toxicity

(continued)

Understanding cardiac arrhythmias *(continued)*

Arrhythmia and features

Ventricular tachycardia

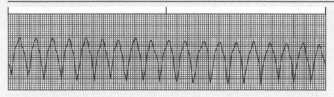

- Ventricular rate 150 to 250 beats per minute; rhythm may be regular or irregular.
- QRS complexes wide, bizarre, and independent of P waves
- P waves not discernible
- May start and stop suddenly

Ventricular fibrillation

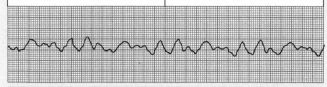

- Ventricular rhythm and rate chaotic and rapid
- QRS complexes wide and irregular; no visible P waves

Asystole

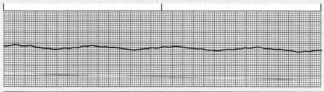

- No atrial or ventricular rate or rhythm
- No discernible P waves, QRS complexes, or T waves

Causes	Treatment
• Myocardial ischemia, MI, or aneurysm; CAD; rheumatic heart disease; mitral valve prolapse; heart failure; cardiomyopathy; ventricular catheters; hypokalemia; hypercalcemia; hypomagnesemia; and pulmonary embolism (PE) • Drug toxicity: digoxin, procainamide, epinephrine, or quinidine • Anxiety	• If regular QRS rhythm, follow ACLS protocol: administer IV amiodarone, procainamide, or sotalol (follow ACLS protocol); if drug is unsuccessful, cardioversion • If irregular QRS rhythm (polymorphic) and QT interval is prolonged, stop medications that may prolong QT interval; correct electrolyte imbalance; administer magnesium; if ineffective, cardioversion • If irregular QRS rhythm (polymorphic) and QT interval is normal, stop medications that may prolong QT interval; correct electrolyte balance; administer amiodarone; if ineffective, cardioversion • If the patient with monomorphic or polymorphic QRS complexes becomes unstable, immediate defibrillation • If pulseless, initiate cardiopulmonary resuscitation (CPR); follow ACLS protocol for defibrillation, endotracheal (ET) intubation, and administration of epinephrine, followed by amiodarone. • Implantable cardioverter–defibrillator (ICD) if recurrent ventricular tachycardia
• Myocardial ischemia, MI, untreated ventricular tachycardia, R-on-T phenomenon, electrolyte imbalances, electric shock, hypoxemia, and hypothermia • Catheter stimulation of ventricle during cardiac catheterization or cardiac pacing • Drug toxicity	• CPR; follow ACLS protocol for defibrillation, ET intubation, and administration of epinephrine, amiodarone. • ICD if risk of recurrent ventricular fibrillation
• Advanced cardiac disease; severe conduction system disturbance; end-stage heart failure; hypoxia, hypokalemia, severe acidosis, electric shock, PE, heart rupture, cardiac tamponade, hyperkalemia	• Continue CPR; follow ACLS protocol for ET intubation, temporary pacing, and administration of epinephrine.

normal, regain AV synchrony, and maintain normal sinus rhythm. Treatments to correct abnormal rhythms include therapy with:

- antiarrhythmic drugs
- electrical conversion with defibrillation and cardioversion
- management of the underlying disorder, such as correction of hypoxia
- temporary or permanent placement of a pacemaker to maintain heart rate
- Valsalva maneuver
- ICD, if indicated
- surgical removal or cryotherapy of an irritable ectopic focus to prevent recurring arrhythmias.

What to do

- Evaluate the patient's ECG frequently for arrhythmia and assess hemodynamic parameters as indicated. Document arrhythmias and notify the healthcare provider immediately.
- When life-threatening arrhythmias develop, rapidly assess the patient's LOC, pulse and respiratory rates, and hemodynamic parameters. Monitor ECG continuously. Be prepared to initiate CPR, if indicated. Follow ACLS protocol to treat specific life-threatening arrhythmias.
- Assess the patient for predisposing factors, such as fluid and electrolyte imbalance, and signs of drug toxicity, especially with digoxin.
- Administer medications as ordered; monitor for adverse effects; and monitor vital signs, hemodynamic parameters (as appropriate), and appropriate laboratory studies. Prepare to assist with or perform cardioversion or defibrillation, if indicated.
- If you suspect drug toxicity, report it to the health care provider immediately and withhold the next dose.
- Prepare the patient for transcutaneous or transvenous pacing, if appropriate.
- Prepare the patient for cardioversion, electrophysiology studies, an angiogram, internal cardiac defibrillator placement, or pacemaker placement as indicated.
- If a temporary pacemaker must be inserted, monitor the patient's pulse rate regularly after insertion and watch for signs of pacemaker failure and decreased cardiac output.

Cardiac contusion

Cardiac contusion refers to the bruising of the myocardium. It's the most common type of injury sustained from blunt trauma to the chest.

What causes it
A cardiac contusion typically results from blunt trauma. The trauma can be related to vehicular collisions or falls. The right ventricle is the most common site of injury because it's located directly behind the sternum.

How it happens
During deceleration injuries, the myocardium strikes the sternum when the heart and aorta move forward. In addition, the aorta may be lacerated by shearing forces. Direct force may also be applied to the sternum, causing injury. Crushing and compressive forces may result in contusion as the heart is compressed between the sternum and vertebral column.

What to look for
Cardiac contusion should be suspected after any blow to the chest. Be alert for these signs and symptoms of trauma:
- shortness of breath
- bruising on the chest
- murmurs
- bradycardia or tachycardia
- precordial chest pain.

And also . . .

Keep these signals in mind as well:
- arrhythmias due to ventricular irritability
- cardiac tamponade
- hemodynamic instability
- pericardial friction rub.

What tests tell you
- ECG will reveal rhythm disturbances, such as premature ventricular contractions, premature atrial contractions, ventricular tachycardia, atrial tachycardia, and ventricular fibrillation, along with nonspecific ST segment or T wave changes occurring within 24 to 48 hours after the injury.
- Echocardiogram will show evidence of abnormal ventricular wall movement and decreased ejection fraction.
- Multiple-gated acquisition scan will show decreased ability of effective heart pumping.
- Cardiac enzyme levels will show elevations of CK-MB to greater than 8% of total creatinine kinase within 3 to 4 hours after the injury.
- Cardiac troponin T and I levels may be elevated as soon as 2 hours after the injury.

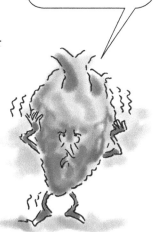

Ventricular irritability is a sure sign of cardiac contusion.

How it's treated

Maintaining hemodynamic stability and adequate cardiac output are key. IV fluid therapy may be necessary. Continuous ECG monitoring is used to detect arrhythmias. Amiodarone or lidocaine may be administered to treat ventricular arrhythmias, and digoxin may be given to treat pump failure. Inotropic agents may be used to assist with improving cardiac output and ejection fraction.

Close watch

The patient with a cardiac contusion must be monitored closely for signs and symptoms of cardiopulmonary compromise because trauma leading to cardiac contusion is commonly associated with pulmonary trauma. Supplemental oxygen therapy may be necessary. If the extent of pulmonary trauma is great, ET intubation and mechanical ventilation may be necessary.

No if hypo

IV morphine may be used to treat severe pain, unless the patient is hypotensive. In the latter case, other less potent analgesics may be used.

What to do

- Assess the patient's cardiopulmonary status at least hourly, or more frequently if indicated, to detect signs and symptoms of possible injury.
- Auscultate breath sounds at least hourly, reporting signs of congestion or fluid accumulation. Evaluate peripheral pulses and capillary refill to detect decreased peripheral tissue perfusion.
- Monitor heart rate and rhythm, heart sounds, and blood pressure every hour for changes; institute hemodynamic monitoring, including CVP, PAOP, and cardiac output as indicated, at least every 1 to 2 hours.
- Administer fluid replacement therapy, including blood component therapy as prescribed, typically to maintain systolic blood pressure above 90 mm Hg.
- Monitor urine output every hour, notifying the health care provider if output is less than 30 mL per hour.
- Institute continuous cardiac monitoring to detect arrhythmias or conduction defects. If arrhythmias appear, administer antiarrhythmic agents as prescribed.
- Assess the patient's degree of pain and administer analgesic therapy as prescribed, monitoring for effectiveness. Position the patient comfortably, usually with the head of the bed elevated 30 to 45 degrees.
- Prepare the patient and family for surgery, if indicated.
- Anticipate transfer of the patient to a CCU when appropriate.

Understanding cardiac tamponade

The pericardial sac, which surrounds and protects the heart, is composed of several layers:
• The fibrous pericardium is the tough, outermost membrane.
• The inner membrane, called the *serous membrane,* consists of the visceral and parietal layers.
• The visceral layer of the heart, also known as the *epicardial layer,* clings to the heart.
• The parietal layer lies between the visceral layer and the fibrous pericardium.

• The pericardial space—between the visceral and parietal layers—contains 10 to 30 mL of pericardial fluid. The fluid lubricates the layers and minimizes friction when the heart contracts.

In cardiac tamponade (shown as follows), blood or fluid fills the pericardial space, compressing the heart chambers, increasing intracardiac pressure, and obstructing venous return. As blood flow into the ventricles decreases, so does cardiac output. Without prompt treatment, low cardiac output can be fatal.

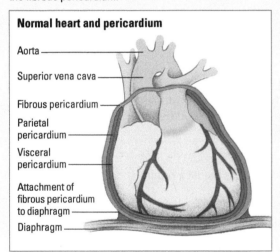

Normal heart and pericardium

Aorta
Superior vena cava
Fibrous pericardium
Parietal pericardium
Visceral pericardium
Attachment of fibrous pericardium to diaphragm
Diaphragm

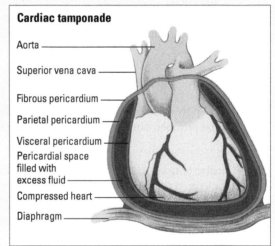

Cardiac tamponade

Aorta
Superior vena cava
Fibrous pericardium
Parietal pericardium
Visceral pericardium
Pericardial space filled with excess fluid
Compressed heart
Diaphragm

Cardiac tamponade

Cardiac tamponade is a rapid, unchecked increase in pressure in the pericardial sac. The increased pressure compresses the heart, impairs diastolic filling, and reduces cardiac output.

Pericardial pressure

The increase in pressure usually results from blood or fluid accumulation in the pericardial sac. Even a small amount of fluid (50 to 100 mL) can cause a serious tamponade if it accumulates rapidly.

If fluid accumulates rapidly, cardiac tamponade requires emergency lifesaving measures to prevent death. A slow accumulation and increase in pressure may not produce immediate symptoms because the fibrous wall of the pericardial sac can gradually stretch to accommodate as much as 1 to 2 L of fluid. (See *Understanding cardiac tamponade.*)

What causes it

Cardiac tamponade may result from:

- viral or postirradiation pericarditis
- acute MI
- chronic renal failure requiring dialysis
- connective tissue disorders (such as rheumatoid arthritis, systemic lupus erythematosus, rheumatic fever, vasculitis, and scleroderma)
- effusion (from cancer, bacterial infections, tuberculosis, and, rarely, acute rheumatic fever)
- hemorrhage due to nontraumatic causes (such as anticoagulant therapy in patients with pericarditis or rupture of the heart or great vessels)
- hemorrhage due to trauma (such as gunshot or stab wounds of the chest)
- idiopathic causes
- drug reaction.

How it happens

In cardiac tamponade, accumulation of fluid in the pericardial sac causes compression of the heart chambers. The compression obstructs blood flow into the ventricles and reduces the amount of blood that can be pumped out of the heart with each contraction.

What to look for

Cardiac tamponade has three classic features known as the *Beck triad*:
1. elevated CVP with jugular vein distention
2. muffled heart sounds
3. pulsus paradoxus (inspiratory drop in systemic blood pressure greater than 15 mm Hg).

That's not all

Other signs include:

- restlessness
- anxiety
- cold, clammy skin
- cyanosis
- diaphoresis
- orthopnea
- decreased arterial pressure, decreased systolic blood pressure, and narrow pulse pressure
- tachycardia and a weak, thready pulse.

What tests tell you

- Chest X-ray shows a slightly widened mediastinum and an enlarged cardiac silhouette.

- ECG may show a low-amplitude QRS complex and electrical alternans or an alternating beat-to-beat change in amplitude of the P wave, QRS complex, and T wave. Generalized ST segment elevation is noted in all leads. An ECG is used to rule out other cardiac disorders; it may reveal changes produced by acute pericarditis.
- PA catheterization indicates increased right atrial pressure, right ventricular diastolic pressure, and CVP.
- Echocardiography may reveal pericardial effusion with signs of right ventricular and atrial compression.
- CT scan or MRI may be used to identify pericardial effusions or pericardial thickening caused by constrictive pericarditis.

How it's treated

The goal of treatment is to relieve intrapericardial pressure and cardiac compression by removing accumulated blood or fluid, which can be done in three different ways:
1. pericardiocentesis (needle aspiration of the pericardial cavity)
2. insertion of a drain into the pericardial sac to drain the effusion
3. surgical creation of an opening called a *pericardial window*.

When pressure is low

If the patient is hypotensive, trial volume loading with crystalloids, such as IV normal saline solution, may be used to maintain systolic blood pressure. An inotropic drug, such as dopamine, may be necessary to improve myocardial contractility until fluid in the pericardial sac can be removed.

Additional treatments

Additional treatment may be necessary, depending on the cause. Examples of such causes and treatments are:
- heparin-induced tamponade—administration of the heparin antagonist protamine sulfate
- traumatic injury—blood transfusion or a thoracotomy to drain reaccumulating fluid or repair bleeding sites
- warfarin-induced tamponade—vitamin K administration.

What to do

- Monitor the patient's cardiovascular status frequently, at least every hour, noting the extent of jugular vein distention, quality of heart sounds, and blood pressure.
- Assess hemodynamic status, including CVP, right atrial pressure, and PAP, and determine cardiac output.
- Monitor for pulsus paradoxus.
- Be alert for ST segment and T wave changes on the ECG. Note rate and rhythm and report evidence of arrhythmias.

Keep an eye on the increase

- Watch closely for signs of increasing tamponade, increasing dyspnea, and arrhythmias; report them immediately.
- Infuse IV solutions and inotropic drugs, such as dopamine, as prescribed to maintain the patient's blood pressure.
- Administer oxygen therapy as needed and assess oxygen saturation levels. Monitor the patient's respiratory status for signs of respiratory distress, such as severe tachypnea and changes in the patient's LOC. Anticipate the need for ET intubation and mechanical ventilation if the patient's respiratory status deteriorates.
- Prepare the patient for pericardiocentesis or thoracotomy.
- If the patient has trauma-induced tamponade, assess for other signs of trauma and institute appropriate care, including the use of colloids, crystalloids, and blood component therapy under pressure or by rapid volume infuser if massive fluid replacement is needed; administration of protamine sulfate for heparin-induced tamponade; and vitamin K administration for warfarin-induced tamponade.
- Assess renal function status closely, monitoring urine output every hour.
- Monitor capillary refill time, LOC, peripheral pulses, and skin temperature for evidence of diminished tissue perfusion.
- Anticipate transfer of the patient to a CCU when appropriate.

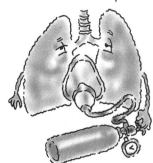

Oxygen therapy is just one aspect of cardiac tamponade treatment.

Heart failure

Heart failure results when the heart can't pump enough blood to meet the metabolic needs of the body. It results in intravascular and interstitial volume overload and poor tissue perfusion. An individual with heart failure experiences reduced exercise tolerance, a reduced quality of life, and a shortened life span.

What causes it

The most common cause of heart failure is CAD, but it also occurs in infants, children, and adults with congenital and acquired heart defects.

How it happens

Heart failure may be classified into four general categories:
1. left-sided heart failure
2. right-sided heart failure
3. systolic dysfunction
4. diastolic dysfunction.

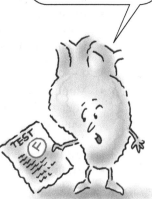

I can't believe failure was an option. I'm in real trouble!

When the left loses its faculties

Left-sided heart failure is a result of ineffective left ventricular contractile function. As the pumping ability of the left ventricle fails, cardiac output drops. Blood is no longer effectively pumped out into the body; it backs up into the left atrium and then into the lungs, causing pulmonary congestion, dyspnea, and activity intolerance. If the condition persists, pulmonary edema and right-sided heart failure may result. Common causes include:
- hypertension
- aortic and mitral valve stenosis
- left ventricular infarction.

When right goes wrong

Right-sided heart failure results from ineffective right ventricular contractile function. When blood isn't pumped effectively through the right ventricle to the lungs, blood backs up into the right atrium and into the peripheral circulation. The patient typically gains weight with fluid accumulation and develops peripheral edema and engorgement of the kidney and other organs. The patient may exhibit hepatomegaly, splenomegaly, and jugular venous distention.

Blame it on the left

Right-sided heart failure may be due to an acute right ventricular infarction or a pulmonary embolus. However, the most common cause is profound backward flow due to left-sided heart failure.

Just can't pump enough

Systolic dysfunction results when the left ventricle can't pump enough blood out to the systemic circulation during systole and the ejection fraction falls. Consequently, blood backs up into the pulmonary circulation and pressure increases in the pulmonary venous system. Cardiac output decreases; weakness, fatigue, and shortness of breath may occur. Causes of systolic dysfunction include MI and dilated cardiomyopathy.

It all goes to swell from here

Diastolic dysfunction results when the ability of the left ventricle to relax and fill during diastole is reduced and the stroke volume falls. Therefore, higher volumes are needed in the ventricles to maintain cardiac output. Consequently, pulmonary congestion and peripheral edema develop. Diastolic dysfunction may occur as a result of left ventricular hypertrophy, hypertension, or restrictive cardiomyopathy. The type of heart failure is less common than heart failure resulting from systolic dysfunction, and treatment isn't as clear.

Compensatory mechanisms

All types of heart failure eventually lead to reduced cardiac output, which triggers compensatory mechanisms that improve cardiac output at the expense of increased ventricular work. These compensatory mechanisms include:

- increased sympathetic activity
- activation of the renin–angiotensin–aldosterone system
- ventricular dilation
- ventricular hypertrophy.

Increased sympathetic activity

Increased sympathetic activity—a response to decreased cardiac output and blood pressure—enhances peripheral vascular resistance, contractility, heart rate, and venous return. Signs of increased sympathetic activity, such as cool extremities and clamminess, may indicate impending heart failure.

Renin–angiotensin–aldosterone system

Increased sympathetic activity also restricts blood flow to the kidneys, causing them to secrete renin, which in turn converts angiotensinogen to angiotensin I. Angiotensin I then becomes angiotensin II—a potent vasoconstrictor. Angiotensin causes the adrenal cortex to release aldosterone, leading to sodium and water retention and an increase in circulating blood volume.

The renal mechanism is helpful; however, if it persists unchecked, it can aggravate heart failure as the heart struggles to pump against the increased volume.

Ventricular dilation

In ventricular dilation, an increase in end-diastolic ventricular volume (preload) causes increased stroke work and stroke volume during contraction. The increased volume stretches cardiac muscle fibers so that the ventricle can accept the increased volume. Eventually, the muscle becomes stretched beyond optimal limits and contractility declines.

Ventricular hypertrophy

In ventricular hypertrophy, an increase in ventricular muscle mass allows the heart to pump against increased resistance to the outflow of blood, improving cardiac output. However, the increased muscle mass also increases the myocardial oxygen requirements.

Compromising situation

An increase in the ventricular diastolic pressure necessary to fill the enlarged ventricle may compromise diastolic coronary blood flow, limiting the oxygen supply to the ventricle and causing ischemia and impaired muscle contractility.

> Check extremities for signs of sympathetic activity. Cold hands could mean impending heart failure.

Counterregulatory substances

In heart failure, counterregulatory substances—prostaglandins and atrial natriuretic factor—are produced in an attempt to reduce the negative effects of volume overload and vasoconstriction caused by the compensatory mechanisms.

Kidneys' contributions

The kidneys release the prostaglandins prostacyclin and prostaglandin E_2, which are potent vasodilators. These vasodilators also act to reduce volume overload produced by the renin–angiotensin–aldosterone system by inhibiting sodium and water reabsorption by the kidneys.

Counteracting hormone

Atrial natriuretic factor is a hormone that's secreted mainly by the atria in response to stimulation of the stretch receptors in the atria caused by excess fluid volume. Atrial natriuretic factor works to counteract the negative effects of sympathetic nervous system stimulation and the renin–angiotensin–aldosterone system by producing vasodilation and diuresis.

What to look for

Early signs and symptoms of left-sided heart failure include:
- fatigue
- nonproductive cough
- orthopnea
- dyspnea
- paroxysmal nocturnal dyspnea.

Later, on the left

Later clinical manifestations of left-sided heart failure may include:
- cool, pale skin
- restlessness and confusion
- displacement of the PMI toward the left anterior axillary line
- hemoptysis
- crackles on auscultation
- S_3 heart sound
- S_4 heart sound
- tachycardia.

On the right side

Clinical manifestations of right-sided heart failure include:
- weight gain
- anorexia, fullness, and nausea
- edema
- ascites or anasarca

- hepatojugular reflux and hepatomegaly
- jugular vein distention
- nocturia
- right upper quadrant pain.

What tests tell you

- Chest X-ray shows increased pulmonary vascular markings, interstitial edema, or pleural effusion and cardiomegaly.
- ECG may indicate hypertrophy, ischemic changes, or infarction and may also reveal tachycardia and extra systoles.
- Laboratory testing may reveal abnormal liver function and elevated BUN and creatinine levels. BNP is a substance secreted from the ventricles or the lower heart chambers in response to pressures in the heart. BNP levels increase in heart failure.
- ABG analysis may reveal hypoxemia from impaired gas exchange and respiratory alkalosis because the patient blows off more carbon dioxide as the respiratory rate increases in compensation.
- Echocardiography may reveal left ventricular hypertrophy, dilation, and abnormal contractility.
- PA monitoring typically demonstrates elevated PAP and PAOP, left ventricular end-diastolic pressure in left-sided heart failure, and elevated right atrial pressure or CVP in right-sided heart failure.
- Radionuclide ventriculography may reveal an ejection fraction less than 40%; in diastolic dysfunction, the ejection fraction may be normal.

How it's treated

The goal of therapy is to improve pump function. Correction of heart failure may involve:

- ACE inhibitors to prohibit remodeling of the left ventricle and slow dilation of the left ventricle. Angiotensin-receptor blockers are used for patients who do not tolerate ACE inhibitors (Urden et al., 2018).
- beta-adrenergic blockers to prevent remodeling in patients with mild to moderate heart failure caused by left ventricular systolic dysfunction
- CABG surgery or angioplasty for patients with heart failure due to CAD
- digoxin for patients with heart failure due to left ventricular systolic dysfunction to increase myocardial contractility, improve cardiac output, reduce the volume of the ventricle, and decrease ventricular stretch
- diuretics to reduce fluid volume overload, venous return, and preload
- diuretics, nitrates, morphine, and oxygen to treat pulmonary edema

- continuous positive airway pressure for patients with sleep apnea to improve cardiac output and ejection fraction and decrease preload and afterload (Ignatavicius et al., 2018).
- heart transplantation in patients receiving aggressive medical treatment but still experiencing limitations or repeated hospitalizations
- lifestyle modifications, such as weight loss (if obese), limited sodium (to 2 g per day) and alcohol intake, reduced fat intake, smoking cessation, stress reduction, and development of an exercise program to reduce symptoms
- other surgery or invasive procedures, such as insertion of an intra-aortic balloon pump (IABP), partial left ventriculectomy, use of a mechanical VAD, and implantation of an ICD or a biventricular pacemaker
- treatment of the underlying cause, if known.

What to do

- Place the patient in Fowler position to maximize chest expansion and give supplemental oxygen, as prescribed or per unit protocol, to ease breathing. Monitor oxygen saturation levels and ABGs as indicated. If respiratory status deteriorates, anticipate the need for ET intubation and mechanical ventilation.
- Institute continuous cardiac monitoring and notify the health care provider of changes in rhythm and rate. If the patient develops tachycardia, administer beta-adrenergic blockers as prescribed; if atrial fibrillation is present, administer anticoagulants or antiplatelet agents, as prescribed, to prevent thrombus formation.
- If the patient develops a new arrhythmia, obtain a 12-lead ECG immediately.
- Monitor hemodynamic status, including cardiac output, cardiac index, and pulmonary and systemic vascular pressures, at least hourly, noting trends.
- Administer medications as ordered. Check the apical heart rate before administering digoxin.

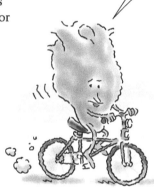

Developing an exercise program is just one lifestyle modification that can reduce symptoms of heart failure.

Pump up the potassium

- Expect to administer electrolyte replacement therapy (especially potassium) after the administration of diuretics to prevent such imbalances as hypokalemia and the arrhythmias that they may cause.
- Assess respiratory status frequently—at least every hour. Auscultate lungs for abnormal breath sounds, such as crackles, wheezes, and rhonchi. Encourage coughing and deep breathing.
- Obtain a baseline weight and observe for peripheral edema.
- Assess hourly urine output. Also, monitor fluid intake, including IV fluids.

Education edge

Teaching about heart failure

For a patient with heart failure, education about the disorder and treatments is essential to prevent complications and minimize the effects of this condition on quality of life. Additionally, a thorough understanding of the condition may help prevent future admission to the emergency department (ED).

Although admission to the ED is commonly filled with activity, it's an opportune time to begin your teaching. Consider these points:

• Explain underlying problems associated with the patient's heart failure and typical signs and symptoms.

• Review the medications prescribed to treat heart failure.

• Review suggested lifestyle changes, including diet and energy conservation measures.

• Teach the patient about avoiding foods high in sodium and provide a list of foods and their sodium content, indicating which to avoid and which to include in the diet.

• Instruct how to replace potassium lost through diuretic therapy (if appropriate) by taking prescribed potassium supplements or eating potassium-rich foods, such as bananas and apricots, and drinking orange juice.

• Encourage the patient to weigh daily and keep a record of weights; urge the patient to report a weight gain or loss of 2 lb (0.9 kg) or more in 3 or 4 days.

• Stress the importance of taking medications as prescribed; instruct the patient in possible adverse effects and signs and symptoms of toxicity.

• Instruct the patient on how to monitor pulse rate; advise the patient to report a pulse rate that is irregular or less than 60 beats per minute.

• Review the danger signs and symptoms to report to the health care provider, such as dizziness, blurred vision, shortness of breath, persistent dry cough, palpitations, increased fatigue, swelling of the ankles, and decreased urine output.

• Encourage adherence to medical follow-up, including checkups and periodic blood tests.

• If applicable, provide information and resources for smoking cessation.

• Organize all activities to provide maximum rest periods. Assess for signs of activity intolerance, such as increased shortness of breath, chest pain, increased arrhythmias, heart rate greater than 120 beats per minute, and ST segment changes, and have the patient stop activity.

• Prepare the patient for surgical intervention or insertion of an IABP or ICD or transfer to the CCU if indicated.

• Begin patient teaching related to heart failure and measures to reduce the risk of complications.

• If applicable, provide patient teaching and resources for smoking cessation. (See *Teaching about heart failure*.)

Hypertensive emergency

A hypertensive emergency, formerly referred to as *hypertensive crisis*, refers to the abrupt, acute, marked increase in blood pressure from the patient's baseline that ultimately leads to acute and rapidly progressing end-organ damage (Urden et al., 2018).

Rapid rise

Typically, in a hypertensive crisis, the patient's diastolic blood pressure is greater than 120 mm Hg. The increased blood pressure value, although important, is probably less important than how rapidly the blood pressure increases.

What causes it

Patients who develop hypertensive crisis may or may not have a history of primary hypertension. Conditions that cause secondary hypertension, such as pheochromocytoma, acute aortic dissection, pregnancy-induced eclampsia, illegal drug use, or Cushing syndrome, may also be responsible (Urden et al., 2018).

How it happens

Arterial blood pressure is a product of total peripheral resistance and cardiac output:

- Cardiac output is increased by conditions that increase heart rate, stroke volume, or both.
- Peripheral resistance is increased by factors that increase blood viscosity or reduce the lumen size of vessels, especially the arterioles.

Faulty mechanisms

Hypertension may result from a disturbance in one of the body's intrinsic mechanisms, including:

- sympathetic nervous system
- antidiuretic hormone
- autoregulation
- renin–angiotensin system.

Up with pressure

The renin–angiotensin system increases blood pressure in several ways.

- Sodium depletion, reduced blood pressure, and dehydration stimulate renin release.
- Renin reacts with angiotensinogen, a liver enzyme, and converts it to angiotensin I, which increases preload and afterload.
- Angiotensin I converts to angiotensin II in the lungs; angiotensin II is a potent vasoconstrictor that targets the arterioles.

- Circulating angiotensin II increases preload and afterload by stimulating the adrenal cortex to secrete aldosterone. This secretion increases blood volume by conserving sodium and water.

Maintaining flow

In autoregulation, several intrinsic mechanisms together change an artery's diameter to maintain tissue and organ perfusion despite fluctuations in systemic blood pressure. These mechanisms include:
- stress relaxation, in which blood vessels gradually dilate when blood pressure increases, reducing peripheral resistance
- capillary fluid shift, in which plasma moves between vessels and extravascular spaces to maintain intravascular volume.

Taking control

Sympathetic nervous system mechanisms control blood pressure. When blood pressure decreases, baroreceptors in the aortic arch and carotid sinuses decrease their inhibition of the medulla's vasomotor center.

Consequent increases in sympathetic stimulation of the heart by norepinephrine increases cardiac output by:
- strengthening the contractile force
- raising the heart rate
- augmenting peripheral resistance by vasoconstriction.

Regulating reabsorption

Stress can also stimulate the sympathetic nervous system to increase cardiac output and peripheral vascular resistance. The release of antidiuretic hormone can regulate hypotension by increasing reabsorption of water by the kidney. In reabsorption, blood plasma volume increases, thus raising blood pressure. In a hypertensive emergency, one or more of these regulating mechanisms is disrupted. (See *What happens in hypertensive emergencies*.)

Strain for the brain

In hypertensive emergency, the blood pressure–regulating mechanism is disturbed, causing cerebral vasodilation. Blood flow increases, causing an increase in pressure and subsequent cerebral edema. The increase in pressure damages the intimal and medial lining of the arterioles.

What to look for

Signs and symptoms of hypertensive emergency may include:
- dizziness
- confusion, somnolence, or stupor
- irritability
- nausea
- vomiting

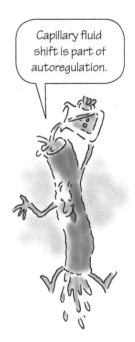

Capillary fluid shift is part of autoregulation.

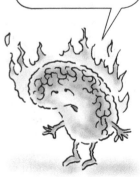

Bad for the heart, bad for the head. Hypertensive crisis can lead to cerebral edema.

What happens in hypertensive emergencies

Hypertensive emergency is a severe rise in arterial blood pressure caused by a disturbance in one or more of the regulating mechanisms. If untreated, hypertensive crisis may result in renal, cardiac, or cerebral complications and, possibly, death. The flowchart outlines the process.

Causes of hypertensive crisis

- Abnormal renal function
- Eclampsia
- Hypertensive encephalopathy
- Intracerebral hemorrhage
- Monoamine oxidase inhibitor interactions
- Myocardial ischemia
- Pheochromocytoma
- Withdrawal of antihypertensive drugs (abrupt)

Prolonged hypertension

Inflammation and necrosis of arterioles

Narrowing of blood vessels

Restriction of blood flow to major organs

Organ damage

Renal
- Decreased renal perfusion
- Progressive deterioration of nephrons
- Decreased ability to concentrate urine
- Increased serum creatinine and blood urea nitrogen
- Increased renal tubule permeability with protein leakage into tubules
- Renal insufficiency
- Uremia
- Renal failure

Cardiac
- Decreased cardiac perfusion
- Coronary artery disease
- Angina or myocardial infarction
- Increased cardiac workload
- Left ventricular hypertrophy
- Heart failure

Cerebral
- Decreased cerebral perfusion
- Increased stress on vessel wall
- Arterial spasm
- Ischemia
- Transient ischemic attacks
- Weakening of vessel intima
- Aneurysm formation
- Intracranial hemorrhage

- anorexia
- edema
- acute retinopathy and hemorrhage, retinal exudates, and papilledema
- angina
- dyspnea on exertion, orthopnea, or paroxysmal nocturnal dyspnea
- possible left ventricular heave palpated at the mitral valve area
- severe, throbbing headache in the back of the head
- S_4 heart sound
- vision loss, blurred vision, or diplopia.

Check the head

If the patient has hypertensive encephalopathy, you may note:
- disorientation
- decreased LOC
- seizures.

Kidney-related consequences

If the hypertensive emergency has affected the kidneys, you may note reduced urine output as well as elevated BUN and creatinine levels.

What tests tell you

- Blood pressure measurement—hypertensive emergencies are defined by acute blood pressure elevations greater than 180/120 mm Hg (Urden et al., 2018).
- RBC count may be decreased secondary to hematuria if the kidneys are involved.
- If the kidneys are involved, BUN may be greater than 20 mg/dL and the serum creatinine level may be greater than 1.3 mg/dL.
- ECG may reveal ischemic changes or left ventricular hypertrophy. ST segment depression and T-wave inversion suggest repolarization problems from endocardial fibrosis associated with left ventricular hypertrophy.
- Echocardiography may reveal increased wall thickness with or without an increase in left ventricle size.
- Chest X-ray may reveal enlargement of the cardiac silhouette with left ventricular dilation or pulmonary congestion and pleural effusions with heart failure.
- Urinalysis results may be normal unless renal impairment occurs; then specific gravity is low (less than 1.010), and hematuria, casts, and proteinuria may also be found.

How it's treated

Treatment of hypertensive emergency immediately focuses on reducing the patient's blood pressure with IV antihypertensive therapy. However, you must take care not to reduce the patient's blood pressure too rapidly because autoregulatory control is impaired.

Slow pressure cuts

The current recommendation is to reduce blood pressure by no more than 25% of the MAP over the first 2 hours. The next several days should bring further reductions. Here are some additional guidelines:

- Sodium nitroprusside, given as an IV infusion and titrated according to the patient's response, is the drug of choice. It has a rapid onset of action, and its effects cease within 10 minutes of stopping the drug (Elliott & Varon, 2018). Thus, if the patient's blood pressure drops too low, stopping the drug enables the blood pressure to increase very quickly.
- Other agents that may be used include labetalol, nitroglycerin, and hydralazine.
- Lifestyle changes may include weight reduction, smoking cessation, exercise, and dietary changes.
- After the acute episode is controlled, maintenance pharmacotherapy to control blood pressure plays a key role.

What to do

- Immediately obtain the patient's blood pressure.
- Institute continuous cardiac and arterial pressure monitoring to assess blood pressure directly; determine the patient's MAP.
- Assess ABGs. Monitor the patient's oxygen saturation level using pulse oximetry; if you're monitoring the patient hemodynamically, assess mixed venous oxygen saturation. Administer supplemental oxygen, as prescribed, based on the findings.
- Administer IV antihypertensive therapy as ordered; titrate IV antihypertensive medications according to the desired response and parameters set by the health care provider.
- If using nitroprusside, protect from the light and titrate the dose based on specified target ranges for systolic and diastolic pressures. Immediately stop the drug if the patient's blood pressure drops below the target range.
- If the patient is receiving nitroprusside therapy, assess for signs and symptoms of cyanide toxicity, such as decreased oxygen saturation, bradycardia, nausea, tinnitus, blurred vision, and delirium. Nitroprusside is metabolized to thiocyanate, which is excreted by the kidneys. Notify the health care provider if cyanide toxicity is suspected.

Much monitoring

- Monitor blood pressure every 1 to 5 minutes while titrating drug therapy and then every 15 minutes to 1 hour as the patient's condition stabilizes.

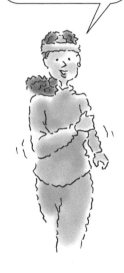

When it comes to reducing blood pressure with IV antihypertensive therapy, slow and steady wins the race: no more than 25% of the MAP over the first 2 hours.

Teaching about hypertensive emergency

Educate the patient about measures to control hypertension to reduce the risk of complications and a recurrence of the emergency. As the patient's condition begins to stabilize and time permits, begin your teaching. Consider these points:
• Explain the underlying events associated with the patient's current hypertensive emergency.
• Review the medications being used to treat this acute condition.
• Reinforce all aspects of blood pressure control, such as diet, medications, and lifestyle changes.
• Stress the need for adherence to medication therapy and frequent medical follow-up.
• Explain the prescribed medication regimen, including dosage, frequency, adverse effects, and when to notify the health care provider.
• Reinforce necessary lifestyle changes and the need for regular exercise.
• Instruct the patient in signs and symptoms associated with possible complications, such as changes in levels of alertness, headache, vision changes, reduced urine output, and weight gain, along with the need to notify the healthcare provider if any occur.

• Continuously monitor ECG and institute treatment as indicated if you find arrhythmias. Auscultate the patient's heart, noting signs of heart failure such as S_3 or S_4 heart sounds.
• Assess the patient's neurologic status frequently—every 15 to 30 minutes initially and then every hour based on the patient's response to therapy.

Check in on output

• Monitor urine output every hour and notify the health care provider if output decreases. Evaluate BUN and serum creatinine levels for changes and monitor daily weights.
• Administer other antihypertensives as prescribed. If the patient is experiencing fluid overload, administer diuretics as prescribed.
• Assess the patient's vision and report changes, such as blurred vision, diplopia, or loss of vision.
• Administer analgesics as prescribed for headache; keep your patient's environment quiet, with low lighting.
• Anticipate transfer of the patient to the CCU as indicated.
• Provide support to the patient and family; begin patient teaching related to the condition and measures to reduce the risk of complications as the patient's condition begins to stabilize. (See *Teaching about hypertensive emergency*.)

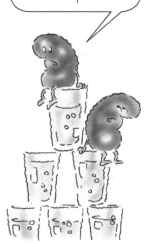

Stay in the know about your patient's urine flow! Less than 0.5 mL/kg/hour means there's a problem.

Quick quiz

1.   Which assessment will the nurse anticipate for a patient who has been admitted with a diagnosis of cardiac tamponade?
   A.   Shortness of breath
   B.   Pulsus paradoxus
   C.   Holosystolic murmur
   D.   Bounding peripheral pulse

Answer: B. Pulsus paradoxus (inspiratory drop in systemic blood pressure greater than 15 mm Hg) is one of the three classic signs of cardiac tamponade. The other classic signs are elevated CVP with jugular vein distention and muffled heart sounds.

2.   A patient receiving IV nitroprusside for treatment of hypertensive emergency develops blurred vision and tinnitus. Which nursing intervention is appropriate?
   A.   Increase the rate of nitroprusside infusion.
   B.   Administer a dose of antiarrhythmic medication, as needed.
   C.   Notify the health care provider.
   D.   Increase the flow rate of supplemental oxygen.

Answer: C. The patient is exhibiting signs and symptoms of cyanide toxicity, which include fatigue, nausea, tinnitus, blurred vision, and delirium. These symptoms would cause the nurse to suspect cyanide toxicity, which can occur with administration of nitroprusside. The nurse should contact the health care provider immediately.

3.   Which assessment finding would the nurse expect to find elevated in a patient admitted with right-sided heart failure?
   A.   CVP
   B.   Left ventricular end-diastolic pressure
   C.   PAOP
   D.   Cardiac output

Answer: A. CVP is elevated in right-sided heart failure.

4.   When performing synchronized cardioversion, the nurse understands that the electrical charge is delivered at which point in the cardiac cycle?
   A.   Initiation of the QRS complex
   B.   During the ST segment
   C.   At the peak of the R wave
   D.   Just before the onset of the P wave

Answer: C. Synchronized cardioversion delivers an electrical charge to the myocardium at the peak of the R wave.

Scoring

☆☆☆ If you answered all four questions correctly, let your heart swell with pride. You're tops when it comes to cardiac emergencies!

☆☆ If you answered three questions correctly, congratulations on all your "heart" work. You're a member of the cardiac emergency team!

☆ If you answered fewer than three questions correctly, don't be heartbroken. Just go back and review the chapter!

Selected references

American Heart Association. (2016). *Advanced cardiovascular life support provider manual* (16th ed.). Dallas, TX: Author.

Baird, M. S. (2016). *Manual of critical care nursing: Nursing interventions and collaborative management* (7th ed.). St. Louis, MO: Elsevier.

Burchum, J. R., & Rosenthal, L. D. (2018). *Lehne's pharmacology for nursing care* (10th ed.). St. Louis, MO: Elsevier.

Elliott, W. J., & Varon, J. (2018). *Drugs used for the treatment of hypertensive emergencies.* Retrieved from https://www.uptodate.com/contents/drugs-used-for-the-treatment-of-hypertensive-emergencies

Garcia, D. A., & Crowther, M. (2019). *Management of bleeding in patients receiving direct oral anticoagulants.* Retrieved from https://www.uptodate.com/contents/management-of-bleeding-in-patients-receiving-direct-oral-anticoagulants

Gibson, M., Carrozza, J., Laham, R., et al. (2018). *Primary percutaneous coronary intervention in acute ST elevation myocardial infarction: Determinants of outcome.* Retrieved from https://www.uptodate.com/contents/primary-percutaneous-coronary-intervention-in-acute-st-elevation-myocardial-infarction-determinants-of-outcome

Huether, S. E., & McCance, K. L. (2016). *Understanding pathophysiology* (6th ed.). St. Louis, MO: Elsevier.

Ignatavicius, D. D., Workman, L., & Rebar, C. (2018). *Medical-surgical nursing: Concepts for interprofessional collaborative care* (9th ed.). St. Louis, MO: Elsevier.

Jaffe, A. S., & Morrow, D. A. (2018). *Troponin testing: Clinical use.* Retrieved from https://www.uptodate.com/contents/troponin-testing-clinical-use

Jarvis, C. (2016). *Physical examination and health assessment* (7th ed.). St. Louis, MO: Elsevier.

Kee, J. L., Hayes, E. R., & McCuistion, L. E. (2015). *Pharmacology: A patient-centered nursing process approach* (8th ed.). St. Louis, MO: Elsevier.

Lilley, L. L., Collins, S. R., & Snyder, J. S. (2017). *Pharmacology and the nursing process* (8th ed.). St. Louis, MO: Elsevier.

Pagana, K. D., & Pagana, T. J. (2018). *Mosby's manual of diagnostic laboratory tests* (6th ed.). St. Louis, MO: Elsevier.

Reeder, G. S., & Kennedy, H. L. (2018). *Diagnosis of acute myocardial infarction.* Retrieved from https://www.uptodate.com/contents/diagnosis-of-acute-myocardial-infarction/print

Sauer, W. H. (2019a). *First degree atrioventricular block.* Retrieved from https://www .uptodate.com/contents/first-degree-atrioventricular-block

Sauer, W. H. (2019b). *Second degree atrioventricular block: Mobitz type II.* Retrieved from https://www.uptodate.com/contents/second-degree-atrioventricular-block -mobitz-type-ii

Sauer, W. H. (2019c). *Third degree (complete) atrioventricular block.* Retrieved from https://www.uptodate.com/contents/third-degree-complete-atrioventricular -block

Urden, L. D., Stacy, K. M., & Lough, M. E. (2018). *Critical care nursing. Diagnosis and management* (8th ed.). St. Louis, MO: Elsevier.

U.S. Food and Drug Administration. (2018). *Drugs@FDA: FDA approved drug products.* Retrieved from https://www.accessdata.fda.gov/scripts/cder/daf/index.cfm

Chapter 5

Respiratory emergencies

Just the facts

In this chapter, you'll learn:

♦ assessment of the respiratory system

♦ respiratory disorders and treatments

♦ diagnostic tests and procedures for respiratory emergencies.

Understanding respiratory emergencies

Respiratory emergencies can be life-threatening and require expert assessment techniques and prompt interventions. Any trauma that alters the integrity of the respiratory system can alter gas exchange. Respiratory emergencies can be caused by obstructions, infections, or injury of the respiratory system.

Assessment

Respiratory assessment is a critical nursing responsibility in the emergency department (ED). Conduct a thorough assessment to detect subtle and obvious respiratory changes.

History

Build your patient's health history by asking short, open-ended questions. Conduct the interview in several short sessions if you have to, depending on the severity of your patient's condition. Ask the family to provide information if the patient is unable.

Cover all the bases

Respiratory disorders may be caused or exacerbated by obesity, smoking, circulatory problems, environmental influences, workplace conditions, and known food or drug allergies, so be sure to ask about these factors.

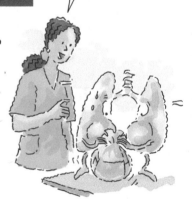

I know respiratory emergencies can be life-threatening, but don't panic! This chapter helps you deal with them.

Current health status

Begin by asking why your patient is seeking care. Many respiratory disorders are chronic, so be sure to ask how the current acute episode compares with the previous episode and which relief measures are helpful and not helpful. Patients with respiratory disorders commonly report concerns such as:
- chest pain
- cough
- shortness of breath
- sleep disturbance
- sputum production
- wheezing
- air hunger.

Chest pain

If the patient has chest pain, ask: Where's the pain? What does it feel like? Is it sharp, stabbing, burning, or aching? Does it move to another area? How long does it last? What causes it? What makes it better?

Pain provocations

Chest pain due to a respiratory problem is usually the result of pleural inflammation, inflammation of the costochondral junctions, soreness of chest muscles because of coughing, or indigestion. Less common causes of pain include rib or vertebral fractures caused by coughing or osteoporosis.

Cough

Ask the patient with a cough: At what time of day do you cough most often? Is the cough productive? If the cough is a chronic problem, has it changed recently? If so, how? What makes the cough better? What makes it worse?

Shortness of breath

Assess your patient's shortness of breath by asking the patient to rate the usual level of dyspnea on a scale of 1 to 10 (1 means no dyspnea and 10 means the worst ever experienced). Then ask the patient to rate the level that day. Other scales grade dyspnea as it relates to activity, such as climbing a set of stairs or walking a city block. (See *Grading dyspnea*, page 202.)

Pillow talk

A patient with orthopnea (shortness of breath when lying down) tends to sleep with the upper body elevated. Ask the patient how many pillows are used for sleep; the answer reflects the severity of the orthopnea. For instance, a patient who uses three pillows can be said to have *three-pillow orthopnea*.

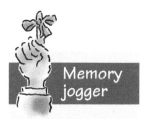

Memory jogger

Use "30-2-CAN DO" for a quick way to determine adequate ABCs.

The adult patient has adequate oxygenation and perfusion or circulation if the patient:
- has fewer than 30 respirations per minute (30)
- is oriented to person and situation (2)
- obeys simple verbal requests (CAN DO).

Don't forget to ask

In addition to using a severity scale, ask: What do you do to relieve the shortness of breath? How well does it usually work?

Sleep disturbance

Sleep disturbances may be related to obstructive sleep apnea or another sleep disorder requiring additional evaluation.

Daytime drowsiness

If the patient reports being drowsy or irritable in the daytime, ask: How many hours of continuous sleep do you get at night? Do you wake up often during the night? Does your family report that you snore or show restlessness during the night?

Sputum production

If a patient produces sputum, ask for an estimate of the amount produced—in teaspoons or some other common measurement. Also ask: What's the color and consistency of the sputum? If sputum is a chronic problem, has it changed recently? If so, how?

Hemoptysis

Hemoptysis may be related to tuberculosis (TB), lung cancer, bronchiectasis, pneumonia, or pulmonary embolism. Ask the patient if coughing produces blood, and if so, how much and how often? What is the character—is it grossly bloody, blood tinged, or blood streaked? To differentiate from hematemesis, hemoptysis is typically frothy, alkaline, and accompanied by sputum.

Wheezing

If a patient wheezes, ask: When do you wheeze? What makes you wheeze? Do you wheeze loudly enough for others to hear it? What helps stop your wheezing?

Previous health status

Look at the patient's health history, being especially watchful for:
- allergies
- respiratory diseases, such as pneumonia and TB
- smoking habit
- exposure to secondhand smoke
- previous operations/hospitalizations.

Ask about current immunizations, such as a flu shot or pneumococcal vaccine. Also determine whether the patient uses respiratory equipment, such as oxygen, nebulizers, or continuous positive airway pressure (CPAP) masks, at home.

Grading dyspnea

To assess dyspnea as objectively as possible, ask your patient to briefly describe how various activities affect breathing. Then document patient response using this grading system:
- *Grade 0*—not troubled by breathlessness except with strenuous exercise
- *Grade 1*—troubled by shortness of breath when hurrying on a level path or walking up a slight hill
- *Grade 2*—walks more slowly than people of the same age on a level path because of breathlessness or has to stop to breathe when walking on a level path at his or her own pace
- *Grade 3*—stops to breathe after walking about 100 yards (91 m) on a level path
- *Grade 4*—too breathless to leave the house or breathless when dressing or undressing.

Family history

Ask the patient whether there is a family history of cancer, sickle cell anemia, heart disease, or chronic illness, such as asthma and emphysema. Determine if the patient lives with anyone who has an infectious disease, such as TB or influenza.

Lifestyle patterns

Ask about the patient's workplace because some jobs, such as coal mining and construction work, expose workers to substances such as asbestos that can cause lung disease.

Also ask about the patient's home, community, and other environmental factors that may influence dealing with respiratory problems. For example, you may ask questions about interpersonal relationships, stress management, and coping methods. Ask about the patient's sex habits or drug use, which may be connected with AIDS-related pulmonary disorders.

Physical examination

In most cases, the physical examination begins after taking the patient's history, although it may be done simultaneously. However, you may not be able to take a complete history if the patient develops an ominous sign such as acute respiratory distress. If your patient is in respiratory distress, establish the priorities of your nursing assessment, progressing from the most critical factors (airway, breathing, and circulation) to less critical factors. (See *Emergency respiratory assessment*, page 204.)

Four steps

Use a systematic approach to detect subtle and obvious respiratory changes. The four steps for conducting a physical examination of the respiratory system are:
1. inspection
2. palpation
3. percussion
4. auscultation.

Back, then front

Examine the back of the chest first, using inspection, palpation, percussion, and auscultation. Always compare one side with the other. Then examine the front of the chest using the same sequence. The patient can lie back when you examine the front of the chest if that's more comfortable.

Emergency respiratory assessment

Begin your assessment with an "across the room look" as the patient approaches triage. If your patient is in acute respiratory distress, immediately assess the ABCs—airway, breathing, and circulation. If these are absent, call for help and start cardiopulmonary resuscitation.

Next, quickly check for these signs of impending crisis:
• Is the patient having trouble breathing?
• Is the patient using accessory muscles to breathe? Look for evidence that the patient is using accessory muscles when breathing, including shoulder elevation, intercostal muscle retraction, and use of scalene and sternocleidomastoid muscles.
• Is there a change in the patient's level of consciousness?
• Is there confusion, anxiety, or agitation?
• Does the patient change body position to ease breathing?
• Does the skin look pale, diaphoretic, or cyanotic?

Setting priorities

If your patient is in respiratory distress, establish priorities for your nursing assessment. Don't assume the obvious. Note positive and negative factors, starting with the most critical factors (the ABCs) and progressing to less critical factors.

During an emergency, you may not have time to go through each step of the nursing process. Use your assessment skills and clinical judgment to gather enough data to answer vital questions. A single sign or symptom has many possible meanings, so gather a group of findings to assess the patient and develop interventions.

Inspection

Make the following observations about the patient as soon as you enter the patient care area and include these observations in your assessment. Note the patient's position on the stretcher. Does the patient appear comfortable? Is the patient sitting up, lying quietly, or shifting about? Watch the respiratory pattern, chest movement, and work of breathing. Are there symptoms of anxiety present? Is the breathing pattern labored or does breathing appear difficult for the patient? Is oxygen required?

Chest inspection

Inspect the patient's chest configuration, tracheal position, chest symmetry, skin condition, nostrils (for flaring), and accessory muscle use.

Beauty in symmetry

Look for chest wall symmetry. Both sides of the chest should be equal at rest and expand equally as the patient inhales.

A new angle

Also, look at the costal angle (the angle between the ribs and the sternum at the point immediately above the xiphoid process). This angle should be less than 90 degrees in an adult. The angle is larger if the chest wall is chronically expanded because of an enlargement of the intercostal muscles, which can happen with chronic obstructive pulmonary disease (COPD).

> Hypertrophy in accessory muscles can be normal in some athletes, but in most patients, it signals respiratory problems.

Muscles in motion

When the patient inhales, the diaphragm should descend and the intercostal muscles should contract. This dual motion causes the abdomen to push out and the lower ribs to expand laterally.

When the patient exhales, the abdomen and ribs return to their resting positions. The upper chest shouldn't move much. Accessory muscles may hypertrophy, indicating frequent use. This may be normal in some athletes, but for most patients, it indicates a respiratory problem, especially when the patient demonstrates pursed lips and flared nostrils when breathing.

Chest wall abnormalities

Inspect for chest wall abnormalities, keeping in mind that a patient with a deformity of the chest wall might have completely normal lungs that could be cramped in the chest. The patient may have a smaller-than-normal lung capacity and limited exercise tolerance.

Raising a red flag

Watch for paradoxical (uneven) movement of the patient's chest wall. Paradoxical movement may appear as an abnormal collapse of part of the chest wall when the patient inhales or an abnormal expansion when the patient exhales. In either case, such uneven movement indicates a loss of normal chest wall function.

Breathing rate and pattern

Assess your patient's respiratory function by determining the rate, rhythm, and quality of respirations.

Count on it

The respiratory pattern should be even, coordinated, and regular, with occasional sighs. The normal ratio of inspiration to expiration (I:E ratio) is about 1:2.

Abnormal respiratory patterns

Apneustic

Apneustic respirations are prolonged gasping inspirations followed by short inefficient expirations. Suspect a lesion on the pons.

Ataxic

Ataxic respirations are a lack of any pattern to the respirations. Suspect a brainstem lesion.

Biot respirations

Biot respirations involve rapid, deep breaths that alternate with abrupt periods of apnea. It's an ominous sign of severe central nervous system (CNS) damage, increased intracranial pressure, meningitis, or encephalitis.

Bradypnea

Bradypneic respirations are slow (less than 10 breaths per minute) and regular. Causes include depression of the respiratory center related to drugs, alcohol or tumor, increased intracranial pressure, carbon dioxide narcosis, or metabolic alkalosis.

Cheyne–Stokes

Cheyne–Stokes respirations are initially shallow but gradually become deeper and deeper; then a period of apnea follows, lasting up to 20 seconds, and the cycle starts again. This respiratory pattern is seen in patients with heart failure, kidney failure, or CNS damage. Cheyne–Stokes respirations can be a normal breathing pattern during sleep in older adult patients.

Kussmaul respirations

Kussmaul respirations are deep, gasping, and rapid (usually greater than 35 breaths per minute). These are due to metabolic acidosis (diabetic ketoacidosis or renal failure).

Tachypnea

Tachypnea is rapid (greater than 30 breaths per minute) and may be related to restrictive lung disease, pneumonia, pleurisy, chest pain, fear, anxiety, or respiratory insufficiency (Potter et al., 2017).

Inspecting related structures
Inspect the patient's skin for cyanosis or clubbing.

Don't be blue

Skin color varies considerably among patients, but a patient with a bluish tint to the skin, nail beds, and mucous membranes is considered cyanotic. Cyanosis, which results when oxygenation to the tissues is poor, is a late sign of hypoxemia.

Finger findings

When you inspect the fingers, assess for clubbing, a sign of long-standing respiratory or cardiac disease. The fingernail normally enters the skin at an angle of less than 180 degrees. When fingernail clubbing occurs, the angle is greater than or equal to 180 degrees.

Palpation

Palpation of the chest provides some important information about the respiratory system and the processes involved in breathing.

Leaky lungs

The chest wall should feel smooth, warm, and dry. Crepitus, which feels like puffed rice cereal crackling under the skin, indicates that air is leaking from the airways or lungs.

Probing palpation pain

Gentle palpation shouldn't cause the patient pain. If the patient reports chest pain, try to find a painful area on the chest wall. Here's a guide to assessing some types of chest pain:
- Painful costochondral joints are typically located at the midclavicular line or next to the sternum.
- A rib or vertebral fracture is quite painful over the fracture.
- Protracted coughing may cause sore muscles.
- A collapsed lung can cause pain in addition to dyspnea.

Feeling for fremitus

Palpate for tactile fremitus (palpable vibrations caused by the transmission of air through the bronchopulmonary system). Fremitus decreases over areas where pleural fluid collects; when the patient speaks softly; and with pneumothorax, atelectasis, and emphysema.

Fremitus is normally increased over the large bronchial tubes and abnormally increased over areas in which alveoli are filled with fluid or exudates, as in pneumonia. (See *Checking for tactile fremitus*, page 208.)

Checking for tactile fremitus

When you check the back of the thorax for tactile fremitus, ask the patient to fold the arms across the chest, as shown here. This movement shifts the scapulae out of the way.

What to do

Check for tactile fremitus by lightly placing your open palms on both sides of the patient's back without touching the patient's back with your fingers, as shown here. Ask the patient to repeat the word "ninety-nine" loudly enough to produce palpable vibrations. Then palpate the front of the chest using the same hand positions.

What the results mean

Vibrations that feel more intense on one side than on the other indicate tissue consolidation on that side. Less intense vibrations may indicate emphysema, pneumothorax, or pleural effusion. Faint or no vibrations in the upper posterior thorax may indicate bronchial obstruction or a fluid-filled pleural space.

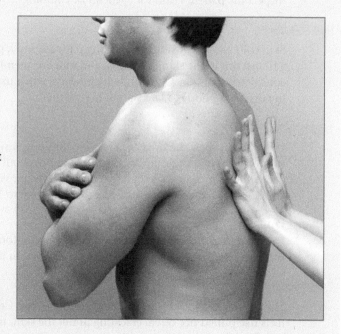

Evaluating symmetry

To evaluate your patient's chest wall symmetry and expansion, place your hands on the front of the chest wall with your thumbs touching each other at the second intercostal space. As the patient inhales deeply, watch your thumbs. They should separate simultaneously and equally to a distance several centimeters away from the sternum. Repeat the measurement at the fifth intercostal space. You may make the same measurement on the back of the chest near the 10th rib (Potter et al., 2017).

Warning signs

The chest may expand asymmetrically if the patient has:

- pneumonia
- atelectasis
- pleural effusion
- pneumothorax
- flail chest
- right mainstem intubation (no movement on the left).

Chest expansion may be decreased at the level of the diaphragm if the patient has:

- respiratory depression
- emphysema
- obesity
- ascites
- atelectasis
- diaphragm paralysis.

Percussion

Percuss the chest to:

- find the boundaries of the lungs
- determine whether the lungs are filled with air, fluid, or solid material
- evaluate the distance the diaphragm travels between the patient's inhalation and exhalation.

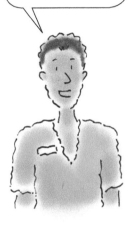

Percuss the chest to determine whether lungs are filled with air, fluid, or solid material.

Sites and sounds

Listen for normal, resonant sounds over most of the chest. In the left front chest wall from the third or fourth intercostal space at the sternum to the third or fourth intercostal space at the midclavicular line, listen for a dull sound because that's the space occupied by the heart. With careful percussion, you can identify the borders of the heart when lung tissue is normal. Resonance resumes at the sixth intercostal space. The sequence of sounds in the back is slightly different. (See *Percussion sequences*, page 210.)

Warning sounds

When you hear hyperresonance during percussion, it means you've found an area of increased air in the lung or pleural space. Expect to hear hyperresonance in patients with:

- acute asthma
- pneumothorax
- bullous emphysema (large holes in the lungs from alveolar destruction).

When you hear abnormal dullness, it means you've found areas of decreased air in the lungs. Expect abnormal dullness in the presence of:

- pleural fluid
- consolidation atelectasis
- tumor.

Detecting diaphragm movement

Percussion also allows you to assess how much the diaphragm moves during inspiration and expiration. The normal diaphragm

Percussion sequences

Follow these percussion sequences to distinguish between normal and abnormal sounds in the patient's lungs. Compare sound variations from one side with the other as you proceed. Carefully describe abnormal sounds you hear and note their locations. (Follow the same sequence for auscultation.)

Anterior

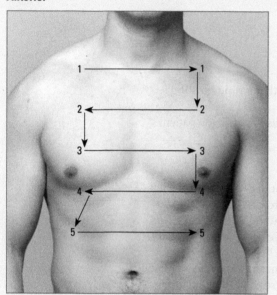

Posterior

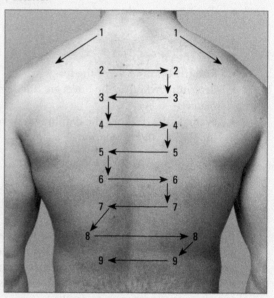

descends 1⅛" (double prime) to 1⅞" (double prime) (3 to 5 cm) when the patient inhales. The diaphragm doesn't move as far in patients with emphysema, respiratory depression, diaphragm paralysis, atelectasis, obesity, or ascites.

Auscultation

As air moves through the bronchi, it creates sound waves that travel to the chest wall. The sound produced by breathing changes as air moves from larger to smaller airways. Sounds also change if they pass through fluid, mucus, or narrowed airways.

Auscultation preparation

Auscultation sites are the same as percussion sites. Using the diaphragm of the stethoscope, listen to a full cycle of inspiration and expiration at each site. Ask the patient to breathe through the mouth if it doesn't cause discomfort; nose breathing alters the pitch of breath sounds.

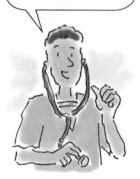

Normally, I'd say that breathing through one's mouth is rude, but when you're auscultating, I say the mouth the merrier!

Qualities of normal breath sounds

Use this chart as a quick reference for the qualities of normal breath sounds.

Breath sound	Quality	Inspiration–expiration ratio	Location
Tracheal	Harsh, high pitched	I < E	Over trachea
Bronchial	Loud, high pitched	I > E	Next to trachea
Bronchovesicular	Medium in loudness and pitch	I = E	Next to sternum, between scapula
Vesicular	Soft, low pitched	I > E	Remainder of lungs

Be firm

To auscultate for breath sounds, press the diaphragm side of the stethoscope firmly against the skin. Remember that if you listen through clothing or chest hair, breath sounds won't be heard clearly and you may hear unusual and deceptive sounds. Ask the patient to take deep breaths through the mouth and listen for at least one full breath at each location. Compare symmetrical areas.

Interpreting breath sounds

Classify each breath sound you auscultate by its intensity, pitch, duration, characteristic, and location. Note whether it occurs during inspiration, expiration, or both.

Normal breath sounds

During auscultation, listen for four types of breath sounds over normal lungs. (See *Locations of normal breath sounds.*) Here's a rundown of the normal breath sounds and their characteristics:
- Tracheal breath sounds, heard over the trachea, are harsh and discontinuous. They're present when the patient inhales or exhales.
- Bronchial breath sounds, usually heard next to the trachea just above or below the clavicle, are loud, high pitched, and discontinuous. They're loudest when the patient exhales.
- Bronchovesicular sounds are medium pitched and continuous. They're best heard over the upper third of the sternum and between the scapulae when the patient inhales or exhales.
- Vesicular sounds, heard over the rest of the lungs, are soft and low pitched. They're prolonged during inhalation and shortened during exhalation (Potter et al., 2017). (See *Qualities of normal breath sounds.*)

Locations of normal breath sounds

These photographs show the normal locations of different types of breath sounds.

Anterior thorax

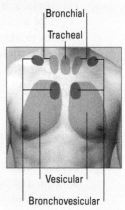

Bronchial

Tracheal

Vesicular

Bronchovesicular

Posterior thorax

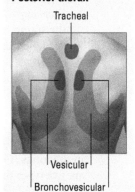

Tracheal

Vesicular

Bronchovesicular

Abnormal breath sounds

Because solid tissue transmits sound better than air or fluid, breath sounds (as well as spoken or whispered words) are louder than normal over areas of consolidation. If pus, fluid, or air fills the pleural space, breath sounds are quieter than normal. If a foreign body or secretions obstruct a bronchus, breath sounds are diminished or absent over lung tissue distal to the obstruction.

Detect the unexpected

Breath sounds heard in an unexpected area are also abnormal. For instance, if you hear bronchial sounds where you expect to hear vesicular sounds, the area you're auscultating might be filled with fluid or exudates, as in pneumonia. The vesicular sounds you expect to hear in those areas are absent because no air is moving through the small airways. Some common abnormal breath sounds are vocal fremitus and adventitious breath sounds.

Vocal fremitus

Vocal fremitus is the sound produced by chest vibrations as the patient speaks. Voice sounds can transmit abnormally over consolidated areas because sound travels well through fluid. There are three common abnormal voice sounds:
1. *Bronchophony*—Ask the patient to say "ninety-nine" or "blue moon." Over normal tissue, the words sound muffled, but over consolidated areas, the words sound unusually loud.
2. *Egophony*—Ask the patient to say "E." Over normal lung tissue, the sound is muffled, but over consolidated areas, it sounds like the letter A.
3. *Whispered pectoriloquy*—Ask the patient to whisper "1, 2, 3." Over normal lung tissue, the numbers are almost indistinguishable. Over consolidated tissue, the numbers sound loud and clear.

Adventitious sounds

Adventitious sounds are abnormal no matter where you hear them in the lungs (Potter et al., 2017). (See *Abnormal breath sounds.*) There are five types of adventitious breath sounds:
1. crackles (rales)
2. wheezes
3. rhonchi
4. stridor
5. pleural friction rub.

Abnormal breath sounds

Here's a quick guide to assessing abnormal breath sounds.

Crackles (rales)

Crackles (rales) are intermittent, non-musical, crackling sounds heard during inspiration. They're classified as *fine* or *coarse* and are common in older adults when small sections of the alveoli don't fully aerate and secretions accumulate during sleep. Alveoli reexpand or pop open when the patient takes deep breaths upon awakening. Fine crackles sound like strands of hair being rubbed between the fingers. Coarse crackles sound like bubbling or gurgling as air moves through secretions in larger airways.

Wheezes

Wheezes are high-pitched sounds caused by blocked airflow and are heard on exhalation or also on inspection as the block increases. Patients may wheeze as a result of asthma, infection, or airway obstruction from a tumor or foreign body.

Rhonchi

Rhonchi are low-pitched, snoring, or rattling sounds heard primarily on exhalation and usually change with coughing.

Stridor

Stridor is a loud, high-pitched sound heard during inspiration.

Pleural friction rub

Pleural friction rub is a low-pitched, grating sound heard during inspiration and expiration and is accompanied by pain.

Diagnostic tests

If your patient's history and the physical examination findings reveal evidence of pulmonary dysfunction, diagnostic tests can identify and evaluate the dysfunction. These tests include:

- bedside testing procedures
- blood and sputum studies
- endoscopy and imaging
- pulmonary angiography.

Pulse oximetry

Pulse oximetry is a relatively simple procedure used to monitor arterial oxygen saturation noninvasively. It's performed intermittently or continuously.

A closer look at pulse oximetry

Oximetry may be intermittent or continuous and is used to monitor arterial oxygen saturation. Normal oxygen saturation levels are 95% to 100% for adults. Lower levels may indicate hypoxemia and warrant intervention.

Interfering factors
Certain factors can interfere with the accuracy of oximetry readings. For example, an elevated bilirubin level may falsely lower oxygen saturation readings, whereas elevated carboxyhemoglobin or methemoglobin levels can falsely elevate oxygen saturation readings.

Certain intravascular substances, such as lipid emulsions and diagnostic intravenous dyes, can also prevent accurate readings. Other interfering factors include excessive light (such as from phototherapy or direct sunlight), excessive patient movement, excessive ear pigment, hypothermia, hypotension, and vasoconstriction.

Some acrylic nails and certain colors of nail polish (blue, green, black, and brown-red) may also interfere with readings.

Keep in mind that pulse oximetry readings may not be reliable in certain instances such as:
- cardiopulmonary arrest
- shock states
- vasoconstrictive medication use
- anemia
- high carbon monoxide levels.

Shedding light on the subject

In this procedure, two diodes send red and infrared light through a pulsating arterial vascular bed such as the one in the fingertip. A photodetector (also called a *sensor* or *transducer*) slipped over the finger measures the transmitted light as it passes through the vascular bed; detects the relative amount of color absorbed by arterial blood; and calculates the saturation without interference from the venous blood, skin, or connective tissue. The percentage expressed is the ratio of oxygen to hemoglobin (Jurbran, 2015). (See *A closer look at pulse oximetry*.)

Note denotation

In pulse oximetry, arterial oxygen saturation values are usually denoted with the symbol SpO_2. Arterial oxygen saturation values that are measured invasively using arterial blood gas (ABG) analysis are denoted by the symbol SaO_2.

Practice pointers

- Place the sensor over the finger or other site—such as the toe, bridge of the nose, or earlobe—so that the light beams and sensors are opposite each other.
- Protect the sensor from exposure to strong light, such as fluorescent lighting, because it interferes with results. Check the sensor site frequently to make sure the device is in place and examine the skin for abrasion and circulatory impairment.
- The pulse oximeter displays the patient's pulse rate and oxygen saturation reading. The pulse rate on the oximeter should correspond to the patient's actual pulse. If the rates don't correspond, the saturation reading can't be considered accurate. You may need to reposition the sensor to obtain an accurate reading.
- Rotate the sensor site at least every 4 hours, following the manufacturer's instructions and your facility's policy for site rotation, to avoid skin irritation and circulatory impairment.
- If oximetry is done properly, the oxygen saturation readings are usually within 2% of ABG values. A normal reading is 95% to 100%.

Poisoning precludes pulse oximetry

- Pulse oximetry isn't used when carbon monoxide (CO) poisoning is suspected because the oximeter doesn't differentiate between oxygen and CO bound to hemoglobin. An ABG analysis should be performed in such cases.

End-tidal carbon dioxide monitoring (capnography)

End-tidal carbon dioxide ($ETCO_2$) monitoring is used to measure the carbon dioxide concentration at end expiration. An $ETCO_2$ monitor may be a separate monitor or part of the patient's bedside hemodynamic monitoring system. Capnography is used to verify endotracheal tube (ETT) placement by measuring the exhaled carbon dioxide at the end of each breath.

Indications for $ETCO_2$ monitoring include:

- monitoring apnea, respiratory function, and patency of the airway in acute airway obstruction
- early detection of hypercapnia, hyperthermia, and changes in carbon dioxide production and elimination with hyperventilation therapy
- assessing effectiveness of such interventions as mechanical ventilation, neuromuscular blockade used with mechanical ventilation, and prone positioning

- monitoring for ETT displacement or obstruction while transporting a patient
- assessing the adequacy of chest compressions during cardiopulmonary resuscitation (CPR)
- monitoring ventilation during procedural sedation
- determining the severity of asthma exacerbation and the effectiveness of interventions.

In-lightened

In $ETCO_2$ monitoring, a photodetector measures the amount of infrared light absorbed by the airway during inspiration and expiration. (Light absorption increases along with carbon dioxide concentration.) The monitor converts these data to a carbon dioxide value and a corresponding waveform or capnogram, if capnography is used.

Crunching the numbers

Values are obtained by monitoring samples of expired gas from an ETT or an oral or nasopharyngeal airway. Although the values are similar, the $ETCO_2$ values are usually 2 to 5 mm Hg lower than the partial pressure of arterial carbon dioxide ($PaCO_2$) value. End exhalation contains the highest carbon dioxide concentration. Normal $ETCO_2$ is 35 to 45 mm Hg.

Capnograms and $ETCO_2$ monitoring reduce the need for frequent ABG sampling.

Practice pointers

- Explain the procedure to the patient and the family.
- Assess the patient's respiratory status, vital signs, oxygen saturation, and $ETCO_2$ readings.
- Observe waveform quality and trends of $ETCO_2$ readings and observe for sudden increases (which may indicate hypoventilation, partial airway obstruction, or respiratory depressant effects from drugs) or decreases (due to complete airway obstruction, a dislodged ETT, or ventilator malfunction). Notify the health care provider of a 10% increase or decrease in readings.

ABG analysis

ABG analysis is useful in assessing respiratory status and acid–base balance. ABGs are a measurement of systemic gas exchange.

ABCs of ABGs

Arterial blood is measured because it reflects how much oxygen is available to peripheral tissues. Together, ABG values tell the story of how well a patient is oxygenated and whether acidosis or alkalosis is developing.

Here's a summary of commonly assessed ABG components and what the findings indicate:

- pH measurement of the hydrogen ion (H^+) concentration is an indication of the blood's acidity or alkalinity.
- $Paco_2$ reflects the adequacy of ventilation of the lungs.
- Partial pressure of arterial oxygen (Pao_2) reflects the body's ability to pick up oxygen from the lungs.
- Bicarbonate (HCO_3^-) level reflects the activity of the kidneys in retaining or excreting bicarbonate.
- Sao_2 is the ratio of actual hemoglobin oxygen content to potential maximum oxygen-carrying capacity of the hemoglobin. (See *Normal ABG values*.)

Valuable values

Here's an interpretation of possible ABG values:

- An Sao_2 value less than 95% represents decreased saturation and may contribute to a low Pao_2 value.
- A pH value above 7.45 (alkalosis) reflects an H^+ deficit; a value below 7.35 (acidosis) reflects an H^+ excess.

A sample scenario

Suppose you find a pH value greater than 7.45 indicating alkalosis. Investigate further by checking the $Paco_2$ value, which is known as the *respiratory parameter*. This value reflects how efficiently the lungs eliminate carbon dioxide. A $Paco_2$ value below 35 mm Hg indicates respiratory alkalosis and hyperventilation.

Next, check the HCO_3^- value called the *metabolic parameter*. An HCO_3^- value greater than 26 mEq/L indicates metabolic alkalosis.

Likewise, a pH value below 7.35 indicates acidosis. A $Paco_2$ value above 45 mm Hg indicates respiratory acidosis; an HCO_3^- value below 22 mEq/L indicates metabolic acidosis.

Seesaw systems

The respiratory and metabolic systems work together to keep the body's acid–base balance within normal limits. For example, if respiratory acidosis develops, the kidneys compensate by conserving HCO_3^-. That's why you expect to see an above-normal HCO_3^- value.

Normal ABG values

Arterial blood gas (ABG) values provide information about the blood's acid–base balance and oxygenation. Normal values are:

- pH: 7.35 to 7.45
- partial pressure of arterial carbon dioxide ($Paco_2$): 35 to 45 mm Hg
- partial pressure of arterial oxygen (Pao_2): 80 to 100 mm Hg
- bicarbonate (HCO_3^-): 22 to 26 mEq/L
- arterial oxygen saturation (Sao_2): 95% to 100%.

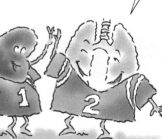

Here's the game plan: If you develop respiratory acidosis, I'll cover you and conserve HCO_3^-. Ready? Break!

Understanding acid–base disorders

This chart provides an overview of selected acid–base disorders.

Disorder and arterial blood gas findings	Possible causes	Signs and symptoms
Respiratory acidosis (excess carbon dioxide retention) pH <7.35 Bicarbonate (HCO_3^-) >26 mEq/L (if compensating) Partial pressure of arterial carbon dioxide ($Paco_2$) >45 mm Hg	• Asphyxia • Central nervous system depression from drugs, injury, or disease • Hypoventilation from pulmonary, cardiac, musculoskeletal, or neuromuscular disease	Diaphoresis, headache, tachycardia, confusion, restlessness, apprehension, flushed face
Respiratory alkalosis (excess carbon dioxide excretion) pH >7.45 HCO_3^- <22 mEq/L (if compensating) $Paco_2$ <35 mm Hg	• Gram-negative bacteremia • Hyperventilation from anxiety, pain, or improper ventilator settings • Respiratory stimulation by drugs, disease, hypoxia, fever, or high room temperature	Rapid, deep respirations; paresthesias; light-headedness; twitching; anxiety; fear
Metabolic acidosis (bicarbonate loss, acid retention) pH <7.35 HCO_3^- <22 mEq/L $Paco_2$ <35 mm Hg (if compensating)	• Bicarbonate depletion from diarrhea • Excessive production of organic acids from hepatic disease, endocrine disorders, shock, or drug intoxication • Inadequate excretion of acids from renal disease	Rapid, deep breathing; fruity breath; fatigue; headache; lethargy; drowsiness; nausea; vomiting; coma (if severe); abdominal pain
Metabolic alkalosis (bicarbonate retention, acid loss) pH >7.45 HCO_3^- >26 mEq/L $Paco_2$ >45 mm Hg (if compensating)	• Excessive alkali ingestion • Loss of hydrochloric acid from prolonged vomiting or gastric suctioning • Loss of potassium from increased renal excretion (as in diuretic therapy) or steroids	Slow, shallow breathing; hypertonic muscles; restlessness; twitching; confusion; irritability; apathy; tetany; seizures; coma (if severe)

Adapted from Ignatavicius, D., Workman, M., & Rebar, C. (2018). *Medical-surgical nursing: Concepts for interprofessional collaborative care* (9th ed.). St. Louis, MO: Elsevier.

Similarly, if metabolic acidosis develops, the lungs compensate by increasing the respiratory rate and depth to eliminate carbon dioxide (Ignatavicius et al., 2018). (See *Understanding acid–base disorders*.)

Practice pointers

- A health care provider, respiratory therapist, or specially trained nurse draws ABG samples, usually from an arterial line if the patient has one. If a percutaneous puncture must be done, choose the site carefully. The most common site is the radial artery, but the brachial or femoral arteries can be used.

- After obtaining the sample, apply pressure to the puncture site for 5 minutes and tape a gauze pad firmly in place. Regularly monitor the site for bleeding and check the arm for signs of complications, such as swelling, discoloration, pain, numbness, and tingling. (See *Obtaining an ABG sample*.)
- Note whether the patient is breathing room air or oxygen. If the patient is on oxygen, document the number of liters. If the patient is receiving mechanical ventilation, document the fraction of inspired oxygen.
- Make sure you remove all air bubbles in the sample syringe because air bubbles also alter results.
- Make sure the sample of arterial blood is kept cold, preferably on ice, and delivered as soon as possible to the laboratory for analysis.

What's in a name?

Modified Allen test: This test is completed before an arterial blood draw and assesses arterial competency.
- Have patient clench the fist.
- Then apply occlusive pressure to both the ulnar and radial arteries to block blood flow to the hand.
- Have the patient relax the hand and check for palm and finger blanching/pallor (if the fingers exhibit good circulation, without blanching, blood flow has not been occluded completely and first steps should be repeated with more pressure applied to the vessels).
- If the patient's hand exhibits signs of blanching/pallor, release the occlusive pressure on the ulnar artery only. This action will determine whether the test is positive or negative.

The results:

Positive: The hand flushes within 5 to 10 seconds. This indicates that the ulnar artery has good blood flow.

Negative: The hand does not flush within 10 seconds. This indicates that ulnar circulation is inadequate or nonexistent (Theodore, 2017).

If the modified Allen test is negative, the arterial stick blood draw should not be completed on that arm. (See *Modified Allen test*, page 220.)

Obtaining an ABG sample

Follow these steps to obtain a sample for arterial blood gas (ABG) analysis:
- After performing a modified Allen test, perform a cutaneous arterial puncture (or, if an arterial line is in place, draw blood from the arterial line).
- Use a heparinized blood gas syringe to draw the sample.
- Eliminate all air from the sample, place it on ice immediately, and transport it for analysis.
- Apply pressure to the puncture site for 5 minutes. If the patient is receiving anticoagulants or has a coagulopathy, hold the puncture site longer than 5 minutes, if necessary.
- Tape a gauze pad firmly over the puncture site. If the puncture site is on the arm, don't tape the entire circumference because this may restrict circulation.

Modified Allen test

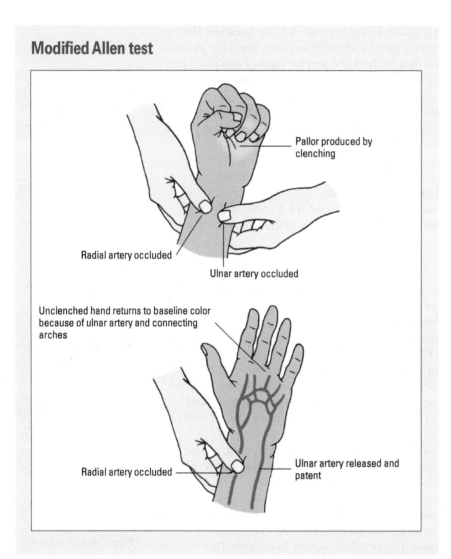

Pallor produced by clenching

Radial artery occluded

Ulnar artery occluded

Unclenched hand returns to baseline color because of ulnar artery and connecting arches

Radial artery occluded

Ulnar artery released and patent

Sputum analysis

Sputum analysis assesses sputum specimens to diagnose respiratory disease, identify the cause of pulmonary infection (including viral and bacterial causes), identify abnormal lung cells, and manage lung disease.

Practice pointers

- When ready to expectorate, instruct the patient to take three deep breaths and force a deep cough.
- Before sending the specimen to the laboratory, make sure it's sputum, not saliva. Saliva has a thinner consistency and more bubbles (froth) than sputum.

Bronchoscopy

Bronchoscopy allows direct visualization of the larynx, trachea, and bronchi through a fiber-optic bronchoscope (a slender, flexible tube with mirrors and a light at its distal end). The flexible fiber-optic bronchoscope is preferred to metal because it's smaller, allows a better view of the bronchi, and carries less risk of trauma.

To remove and evaluate

The purpose of a bronchoscopy is to:
- remove foreign bodies, malignant or benign tumors, mucus plugs, or excessive secretions from the tracheobronchial tree and to control massive hemoptysis
- pass brush biopsy forceps or a catheter through the bronchoscope to obtain specimens for cytologic evaluation.

Practice pointers
- The patient may be premedicated with atropine to dry secretions and a mild sedative or antianxiety agent such as midazolam to help with relaxation. Before insertion of the bronchoscope, a topical anesthetic is applied to the oropharynx, nasopharynx, larynx, vocal cords, and trachea to suppress the cough reflex and prevent gagging.
- The health care provider introduces the bronchoscope tube through the patient's nose or mouth into the airway. Various ports on the bronchoscope allow for suctioning, oxygen administration, and biopsies during the procedure. Monitor vital signs, oxygen saturation levels (with pulse oximetry), and heart rhythm throughout the procedure.
- After the procedure, the patient is positioned on the side or may have the head of the bed elevated 30 degrees until the gag reflex returns. Assess respiratory status and monitor vital signs, oxygen saturation levels, and heart rhythm. Report signs and symptoms of respiratory distress, such as dyspnea, laryngospasm, or hypoxemia.
- Monitor cardiac status frequently for changes in heart rate or rhythm. Report any tachycardia or evidence of arrhythmia.
- If the patient isn't intubated, assess for return of the gag, cough, and swallow reflexes.

Chest X-ray

During chest radiography (commonly known as *chest X-ray*), X-ray beams penetrate the chest and react on specially sensitized film. Because normal pulmonary tissue is radiolucent, such abnormalities as infiltrates, foreign bodies, fluid, and tumors appear dense on the film. This verifies the placement of ETT, central venous catheters, and chest tubes.

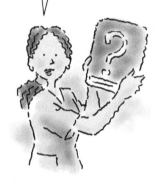

Comparing two chest X-rays can paint a better picture of respiratory change than looking at just one.

More is better

A chest X-ray is most useful when compared with the patient's previous films, allowing the radiologist to detect changes. By themselves, chest X-rays may not provide definitive diagnostic information. For example, they may not reveal mild to moderate obstructive pulmonary disease. However, they can show the location and size of lesions and can also be used to identify structural abnormalities that influence ventilation.

X-ray vision

Examples of abnormalities visible on X-ray include:
- fibrosis
- infiltrates
- atelectasis
- pneumothorax.

Practice pointers
- When a patient in the ED can't be moved, chest X-ray is commonly performed at the bedside.
- Make sure that female patients of childbearing age wear a lead apron. Males should have protection for the testes. Both males and females should wear lead thyroid protection.

Magnetic resonance imaging

Magnetic resonance imaging (MRI) is a noninvasive test that employs a powerful magnet, radio waves, and a computer. It's used to diagnose respiratory disorders by providing high-resolution, cross-sectional images of lung structures and by tracing blood flow.

View that's see-through

The greatest advantage of MRI is that it enables you to "see through" bone and delineate fluid-filled soft tissue in great detail without using ionizing radiation or contrast media. It's used to distinguish tumors from other structures such as blood vessels.

Practice pointers

- All metal objects must be removed from the patient before entering the scanning room. (See *MRI and metals don't mix.*)
- If the patient is claustrophobic, sedation can be used before the test.
- Tell the patient that the test usually takes 15 to 30 minutes. Some facilities can perform open MRIs, which are more tolerable for patients who are claustrophobic.

Thoracic computed tomography scan

Thoracic computed tomography (CT) scan provides cross-sectional views of the chest by passing an X-ray beam from a computerized scanner through the body at different angles and depths. A contrast agent is sometimes used to highlight blood vessels and allow greater visual discrimination.

CT in 3-D

Thoracic CT scan provides a three-dimensional image of the lung, allowing the health care provider to assess abnormalities in the configuration of the trachea or major bronchi and evaluate masses or lesions, such as tumors and abscesses, and abnormal lung shadows.

Practice pointers

- Confirm that the patient isn't allergic to iodine or shellfish. A patient with these allergies may have an adverse reaction to the contrast medium. Diphenhydramine (Benadryl) and prednisone may be administered, as prescribed, before the test to reduce the risk of a reaction to the dye.
- If a contrast medium is used, explain that it's injected into the existing intravenous (IV) line or that a new line may be inserted.
- Explain to the patient that there may be a flushing sensation or a metallic or salty taste in the mouth when the contrast medium is injected.
- Explain that the CT scanner circles around the patient for 10 to 30 minutes, depending on the procedure.
- Instruct the patient to lie still during the test.
- Inform the patient that the contrast medium may discolor the urine for 24 hours.
- Encourage oral fluid intake to flush the contrast medium out of the patient's system unless it's contraindicated or the patient is on nothing-by-mouth status. The health care provider may prescribe an increase in the rate of IV fluid infusion.

MRI and metals don't mix

Before undergoing magnetic resonance imaging (MRI), make sure the patient does not have a pacemaker or surgically implanted joint, pin, clip, valve, or pump containing metal. Such objects could be attracted to the strong MRI magnet.

Ask your patient if there is a history of working with metals or if he or she has ever had metal in the eyes. (Some facilities have a checklist that covers all pertinent questions regarding metals, clips, pins, pacemakers, and other devices.) If such a device or metal is present, the test can't be done.

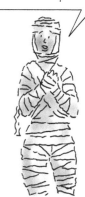

CT scanner and MRI equipment can make some patients feel claustrophobic.

Ventilation–perfusion scan

A ventilation–perfusion ($\dot{V}/\dot{Q}$) scan is used to:
- evaluate $\dot{V}/\dot{Q}$ mismatch
- detect pulmonary embolus
- evaluate pulmonary function, especially in patients with marginal lung reserves.

Although it's less reliable than pulmonary angiography, $\dot{V}/\dot{Q}$ scanning carries fewer risks.

Two-tined test

A $\dot{V}/\dot{Q}$ scan has two parts:
1. During the ventilation portion of the test, the patient inhales the contrast medium gas; ventilation patterns and adequacy of ventilation are noted on the scan.
2. During the perfusion scan, the contrast medium is injected intravenously and the pulmonary blood flow to the lungs is visualized.

$\dot{V}/\dot{Q}$ caveat

$\dot{V}/\dot{Q}$ scans aren't commonly used for patients on mechanical ventilators because the ventilation portion of the test is difficult to perform. (Pulmonary angiography is the preferred test for a critically ill patient with a suspected pulmonary embolus.)

Practice pointers
- Explain the test to the patient and family, telling them who will perform the test and where it's done.
- Like pulmonary angiography, a $\dot{V}/\dot{Q}$ scan requires the injection of a contrast medium. Confirm that the patient doesn't have an allergy to the contrast material.
- Explain to the patient that the test has two parts. During the ventilation portion, a mask is placed over the patient's mouth and nose, and the patient breathes in the contrast medium gas mixed with air while the scanner takes pictures of his lungs. For the perfusion portion, the patient is placed in a supine position on a movable table as the contrast medium is injected into the IV line while the scanner again takes pictures of the lungs.
- After the procedure, maintain bed rest as ordered and monitor the patient's vital signs, oxygen saturation levels, and heart rhythm.
- Monitor for adverse reactions to the contrast medium, which may include restlessness, tachypnea and respiratory distress, tachycardia, urticaria, and nausea and vomiting. Keep emergency equipment nearby in case of a reaction.

Pulmonary angiography

Pulmonary angiography, also called *pulmonary arteriography*, allows radiographic examination of the pulmonary circulation.

After injecting a radioactive contrast dye through a catheter inserted into the pulmonary artery or one of its branches, a series of X-rays is taken to detect blood flow abnormalities, possibly caused by embolus or pulmonary infarction.

More reliable, more risks

- Pulmonary angiography yields more reliable results than a $\dot{V}/\dot{Q}$ scan but carries higher risks for certain conditions such as cardiac arrhythmias (especially ventricular arrhythmias caused by myocardial irritation from passage of the catheter through the heart chambers).
- It may be the health care provider's preferred test to evaluate pulmonary circulation, especially if the patient is on a ventilator.

Practice pointers

- Explain the procedure to the patient and family and answer their questions. Tell them who performs the test, where it's done, and how long it takes.
- Confirm that the patient isn't allergic to shellfish or iodine. Notify the health care provider if the patient has such an allergy because the patient may have an adverse reaction to the contrast medium. Diphenhydramine (Benadryl) and prednisone may be administered, as prescribed, before the test to reduce the risk of a reaction to the dye.
- Preprocedure testing should include evaluation of renal function (by serum creatinine levels and blood urea nitrogen [BUN] levels) and potential risk of bleeding (by prothrombin time, partial thromboplastin time, and platelet count). Notify the health care provider of abnormal results.
- Instruct the patient to lie still for the procedure.
- Explain that there will likely be a flushing sensation in the face as the dye is injected.

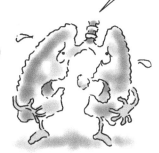

Whew! Is it hot in here, or is it just the dye from my pulmonary angiography?

Postprocedure procedures

- Maintain bed rest as ordered and monitor the patient's vital signs, oxygen saturation levels, and heart rhythm.
- Keep a sandbag or femoral/radial compression device over the catheter insertion site as prescribed or according to unit protocols.
- Check the pressure dressing for signs of bleeding. Monitor the patient's peripheral pulse in the arm or leg used for catheter insertion (and mark the site). Check the temperature, color, and sensation of the extremity and compare with the opposite side.

- Unless contraindicated, encourage the patient to drink more fluids to flush the dye or contrast medium from the system or increase the IV flow rate as prescribed.
- Check serum creatinine and BUN levels after the procedure because the contrast medium can cause acute kidney injury.
- Monitor for adverse reactions to the contrast medium, which may include restlessness, tachypnea and respiratory distress, tachycardia, facial flushing, urticaria, and nausea and vomiting. Keep emergency equipment nearby in case of a reaction.

Treatments

Respiratory disorders interfere with airway clearance, breathing patterns, and gas exchange. If not corrected, they can adversely affect many other body systems and can be life-threatening. Treatments for patients with respiratory disorders include drug therapy, inhalation therapy, and surgery.

Drug therapy

Drugs are used for airway management in patients with such disorders as acute respiratory failure, acute respiratory distress syndrome (ARDS), asthma, emphysema, and chronic bronchitis. Some types of drugs commonly seen in the ED include anti-inflammatory agents, bronchodilators, neuromuscular blocking agents, and sedatives.

Anti-inflammatory agents

Anti-inflammatory agents (corticosteroids) are used to reduce bronchial inflammation.

Reversing obstruction

Corticosteroids are the most effective anti-inflammatory agents used to treat patients with reversible airflow obstruction. They work by suppressing immune responses and reducing inflammation.

Systemic drugs, such as dexamethasone, methylprednisolone (Medrol), and prednisone, are given to manage an acute respiratory event, such as acute respiratory failure or exacerbation of COPD. These drugs are initially given intravenously; when the patient stabilizes, the dosage is tapered and oral dosing may be substituted.

Patients with asthma commonly use inhaled steroids, such as beclomethasone (QVAR), budesonide (Pulmicort), flunisolide (Aerospan), and fluticasone (Flovent). These agents also work by suppressing immune response and reducing airway inflammation. (See *Understanding corticosteroids*.)

Understanding corticosteroids

Use this table to learn about the indications, adverse reactions, and practice pointers associated with steroids.

Drug	Indications	Adverse reactions	Practice pointers
Systemic steroids Dexamethasone, methylprednisolone (Solu-Medrol, Medrol), prednisone	• Anti-inflammatory for acute respiratory failure, acute respiratory distress syndrome, and acute exacerbation of chronic obstructive pulmonary disease • Anti-inflammatory and immunosuppressant for asthma	• Arrhythmias • Circulatory collapse • Edema • Heart failure • Pancreatitis • Peptic ulcer • Thromboembolism • Infection • Steroid psychosis	• Use cautiously in patients with recent myocardial infarction, hypertension, renal disease, and gastrointestinal ulcer. • Monitor blood pressure and blood glucose levels.
Inhaled steroids Beclomethasone (QVAR), budesonide (Pulmicort), flunisolide (Aerospan), fluticasone (Flovent)	• Long-term asthma control	• Bronchospasm • Dry mouth • Hoarseness • Oral candidiasis • Wheezing	• Don't use for treatment of acute asthma attack. • Use a spacer to reduce adverse effects. • Rinse the patient's mouth after use to prevent oral fungal infection.

Adapted from American College of Allergy, Asthma & Immunology. (2014). Asthma treatment. Retrieved from https://acaai.org/asthma/asthma-treatment; and Fanta, C. H. (2018). Management of acute exacerbations of asthma in adults. Retrieved from https://www.uptodate.com/contents/management-of-acute-exacerbations-of-asthma-in-adults

Bronchodilators

Bronchodilators relax bronchial smooth muscle and treat patients with bronchospasm. Here's how some types of bronchodilators are used:

- Short-acting inhaled beta$_2$-adrenergic agonists such as albuterol and levalbuterol (Xopenex) are used to relieve acute symptoms in asthma and bronchospasm.
- Long-acting inhaled beta$_2$-adrenergic agonists include salmeterol (Serevent) and formoterol (Perforomist). These agents are typically used for long-term management and not for acute symptoms due to slower onset (Ignatavicius et al., 2018).
- Epinephrine acts on alpha- and beta-adrenergic receptors. It's used to relieve anaphylactic, allergic, and other hypersensitivity reactions. Its beta-adrenergic effects relax bronchial smooth muscle and relieve bronchospasm.
- Anticholinergic agents, such as ipratropium (Atrovent), act by inhibiting the action of acetylcholine at bronchial smooth-muscle receptor sites and thus produce bronchodilation. A combination therapy of ipratropium and albuterol (Combivent) may also be used (ACAAI, 2014; Fanta, 2018). (See *Understanding bronchodilators*, page 228.)

Spontaneous conversations need quick wit; spontaneous breathing efforts need neuromuscular blocking agents if they hamper ventilator function.

Understanding bronchodilators

Use this table to learn about the indications, adverse reactions, and practice pointers associated with bronchodilators.

Drug	Indications	Adverse reactions	Practice pointers
Beta₂-adrenergic agonists			
Albuterol	• Short-acting relief of acute symptoms with asthma and bronchospasm	• Hyperactivity • Palpitations • Paradoxical bronchospasm • Tachycardia • Tremor	• Warn the patient about the possibility of paradoxical bronchospasm. If it occurs, stop the drug and seek medical treatment. • An older adult patient may require a lower dose. • Monitor respiratory status, vital signs, and heart rhythm.
Salmeterol (Serevent), Formoterol (Perforomist)	• Maintenance treatment to prevent or decrease wheezing in asthma and chronic obstructive pulmonary disease	• Hoarseness • Headache • Dry mouth • Rapid heartbeat	• Use as an adjunctive therapy. • Should not be used for the treatment of acute symptoms • Not a substitute for corticosteroids
Levalbuterol (Xopenex)	• Relief of acute symptoms with asthma and bronchospasm	• Palpitations • Headache • Insomnia • Dry mouth • Nausea	• Like other beta-agonists, can produce paradoxical bronchospasm • Use cautiously in patients with cardiovascular disorders. • Monitor respiratory status, vital signs, and heart rhythm.
Alpha-/beta-adrenergic agonist			
Epinephrine	• Relaxation of bronchial smooth muscle through stimulation of beta₂-adrenergic receptors; used for bronchospasm, hypersensitivity reaction, anaphylaxis, and asthma	• Palpitations • Tachycardia • Ventricular fibrillation • Seizure • Increased blood pressure	• Use cautiously in older adult patients and those with long-standing asthma and emphysema with degenerative heart disease. • Monitor respiratory status, vital signs, and heart rhythm. • This drug is contraindicated in patients with angle-closure glaucoma, coronary insufficiency, and cerebral arteriosclerosis.
Anticholinergic agents			
Ipratropium (Atrovent)	• Blocks muscarinic receptors; this allows the muscle around the airways to relax and the airways to open; used to treat bronchospasm associated with chronic bronchitis, asthma, and emphysema	• Bronchospasm • Chest pain • Nervousness • Palpitations	• Because of delayed onset of bronchodilation, this drug isn't recommended for acute respiratory distress. • Use cautiously in patients with angle-closure glaucoma, bladder neck obstruction, and prostatic hypertrophy. • Monitor respiratory status, vital signs, and heart rhythm.

Adapted from American College of Allergy, Asthma & Immunology. (2014). Asthma treatment. Retrieved from https://acaai.org/asthma/asthma-treatment; and Fanta, C. H. (2018). Management of acute exacerbations of asthma in adults. Retrieved from https://www.uptodate.com/contents/management-of-acute-exacerbations-of-asthma-in-adults

Neuromuscular blocking agents

Patients on mechanical ventilation may require neuromuscular blocking agents to eliminate spontaneous breathing efforts that can interfere with the ventilator's function. Neuromuscular blocking agents cause paralysis without altering the patient's level of consciousness (LOC) (Bortle, 2017; Caro, 2018). (See *Understanding neuromuscular blocking agents*, page 230.)

Sedatives

Benzodiazepines, such as midazolam (Versed) and lorazepam (Ativan), are used for conscious sedation and preoperative sedation to reduce anxiety in patients undergoing diagnostic or surgical procedures.

These drugs are also used to relieve anxiety and promote sedation in patients on mechanical ventilators, especially those receiving neuromuscular blocking agents. Such agents cause paralysis without altering the LOC, which—without sedation—is frightening for the patient (Bortle, 2017). (See *Understanding sedatives*, page 232.)

Inhalation therapy

Inhalation therapy employs carefully controlled ventilation techniques to help the patient maintain optimal ventilation in the event of respiratory failure. Techniques include aerosol treatments, CPAP, endotracheal (ET) intubation, mechanical ventilation, and oxygen therapy.

Aerosol treatments

Aerosol therapy is a means of administering medication into the airways. The administration method can use handheld nebulizers or metered-dose inhalers. These devices deliver topical medications to the respiratory tract, producing local and systemic effects. The mucosal lining of the respiratory tract absorbs the inhalant almost immediately.

Common inhalants are bronchodilators, used to improve airway patency and facilitate mucus drainage; mucolytics, which attain a high local concentration to liquefy tenacious bronchial secretions; and corticosteroids, used to decrease inflammation.

Nursing considerations

- Monitor the patient's response to the medication.
- Check pulse oximetry after the treatment and document any changes.
- Assess patient's breath sounds and document findings before and after treatment.

(*Text continues on page 234.*)

Understanding neuromuscular blocking agents

Use this table to learn about the indications, adverse reactions, and practice pointers associated with neuromuscular blocking agents.

Drug	Indications	Adverse reactions	Practice pointers
Depolarizing			
Succinylcholine (Anectine)	• Adjunct to general anesthesia to aid endotracheal (ET) intubation • Induction of skeletal muscle paralysis during surgery or mechanical ventilation	• Bradycardia, arrhythmias, cardiac arrest • Malignant hyperthermia, increased intraocular pressure, flushing • Postoperative muscle pain • Respiratory depression, apnea, bronchoconstriction	• This drug is contraindicated in patients with histories of malignant hyperthermia, myopathies associated with creatinine phosphokinase, acute angle-closure glaucoma, and penetrating eye injuries. • Contraindicated in patients with significant hyperkalemia • Monitor the patient for histamine release and resulting hypotension and flushing.
Nondepolarizing			
Atracurium	• Adjunct to general anesthesia, to facilitate ET intubation, and to provide skeletal muscle relaxation during surgery or mechanical ventilation	• Anaphylaxis • Flushing, bradycardia • Prolonged, dose-related apnea, bronchospasm, laryngospasm	• This drug doesn't affect consciousness or relieve pain. Be sure to keep the patient sedated. • Have emergency respiratory support readily available. • This drug has little or no effect on heart rate and doesn't counteract or reverse the bradycardia caused by anesthetics or vagal stimulation. Thus, bradycardia is seen more frequently with atracurium than with other neuromuscular blocking agents. Pretreatment with anticholinergics (atropine or glycopyrrolate) is advised. • Use drug only if ET intubation, administration of oxygen under positive pressure, artificial respiration, and assisted or controlled ventilation are immediately available. • Use a peripheral nerve stimulator to monitor responses during critical care unit administration; it may be used to detect residual paralysis during recovery and to avoid atracurium overdose.

Understanding neuromuscular blocking agents *(continued)*

Drug	Indications	Adverse reactions	Practice pointers
Nondepolarizing *(continued)*			
Pancuronium	• Adjunct to anesthesia to induce skeletal muscle relaxation, facilitate intubation and ventilation, and weaken muscle contractions in induced seizures	• Allergic or idiosyncratic hypersensitivity reactions • Prolonged, dose-related respiratory insufficiency or apnea • Residual muscle weakness	• If using succinylcholine, allow its effects to subside before giving pancuronium. • Don't mix in same syringe or give through same needle with barbiturates or other alkaline solutions. • Large doses may increase the frequency and severity of tachycardia. • Monitor electrocardiogram (ECG) and vital signs throughout administration.
Rocuronium	• Adjunct to anesthesia, to facilitate intubation, and to provide skeletal muscle relaxation during surgery or mechanical ventilation	• Anaphylaxis • Bronchospasm • Blood pressure fluctuations • Residual paralysis	• This drug does not affect consciousness, thinking, or relieve pain. Be sure to keep the patient sedated. Have emergency respiratory support readily available. • Use drug only if ET intubation, administration of oxygen under positive pressure, artificial respiration, and assisted or controlled ventilation are immediately available. • Monitor ECG and vital signs throughout administration. • Pay particular attention to blood pressure because this drug can cause marked fluctuations in both directions. • Due to a longer half-life, monitor the patient for muscle weakness and respiratory distress after stopping the infusion.
Vecuronium (Norcuron)	• Adjunct to anesthesia, to facilitate intubation, and to provide skeletal muscle relaxation during surgery or mechanical ventilation	• Bronchospasm • Rash • Prolonged, dose-related respiratory insufficiency or apnea	• Administer by rapid intravenous (IV) injection or IV infusion. Don't give intramedullary. • Recovery time may double in patients with cirrhosis or cholestasis. • Assess baseline serum electrolyte levels, acid–base balance, and renal and hepatic function before administration. • Monitor ECG and vital signs throughout administration.

Adapted from Bortle, C. D. (2017). *Drugs to aid intubation*. Retrieved from https://www.merckmanuals .com/professional/critical-care -medicine/respiratory-arrest/drugs-to-aid-intubation; and Caro, D. (2018). *Neuromuscular blocking agents for rapid sequence intubation in adults outside of the operating room*. Retrieved from https://www.uptodate.com/contents/neuromuscular-blocking-agents -nmbas-for-rapid-sequence-intubation-in-adults-outside-of-the-operating-room

Understanding sedatives

Use this table to learn about the indications, adverse reactions, and practice pointers associated with sedatives.

Drug	Indications	Adverse reactions	Practice pointers
Etomidate (Amidate)	• Induction and maintenance of sedation in mechanically ventilated patients • Adjunct sedation for short operative procedures	• Myoclonus (temporary skeletal movements) • Hyperventilation • Blood pressure fluctuations • Adrenal suppression	• Use with caution in patients with hepatic and renal impairment. • Monitor electrocardiogram (ECG) and vital signs throughout administration. • This medication is highly irritating. Avoid administration in small veins. • Administer intravenous (IV) push over 1 minute. • Continue monitoring patient after drug discontinuation until respiratory and neurologic status are stabilized.
Fentanyl (Sublimaze)	• Sedation and analgesia prior to rapid sequence intubation • Analgesia and/or maintenance of sedation for mechanically ventilated patients • Analgesia for moderate to severe pain	• Respiratory depression • Laryngospasm • Hypotension • "Rigid chest" syndrome	• Monitor ECG and vital signs throughout administration. • Be aware of risk for "rigid chest" syndrome immediately after administration for intubation. Patient may become apneic and can be hard to ventilate. This can be remedied by administering succinylcholine. • Administer intramuscularly or intravenously slowly over 1 to 2 minutes to decrease risk for "rigid chest" syndrome.
Ketamine (Ketalar)	• Induction and maintenance of sedation in mechanically ventilated patients • Anesthetic for short operative procedures • Analgesic when patient is opioid intolerant	• Laryngospasm • Hallucinations	• Monitor ECG and vital signs throughout administration. • Monitor neurologic status both during and after drug discontinuation. • Ensure airway support if being used for procedure without intubation. • Administer slow IV push over at least 1 minute. Rapid administration may cause respiratory depression and hypotension.

Understanding sedatives *(continued)*

Drug	Indications	Adverse reactions	Practice pointers
Lorazepam (Ativan)	• Useful for long-term sedation following intubation • Anxiety, tension, agitation, irritability—especially in anxiety neuroses or organic (especially gastrointestinal or cardiovascular) disorders • Status epilepticus	• Drowsiness • Muscle weakness • Acute withdrawal syndrome (long-term use)	• This drug is contraindicated in patients with acute angle-closure glaucoma. • Use cautiously in patients with pulmonary, renal, or hepatic impairment and in older adults, acutely ill, or debilitated patients. • Parenteral lorazepam appears to possess potent amnesic effects. • For IV administration, dilute lorazepam with an equal volume of a compatible diluent, such as dextrose 5% in water (D_5W), sterile water for injection, or normal saline solution. • Inject the drug directly into a vein or into the tubing of a compatible IV infusion, such as normal saline solution or D_5W solution. The rate of lorazepam IV injection shouldn't exceed 2 mg/minute. Have emergency resuscitative equipment available when administering IV. • Monitor liver function studies to prevent cumulative effects and ensure adequate drug metabolism.
Midazolam (Versed)	• Preoperative sedation (to induce sleepiness or drowsiness and relieve apprehension) • Conscious sedation • Continuous infusion for sedation of intubated and mechanically ventilated patients as a component of anesthesia or during treatment in a critical care setting • Sedation and amnesia before diagnostic, therapeutic, or endoscopic procedures or before induction of anesthesia	• Apnea • Cardiac arrest • Respiratory depression • Hiccups • Nausea • Pain • Respiratory arrest	• This drug is contraindicated in patients with acute angle-closure glaucoma and in those experiencing shock, coma, or acute alcohol intoxication. • Use cautiously in patients with uncompensated acute illnesses, in older adults or debilitated patients, and in patients with myasthenia gravis or neuromuscular disorders and pulmonary disease. • Closely monitor cardiopulmonary function; continuously monitor patients who have received midazolam to detect potentially life-threatening respiratory depression. • Have emergency respiratory equipment readily available. Laryngospasm and bronchospasm, although rare, may occur. • Solutions compatible with midazolam include D_5W, normal saline solution, and lactated Ringer solution.

(continued)

Understanding sedatives *(continued)*

Drug	Indications	Adverse reactions	Practice pointers
Propofol (Diprivan)	• Induction and maintenance of sedation in mechanically ventilated patients	• Apnea • Bradycardia • Hyperlipidemia • Hypotension	• This drug is contraindicated in patients hypersensitive to propofol or components of the emulsion, including soybean oil, egg lecithin, and glycerol. • Because the drug is administered as an emulsion, administer cautiously to patients with a disorder of lipid metabolism (such as pancreatitis, primary hyperlipoproteinemia, and diabetic hyperlipidemia). Use cautiously if the patient is receiving lipids as part of a total parenteral nutrition infusion; IV lipid dose may need to be reduced. • Use cautiously in older adults or debilitated patients and in those with circulatory disorders. • Although the hemodynamic effects of this drug can vary, its major effect in patients maintaining spontaneous ventilation is arterial hypotension (arterial pressure can decrease as much as 30%) with little or no change in heart rate and cardiac output. However, significant depression of cardiac output may occur in patients undergoing assisted or controlled positive pressure ventilation. • Don't mix propofol with other drugs or blood products. If dilution is necessary, use only D_5W and don't dilute to a concentration of less than 2 mg/mL.

Adapted from Bortle, C. D. (2017). *Drugs to aid intubation.* Retrieved from https://www.merckmanuals .com/professional/critical-care -medicine/respiratory-arrest/drugs-to-aid-intubation

Continuous positive airway pressure

As its name suggests, CPAP ventilation maintains positive pressure in the airways throughout the patient's respiratory cycle. Originally delivered only with a ventilator, CPAP may now be delivered to intubated or nonintubated patients through an artificial airway, a mask, or nasal prongs by means of a ventilator or a separate high-flow generating system. (See *Using CPAP.*)

Goes with the flows

CPAP is available as a continuous flow system and a demand system. In the continuous flow system, an air–oxygen blend flows through a humidifier and a reservoir bag into a T-piece. In the demand system, a valve opens in response to the patient's inspiratory flow.

Using CPAP

This illustration shows the continuous positive airway pressure (CPAP) apparatus used to apply positive pressure to the airway to prevent obstruction during inspiration in patients with sleep apnea.

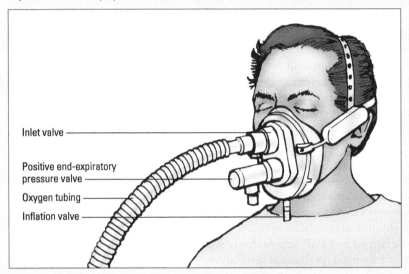

Inlet valve

Positive end-expiratory pressure valve

Oxygen tubing

Inflation valve

Other talents

In addition to treating respiratory distress syndrome, CPAP has been used successfully in pulmonary edema, pulmonary embolus, bronchiolitis, fat embolus, pneumonitis, viral pneumonia, and postoperative atelectasis. In mild to moderate cases of these disorders, CPAP provides an alternative to intubation and mechanical ventilation. It increases the functional residual capacity by distending collapsed alveoli, which improves PaO_2 and decreases intrapulmonary shunting and oxygen consumption. It also reduces the work of breathing.

Through the nose

Nasal CPAP has proved successful for long-term treatment of obstructive sleep apnea. This type of CPAP provides high-flow compressed air directly into a mask that covers only the patient's nose. The pressure supplied through the mask serves as a back-pressure splint, preventing the unstable upper airway from collapsing during inspiration.

Not so positive

CPAP may cause gastric distress if the patient swallows air during the treatment (most common when CPAP is delivered without intubation). The patient may feel claustrophobic. Because mask CPAP can also cause nausea and vomiting, it shouldn't be used in patients who are unresponsive or at risk for vomiting and aspiration. In rare cases, CPAP causes barotrauma or lowers cardiac output (Pinto & Sharma, 2019).

Nursing considerations
- If the patient is intubated or has a tracheostomy, you can accomplish CPAP with a mechanical ventilator by adjusting the settings.
- Assess vital signs and breath sounds during CPAP.
- If CPAP is prescribed for delivery through a mask, a respiratory therapist usually sets up the system and fits the mask. The mask should be transparent and lightweight, with a soft, pliable seal. A tight seal isn't required as long as pressure can be maintained.
- Obtain ABG results and bedside pulmonary function studies as prescribed to establish a baseline.

After the fact
- Check for decreased cardiac output and blood pressure, which may result from increased intrathoracic pressure associated with CPAP.
- Watch closely for changes in respiratory rate and pattern. Uncoordinated breathing patterns may indicate severe respiratory muscle fatigue that can't be helped by CPAP. Report this to the health care provider; the patient may need mechanical ventilation.
- Check the CPAP system for pressure fluctuations.
- Keep in mind that high airway pressures increase the risk of pneumothorax, so monitor for chest pain and decreased breath sounds.
- Use oximetry to monitor oxygen saturation.
- Check closely for air leaks around the mask near the eyes (an area difficult to seal); escaping air can dry the eyes, causing conjunctivitis or other problems.

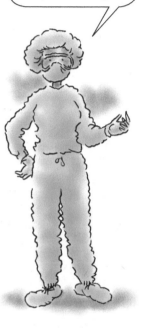

Careful—CPAP masks can leak air around the eyes and cause conjunctivitis. This mask won't do me any harm, though.

ET intubation
ET intubation involves insertion of a tube into the lungs through the mouth or nose to establish a patent airway. It protects patients from aspiration by sealing off the trachea from the digestive tract and permits removal of tracheobronchial secretions in patients who can't cough effectively. ET intubation also provides a route for mechanical ventilation.

Conversation stopper
Drawbacks of ET intubation are that it bypasses normal respiratory defenses against infection, reduces cough effectiveness, may be uncomfortable, and prevents verbal communication.

Potential complications of ET intubation include:
- aspiration of blood, secretions, or gastric contents
- bronchospasm or laryngospasm
- cardiac arrhythmias

- hypoxemia (if attempts at intubation are prolonged or oxygen delivery interrupted)
- injury to the lips, mouth, pharynx, or vocal cords
- tooth damage or loss
- tracheal stenosis, erosion, and necrosis.

Open up

In orotracheal intubation, the oral cavity is used as the route of insertion. This route is preferred in emergency situations because it's easier and faster. However, maintaining exact tube placement is more difficult because the tube must be well secured to avoid kinking and prevent bronchial obstruction or accidental extubation. It's also uncomfortable for conscious patients because it stimulates salivation, coughing, and retching.

Be quick about it

Rapid sequence intubation (RSI) is the standard of care for ET intubation. RSI minimizes the complications of ET intubation, such as airway trauma and aspiration, and is more comfortable for the patient (Brown & Sakles, 2017). (See *The seven Ps of RSI*, page 238.)

Not for everyone

Orotracheal intubation is contraindicated in patients with orofacial injuries, acute cervical spinal injury, and degenerative spinal disorders.

Through the nose

Oral ET intubation is the preferred method of airway management in patients who are apneic. However, nasal intubation may be an alternative if the oral route is contraindicated. In nasal intubation, a nasal passage is used as the route of insertion. Nasal intubation is preferred for elective insertion when the patient is capable of spontaneous ventilation for a short period.

A conscious choice

Nasal intubation is more comfortable than oral intubation and is typically used in conscious patients who are at risk for imminent respiratory arrest or who have cervical spinal injuries. It's contraindicated in patients with facial or basilar skull fractures.

Difficult and damaging

Although it's more comfortable than oral intubation, nasal intubation is more difficult to perform. Because the tube passes blindly through the nasal cavity, it causes more tissue damage, increases the risk of infection by nasal bacteria introduced into the trachea, and increases the risk of pressure necrosis of the nasal mucosa.

The seven Ps of RSI

Rapid sequence intubation (RSI) is used to rapidly produce optimal conditions for intubation in emergency situations, especially for difficult patients. Seven steps are outlined below.

1. Prepare
• Ensure at least two intravenous access sites.
• Administer oxygen (O_2).
• Institute cardiac and oxygenation saturation monitoring.
• Prepare medications and equipment.

2. Preoxygenate
• Administer 100% O_2 for 5 minutes using a tight-fitting mask with reservoir.

3. Pretreatment
• Administer a sedating agent, such as etomidate (Amidate), propofol (Diprivan), Midazolam (Versed), or ketamine (Ketalar).
• Administer additional drugs to minimize the effects of intubation, such as fentanyl (Sublimaze) or lidocaine (to prevent increased intracranial pressure).

4. Paralysis
• Administer a neuromuscular blocking agent, such as succinylcholine, rocuronium (Zemuron), or vecuronium (Norcuron).
• Begin or continue to administer mechanical ventilation.

5. Protection and position
• The patient's head and neck should be positioned for optimal visualization of the airway.
• Although it has become increasingly controversial, cricoid pressure (Sellick maneuver) can be used to prevent aspiration (Salem et al., 2017).
• The patient is intubated.
• Once in place in the trachea, the cuff on the end of the endotracheal tube (ETT) is inflated.

6. Placement and proof
• ETT placement is verified by observation, auscultation, end-tidal carbon dioxide ($ETco_2$) detector, and chest X-ray.

7. Postintubation management
• Note measurement/level of ETT at teeth.
• Secure the ETT using tape or a commercial device.
• Maintain continuous $ETco_2$ monitoring.
• Continue sedation or paralysis as indicated.
• Monitor the patient's response, including vital signs, arterial blood gas values, cardiac monitor, and arterial oxygen saturation.

Nursing considerations
• If possible, explain the procedure to the patient and family.
• Obtain the correct size of ETT. The typical size for an oral ETT is 7.5 mm (indicates the diameter of the lumen) for women and 8 mm for men.
• Administer medication, as prescribed, to decrease respiratory secretions, induce amnesia and/or analgesia, and help calm and relax the conscious patient.
• Remove dentures and bridgework, if present.

Confirm ETT placement

- Assess bilateral chest excursion.
- Auscultate bilateral breath sounds.
- Use capnography to confirm consistent exhalation of carbon dioxide.
- Auscultate over epigastrium; air movement should not be heard.
- Confirm tube positioning by chest X-ray—the distal tip of the tube should be 3 to 5 cm above the tracheal carina.
- Secure the ETT in place to minimize pressure across the face.
- Note the depth marking on the side of the tube.
- Follow standard precautions and suction through the ETT because the patient's condition indicates to clear secretions and prevent mucus plugs from obstructing the tube.
- After suctioning, use a handheld resuscitation bag to hyper-oxygenate the patient who's being maintained on a ventilator. (See *Understanding manual ventilation*, page 240.)
- If available, use a closed tracheal suctioning system, which permits the ventilated patient to remain on the ventilator during suctioning.

Mechanical ventilation

Mechanical ventilation involves the use of a machine to move air into a patient's lungs. Mechanical ventilators use positive or negative pressure to ventilate patients.

When to ventilate

Indications for mechanical ventilation include:
- acute respiratory failure due to ARDS, pneumonia, acute exacerbations of COPD, pulmonary embolus, heart failure, trauma, tumors, or drug overdose
- respiratory center depression due to stroke, brain injury, or trauma
- neuromuscular disturbances caused by neuromuscular diseases, such as Guillain–Barré syndrome, multiple sclerosis, and myasthenia gravis; trauma, including spinal cord injury; or CNS depression.

Accentuate the positive

Positive pressure ventilators exert positive pressure on the airway, which causes inspiration while increasing tidal volume (V_T). A high-frequency ventilator uses high respiratory rates and low V_T to maintain alveolar ventilation.

The inspiratory cycles of these ventilators may be adjusted for volume, pressure, or time:
- A volume-cycled ventilator (the type used most commonly) delivers a preset volume of air each time regardless of the amount of lung resistance.

Understanding manual ventilation

A handheld resuscitation bag is an inflatable device that can be attached to a face mask or directly to a tracheostomy or endotracheal tube (ETT) to allow manual delivery of oxygen or room air to the lungs of a patient who is unable to breathe on his or her own.

Although usually used in an emergency, manual ventilation can also be performed while the patient is disconnected temporarily from a mechanical ventilator (such as during a tubing change), during transport, or before suctioning. In such instances, use of the handheld resuscitation bag maintains ventilation. Oxygen administration with a resuscitation bag can help improve a compromised cardiorespiratory system.

Ventilation guidelines

To manually ventilate a patient with an ETT or tracheostomy tube, follow these guidelines:
• If oxygen is readily available, connect the handheld resuscitation bag to the oxygen. Attach one end of the tubing to the bottom of the bag and the other end to the nipple adapter on the flowmeter of the oxygen source.
• Turn on the oxygen and adjust the flow rate according to the patient's condition.

• Before attaching the handheld resuscitation bag, suction the ETT or tracheostomy tube to remove any secretions that may obstruct the airway.
• Remove the mask from the ventilation bag and attach the handheld resuscitation bag directly to the tube.
• Keeping your nondominant hand on the connection of the bag to the tube, exert downward pressure to seal the mask against his face. For an adult patient, use your dominant hand to compress the bag every 5 seconds to deliver approximately 1 L of air.

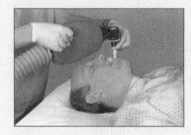

• Deliver breaths with the patient's own inspiratory effort if any are present. Don't attempt to deliver a breath as the patient exhales.
• Observe the patient's chest to ensure that it rises and falls with each bag compression. If ventilation fails to occur, check the connection and

the patency of the patient's airway; if necessary, reposition the head and suction.
• Be alert for possible underventilation, which commonly occurs because the handheld resuscitation bag is difficult to keep positioned while ensuring an open airway. In addition, the volume of air delivered to the patient varies with the type of bag used and the hand size of the person compressing the bag. An adult with a small- or medium-sized hand may not consistently deliver 1 L of air. For these reasons, have someone assist with the procedure, if possible.
• Keep in mind when the patient is not intubated, that air is forced into the patient's stomach with manual ventilation, placing the patient at risk for aspiration of vomitus (possibly resulting in pneumonia) and gastric distention.
• Record the date and time of the procedure, reason and length of time the patient was disconnected from mechanical ventilation and received manual ventilation, any complications and the nursing action taken, and the patient's tolerance of the procedure.

• A pressure-cycled ventilator generates flow until the machine reaches a preset pressure regardless of the volume delivered or the time required to achieve the pressure.
• A time-cycled ventilator generates flow for a preset amount of time. Several different modes of ventilatory control are found on the ventilator. The choice of mode depends on the patient's respiratory condition.

Nursing considerations

- Provide emotional support to the patient during all phases of mechanical ventilation to reduce anxiety and promote successful treatment. Even if the patient is unresponsive, continue to explain all procedures and treatments.
- Work with your respiratory therapy staff to monitor the patient and provide ventilatory and ventilator support.

Be alarmed

- Make sure the ventilator alarms are on at all times to alert you to potentially hazardous conditions and changes in the patient's status. If an alarm sounds and the problem can't be easily identified, disconnect the patient from the ventilator and use a handheld resuscitation bag to ventilate him or her.
- Depending on the patient's status, assess cardiopulmonary status frequently per department or facility protocols. Assess vital signs and auscultate breath sounds. Monitor pulse oximetry or $ETco_2$ levels and hemodynamic parameters as ordered. Monitor intake and output and assess for fluid volume excess or dehydration.
- Administer a sedative or neuromuscular blocking agent, as ordered, to relax the patient or eliminate spontaneous breathing efforts that can interfere with the ventilator's action.

Be extra vigilant

- Remember that the patient receiving a neuromuscular blocking agent requires close observation because he or she cannot breathe or communicate. In addition, if the patient is receiving a neuromuscular blocking agent, make sure he or she also receives a sedative and analgesia. Neuromuscular blocking agents cause paralysis without altering the patient's LOC or sensation. Reassure the patient and family that the paralysis is temporary.

Oxygen therapy

In oxygen therapy, oxygen is delivered by mask or nasal prongs to prevent or reverse hypoxemia and reduce the workload of breathing.

Fully equipped

Choice of delivery device depends on the patient's condition and the required fraction of inspired oxygen. High-flow systems, such as Venturi masks and ventilators, deliver a precisely controlled air–oxygen mixture. Low-flow systems, such as nasal prongs or masks, allow variation in the oxygen percentage delivery based on the patient's respiratory pattern.

Concentrate on concentration

Nasal cannula delivers oxygen at flow rates from 0.5 to 8 L/minute. Masks deliver up to 100% oxygen concentrations but can't be used to deliver controlled oxygen concentrations.

Nursing considerations

- Humidify oxygen to help prevent drying of mucous membranes and secretions. However, humidity isn't added with Venturi masks because water can block the Venturi jets.
- Assess for signs of hypoxia, including decreased LOC, tachycardia, arrhythmias, diaphoresis, restlessness, altered blood pressure or respiratory rate, clammy skin, and cyanosis. If these occur, notify the health care provider, obtain pulse oximetry readings, and check the oxygen equipment to see if it's malfunctioning.
- Use a low flow rate if your patient has COPD. However, don't use a simple face mask because low flow rates won't flush carbon dioxide from the mask and the patient will rebreathe carbon dioxide. Watch for alterations in LOC, heart rate, and respiratory rate, which may signal carbon dioxide narcosis or worsening hypoxemia (Torrey, 2018).

Surgery

If drugs or other therapeutic modes fail to maintain the patient's airway patency and protect healthy tissues from disease, surgery may be necessary. Some types of respiratory surgeries are chest tube insertion and tracheotomy.

Chest tube insertion

Chest tube insertion may be needed when treating patients with pneumothorax, hemothorax, empyema, pleural effusion, or chylothorax. The tube, which is inserted into the pleural space, allows blood, fluid, pus, or air to drain and allows the lung to reinflate. Most chest tubes are placed at the fourth or fifth intercostal space in the anterior axillary line. This site allows for drainage of blood and air.

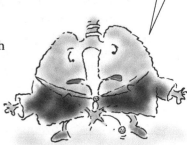

Chest tube insertion gives me the chance to reinflate— maybe a little TOO much this time!

Gotta have some negative pressure

The tube restores negative pressure to the pleural space through an underwater seal drainage system. The water in the system prevents air from being sucked back into the pleural space during inspiration. If a leak through the bronchi can't be sealed, suction applied to the underwater seal system removes air from the pleural space faster than it can collect.

Nursing considerations

After chest tube insertion

- Assess respiratory function and obtain vital signs and oxygen saturation levels immediately after insertion. Routinely assess chest tube function, including fluctuation of drainage, in the tubing; amount of output; color of drainage; and presence or absence of air leak. Notify the health care provider immediately if the amount of drainage is greater than 200 mL in 1 hour (indicates bleeding).
- The fluid in the water seal chamber typically rises on inspiration and decreases on expiration. However, if the patient is receiving positive pressure ventilation, the opposite is normal.
- Avoid creating dependent loops, kinks, or pressure in the tubing. Don't lift the drainage system above the patient's chest because fluid may flow back into the pleural space. Keep two rubber-tipped clamps at the bedside to clamp the chest tube if the system cracks or to locate an air leak in the system. (See *Checking for chest tube leaks*.)
- If the drainage collection chamber fills, replace it according to your facility's policy. To do so, double clamp the chest tube close to the insertion site (using two clamps facing in opposite directions), exchange the system, remove the clamps, and retape the connection.
- To prevent a tension pneumothorax (which can result when clamping stops air and fluid from escaping), never leave the chest tube clamped for more than 1 minute.
- Notify the health care provider immediately if the patient develops cyanosis, rapid or shallow breathing, subcutaneous emphysema, chest pain, or excessive bleeding.

Tracheotomy

A tracheotomy is a surgical procedure that creates an opening into the trachea called a *tracheostomy*. This opening allows insertion of an indwelling tube to keep the patient's airway open. The tracheostomy tube may be made of plastic, polyvinyl chloride, or metal and comes in various sizes, lengths, and styles, depending on the patient's needs. A patient receiving mechanical ventilation needs a cuffed tube to prevent backflow of air around the tube. A cuffed tracheostomy tube also prevents an unconscious or a paralyzed patient from aspirating food or secretions.

Checking for chest tube leaks

When trying to locate a leak in your patient's chest tube system, try:
- briefly clamping the tube at various points along its length, beginning at the tube's proximal end and working down toward the drainage system
- paying special attention to the seal around the connections
- pushing any loose connections back together and taping them securely.

Bubble may mean trouble

The bubbling of the system stops when a clamp is placed between an air leak and the water seal. If you clamp along the tube's entire length and the bubbling doesn't stop, you probably need to replace the drainage unit because it may be cracked.

Emergency or planned procedure

In emergency situations, such as foreign body obstruction and laryngeal edema with anaphylactic shock, tracheotomy may be done at the bedside.

Nursing considerations

- Before an emergency tracheotomy, briefly explain the procedure to the patient and family as time permits and quickly obtain supplies or a tracheotomy tray.
- Ensure that samples for ABG analysis and other diagnostic tests have been completed and that the patient or a responsible family member has signed a consent form.

Afterward

- After the procedure, assess the patient's respiratory status, breath sounds, oxygen saturation levels, vital signs, and heart rhythm. Note any crackles, rhonchi, wheezes, or diminished breath sounds.
- Assess the patient for such complications as hemorrhage, edema into tracheal tissue causing airway obstruction, aspiration of secretions, hypoxemia, and introduction of air into surrounding tissue causing subcutaneous emphysema.
- Document the procedure; the amount, color, and consistency of secretions, stoma, and skin conditions; the patient's respiratory status; the duration of any cuff deflation; and cuff pressure readings with inflation.

Common disorders

Some common respiratory disorders seen in the ED include airway obstruction, inhalation injuries, pneumothorax, status asthmaticus, and submersion injury.

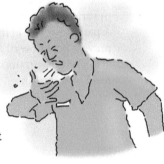

If coughing doesn't clear the airway, the patient may have an obstruction.

Airway obstruction

The body uses coughing as its main mechanism to clear the airway. Yet, coughing may not clear the airway during some disease states or even under normal, healthy conditions if an obstruction is present.

Upper airway obstruction is an interruption in the flow of air through the nose, mouth, pharynx, or larynx. Obstruction of the upper airway is considered a life-threatening situation; if not recognized early, it will progress to respiratory arrest. Respiratory arrest will lead to cardiac arrest, which requires CPR.

What causes it

A patient's airway can become obstructed or compromised by vomitus; food; edema; or the tongue, teeth, or saliva. Although there are several causes of upper airway obstruction, the most common cause is the tongue. Because muscle tone decreases when a person is unconscious or unresponsive, the potential for the tongue and epiglottis to obstruct the airway increases. Partial airway obstruction is commonly caused by edema or a small foreign object that doesn't completely obstruct the airway.

It's anatomical

The presence of edema—edema of tongue (caused by trauma), laryngeal edema, and smoke inhalation edema—in anatomical structures of the upper airway can lead to an upper airway obstruction. Other potential causes of airway obstruction include:
- anaphylaxis
- aspiration of a foreign object
- burns to the head, face, or neck area
- cerebral disorders (stroke)
- croup
- epiglottitis
- laryngospasms
- peritonsillar or pharyngeal abscesses
- tenacious secretions in the airway
- trauma of the face, trachea, or larynx
- tumors of the head or neck.

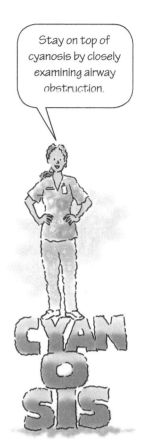

Stay on top of cyanosis by closely examining airway obstruction.

How it happens

In airway obstructions, the patient is partially able or not able to take in oxygen through inhalation. Hypoxemia results the longer the obstruction remains.

What to look for

Prompt detection and intervention can prevent a partial airway obstruction from progressing to a complete airway obstruction. Signs of a partial airway obstruction include restlessness, agitation and anxiety, diaphoresis, tachycardia, coughing, stridor, respiratory distress, and elevated blood pressure. Patients with a partial obstruction may also experience no symptoms. With a complete airway obstruction, the following symptoms may be observed:
- universal choking sign—patient clutches throat with hands
- inability to speak
- sudden onset of choking or gagging

- stridor
- cyanosis
- wheezing, whistling, or any other unusual breath sound that indicates breathing difficulty
- diminished breath sounds (bilateral or unilateral)
- sense of impending doom
- progression to unconsciousness.

What tests tell you

Physical examination may indicate decreased breath sounds. Tests aren't usually necessary to diagnose an upper airway obstruction but may include X-rays (particularly a chest X-ray), bronchoscopy, and laryngoscopy. If there are persistent symptoms of an upper airway obstruction, a chest X-ray, neck X-rays, laryngoscopy, or CT scan may be ordered to rule out the presence of a tumor, foreign body, or infection.

How it's treated

- Rapid assessment of airway patency, breathing, and circulation are foremost. (See *Opening an obstructed airway.*)
- Promptly assess the obstruction's cause. When an obstruction relates to the tongue or an accumulation of tenacious secretions, place the head in a slightly extended position and insert an oral airway.
- Promptly remove objects visible in the mouth with suction, fingers, or Magill forceps.
- If the patient can breathe (partial obstruction), encourage sitting forward and coughing to relieve the obstruction. However, be aware that this might worsen the obstruction and may totally occlude the airway.
- If unable to reach or remove object and complete obstruction is present, administer abdominal thrusts.
- ET intubation and removal of the foreign object during insertion of the laryngoscope enables visualization of the obstruction.
- If an oral or ET airway doesn't provide ventilation, emergency cricothyroidotomy is indicated (Ignatavicius et al., 2018).

What to do

- Assess for the cause of the obstruction.
- Assess the patient's breath sounds bilaterally.
- Monitor oxygen saturation (using pulse oximetry) and cardiac rhythm continuously.

Opening an obstructed airway

To open an obstructed airway, use the head-tilt, chin-lift maneuver or the jaw-thrust maneuver as described here.

Head-tilt, chin-lift maneuver

In many cases of airway obstruction, the muscles controlling the patient's tongue have relaxed, causing the tongue to obstruct the airway. If the patient doesn't appear to have a neck injury, use the head-tilt, chin-lift maneuver to open his airway. Use these four steps to carry out this maneuver:

1. Place your hand that's closest to the patient's head on the forehead.
2. Apply firm pressure—firm enough to tilt the patient's head back.
3. Place the fingertips of your other hand under the bony portion of the patient's lower jaw, near the chin.
4. Lift the patient's chin. Be sure to keep the mouth partially open (as shown at right). Avoid placing your fingertips on the soft tissue under the patient's chin because this may inadvertently obstruct the airway you're trying to open.

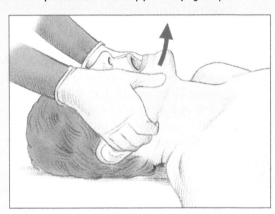

Using the jaw-thrust maneuver

If you suspect a neck injury, use the jaw-thrust maneuver to open the patient's airway. Use these four steps to carry out this maneuver:

1. Kneel at the patient's head with your elbows on the ground.
2. Rest your thumbs on the patient's lower jaw near the corners of his mouth, pointing your thumbs toward his feet.
3. Place your fingertips around the lower jaw.
4. To open the airway, lift the lower jaw with your fingertips (as shown at right).

- Continually assess for stridor, cyanosis, and changes in LOC and notify the health care provider immediately if any of these changes occur.
- Prepare for ET intubation if an airway can't be established.
- Prepare for a cricothyroidotomy if the patient's ventilation isn't established by oral or ET intubation.
- Anticipate cardiac arrest if the obstruction isn't cleared promptly.
- Monitor chest X-ray and ABG results after the obstruction is relieved.

Inhalation injuries

Inhalation injuries result from trauma to the pulmonary system after inhalation of toxic substances or inhalation of gases that are nontoxic but interfere with cellular respiration. Inhaled exposure forms include fog, mist, fume, dust, gas, vapor, or smoke. Inhalation injuries commonly accompany burns.

> Fog, fumes, dust, gas—you name it! If it floats, it can probably cause inhalation injury.

What causes it

There are many causes of inhalation injuries, including CO poisoning and chemical and thermal inhalation.

Carbon monoxide poisoning

CO is a colorless, odorless, tasteless gas produced as a result of combustion and oxidation. Inhaling small amounts of this gas over a long period of time (or inhaling large amounts in a short period of time) can lead to poisoning. CO is considered a chemical asphyxiant. Accidental poisoning can result from exposure to heaters; smoke from a fire; or use of a gas lamp, gas stove, or charcoal grill in a small, poorly ventilated area.

Chemical inhalation

A wide variety of gases may be generated when materials burn. The acids and alkalis produced in the burning process can produce chemical burns when inhaled. The inhaled substances can reach the respiratory tract as insoluble gases and lead to permanent damage. Synthetic materials also produce gases that can be toxic. Plastic material has the ability to produce toxic vapors when heated or burned.

> Accidental carbon monoxide poisoning can make any barbeque blue, so make sure to grill in a well-ventilated area.

Inhaling unburned chemicals in a powder or liquid form can also cause pulmonary damage. Such substances as ammonia, chlorine, sulfur dioxide, and hydrogen chloride are considered pulmonary irritants.

Thermal inhalation

Pulmonary complications remain the leading cause of death following thermal inhalation trauma. This type of trauma is commonly caused by the inhalation of hot air or steam. The mortality rate increases from 8% to nearly 35% when inhalation injury accompanies burns of the skin (Monteiro et al., 2017). This type of injury should be suspected when the circumstances associated with the patient's injuries involve flames in a confined area, even if burns on the surface of the patient's skin aren't visible.

Other complications

Pulmonary complications can arise from tight eschar formation on the chest from circumferential chest burns. The eschar can restrict chest movement or can impair ventilation from compression of the anatomical structures of the throat and neck. Visual assessment of the chest will reveal the ease of respirations, depth of chest movement, rate of respirations, and respiratory effort.

How it happens

Carbon monoxide poisoning

There are several gases (such as CO and hydrogen cyanide) that are nontoxic to the respiratory system directly yet interfere with cellular respiration. CO has a greater attraction to hemoglobin than oxygen. When CO enters the blood, it binds with the hemoglobin to form carboxyhemoglobin. Carboxyhemoglobin reduces the oxygen-carrying capacity of hemoglobin. This reduction results in decreased oxygenation to the cells and tissues.

Chemical inhalation

Irritating gases (chlorine, hydrogen chloride, nitrogen dioxide, phosgene, and sulfur dioxide) commonly combine with water in the lungs to form corrosive acids. These acids cause denaturation of proteins, cellular damage, and edema of the pulmonary tissues. Smoke inhalation injuries generally fall into this category. Chemical burns to the airway are similar to burns on the skin, except that they're painless. The tracheobronchial tree is insensitive to pain. The inhalation of small quantities of noxious chemicals can also damage the alveoli and bronchi.

Thermal inhalation

Inhaled hot air or steam is rapidly cooled by the upper airway. Because the hot air or steam is confined to this area, the upper airway suffers the greatest damage. Inhaled hot air or steam can also injure the lower respiratory tract because water holds heat better than dry air. Even so, this injury is rare because reflexive closure of the vocal cords and laryngeal spasm commonly prevent full inhalation of the hot air or steam.

What to look for

Physical findings with an inhalation injury vary depending on the gas or substance inhaled and the duration of the exposure.

Carbon monoxide poisoning

Carboxyhemoglobin reduces the oxygen-carrying capacity of hemoglobin. This reduction commonly causes the patient's face to turn bright red and the lips cherry red. The symptoms of CO poisoning vary with the concentration of carboxyhemoglobin. (See *Oxygen saturation in CO poisoning.*)

When it's a little . . .

Mild poisoning generally indicates a CO level from 11% to 20%. Symptoms at this concentration commonly include:
- slight shortness of breath
- headache
- decreased visual acuity
- decreased cerebral function
- poor coordination.

When it's a lot . . .

Moderate poisoning indicates a CO level from 21% to 41%. Symptoms at this concentration include:
- altered mental status
- impaired judgment
- confusion
- headache
- tinnitus
- dizziness
- drowsiness
- irritability
- nausea
- changes in skin color
- electrocardiogram (ECG)
- tachycardia
- hypotension
- stupor.

And when it's way too much . . .

Severe poisoning is defined as a level of CO from 42% to 60%. Symptoms include:
- convulsions
- coma
- generalized instability.
  In the final stage (fatal poisoning), the CO level reaches 61% to 80% and results in death (O'Malley, 2018).

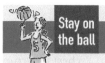

Stay on the ball

Oxygen saturation in CO poisoning

When assessing for carbon monoxide (CO) poisoning, be aware that pulse oximetry devices measure oxygenated and deoxygenated hemoglobin but don't measure dysfunctional hemoglobin such as carboxyhemoglobin. Therefore, the oxygen saturation levels in the presence of CO poisoning will be within normal ranges because the carboxyhemoglobin levels aren't measured.

Chemical inhalation

The most common effects of smoke or chemical inhalation include atelectasis, pulmonary edema, and tissue anoxia. Respiratory distress usually occurs early in the course of smoke inhalation secondary to hypoxia. Patients also exhibiting no respiratory difficulties may suddenly develop respiratory distress. Intubation and mechanical ventilation equipment should be available for immediate use.

Thermal inhalation

The entire respiratory tract has the potential to be damaged by thermal inhalation injury; however, injury rarely progresses to the lungs. Ulcerations, erythema, and edema of the mouth and epiglottis are the initial symptoms of this type of injury. Edema may rapidly progress to upper airway obstruction. You may also note stridor, wheezing, crackles, increased secretions, hoarseness, and shortness of breath. Direct thermal injury to the upper airway yields burns of the face and lips, burned nasal hairs, and laryngeal edema.

"Hoarse"-ness is a common symptom of thermal inhalation . . . just like the silence I'm hearing now is a common symptom of bad puns.

What tests tell you

Initial laboratory studies commonly include electrolytes, liver function studies, BUN and creatinine, and a complete blood count (CBC). Obtaining these studies will provide baseline data for analysis. ABG analysis will provide valuable information on the acid–base status, ventilation, and oxygenation status of the patient. In patients with suspected CO poisoning, a carboxyhemoglobin level will be obtained. Cardiac monitoring detects ischemic changes, and ECG and chest X-ray should be evaluated. A depressed ST segment on ECG is a common finding in the moderate stage of CO poisoning.

How it's treated

- Assessment of the patient's airway, breathing, and circulation is the first step.
- Obtain a history of the exposure and attempt to identify the toxic agent of exposure.
- Immediately provide oxygen to the patient. Intubation and mechanical ventilation may be required if the patient demonstrates severe respiratory distress or an altered mental state.
- Upper airway edema requires emergent ET intubation.
- Bronchodilators, antibiotics, and IV fluids may be prescribed.
- The preferred treatment for CO poisoning is administering 100% humidified oxygen and continuing until carboxyhemoglobin levels fall to the nontoxic range of 10%.
- Chest physical therapy may assist in the removal of necrotic tissue.

- Although its use has become increasingly controversial, the use of a hyperbaric oxygen chamber for CO poisoning is a tool that can be used in severe cases.
- Fluid resuscitation is an important component of managing inhalation injury. However, careful monitoring of fluid status is essential because of the risk of pulmonary edema.

What to do

- Remove the patient's clothing, but take care to prevent self-contamination from the toxic substance if the clothing has possibly been exposed to it.
- Establish IV access for medication, blood products, and fluid administration.
- Obtain laboratory specimens to evaluate ventilation, oxygenation, and baseline values.
- Obtain chest X-ray, ECG, and pulmonary function studies.
- Implement cardiac monitoring to assess for ischemic changes or arrhythmias.
- Monitor for signs of pulmonary edema that may accompany fluid resuscitation.
- In the event of bronchospasms, provide oxygen, bronchodilators via a nebulizer, and, possibly, aminophylline.
- Monitor fluid balance and intake and output closely.
- Administer antibiotics as prescribed.
- Assess lung sounds frequently and notify the health care provider immediately of changes in those sounds or oxygenation.
- Provide a supportive and educative environment for the patient and family. (See *Inhalation injury in children.*)
- Monitor laboratory studies for changes that may indicate multisystem complications.

Submersion injury

Submersion injuries refer to surviving—at least temporarily—the physiologic effects of hypoxemia and acidosis that result from submersion in fluid. Hypoxemia and acidosis are the primary problems in victims of submersion injury. Although we know that unintentional drowning claims nearly 4,000 lives annually in the United States, no statistics are available for submersion injury incidents (Centers for Disease Control and Prevention, 2016).

What causes it?

Submersion injuries result from an inability to swim, panic, a boating accident, a heart attack, a blow to the head while in the water, heavy drinking before swimming, or a suicide attempt.

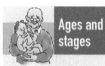

Ages and stages

Inhalation injury in children

It's essential that your care of a child with inhalation injury addresses the emotional and psychological needs of the child and the family. Initially, care will focus on oxygenating, stabilizing the child, and managing the physical components of the injury. However, your care must eventually encompass the psychological needs of the frightened child and the emotional needs of the parents.

Parents may have feelings of guilt if the injury could have been prevented or even if it couldn't. Be sure to provide information to the parents about the child's condition, prognosis, treatment plan, and discharge needs. In addition to ongoing communication, psychological intervention may be needed to discuss feelings of guilt, emotional stress, or fears of the parent and child.

Submersion injuries take three forms:

- *dry*, in which the victim doesn't aspirate fluid but suffers respiratory obstruction or asphyxia
- *wet*, in which the victim aspirates fluid and suffers from asphyxia or secondary changes due to fluid aspiration
- *secondary*, in which the victim suffers a recurrence of respiratory distress (usually aspiration pneumonia or pulmonary edema) within minutes or 1 to 2 days after a submersion injury incident.

How it happens

Regardless of the tonicity of the fluid aspirated, hypoxemia is the most serious consequence of submersion injury, followed by metabolic acidosis. Other consequences depend on the kind of water aspirated.

After freshwater aspiration, changes in the character of lung surfactant result in exudation of protein-rich plasma into the alveoli. These changes, plus increased capillary permeability, lead to pulmonary edema and hypoxemia. (See *Physiologic changes in submersion injuries*, page 254.)

After saltwater aspiration, the hypertonicity of seawater exerts an osmotic force that pulls fluid from pulmonary capillaries into the alveoli. The resulting intrapulmonary shunt causes hypoxemia. In addition, the pulmonary capillary membrane may be injured and induce pulmonary edema. In each kind of submersion injury, pulmonary edema and hypoxemia take place secondary to aspiration.

What to look for

Submersion injury victims can display a host of clinical problems, including:

- fever
- confusion
- unconsciousness
- irritability
- lethargy
- restlessness
- substernal chest pain
- shallow or gasping respirations
- cough that produces a pink, frothy fluid
- vomiting
- abdominal distention
- apnea
- asystole
- bradycardia
- tachycardia.

Physiologic changes in submersion injuries

This flowchart shows the primary cellular alterations that occur during submersion injuries. Separate pathways are shown for saltwater and freshwater incidents. Hypothermia presents a separate pathway that may preserve neurologic function by decreasing the metabolic rate. All pathways lead to diffuse pulmonary edema.

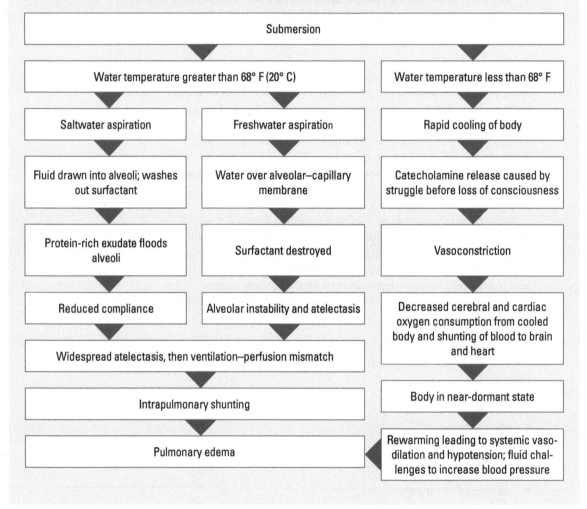

What tests tell you

Diagnosis requires a history of submersion injury, including the type of water aspirated, along with characteristic features and auscultation of crackles and rhonchi.

ABG analysis shows decreased oxygen content, low bicarbonate levels, and low pH. Electrolyte levels may be elevated or decreased, depending on the type of water aspirated. Leukocytosis may occur. ECG shows arrhythmias and waveform changes.

How it's treated

- Emergency treatment begins with CPR and administration of 100% oxygen.
- If hypothermia is an issue, measures must be taken to warm the patient.
- Ongoing support and monitoring of circulation and oxygenation should be maintained, and hemodynamic monitoring should be instituted.

What to do

- Stabilize the patient's neck in case there is a cervical injury.
- Assess for a patent airway and be prepared to administer high-flow oxygen and assist with ET intubation.
- Assess the patient's core body temperature and be prepared to institute rewarming as necessary.
- Continue CPR, intubate the patient, and provide respiratory assistance, such as mechanical ventilation with positive end-expiratory pressure (PEEP), if needed.
- Assess ABG and pulse oximetry values.
- If the patient's abdomen is distended, insert a nasogastric tube. (Intubate the patient first if unconscious.)
- Start IV lines and insert an indwelling urinary catheter.
- Give medications as ordered; drug treatment for near-drowning victims is controversial. Such treatment may include sodium bicarbonate for acidosis, corticosteroids and osmotic diuretics for cerebral edema, antibiotics to prevent infections, and bronchodilators to ease bronchospasms.
- Observe for pulmonary complications and signs of delayed drowning (confusion, substernal pain, adventitious breath sounds). Suction often. Pulmonary artery catheters may be useful in assessing cardiopulmonary status.
- Monitor vital signs, intake and output, and peripheral pulses.
- Check for skin perfusion and watch for signs of infection.
- To facilitate breathing, raise the head of the bed slightly.
- Prepare to administer prophylactic antibiotics as needed.
- Correct acid–base imbalances.
- Prepare the patient for transfer to a critical care unit or, if patient is a child, to a pediatric unit or facility.

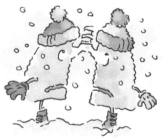

Make sure to check the submersion injury patient's core body temperature to assess for hypothermia.

Pneumothorax

Pneumothorax is an accumulation of air in the pleural cavity that leads to partial or complete lung collapse. The amount of air trapped in the intrapleural space determines the degree of lung collapse. In some cases, venous return to the heart is impeded, causing a life-threatening condition called *tension pneumothorax*.

Pneumothorax can be classified as *traumatic* or *spontaneous*. Traumatic pneumothorax may be further classified as *open* or *closed*. (Note that an open, or penetrating, *wound* may cause closed pneumothorax.) Spontaneous pneumothorax, which is also considered closed, is most common in older patients with COPD but can appear in young, healthy patients as well.

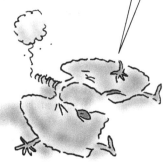

Air plus pleural cavity equals partial or complete lung collapse.

What causes it

The causes of pneumothorax vary according to classification.

Traumatic pneumothorax

Traumatic pneumothorax may be open or closed.

Open book

Causes of open pneumothorax include:
- penetrating chest injury (stab or gunshot wound)
- insertion of a central venous catheter
- thoracentesis or closed pleural biopsy
- transbronchial biopsy
- chest surgery.

Closed call

Causes of closed pneumothorax include:
- blunt chest trauma
- interstitial lung disease such as eosinophilic granuloma
- tubercular or cancerous lesions that erode into the pleural space
- air leakage from ruptured blebs
- rupture resulting from barotrauma caused by high intrathoracic pressures during mechanical ventilation.

Spontaneous pneumothorax

Spontaneous pneumothorax occurs in the absence of trauma and is usually caused by the rupture of a subpleural bleb (a small cystic space) at the surface of a lung. It commonly occurs in tall, healthy young males with no apparent lung disease. Risk factors include cigarette smoking, possible familial propensity, Marfan syndrome, mitral valve disease, and changes in atmospheric pressure.

Tension pneumothorax

Causes of tension pneumothorax include:
- penetrating chest wound treated with an airtight dressing
- fractured ribs
- mechanical ventilation
- chest tube occlusion or malfunction
- high-level PEEP that causes alveolar blebs to rupture.

How it happens

Traumatic pneumothorax

Open pneumothorax results from atmospheric air flowing directly into the pleural cavity (under negative pressure). As the air pressure in the pleural cavity becomes positive, the lung on the affected side collapses, causing decreased total lung capacity. As a result, the patient develops an imbalance that leads to hypoxia.

Closed pneumothorax results when an opening is created between the intrapleural space and the parenchyma of the lung. Air enters the pleural space from within the lung, causing increased pleural pressure and preventing lung expansion during inspiration.

Spontaneous pneumothorax

In spontaneous pneumothorax, the rupture of a subpleural bleb causes air leakage into the pleural spaces, which causes the lung to collapse. Hypoxia results from decreased total lung capacity, vital capacity, and lung compliance.

Tension pneumothorax

Tension pneumothorax results when air in the pleural space is under higher pressure than air in the adjacent lung. (See *Understanding tension pneumothorax*, page 258.) Here's what happens:

- Air enters the pleural space from the site of pleural rupture, which acts as a one-way valve. Thus, air enters the pleural space on inspiration but can't escape as the rupture site closes on expiration.
- More air enters with each inspiration, and air pressure begins to exceed barometric pressure.
- The air pushes against the recoiled lung, causing compression atelectasis, and pushes against the mediastinum, compressing and displacing the heart and great vessels.
- The mediastinum eventually shifts away from the affected side, affecting venous return and putting ever greater pressure on the heart, great vessels, trachea, and contralateral lung. Without immediate treatment, this emergency can rapidly become fatal.

I try my best to hang loose—tension just isn't my thing and neither is tension pneumothorax.

What to look for

Assessment findings depend on the severity of the pneumothorax. Spontaneous pneumothorax that releases a small amount of air into the pleural space may cause no signs or symptoms. Generally, tension pneumothorax causes the most severe respiratory signs and symptoms.

Understanding tension pneumothorax

In tension pneumothorax, air accumulates in the pleural space and can't escape. As intrapleural pressure increases, the lung on the affected side collapses.

On inspiration, the mediastinum shifts toward the unaffected lung, impairing ventilation.

On expiration, the mediastinal shift distorts the vena cava and reduces venous return.

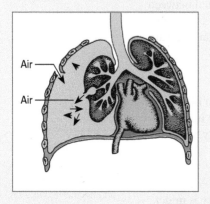

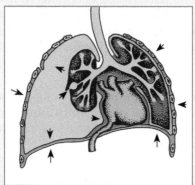

Every breath hurts

Your patient's history reveals sudden, sharp, pleuritic chest pain. The patient may report that chest movement, breathing, and coughing exacerbate the pain. The patient may also report shortness of breath.

Further findings

Inspection reveals asymmetric chest wall movement with overexpansion and rigidity on the affected side. The skin may be cool, clammy, and cyanotic. Palpation of the chest wall may reveal crackling beneath the skin (subcutaneous emphysema) and decreased vocal fremitus.

In addition, percussion may reveal hyperresonance on the affected side. Auscultation may disclose decreased or absent breath sounds on the affected side. Vital signs may follow the pattern of respiratory distress seen with respiratory failure.

Did we mention the tension?

Tension pneumothorax also causes:
- distended jugular veins as a result of high intrapleural pressure, mediastinal shift, and increased cardiovascular pressure
- hypotension and tachycardia due to decreased cardiac output
- tracheal deviation to the opposite side (a late sign).

What tests tell you
- Chest X-rays reveal air in the pleural space and a mediastinal shift, which confirm pneumothorax.
- ABG analysis reveals hypoxemia, usually with elevated $PaCO_2$ and normal bicarbonate ion levels in the early stages.
- ECG may reveal decreased QRS amplitude, precordial T-wave inversion, and rightward shift of the frontal QRS axis.

How it's treated
Treatment of pneumothorax depends on the cause and severity.

With trauma

Open or closed pneumothorax may necessitate surgical repair of affected tissues, followed by chest tube placement with an underwater seal.

With less lung collapse

Spontaneous pneumothorax with less than 2 to 3 cm between the lung and the chest wall, no signs of increased pleural pressure, and no dyspnea or indications of physiologic compromise may be corrected with:
- oxygen administration to improve respiratory status
- monitoring of vital signs to detect physiologic compromise.

With more lung collapse

Lung collapse greater than 3 cm between the lung and the chest wall may necessitate other measures, including:
- aspiration of air from the intrapleural space with a large-bore needle attached to a syringe to restore negative pressure within the pleural space
- placing a chest tube in the fourth or fifth intercostal space in the midclavicular line to reexpand the lung by restoring negative intrapleural pressure
- connecting the chest tube to an underwater seal or a low-pressure suction to reexpand the lung.

With tension

Treatment for tension pneumothorax typically involves:
- analgesics to promote comfort and encourage deep breathing and coughing
- immediate large-bore needle insertion into the pleural space through the second intercostal space to reexpand the lung, followed by insertion of a chest tube if large amounts of air escape through the needle after insertion (Light, 2018).

What to do

- Assess the patient's respiratory status, including auscultation of bilateral breath sounds.
- Monitor oxygen saturation levels closely for changes; obtain ABG analysis as ordered.
- Monitor hemodynamic parameters frequently, as appropriate and indicated. Anticipate the need for cardiac monitoring because hypoxemia can predispose the patient to arrhythmias.
- Initiate and maintain vascular access.
- Watch for complications, signaled by pallor, gasping respirations, and sudden chest pain.
- Carefully monitor vital signs at least every hour for indications of shock, increasing respiratory distress, or mediastinal shift. If your patient's respiratory status deteriorates, anticipate the need for ET intubation and mechanical ventilation and assist as necessary.
- Assist with chest tube insertion and connect to suction as ordered. Monitor your patient for possible complications associated with chest tube insertion.
- Maintain bed rest in high Fowler position.

Status asthmaticus

Status asthmaticus is a life-threatening situation resulting from severe asthma exacerbation. It begins with impaired gas exchange and—without rapid intervention—may lead to respiratory failure and, eventually, death. Ominous signs indicating the need for ET intubation include:

- "silent chest"—indicating minimal airflow
- fatigue and decreasing LOC
- hypoxemia, hypercapnia, or metabolic acidosis.

Asthma overview

Asthma is a chronic reactive airway disorder involving episodic, reversible airway obstruction and hyperresponsiveness of the airway to multiple stimuli. It results from bronchospasms, increased mucus secretion, and mucosal edema. If left untreated or if the patient doesn't respond to drug therapy after 24 hours, status asthmaticus is diagnosed.

Making things worse

Asthma exacerbations are acute or subacute episodes of worsening shortness of breath, coughing, and wheezing, with measurable decreases in expiratory airflow.

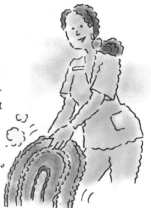

Look at it this way—you aren't spring cleaning, you're reducing the risk of atopic asthma.

What causes it

Sensitivity to specific external allergens is the leading cause. Incidence is highest with chronic exposure to the allergens. Internal, nonallergenic factors, such as genetic factors and stress, may also lead to asthma.

Outside factors

Atopic (or *allergic*) asthma begins in childhood. Patients are typically sensitive to specific external allergens. Allergens that can trigger an asthma attack include pollen, animal dander, house dust or mold, and kapok or feather pillows.

Atopic or allergic asthma in childhood is commonly accompanied by other hereditary allergies, such as eczema and allergic rhinitis.

Factors within

Patients with nonallergic (or *nonatopic*) asthma react to internal, nonallergenic factors. Nonallergic factors that can trigger an asthma attack include irritants, emotional stress, fear or anger, infection, fatigue, endocrine changes, temperature variations, humidity variations, exposure to noxious fumes, anxiety, coughing or laughing, and genetic factors. Most episodes take place after a severe respiratory tract infection, especially in adults.

Constricting factors

Other situations can cause asthma or asthma-like symptoms including cold air; exercise; psychological stress; drugs such as aspirin, beta-adrenergic blockers, and nonsteroidal anti-inflammatory drugs; sensitivity to allergens and pollutants; exposure to tartrazine; and viral infections.

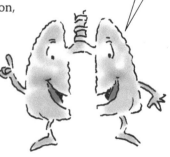

Irritants in the workplace—and no, the guy who hogs the copier doesn't count—can exacerbate existing asthma.

Irritants in the workplace

Many adults acquire an allergic form of asthma or exacerbation of existing asthma from exposure to agents in the workplace. Irritants include chemicals in flour, acid anhydrides, and excreta of dust mites in carpet.

Genetic messes

Asthma is associated with two genetic influences:
1. ability to develop asthma because of an abnormal gene (atopy)
2. tendency to develop hyperresponsive airways (without atopy).

A potent mix

Environmental factors interact with inherited factors to cause asthmatic reactions with associated bronchospasms.

How it happens

Status asthmaticus begins with an asthma attack. In asthma, bronchial linings overreact to various stimuli, causing episodic smooth muscle spasms that severely constrict the airways. Here's how asthma develops into status asthmaticus:

- Immunoglobulin E (IgE) antibodies attached to histamine-containing mast cells and receptors on cell membranes initiate intrinsic asthma attacks.
- When exposed to an antigen, such as pollen, the IgE antibody combines with it.
- On subsequent exposure to the antigen, mast cells degranulate and release mediators.
- Mast cells in the lung are stimulated to release histamine and the slow-reacting substance of anaphylaxis.

Attachment disorder

- Histamine attaches to receptor sites in the larger bronchi, where it causes swelling in smooth muscles.
- Mucous membranes become inflamed, irritated, and swollen. The patient may experience dyspnea, prolonged expiration, and increased respiratory rate.
- Leukotrienes attach to receptor sites in the smaller bronchi and cause local swelling of the smooth muscle.
- Leukotrienes also cause prostaglandins to travel by way of the bloodstream to the lungs, where they enhance the effect of histamine. A wheeze may be audible during coughing—the higher the pitch, the narrower the bronchial lumen.
- Histamine stimulates the mucous membranes to secrete excessive mucus, further narrowing the bronchial lumen.

A not-so-good goblet

- Goblet cells secrete viscous mucus that's difficult to cough up, resulting in coughing, rhonchi, higher pitched wheezing, and increased respiratory distress. Mucosal edema and thickened secretions further block the airways.
- On inhalation, the narrowed bronchial lumen can still expand slightly, allowing air to reach the alveoli. On exhalation, increased intrathoracic pressure closes the bronchial lumen completely. Air enters but can't escape.
- When status asthmaticus occurs, hypoxemia worsens and the expiratory rate and volume decrease even further.
- Obstructed airways impede gas exchange and increase airway resistance. The patient works to breathe.

- As breathing and hypoxemia tire the patient, the respiratory rate drops to normal, $PaCO_2$ levels rise, and the patient hypoventilates from exhaustion.
- Respiratory acidosis develops as $PaCO_2$ increases.
- The situation becomes life-threatening when no air is audible on auscultation (a silent chest) and $PaCO_2$ rises to over 70 mm Hg.
- Without treatment, the patient experiences acute respiratory failure (McCance & Huether, 2019).

What to look for

A patient who comes to the ED during a suspected asthma attack will demonstrate:

- absent or minimal wheezing
- inability to speak more than a few words before pausing for breath
- fatigue
- decreasing LOC
- inability to lay flat
- pulsus paradoxus greater than 20 mm Hg
- long expiratory phase
- SpO_2 less than 90%
- hypoxemia
- hypercarbia (elevated $PaCO_2$)
- metabolic acidosis
- increased respiratory rate (rapid shallow breaths)
- use of accessory muscles
- chest wall retractions
- cyanosis (a late sign and usually unreliable).

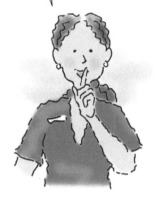

One instance where silence isn't golden: when it's in your patient's chest and means the asthma attack has become life-threatening.

What tests tell you

- Pulmonary function tests reveal decreased vital capacity and increased total lung and residual capacities during an acute attack. Peak and expiratory flow rate measurements are less than 70% of baseline.
- Pulse oximetry commonly shows that oxygen saturation is less than 90%.
- Chest X-ray may show hyperinflation with areas of atelectasis and flat diaphragm due to increased intrathoracic volume.
- ABG analysis reveals decreasing PaO_2 and increasing $PaCO_2$.
- ECG shows sinus tachycardia during an attack.
- Sputum analysis may indicate increased viscosity, mucus plugs, presence of Curschmann spirals (casts of airways), Charcot–Leyden crystals, and eosinophils. Culture may disclose causative organisms if infection is the trigger.

- CBC with differential shows an increased eosinophil count secondary to inflammation and an elevated white blood cell count and granulocyte count if an acute infection is present (McCance & Huether, 2019).

How it's treated

In acute status asthmaticus, the patient is monitored closely for respiratory failure. Oxygen, magnesium sulfate (IV), corticosteroids, and nebulized bronchodilators and anticholinergics may be ordered. The patient may be intubated and placed on mechanical ventilation if $Paco_2$ increases or if he experiences respiratory arrest.

Treatment may include the use of:

- humidified oxygen to correct dyspnea, cyanosis, and hypoxemia and to maintain an oxygen saturation greater than 92%
- intubation followed by mechanical ventilation, which is necessary if the patient doesn't respond to initial ventilatory support and drugs or develops respiratory failure

Bucking bronchos

- bronchodilators, such as levalbuterol and albuterol, to decrease bronchoconstriction, reduce bronchial airway edema, and increase pulmonary ventilation
- anticholinergics to increase the effects of bronchodilators
- corticosteroids, such as methylprednisolone (Solu-Medrol), to decrease bronchoconstriction, reduce bronchial airway edema, and increase pulmonary ventilation
- magnesium sulfate (IV) is recommended in patients who have status asthmaticus that does not respond to other agents; this agent is thought to relax smooth muscle and therefore decrease bronchoconstriction
- mast cell stabilizers, such as cromolyn and nedocromil, in patients with atopic asthma who have seasonal disease because, when given prophylactically, they block the acute obstructive effects of antigen exposure by inhibiting the degranulation of mast cells, thereby preventing the release of chemical mediators responsible for anaphylaxis (Fanta, 2018)
- relaxation exercises to increase circulation and aid recovery from an asthma attack.

What to do

- Monitor Spo_2.
- Monitor ABGs as indicated.
- Provide supplemental oxygen.

- Administer bronchodilators.
- Establish and maintain vascular access.
- Prepare for possible ET intubation.
- Assess the patient's respiratory status, especially if the patient isn't intubated.
- Check the respiratory rate.
- Auscultate for breath sounds.
- Monitor oxygen saturation.
- Assess the patient's mental status for confusion, agitation, or lethargy.
- Assess the patient's heart rate and rhythm.
- Initiate cardiac monitoring, and be alert for cardiac arrhythmias related to bronchodilator therapy or hypoxemia.
- Obtain ordered tests and report results promptly.
- When the acute phase is over, position the patient for maximum comfort, usually in semi-Fowler position. Encourage coughing to clear secretions.
- Offer emotional support and reassurance (Ignatavicius et al., 2018).

Quick quiz

1. A 55-year-old patient comes to the ED with a history of asthma. The patient is breathing rapidly and has a pulse oximetry reading of 91%. What type of acid–base imbalance will the nurse anticipate?

    A. Respiratory acidosis
    B. Respiratory alkalosis
    C. Metabolic acidosis
    D. Metabolic alkalosis

Answer: B. Respiratory alkalosis. Hyperventilation related to hypoxia and pneumonia causes the acid component to be blown off, resulting in respiratory alkalosis.

2. Abnormal dullness during percussion indicates an area of decreased air in the lung or pleural space and may be associated with:

    A. pneumothorax.
    B. acute asthma.
    C. pleural effusion.
    D. bullous emphysema.

Answer: C. Pleural effusion is composed of liquid. Therefore, abnormal dullness can be heard during percussion over the area.

3.   A patient arrives in the ED with severe asthma symptoms. What medication will the nurse anticipate in the immediate emergency care of this patient?
   A.   Albuterol
   B.   Fluticasone
   C.   Budesonide
   D.   Salmeterol

Answer: A. Albuterol is a bronchodilator that opens airways very quickly. Although all the drugs listed are helpful in treating asthma, albuterol is most useful in an asthma emergency.

4.   A patient presents to the ED with diabetic ketoacidosis (DKA), a respiratory rate of 36 breaths per minute, and gasping for breath. What type of respirations is the patient experiencing?
   A.   Cheyne–Stokes
   B.   Kussmaul
   C.   Ataxic
   D.   Biot

Answer: B. Kussmaul respirations are deep, gasping, and rapid. These respirations are related to metabolic acidosis caused by DKA.

5.   RSI is used to rapidly produce optimal conditions for intubation in emergency situations. Which of the following drugs is a neuro-muscular blocking agent used in RSI?
   A.   Propofol
   B.   Midazolam
   C.   Etomidate
   D.   Succinylcholine

Answer: D. Succinylcholine is a depolarizing skeletal muscle relax-ant that is used as a neuromuscular blocking agent to help facilitate RSI.

6.   Which can interfere with oxygen saturation readings when utiliz-ing pulse oximetry?
   A.   Low blood glucose level
   B.   Low bilirubin level
   C.   Elevated carboxyhemoglobin
   D.   Fever

Answer: C. Carboxyhemoglobin is created when red blood cells are exposed to carbon monoxide. Pulse oximetry isn't used when CO poisoning is suspected because the oximeter doesn't differentiate between oxygen and carbon monoxide bound to hemoglobin.

Scoring

☆☆☆   If you answered all six questions correctly, breathe a big sigh of relief. You're a respiratory mastermind!

☆☆   If you answered four or five questions correctly, don't wait to exhale. You're an inspiration!

☆   If you answered fewer than four questions correctly, you're on the verge of expiration. Take a deep breath and dive back into the chapter!

Selected references

American College of Allergy, Asthma & Immunology. (2014). *Asthma treatment*. Retrieved from https://acaai.org/asthma/asthma-treatment

Bortle, C. D. (2017). *Drugs to aid intubation*. Retrieved from https://www.merckmanuals .com/professional/critical-care-medicine/respiratory-arrest/drugs-to-aid -intubation

Brown, C. A., & Sakles, J. C. (2017). *Rapid sequence intubation for adults outside the operating room*. Retrieved from https://www.uptodate.com/contents/rapid-sequence -intubation-for-adults-outside-the-operating-room

Caro, D. (2018). *Neuromuscular blocking agents for rapid sequence intubation in adults outside of the operating room*. Retrieved from https://www.uptodate.com/contents /neuromuscular-blocking-agents-nmbas-for-rapid-sequence-intubation-in -adults-outside-of-the-operating-room

Centers for Disease Control and Prevention. (2016). *Unintentional drowning: Get the facts*. Retrieved from https://www.cdc.gov/homeandrecreationalsafety/water -safety/waterinjuries-factsheet.html

Fanta, C. H. (2018). *Management of acute exacerbations of asthma in adults*. Retrieved from https://www.uptodate.com/contents/management-of-acute- exacerbations-of-asthma-in-adults

Ignatavicius, D., Workman, M., & Rebar, C. (2018). *Medical-surgical nursing: Concepts for interprofessional collaborative care* (9th ed.). St. Louis, MO: Elsevier.

Jurbran, A. (2015). Pulse oximetry. *Critical Care, 19*, 272. doi:10.1186/s13054-015-0984-8

Light, R. W. (2018). *Primary spontaneous pneumothorax in adults*. Retrieved from https:// www.uptodate.com/contents/primary-spontaneous-pneumothorax-in-adults

McCance, K., & Huether, S. (2019). *Pathophysiology: The biologic basis for disease in adults and children* (8th ed.). St. Louis, MO: Elsevier.

Monteiro, D., Silva, I., Egipto, P., et al. (2017). Inhalation injury in a burn unit: A retrospective review of prognostic factors. *Annals of Burns and Fire Disasters, 30*(2), 121–125.

O'Malley, G. F. (2018). *Carbon monoxide poisoning*. Retrieved from https://www.merck manuals.com/professional/injuries-poisoning/poisoning/carbon-monoxide -poisoning

Pinto, V. L., & Sharma, S. (2019). *Continuous positive airway pressure (CPAP)*. Retrieved from https://www.ncbi.nlm.nih.gov/books/NBK482178/

Potter, P., Perry, A., Stockert, P., et al. (2017). *Fundamentals of nursing* (9th ed.). St. Louis, MO: Elsevier.

Salem, R. M., Khorasani, A., Zeidan, A., et al. (2017). Cricoid pressure controversies: Narrative review. *Anesthesiology, 126*(4), 738–752. doi:10.1097/ALN .0000000000001489

Theodore, A. (2017). *Arterial blood gases.* Retrieved from https://www.uptodate.com /contents/arterial-blood-gases

Torrey, S. B. (2018). *Continuous oxygen delivery systems for infants, children, and adults.* Retrieved from https://www.uptodate.com/contents/continuous-oxygen-delivery -systems-for-infants-children-and-adults

Chapter 6

Gastrointestinal emergencies

Just the facts

In this chapter, you'll learn:

◆ emergency assessment of the gastrointestinal (GI) system

◆ diagnostic tests and procedures for GI emergencies

◆ GI disorders in the emergency department and their treatments.

Understanding GI emergencies

Being able to identify subtle changes in a patient's gastrointestinal (GI) system can mean the difference between effective and ineffective emergency care. GI signs and symptoms can have many baffling causes. When your patient comes to the emergency department (ED) with a GI emergency, your assessment can be used to determine whether the patient's signs and symptoms are related to a current medical problem or indicate a new problem.

When faced with an emergency involving the GI system, you must assess the patient thoroughly and stay alert for subtle changes that may indicate a potential deterioration in the patient's condition. A thorough assessment forms the basis for your interventions, which then must be instituted quickly to minimize what can be life-threatening risks to the patient.

Assessment

The initial goal is to determine if the patient needs immediate intervention. Unless the patient requires immediate stabilizing treatment, begin by taking a thorough health history. Then assess further by conducting a thorough physical examination using inspection, auscultation, palpation, and percussion.

If you are unable to interview the patient because of the condition, you may gather history information from the patient's medical record. In some cases, you may need to ask the patient's family or the emergency medical response team that transported the patient to the ED.

Health history

Begin by introducing yourself and explaining what happens during the health history and physical examination. Then obtain information about the patient's chief concern, medications used, family history, and lifestyle patterns. Conduct this part of the assessment as privately as possible because the patient may feel embarrassed when talking about GI function (Penner & Fishman, 2019).

> A patient may be embarrassed to talk about GI function, so make your health history assessment as private as possible.

Chief concern

A patient with a GI problem may report:
- altered bowel habits
- heartburn
- nausea
- pain
- vomiting.

To investigate these and other signs and symptoms, ask about the onset, duration, and severity of each. Inquire about the location of the pain, precipitating factors, alleviating factors, and associated symptoms (Penner & Fishman, 2019; Velissaris et al., 2017). (See *Asking the right questions*.)

Previous health status

To determine if the patient's problem is new or recurring, ask about GI illnesses, such as an ulcer, gallbladder disease, inflammatory bowel disease, and GI bleeding. Also ask if the patient has had abdominal surgery or trauma.

Further questions

Ask the patient additional questions, such as:
- Are you allergic to any foods or medications?
- Have you noticed a change in the color, amount, and appearance of your stool? Have you ever seen blood in your stool?
- Have you recently traveled abroad? (This question applies if the patient seeks care for diarrhea because diarrhea, hepatitis, and parasitic infections can result from ingesting contaminated food or water.)
- Have any members of your household experienced similar symptoms? (This question establishes whether symptoms are likely to be from a common exposure to contaminated food or water, or viral.)
- Ask about dental history. Poor dentition may impair the patient's ability to chew and swallow food.

> Ask about travel—sometimes a patient returns from abroad with diarrhea, hepatitis, or parasites as souvenirs!

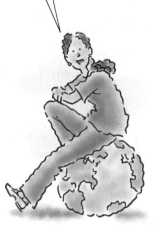

Asking the right questions

When assessing a patient with gastrointestinal-related signs and symptoms, be sure to ask the right questions. To establish a baseline for comparison, ask about the patient's current state of health, including questions about the onset, duration, quality, severity, and location of problems as well as precipitating factors, alleviating factors, and associated symptoms.

Onset

How did the problem start? Was it gradual or sudden? With or without previous symptoms? What was the patient doing when the symptom was first noticed? If the patient reports diarrhea, ask if the patient had been traveling. If so, when and where?

Duration

When did the problem start? Has the patient had the problem before? Does the patient have a history of abdominal surgery? If yes, when? If the patient is in pain, find out when the problem began. Is the pain continuous, intermittent, or colicky (cramp-like)?

Quality

Ask the patient to describe the problem. Ask if this has happened before. Was it diagnosed? If the patient reports pain, find out whether the pain feels sharp, dull, aching, or burning.

Severity

Ask the patient to describe how bad the problem is—for example, have the patient rate it on a pain scale of 0 to 10. Does it keep the patient from normal activities? Has it improved or worsened since it was first noticed? Does it wake the patient at night? If the patient is in pain, is the patient doubled over or in fetal position?

Location

Where does the patient feel the problem? Does it spread, radiate, or shift? Ask the patient to point to where the pain is located.

Precipitating factors

Does anything seem to bring on the problem? What makes it worse? Does it occur at the same time each day or with certain positions? Does the patient notice it after eating or drinking certain foods or after certain activities?

Alleviating factors

Does anything relieve the problem? Does the patient take any prescribed or over-the-counter medications for relief? Has the patient tried anything else for relief?

Associated symptoms

Are there any other symptoms associated with the problem the patient is experiencing? Is there any nausea, vomiting, dry heaves, diarrhea, constipation, bloating, or flatulence? Has the patient lost appetite or lost or gained any weight? If so, how much? When was the patient's last bowel movement? Was it unusual? Ask if the patient has seen stool changes or stool or vomitus with blood and mucus. Has the patient's stool changed in size or color or included mucus? Ask if the patient is able to eat normally and hold down foods and liquids. Also ask about alcohol consumption.

Medications used

Ask the patient what medications are being taken, including over-the-counter medications. Several drugs, including aspirin, sulfonamides, nonsteroidal anti-inflammatory drugs (NSAIDs), analgesics (including narcotic analgesics that may cause constipation), and some antihypertensives, can cause nausea, vomiting, diarrhea, constipation, and other GI problems. Be sure to ask about laxative use because habitual laxative intake can cause constipation.

Family history

Because some GI disorders are hereditary, ask the patient if any family members have had a GI disorder, including:

- alcoholism
- colon cancer
- Crohn disease
- diabetes
- stomach ulcer
- celiac disease
- ulcerative colitis.

Lifestyle patterns

Psychological and sociologic factors can profoundly affect health. To determine factors that may have contributed to your patient's problem, ask about the patient's occupation, home life, financial situation, stress level, and recent life changes.

Be sure to ask about alcohol, illegal drug, caffeine, and tobacco use as well as food consumption, exercise habits, and oral hygiene. Also ask about sleep patterns, such as hours of sleep and whether sleep is restful.

Specific questions for women should include sexual history, menstrual history, and contraception use.

Cultural factors may affect a patient's dietary habits, so ask about any dietary restrictions the patient has, such as following a vegetarian diet.

Physical examination

Physical examination of the GI system usually includes vital signs and evaluation of the mouth, abdomen, liver, rectum, and spleen. Before beginning your examination, explain the techniques you'll be using and warn the patient that some procedures might be uncomfortable. Perform the examination in a private, quiet, warm, and well-lighted room.

Assessing the mouth

Use inspection and palpation to assess the oral cavity:

- First, inspect the patient's mouth and jaw for asymmetry and swelling. Check the patient's bite, noting malocclusion from an overbite or underbite. If the patient has dentures, do they fit? Are they intact or broken?
- Inspect the inner and outer lips, teeth, and gums with a penlight. Note bleeding; gum ulcerations; and missing, displaced, or broken teeth. Palpate the gums for tenderness and the inner lips and cheeks for lesions.

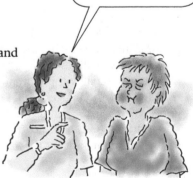

There's no need to hold back; unusual breath odors are common in patients with GI emergencies.

- Assess the tongue, checking for coating, tremors, swelling, and ulcerations. Note unusual breath odors.
- Lastly, examine the pharynx, looking for uvular deviation, tonsillar abnormalities, lesions, plaques, and exudate.

Assessing the abdomen

To ensure an accurate assessment, be sure to:
- drape the patient appropriately
- keep the room warm because chilling can cause abdominal muscles to tense
- warm your hands and the stethoscope
- speak softly and encourage the patient to perform breathing exercises or use imagery during uncomfortable procedures
- assess painful areas last to avoid making the patient tense (Velissaris et al., 2017).

In order, please

The GI system requires abdominal auscultation before percussion and palpation because the latter can alter intestinal activity and bowel sounds. So, when assessing the abdomen, perform the four basic steps in the following sequence (Penner & Fishman, 2019):
1. inspection
2. auscultation
3. percussion
4. palpation.

Abdominal inspection

Before inspecting the abdomen, mentally divide it into four quadrants. (See *Identifying abdominal landmarks*, page 274.)

General inspection

Begin by performing a general inspection of the patient:
- Observe the skin, oral mucosa, nail beds, and sclera for jaundice or signs of anemia.
- Observe the patient's position. Is the patient immobile or writhing in pain?
- Observe the abdomen for symmetry, checking for bumps, bulges, or masses. A bulge may indicate bladder distention or hernia.
- Note the patient's abdominal shape and contour. The abdomen should be flat to rounded in people of average weight. A protruding abdomen may be caused by obesity, pregnancy, ascites, or abdominal distention. A slender person may have a slightly concave abdomen.

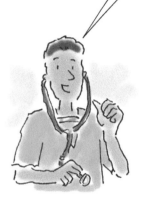

Keeping the room, your hands, and your stethoscope warm can ease patient discomfort during abdominal examination.

The cause of abdominal bulge is pretty obvious here, but in other patients, it may be due to distention or hernia.

Identifying abdominal landmarks

To aid accurate abdominal assessment and documentation of findings, you can mentally divide the patient's abdomen into regions. Use the quadrant method—the easiest and most commonly used method—to divide the abdomen into four equal regions using two imaginary perpendicular lines crossing above the umbilicus.

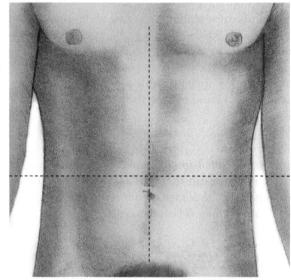

Right upper quadrant
- Liver and gallbladder
- Pylorus
- Duodenum
- Head of pancreas
- Hepatic flexure of colon
- Portions of ascending and transverse colon

Left upper quadrant
- Left liver lobe
- Stomach
- Body of pancreas
- Splenic flexure of colon
- Portions of transverse and descending colon

Right lower quadrant
- Cecum and appendix
- Portion of ascending colon
- Lower portion of right kidney
- Bladder (if distended)

Left lower quadrant
- Sigmoid colon
- Portion of descending colon
- Lower portion of left kidney
- Bladder (if distended)

To striae or not to striae

- Next, inspect the abdominal skin, which normally appears smooth and intact. Striae, or stretch marks, can be caused by pregnancy, excessive weight gain, or ascites. New striae are pink or blue; old striae are silvery white. In patients with darker skin, striae may be dark brown. Note dilated veins. Record the length of any surgical scars on the abdomen.
- Note abdominal movements and pulsations. Usually, waves of peristalsis aren't visible unless the patient is very thin, in which case they may be visible as slight wavelike motions. Marked visible rippling may indicate bowel obstruction; report it immediately. In a thin patient, pulsation of the aorta is visible in the epigastric area. Marked pulsations may occur with hypertension, aortic insufficiency, and other conditions causing widening pulse pressure.

Abdominal auscultation

Auscultation provides information about bowel motility and the underlying vessels and organs.

Follow the clock

Use a stethoscope to auscultate for bowel and vascular sounds. Lightly place the stethoscope diaphragm in the right lower quadrant, slightly below and to the right of the umbilicus.

Do you hear what I hear?

Auscultate in a clockwise fashion in each of the four quadrants, spending at least 2 minutes in each area. Note the character and quality of bowel sounds in each quadrant. In some cases, you may need to auscultate for 5 minutes before you hear sounds. Be sure to allow enough time to listen in each quadrant before you decide that bowel sounds are absent.

Tube tip

Before auscultating the abdomen of a patient with a nasogastric (NG) tube or other abdominal tube connected to suction, briefly clamp the tube or turn off the suction. Suction noises can obscure or mimic actual bowel sounds.

The gurgling, the splashing—nothing makes me happier than a normal bowel sound!

Sound class

Bowel sounds are classified as normal, hypoactive, or hyperactive:
- *Normal* bowel sounds are high-pitched, gurgling noises caused by air mixing with fluid during peristalsis. The noises vary in frequency, pitch, and intensity and occur irregularly from 5 to 34 times per minute. They're loudest before mealtimes. Borborygmus, or stomach growling, is the loud, gurgling, splashing sound heard over the large intestine as gas passes through it.
- *Hypoactive* bowel sounds are heard infrequently. They're associated with ileus, bowel obstruction, or peritonitis and indicate diminished peristalsis. Paralytic ileus, torsion of the bowel, or use of opioids and other medications can decrease peristalsis.
- *Hyperactive* bowel sounds are loud, high-pitched, tinkling sounds that occur frequently and may be caused by diarrhea, constipation, or laxative use.

Sound off

Next, use the bell of the stethoscope to auscultate for vascular sounds. Normally, you should detect no vascular sounds. Note a bruit, venous hum, or friction rub. (See *Interpreting abnormal abdominal sounds*, page 276.)

Interpreting abnormal abdominal sounds

This chart lists abnormal abdominal sounds along with the location and possible cause of each.

Sound and description	Location	Possible cause
Abnormal bowel sounds		
Hyperactive sounds (unrelated to hunger)	Any quadrant	Diarrhea, laxative use, or early intestinal obstruction
Hypoactive and then absent sounds	Any quadrant	Intestinal fluid and air under tension in a dilated bowel
High-pitched tinkling sounds	Any quadrant	Paralytic ileus or peritonitis
High-pitched rushing sounds coinciding with abdominal cramps	Any quadrant	Intestinal obstruction
Systolic bruits		
Vascular blowing sounds resembling cardiac murmurs	Over abdominal aorta	Partial arterial obstruction or turbulent blood flow
	Over renal artery	Renal artery stenosis
	Over iliac artery	Iliac artery obstruction
Venous hum		
Continuous, medium-pitched tone created by blood flow in a large engorged vascular organ such as the liver	Epigastric and umbilical regions	Increased collateral circulation between portal and systemic venous systems, such as in cirrhosis
Friction rub		
Harsh, grating sound like two pieces of sandpaper rubbing together	Over liver and spleen	Inflammation of the peritoneal surface of the liver, such as from a tumor or splenic infarct from an interruption in oxygen supply to the spleen

Abdominal percussion

Use abdominal percussion to determine the size and location of abdominal organs and detect excessive accumulation of fluid and air. Begin percussion in the right lower quadrant and proceed clockwise, covering all four quadrants. Keep the approximate locations of the patient's organs in mind as you progress. Use direct or indirect percussion:

- In *direct* percussion, strike your hand or finger directly over the patient's abdomen.
- With *indirect* percussion, use the middle finger of your dominant hand or a percussion hammer to strike a finger resting on the patient's abdomen.

Percussion precaution

Don't percuss the abdomen of a patient with an abdominal aortic aneurysm or a transplanted abdominal organ. Doing so can precipitate a rupture or organ rejection.

Tympany and dullness

Normally, you should hear two sounds during percussion of the abdomen: tympany and dullness. When you percuss over hollow organs, such as an empty stomach or bowel, you should hear a clear, hollow sound like a drum beating. This sound, *tympany*, predominates because air is normally present in the stomach and bowel. The degree of tympany depends on the amount of air and gastric dilation.

When you percuss over solid organs, such as the liver, kidney, or feces-filled intestines, the sound changes to dullness. Note where percussed sounds change from tympany to dullness, which may indicate a solid mass or enlarged organ.

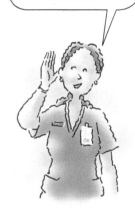

Tympany should be the predominant sound you hear when percussing the abdomen.

Abdominal palpation

Abdominal palpation includes light and deep touch to determine the size, shape, position, and tenderness of major abdominal organs and detect masses and fluid accumulation. Palpate all four quadrants, leaving painful and tender areas for last.

Light palpation

Use light palpation to identify muscle resistance or guarding and tenderness as well as the location of some superficial organs. To do so, gently press your fingertips ½″ to ¾″ (1.5 to 2 cm) into the abdominal wall. Use the lightest touch possible because too much pressure blunts your sensitivity.

Rebound tenderness

To test for rebound tenderness, help the patient into a supine position with knees flexed to relax the abdominal muscles. Place your hands gently on the right lower quadrant at McBurney point (located about midway between the umbilicus and the anterior superior iliac spine). Slowly and deeply dip your fingers into the area and then release the pressure in a quick, smooth motion. Pain on release—rebound tenderness—is a positive sign. The pain may radiate to the umbilicus.

Caution: To minimize the risk of rupturing an inflamed appendix, don't repeat this maneuver.

Deep palpation

The use of deep palpation by pressing the fingertips of both hands about 1½″ (3.5 cm) into the abdominal wall is usually reserved for the health care provider or advanced practice nurse. Deep palpation can help with diagnosis by eliciting pain and/or palpating organs.

Assessing the liver

You can estimate the size and position of the liver through percussion and palpation.

Percussing the liver

Begin percussing the abdomen along the right midclavicular line, starting below the level of the umbilicus. Move upward until the percussion notes change from tympany to dullness, usually at or slightly below the costal margin. Mark the point of change with a felt-tip pen.

Then percuss downward along the right midclavicular line, starting above the nipple. Move downward until percussion notes change from normal lung resonance to dullness, usually at the fifth to seventh intercostal space. Again, mark the point of change with a felt-tip pen. Estimate liver size by measuring the distance between the two marks.

Anatomic landmarks for liver percussion

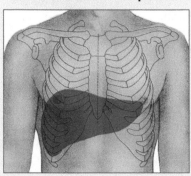

Hand position for liver percussion

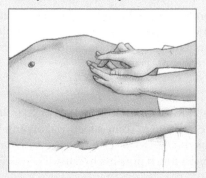

Percussion discussion

Percussing the liver allows you to estimate its size. Hepatomegaly is commonly associated with hepatitis and other liver disease. Liver borders may be obscured and difficult to assess. (See *Percussing the liver*.)

Palpation problem

It's usually impossible to palpate the liver in an adult patient. If palpable, the liver border feels smooth and firm, with a rounded, regular edge. A palpable liver may indicate hepatomegaly. To palpate for hepatomegaly:
1. Start at the lower left quadrant.
2. Have the patient take a deep breath and hold it while you palpate using the tips of your fingers.
3. Slowly move your hand up toward the costal margin and palpate while the patient exhales.

Assessing the rectum

If your patient is aged 40 or older, a rectal examination may be part of your GI assessment. Explain the procedure to reassure the patient.

To perform a rectal examination, first inspect the perianal area following these steps:

- Put on gloves and spread the buttocks to expose the anus and surrounding tissue, checking for fissures, lesions, scars, inflammation, discharge, rectal prolapse, and external hemorrhoids.
- Ask the patient to strain as if having a bowel movement; this may reveal internal hemorrhoids, polyps, or fissures.

Supporting role in rectal examinations

After examining the perianal area, palpate the rectum (the nurse's role in this procedure may be supportive only, i.e., having supplies):

- Apply a water-soluble lubricant to your gloved index finger. Tell the patient to relax. Explain pressure may be felt but it should not be painful.
- Insert your finger into the rectum toward the umbilicus. To palpate, rotate your finger. The walls should feel soft and smooth without masses, fecal impaction, or tenderness.
- Remove your finger from the rectum and inspect the glove for stool, blood, or mucus. Test fecal material adhering to the glove for occult blood using a guaiac test.

Assessing the spleen

- Unless the spleen is enlarged, it isn't palpable. The health care provider or nurse practitioner may attempt to palpate the spleen. The health care provider will stand on the patient's right side using the left hand to support the patient's posterior left lower rib cage and ask the patient to take a deep breath. Then with the right hand on the patient's abdomen, the health care provider will press up and in toward the spleen.

Diagnostic tests

Many tests provide information to guide your care of a patient with a GI emergency. Even if you don't participate in testing, you should know why the test was ordered; what the results mean; and what your responsibilities are before, during, and after the test. Diagnostic tests commonly ordered include abdominal X-ray, colonoscopy, computed tomography (CT) scan, esophagogastroduodenoscopy (EGD), fecal studies, liver-spleen scan, magnetic resonance imaging (MRI), ultrasound, and peritoneal fluid analysis.

Abdominal X-ray

An abdominal X-ray, also called *flat plate of the abdomen* or *kidney–ureter–bladder radiography*, is used to detect and evaluate tumors, kidney stones, abnormal gas collection, and other abdominal disorders. The test consists of two plates: one taken with the patient supine and the other taken while the patient stands.

Reading the rays

On X-ray, air appears black, fat appears gray, and bone appears white. Although a routine X-ray doesn't reveal most abdominal organs, it does show the contrast between air and fluid. For example, intestinal blockage traps large amounts of detectable fluids and air inside organs. When an intestinal wall tears, air leaks into the abdomen and becomes visible on X-ray.

Practice pointers

- Explain the procedure to the patient.
- Radiography requires no special pretest or posttest care. It's usually done at the bedside using portable X-ray equipment.

Colonoscopy

Colonoscopy, also referred to as *lower GI endoscopy*, is used to:
- diagnose inflammatory and ulcerative bowel disease
- pinpoint lower GI bleeding
- detect lower GI abnormalities, such as tumors, polyps, hemorrhoids, and abscesses.

Practice pointers

- Explain the procedure and its purpose and tell the patient an intravenous (IV) premedication and conscious sedation for the procedure will be given.
- Make sure that an informed consent form has been signed.
- Check the time that the patient last ate; if possible, withhold all fluids and food for at least 6 to 8 hours before the test.
- Assist with bowel preparation as indicated.
- To decrease the risk of aspiration in a patient receiving electrolyte lavage solution through an NG tube, ensure proper tube placement and elevate the head of the bed or assist the patient into the side-lying position. Have suction equipment available. (See *Lavage: Increased risk in older adult patients*.)
- Warn the patient an urge to defecate may occur when the scope is inserted; encourage slow, deep breathing through the mouth, as appropriate.

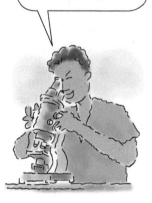

Colonoscopy provides a direct view of visceral linings using fiber optics. Good thing the instruments used are a lot smaller than this!

- Initiate an IV line if one isn't already in place for a patient who will be receiving conscious sedation.
- Obtain the patient's baseline vital signs and oxygen saturation levels. Monitor cardiac rhythm.
- Administer medications as ordered, such as midazolam for sedation. Provide supplemental oxygen as ordered.
- During the procedure, monitor the patient's vital signs, airway patency, oxygen saturation, cardiac rhythm, skin color, abdominal distention, level of consciousness (LOC), and pain tolerance.

Postprocedure

- After the procedure, assess your patient's vital signs and cardiopulmonary status, breath sounds, oxygen saturation, and LOC every 15 minutes for the first hour, every 30 minutes for the next hour, and then hourly until the patient stabilizes.
- Administer supplemental oxygen as ordered and as indicated by oxygen saturation levels.
- Watch for adverse effects of sedation, such as respiratory depression, apnea, hypotension, excessive diaphoresis, bradycardia, and laryngospasm. Notify the health care provider if any occur.
- Assess the patient's stool for evidence of frank or occult bleeding.
- Monitor the patient for signs and symptoms of perforation, such as vomiting, severe abdominal pain, abdominal distention or rigidity, and fever. Notify the health care provider if any occur.
- Document the procedure, interventions, and assessment findings.

Ages and stages

Lavage: Increased risk in older adult patients

Older adult patients are at increased risk for experiencing adverse effects from lavage solution, including nausea, vomiting, abdominal cramps, abdominal fullness, dizziness, and fluid and electrolyte imbalances. What's more, older adult patients may have difficulty ingesting the required amount of solution because of these adverse effects.

CT scan

In a CT scan, a computer translates multiple X-ray beams into three-dimensional oscilloscope images of the patient's biliary tract, liver, and pancreas. The test can be done with or without a contrast medium, but contrast is preferred unless the patient is allergic to contrast media.

Scads of scans

CT scan is used to:
- distinguish between obstructive and nonobstructive jaundice
- identify abscesses, cysts, hematomas, tumors, and pseudocysts
- evaluate the cause of weight loss and look for occult malignancy
- diagnose and evaluate pancreatitis.

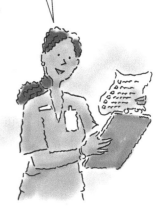

CT scans evaluate everything from A to P—abscesses to pancreatitis—and more.

Practice pointers

- Explain the procedure to the patient and tell the patient to lie still, relax, and breathe normally during the test. Explain that if the health care provider orders an IV contrast medium, the patient may experience discomfort from the needle puncture and a localized feeling of warmth on injection.
- Ascertain when the patient last ate or drank; restrict food and fluids as soon as possible, but continue any drug regimen as ordered.
- Confirm if the patient has an allergy to iodine or shellfish. If the patient has a seafood or dye allergy, the patient may be premedicated with drugs containing prednisone and diphenhydramine as ordered to reduce the risk of a reaction to the dye. Report immediately any adverse reactions, such as nausea, vomiting, dizziness, headache, and urticaria.
- If the patient is on nothing-by-mouth (NPO) status, increase the IV fluid rate as ordered after the procedure to flush the contrast medium from the patient's system. Monitor serum creatinine and blood urea nitrogen levels for signs of acute renal failure, which may be caused by the contrast medium.

Ultrasound

Abdominal ultrasound uses high-frequency sound waves to produce two-dimensional images of the body's soft tissues, which are used for a variety of clinical applications, including diagnosis and guidance of treatment procedures. Ultrasound does not use ionizing radiation to produce images, and, in comparison to other diagnostic imaging modalities, it is inexpensive, safe, fast, and versatile, often being done at the bedside.

Practice pointers
Before the procedure

- Explain the procedure and its purpose to the patient.
- Initiate or maintain NPO status.
- Determine the need for a full urinary bladder and inform patient accordingly.

EGD

EGD, also called *upper GI endoscopy*, is used to identify abnormalities of the esophagus, stomach, and small intestine, such as esophagitis, inflammatory bowel disease, Mallory–Weiss syndrome, lesions, tumors, gastritis, and polyps.

EGD focuses on the esophagus, stomach, and small intestine.

Practice pointers

Before the procedure

- Explain the procedure and its purpose to the patient.
- Tell the patient that an IV premedication and conscious sedation will be administered during the procedure as well as a local anesthetic spray for the patient's mouth and nose.
- Make sure that an informed consent form has been signed.
- Insert an NG tube to aspirate contents and minimize the risk of aspiration.
- Make sure that the patient's dentures and eyeglasses are removed before the test.
- If the procedure is to be performed at the bedside, have the necessary equipment available for the procedure and initiate an IV line if one isn't already in place.
- Monitor the patient before and throughout the procedure, including airway patency, vital signs, oxygen saturation, cardiac rhythm, abdominal distention, LOC, and pain tolerance.

After the procedure

- Monitor the patient's vital signs, oxygen saturation, cardiac rhythm, and LOC.
- Administer oxygen therapy as ordered.
- Place the patient in a side-lying position with the head of the bed flat until sedation wears off.
- Withhold all food and fluids until the patient's gag reflex returns. After it does, offer ice chips and sips of water, gradually increasing the patient's intake as tolerated and allowed.
- Observe for adverse effects of sedation, such as respiratory depression, apnea, hypotension, excessive diaphoresis, bradycardia, and laryngospasm. Notify the health care provider if any occur.
- Monitor the patient for signs and symptoms of perforation, such as difficulty swallowing, pain, fever, and bleeding indicated by black stools or bloody vomitus.
- Document the procedure, interventions, and assessment findings.

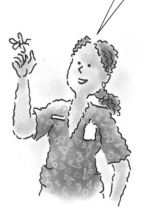

Remember to keep an eye out for adverse effects of sedation.

Fecal studies

Normal stool appears brown and formed but soft. These abnormal findings may indicate a problem:

- Narrow, ribbonlike stool signals spastic or irritable bowel, partial bowel obstruction, or rectal obstruction.
- Constipation may be caused by diet or medications.
- Diarrhea may indicate spastic bowel or viral infection.

- Mixed with blood and mucus, soft stool can signal bacterial infection; mixed with blood or pus, colitis.
- Yellow or green stool suggests severe, prolonged diarrhea; black stool suggests GI bleeding or intake of iron supplements or raw-to-rare meat. Tan or white stool shows hepatic duct or gallbladder duct blockage, hepatitis, or cancer. Red stool may signal colon or rectal bleeding; however, drugs and foods can also cause this coloration.
- Most stools contain 10% to 20% fat. A higher fat content can turn stool pasty or greasy, a possible sign of intestinal malabsorption or pancreatic disease.

Practice pointers

- Collect the stool specimen in a clean, dry container and immediately send it to the laboratory.
- Don't use stool that has been in contact with toilet bowl water or urine.
- Use commercial fecal occult blood slides as a simple method of testing for blood in stool. Follow package directions because certain medications and foods can interfere with test results.

MRI

MRI is used to examine the liver and abdominal organs. It's useful in evaluating liver disease by characterizing tumors, masses, or cysts found on previous studies. An image is generated by energizing protons in a strong magnetic field. Radio waves emitted as protons return to their former equilibrium and are recorded. No ionizing radiation transmits during the scan.

MRI mire

Disadvantages of MRI include the closed, tubelike space required for the scan. Newer MRI centers offer a less confining "open MRI" scan. In addition, the test can't be performed on patients with implanted metal prostheses or devices. If time is of the essence, an MRI may not be used due to the procedure taking 30 minutes to 1 hour.

Practice pointers

- Explain the procedure to the patient and stress the need to remove metal objects such as jewelry before the procedure.
- Explain to the patient to lie still for 1 to 1.5 hours for the procedure.
- Generally, you'll accompany the patient to the MRI suite. If the patient becomes claustrophobic during the test, administer mild sedation as ordered.

Peritoneal fluid analysis

Peritoneal fluid analysis includes examination of gross appearance; erythrocyte and leukocyte counts; cytologic studies; microbiological studies for bacteria and fungi; and determinations of protein, glucose, amylase, ammonia, and alkaline phosphatase levels.

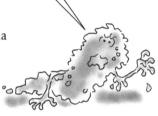

Bacteria like me can find a home in peritoneal fluid, but after peritoneal fluid analysis, I might get evicted.

Peritoneal through paracentesis

Abdominal paracentesis is a bedside procedure involving aspiration of fluid from the peritoneal space through a needle, trocar, or cannula inserted in the abdominal wall.

Paracentesis is used to:
- diagnose and treat massive ascites resistant to other therapy
- detect intra-abdominal bleeding after traumatic injury
- obtain a peritoneal fluid sample for laboratory analysis
- decrease intra-abdominal pressure and alleviate dyspnea.

Practice pointers
- Explain the procedure to the patient.
- Make sure that an informed consent form has been signed.
- Instruct the patient to empty his or her bladder. Usually, an indwelling urinary catheter is inserted.
- Record the patient's baseline vital signs, weight, and abdominal girth. Indicate the abdominal area measured with a felt-tipped marking pen.

During . . .

- The trocar is inserted with the patient supine. After insertion, assist the patient to sit up in bed. (See *Positioning for abdominal paracentesis*, page 286.)
- Remind the patient to remain as still as possible during the procedure.
- Throughout the procedure, monitor the patient's vital signs, oxygen saturation, and cardiac rhythm every 15 minutes and observe for tachycardia, hypotension, dizziness, pallor, diaphoresis, and increased anxiety, especially if the health care provider aspirates more than 1,500 mL of peritoneal fluid at one time.
- If the patient shows signs of hypovolemic shock, slow the drainage rate by raising the collection container vertically, so it's closer to the height of the needle, trocar, or cannula. Stop the drainage if necessary. Limit aspirated fluid to between 1,500 and 2,000 mL.
- After the health care provider removes the needle, trocar, or cannula and, if necessary, sutures the incision, apply a dry sterile pressure dressing.

Positioning for abdominal paracentesis

When positioning a patient for abdominal paracentesis, help the patient to sit up in bed or allow the patient to sit on the edge of the bed with additional support for the patient's back and arms.

In this position, gravity causes fluid to accumulate in the lower abdominal cavity. The internal organs provide counter-resistance and pressure to aid fluid flow.

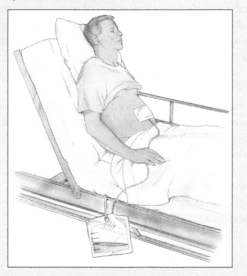

. . . and after

After the procedure

- Monitor the patient's vital signs, oxygen saturation, and cardiac rhythm and check the dressing for drainage every 15 minutes for the first hour, every 30 minutes for the next 2 hours, every hour for 4 hours, and then every 4 hours for 24 hours.
- Observe the patient for signs of hemorrhage or shock, such as hypotension, tachycardia, pallor, and excessive diaphoresis. These signs may indicate puncture of the inferior epigastric artery, hematoma of the anterior cecal wall, or rupture of the iliac vein or bladder. Observe for hematuria.
- Observe the patient for signs of a perforated intestine, such as increasing pain or abdominal tenderness.
- Document the procedure and record the patient's weight and abdominal girth to detect recurrent ascites.

Treatments

GI emergencies present many treatment challenges because they stem from various mechanisms occurring separately or simultaneously, including tumors, hyperactivity and hypoactivity, malabsorption, infection and inflammation, vascular disorders, intestinal obstruction, and degenerative disease. Treatment options include drug therapy and GI intubation.

Drug therapy

Drug therapy may be used for such disorders as acute GI bleeding, peptic ulcer disease, and hepatic failure. Some of the most commonly used drugs in critical care include ammonia detoxicants, antacids, antidiuretic hormone, antiemetics, histamine-2 (H_2) receptor antagonists, and proton pump inhibitors.

How fast?

Some of these drugs, such as antacids and antiemetics, provide relief immediately. Other drugs, such as ammonia detoxicants and H_2-receptor antagonists, may take several days or longer to alleviate the problem. (See *Watch out for sedatives* and *Common GI drugs*, page 288.)

GI intubation

NG and other specialized tubes may be used in treating the patient with acute intestinal obstruction, bleeding, esophageal varices, or another GI dysfunction.

Gastric lavage

Gastric lavage may be an emergency treatment for the patient with GI hemorrhage caused by peptic ulcer disease or ruptured esophageal or gastric varices and as emergency treatment for some drug overdoses. It involves intubation with a large-bore, single- or double-lumen tube; instillation of irrigating fluid; and aspiration of gastric contents.

Rarely seen

Complications are rare and include:
- bradycardia
- electrolyte imbalance or metabolic acidosis
- fluid overload
- vomiting and aspiration.

Nursing considerations
- Explain the procedure to the patient.
- Determine the length of the tube for insertion. (See *Measuring NG tube length*, page 290.)

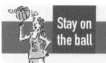

Stay on the ball

Watch out for sedatives

Administer sedatives cautiously in a patient with underlying liver disease. Be sure to establish a baseline for the patient's level of consciousness (LOC) before administering the medication to ensure valid assessments of the patient's LOC after the medication has been given.

Common GI drugs

This chart lists common gastrointestinal (GI) drugs along with their indications and adverse reactions.

Drugs	Indications	Adverse reactions
Ammonia detoxicant		
Lactulose	• To prevent and treat portosystemic encepha-lopathy in patients with severe hepatic disease (increasing clearance of nitrogenous products and decreasing serum ammonia levels through laxative effects) • Laxative to treat constipation	Abdominal cramps, diarrhea, flatulence
Antacids		
Aluminum hydroxide	• Antacid used for heartburn, acid indigestion, and adjunct therapy with peptic ulcer disease	Constipation, intestinal obstruction, encephalopathy
Aluminum hydroxide and magnesium hydroxide (Maalox)	• Antacid used for heartburn, acid indigestion, and adjunct therapy with peptic ulcer disease	Diarrhea, hypermagnesemia in patients with severe renal impairment
Calcium carbonate (Caltrate)	• Antacid used for heartburn, acid indigestion, and adjunct therapy with peptic ulcer disease • Calcium supplement	Nausea, vomiting, possibly hypercalcemia (with excessive use)
Antidiuretic hormone		
Vasopressin	• Administered intravenously or intra-arterially to decrease splanchnic blood flow, reducing portal pressure; for treatment in acute GI	Cardiac ischemia, chest pain, hyperten-sion, acute heart failure, dysrhythmias, bowel ischemia and cerebrovascular accident (Urden et al., 2018)
Antiemetics		
Ondansetron (Zofran)	• Prevention and treatment of postoperative nau-sea and vomiting and in conjunction with cancer chemotherapy	Diarrhea, arrhythmias, electrocar-diogram changes (prolonged PR and QT intervals and widened QRS complex), liver test abnormalities, pruritus
Metoclopramide (Reglan)	• Prevention and treatment of postoperative nau-sea and vomiting and in conjunction with cancer chemotherapy • Delayed gastric emptying secondary to diabetic gastroparesis	Restlessness, anxiety, depression, sui-cidal ideation, seizures, bradycardia, bronchospasm, transient hypertension

Common GI drugs *(continued)*

Drugs	Indications	Adverse reactions
Histamine-2 receptor antagonists		
Famotidine (Pepcid)	• Treatment of duodenal and gastric ulcers, gastroesophageal reflux disease (GERD), and Zollinger–Ellison syndrome • Prevention of gastric stress ulcers	Headache, palpitations, diarrhea, constipation
Ranitidine (Zantac)	• Treatment of duodenal and gastric ulcers, GERD, and Zollinger–Ellison syndrome • Prevention of gastric stress ulcers	Malaise, reversible confusion, depression or hallucinations, blurred vision, jaundice, leukopenia, angioedema
Proton pump inhibitors		
Lansoprazole (Prevacid), omeprazole (Prilosec), pantoprazole (Protonix)	• Treatment of duodenal and gastric ulcers, erosive esophagitis, GERD, Zollinger–Ellison syndrome, and *Helicobacter pylori* eradication • Prophylaxis for gastric stress ulcer (in critically ill patients)	Diarrhea, abdominal pain, nausea, constipation, chest pain, dizziness, hyperglycemia

Adapted from Aggarwal, A., & Bhatt, M. (2014). Commonly used gastrointestinal drugs. *Handbook of Clinical Neurology*, 120, 633–643. doi:10.1016/B978-0-7020-4087-0.00043-7; Burchum, J., & Rosenthal, L. (2019). *Lehne's pharmacology for nursing care* (10th ed.). St. Louis, MO: Elsevier; and Urden, L., Stacy, K., & Lough, M. (2018). *Critical care nursing: Diagnosis and management* (8th ed.). St. Louis, MO: Elsevier.

- Lubricate the end of the tube with a water-soluble lubricant and insert it into the patient's mouth or nostril as ordered. Advance the tube through the pharynx and esophagus and into the stomach.
- Check the tube for placement by attaching a piston or bulb syringe and aspirating stomach contents. Examine the aspirate and place a small amount on the pH test strip. Probability of gastric placement is increased if the aspirate has a typical gastric fluid appearance (grassy-green, clear and colorless with mucus shreds, or brown) and has a pH of less than or equal to 5. (Follow your facility policy for checking placement.)
- When the tube is in place, lower the head of the bed to 15 degrees and reposition the patient on the left side, if possible.
- Fill the syringe with 30 to 50 mL of irrigating solution and begin instillation. Instill about 250 mL of fluid, wait 30 seconds, and then begin to withdraw the fluid into the syringe. If you can't withdraw any fluid, allow the tube to drain into an emesis basin.
- If the health care provider orders a vasoconstrictor to be added to the irrigating fluid, wait for the prescribed period before withdrawing fluid to allow absorption of the drug into the gastric mucosa.

Don't worry, I'll be back. I know it means trouble when the fluid return doesn't at least equal the fluid instilled during lavage.

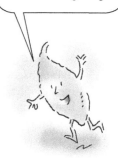

Measuring NG tube length

To determine how long the nasogastric tube must be to reach the stomach, hold the end of the tube at the tip of the patient's nose. Extend the tube to the patient's earlobe and then down to the xiphoid process.

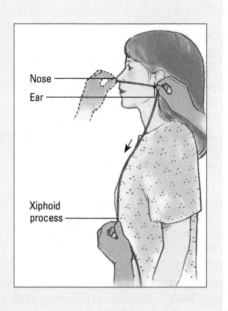

Nose

Ear

Xiphoid process

Fluid watch

- Carefully measure and record fluid return. If the volume of fluid return doesn't at least equal the amount of fluid instilled, abdominal distention and vomiting result.
- Continue lavage until return fluid is clear or as ordered. Remove the tube or secure it as ordered. If appropriate, send lavage specimens to the laboratory for toxicology studies and send gastric contents for pH and guaiac studies.
- Never leave the patient alone during gastric lavage.
- Monitor the patient's cardiac rhythm and observe for possible complications, such as bradycardia, hypovolemia, vomiting, and aspiration.
- Monitor the patient's vital signs and oxygen saturation every 30 minutes until the patient's condition stabilizes.
- Document the procedure and any appropriate interventions.

Multilumen esophageal tube placement

In esophagogastric tamponade, an emergency treatment, a multilumen esophageal tube is inserted to control esophageal or gastric hemorrhage resulting from ruptured varices. It's usually a tentative measure until sclerotherapy can be done. (See *Comparing esophageal tubes.*)

Comparing esophageal tubes

There are three common types of esophageal tubes: the Linton tube, the Minnesota esophagogastric tamponade tube, and the Sengstaken–Blakemore tube.

Linton tube

The Linton tube, a three-lumen, single-balloon device, has ports for esophageal and gastric aspiration. Because the tube doesn't have an esophageal balloon, it isn't used to control bleeding for esophageal varices.

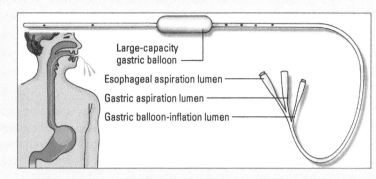

Large-capacity gastric balloon

Esophageal aspiration lumen

Gastric aspiration lumen

Gastric balloon-inflation lumen

Minnesota esophagogastric tamponade tube

The Minnesota esophagogastric tamponade tube has four lumens and two balloons. It has pressure-monitoring ports for both balloons.

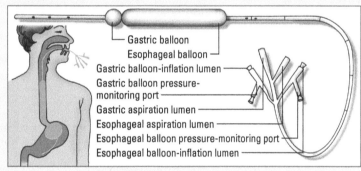

Gastric balloon

Esophageal balloon

Gastric balloon-inflation lumen

Gastric balloon pressure-monitoring port

Gastric aspiration lumen

Esophageal aspiration lumen

Esophageal balloon pressure-monitoring port

Esophageal balloon-inflation lumen

Sengstaken–Blakemore tube

The Sengstaken–Blakemore tube, a three-lumen device with esophageal and gastric balloons, has a gastric aspiration port that allows drainage from below the gastric balloon and is also used to instill medication.

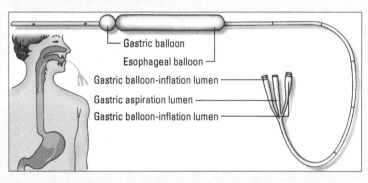

Gastric balloon

Esophageal balloon

Gastric balloon-inflation lumen

Gastric aspiration lumen

Gastric balloon-inflation lumen

The tube is inserted through a nostril, or sometimes the mouth, and then passed into the stomach. The tube's esophageal and gastric balloons are inflated to exert pressure on the varices to stop bleeding, whereas a lumen allows esophageal and gastric contents to be aspirated. Balloon inflation for longer than 48 hours may cause pressure necrosis, which can lead to further hemorrhage. Follow your facility's policy and procedure for balloon inflation and deflation.

Nursing considerations
Before the procedure
- Describe the procedure to the patient. Explain that a helmet may be used to apply traction to keep balloon pressure at the gastro-esophageal junction. Place the patient in semi-Fowler position. (If unconscious, place the patient on the left side, with the head of the bed elevated to 15 degrees.) An unresponsive patient may also require endotracheal intubation.
- Tape a pair of scissors to the head of the bed in case of acute respiratory distress.
- Check tube balloons for air leaks and patency before insertion.
- Never leave the patient alone during tamponade.

When it's done

After the procedure
- Closely monitor the patient's condition and lumen pressure. If the pressure changes or decreases, check for bleeding and notify the health care provider immediately.
- Monitor the patient's cardiac rhythm, vital signs, and oxygen saturation every 30 to 60 minutes. A change may indicate new bleeding.
- Monitor the patient's respiratory status and observe for respiratory distress. If respiratory distress develops, have someone notify the health care provider. If the airway is obstructed, cut both balloon ports and remove the tube. Notify the health care provider immediately.
- Maintain suction on the ports. Irrigate the gastric aspiration port to prevent clogging.
- Deflate the esophageal balloon for about 30 minutes every 12 hours or according to your facility's policy and procedure.
- Observe the patient for signs of esophageal rupture, such as shock, increased respiratory difficulty, and increased bleeding. Notify the health care provider if such signs are present.
- Keep the patient warm, comfortable, and as still as possible.

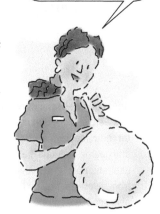

Check your facility's policy for how often you should deflate the patient's esophageal balloon.

Nasoenteric decompression tube
The nasoenteric decompression tube is used to aspirate intestinal contents for analysis and to correct intestinal obstruction. It's inserted nasally and advanced beyond the stomach into the intestinal

Common nasoenteric decompression tubes

The type of nasoenteric decompression tube chosen for your patient will depend on the size of the patient and nostrils, the estimated duration of intubation, and the reason for the procedure.

Most tubes are impregnated with a radiopaque mark so that placement can easily be confirmed by X-ray or another imaging technique. Among the most commonly used types of nasoenteric tubes are the Levin and Salem–Sump. (There are other tubes available, but the two listed here are the most commonly used in the emergency department.)

Levin

The Levin tube is a single-lumen tube. It may be used to relieve bowel obstructions and to aspirate intestinal contents.

Salem–Sump

The Salem–Sump tube is a double-lumen tube. It is primarily used for decompression and aspiration. It may also be used to install medications or fluids. The advantage of the Salem–Sump tube is the second lumen allows for continuous suctioning with minimal to no damage to the mucosal lining.

tract. The tube may also prevent nausea, vomiting, and abdominal distention after GI surgery. (See *Common nasoenteric decompression tubes.*)

Nursing considerations

The patient with a nasoenteric decompression tube needs special care and continuous monitoring to:

- ensure tube patency
- maintain suction and bowel decompression
- detect such complications as fluid and electrolyte imbalance.

Dealing with obstruction

If your patient's tube appears to be obstructed, follow your facility's policy and procedure and notify the health care provider if you're unable to restore patency. The health care provider may order such measures as those described here to restore patency quickly and efficiently:

- First, disconnect the tube from suction and irrigate with normal saline solution. Use gravity flow to help clear the obstruction unless otherwise ordered.
- If irrigation doesn't reestablish patency, the tube may be obstructed by its position against the gastric mucosa. Tug slightly on the tube to move it away from the mucosa.
- If gently tugging doesn't work, the tube may be kinked and need additional manipulation. However, don't reposition or irrigate a tube in a patient who had GI surgery, in one who had the tube inserted during surgery (because this may disturb new sutures), or in a patient who was difficult to intubate.

Common disorders

GI disorders commonly encountered in the ED include abdominal trauma, acute GI bleeding, appendicitis, cholecystitis, and diverticulitis.

Abdominal trauma

Abdominal trauma accounts for approximately one-fourth of all trauma events and is associated with a high rate of morbidity and mortality. It can occur as a single event or be associated with multiple injuries, further compounding their seriousness.

What causes it

Abdominal trauma is commonly classified as *penetrating* or *blunt*, depending on the type of injury.

An explosive situation

Penetrating abdominal trauma involves an injury by a foreign object, such as a knife (the most common cause of stabbing injury), bullet (the most common cause of missile injury), pitchfork, or other pointed object that penetrates the abdomen.

Typically, penetrating abdominal trauma is fairly limited, usually involving isolated organs and lacerated tissues. In some cases, however, extensive tissue damage can occur if a bullet explodes in the abdominal cavity.

To put it bluntly

Blunt abdominal trauma results from sudden compression or positive pressure inflicted by a direct blow to the organ and surrounding tissue. Blunt abdominal trauma commonly occurs in motor vehicle collisions, assaults, and falls. Of these, blunt abdominal trauma from motor vehicle collisions is the most common.

Blunt abdominal trauma can cause extensive injury to the peritoneum and abdominal organs. The liver and spleen are the two organs most commonly injured from blunt abdominal trauma. The other organs, such as the stomach, intestines, and pancreas, as well as the diaphragm and vascular structures, can also be injured, although these injuries are less common.

Blunt abdominal trauma is commonly caused by car collisions and commonly affects the liver. Now I'm uncommonly scared to drive.

How it happens

Injuries to the abdomen usually involve one or more of these conditions:

- hypovolemia resulting from massive fluid or blood loss, especially if the spleen is injured
- hypoxemia resulting from damage to the diaphragm or associated chest trauma
- respiratory or cardiac failure resulting from associated chest injury.

Tissue damage caused by penetrating trauma, such as an impaled object or foreign body, is related to the object size as well as the depth and velocity of penetration. For example, penetrating abdominal trauma from a bullet has many variables; the extent of injury depends on the distance at which the weapon was fired, the type of ammunition, the velocity of the ammunition, and the entrance and (if present) exit wounds.

Other considerations

Additional factors to consider when assessing the extent of abdominal trauma from a bullet include type of weapon; caliber, barrel, and length of the gun; and powder composition. An intact bullet causes less damage than a bullet that explodes on impact. A bullet that explodes within the abdomen may break up and scatter fragments, burn tissue, fracture bone, disrupt vascular structures, or cause a bullet embolism.

Trauma physics

Injury resulting from blunt abdominal trauma is related to the amount of force, compression, and cavitation. Blunt force that strikes the abdomen at high velocity transfers that force to underlying organs and tissue. The direct impact of force is transmitted internally and the energy dissipates to internal structures.

Think of "the FCC"—force, compression, and cavitation—as you evaluate blunt trauma's impact.

Buckle up

Recently, seat belts have been associated with a blunt abdominal trauma. Referred to as "seat belt syndrome," abdominal injury in a motor vehicle collision in which the patient was wearing a seat belt can involve injuries to the large and small intestines, liver, spleen, abdominal vessels, and, possibly, the lumbar spine.

Stay on the ball

Identifying injuries to the liver and spleen

The liver and spleen are the two organs most commonly injured from abdominal trauma.

Spleen signs

When performing your assessment, suspect injury to the spleen if your patient:
- has a history of blunt trauma to the left upper quadrant
- reports pain or exhibits bruising in the left upper quadrant
- demonstrates a positive Kehr sign (evidence of left shoulder pain due to irritation of the diaphragm with blood from the peritoneum).

Liver look-fors

Suspect a liver injury if your patient:
- has a history of direct trauma to the right upper quadrant (between the eighth rib and central abdominal area)
- has pain or bruising over the right upper quadrant
- reports referred pain to the right shoulder
- demonstrates hemodynamic instability.

Memory jogger

To help remember what information to obtain during assessment of the patient with abdominal trauma, use the acronym SAMPLE:

Signs and symptoms

Allergies

Medications

Past medical history

Last meal

Events leading to injury.

What to look for

Assessment findings may vary based on the type and extent of abdominal trauma. In some cases, the patient may be asymptomatic, especially if the trauma occurred days or weeks before the patient arrives at the ED. In other situations, the patient may have multiple injuries and a severely compromised status that require immediate intervention.

Have a look-see

When assessing the patient with abdominal trauma, be alert for:
- bruising, abrasions, and lacerations of the abdomen (See *Identifying injuries to the liver and spleen.*)
- bruising along the area of the seat belt line
- positive Grey Turner sign (purplish discoloration along the flank) or Cullen sign (purplish discoloration around the umbilicus)
- obvious wounds, such as gunshot wounds or stab wounds
- change in bowel sounds (The presence of bowel sounds in the chest suggests diaphragmatic rupture and should be reported immediately.)
- pain, rigidity, tenderness, or guarding on palpation.

What tests tell you

Diagnostic testing depends on the patient's condition and extent of injuries. In addition, diagnostic tests performed are based on the area affected by the trauma. Some possible diagnostic tests include:

- peritoneal lavage to detect blood in the peritoneal cavity
- CT scan, which may reveal hemorrhage, hematomas, or skeletal injuries
- ultrasonography, which may show free fluid in the abdominal cavity
- abdominal and chest X-rays to detect fluid, free air, ileus, or rupture of the diaphragm
- pelvic X-rays, which may demonstrate bony abnormalities.
  Other tests that may be performed include:
- arterial blood gas (ABG) analysis to evaluate respiratory and acid–base status
- complete blood count (CBC) to evaluate degree of blood loss
- coagulation studies to determine the patient's clotting ability
- serum electrolyte levels to determine possible imbalances.

How it's treated

Treatment of abdominal trauma focuses on immediately stabilizing the patient; assessing and maintaining the patient's airway, breathing, circulation, disability, and exposure and environment (ABCDE) (see *Primary assessment of the trauma patient* in Chapter 1); assessing LOC; and preparing the patient for transport and possible surgery.

If the patient has a wound, treatment may include controlling bleeding, usually by applying firm, direct pressure and cleaning the wound. Pain medication and antibiotic therapy are instituted as indicated. In addition, IV therapy is started to ensure fluid balance and maintain the patient's hemodynamic status.

What to do

- Assess the patient's ABCDE and initiate emergency measures, if necessary; administer supplemental oxygen as ordered.
- Monitor vital signs and note significant changes.
- Assess oxygen saturation and cardiac rhythm for arrhythmias. Assess neurologic status, including LOC and pupillary and motor response.
- Obtain blood studies, including type and cross-match.
- Insert two large-bore IV catheters and infuse normal saline or lactated Ringer solution as ordered.
- Quickly and carefully assess the patient for other areas of trauma.
- Assess wounds and provide wound care as appropriate. Cover open wounds and control bleeding by applying pressure.
- Assess for increased abdominal distention.
- Administer blood products as appropriate.

- Monitor for signs of hypovolemic shock.
- Provide pain medication, as appropriate.
- Prepare the patient and family for diagnostic testing and possible surgery.
- Provide reassurance and education to the patient and family.

Acute GI bleeding

GI bleeding can occur anywhere along the GI tract. Although GI bleeding stops spontaneously in most patients, acute bleeding accounts for significant morbidity and mortality.

Maybe multiple morbidities

Many patients who require emergency care experience upper GI bleeding. Additionally, they may have underlying comorbidities that contribute to the risk of upper GI bleeding, such as:
- coronary artery disease
- history of myocardial infarction
- renal failure
- history of chronic liver damage secondary to alcohol abuse or hepatitis
- history of radiation therapy
- chronic pain condition, such as arthritis, requiring treatment with NSAIDs.

What causes it

Upper GI bleeding includes bleeding in the esophagus, stomach, and duodenum. Bleeding below the Treitz ligament is considered lower GI bleeding; the most common site is in the colon.

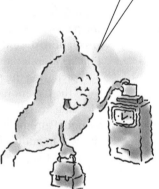

Most GI bleeding clocks out on its own, but the kind that sticks around carries a risk of morbidity and mortality.

Upper causes

Causes of upper GI bleeding include:
- angiodysplasias
- arteriovenous malformations (AVMs)
- erosive gastritis
- esophagitis
- Mallory–Weiss tear
- peptic ulcer disease
- rupture of esophageal varices.

Lower causes

The most common causes of lower GI bleeding include:
- AVMs
- diverticulitis
- hemorrhoids

- inflammatory bowel disease
- neoplasm
- polyps.

How it happens

In GI bleeding, the patient experiences a loss of circulating blood volume, regardless of the cause of bleeding. Because the arterial blood supply near the stomach and esophagus is extensive, bleeding can lead to a rapid loss of large amounts of blood, subsequent hypovolemia, and shock. Here's what else happens:

- Loss of circulating blood volume leads to a decreased venous return.
- Cardiac output and blood pressure decrease, causing poor tissue perfusion. In response, the body compensates by shifting interstitial fluid to the intravascular space.
- The sympathetic nervous system is stimulated, resulting in vasoconstriction and increased heart rate.
- The renin–angiotensin–aldosterone system is activated, leading to fluid retention and increasing blood pressure.
- If blood loss continues, cardiac output decreases, leading to cellular hypoxia. Eventually, all organs fail due to hypoperfusion.

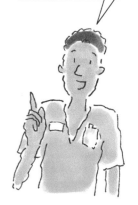

No matter what the cause, too much GI blood loss can lead to hypovolemia and shock.

What to look for

Because GI bleeding can occur anywhere along the GI tract, assessment is crucial to determine the level and possible location of bleeding.

Source signs

The appearance of blood in tube drainage, vomitus, and stool indicates the source of GI bleeding:

- *Hematemesis* (bright red blood in NG tube drainage or vomitus) typically indicates an upper GI source. However, if the blood has spent time in the stomach where it was exposed to gastric acid, the drainage or vomitus resembles coffee grounds.
- *Hematochezia* (bright red blood from the rectum) typically indicates a lower GI source of bleeding. It may also suggest an upper GI source if the transit time through the bowel was rapid.
- *Melena* (black, tarry, sticky stool) usually indicates an upper GI bleeding source. However, it can result from bleeding in the small bowel or proximal colon.

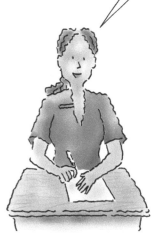

Thirty percent of total blood volume is GI bleeding's critical calculation. A patient losing more than that may go into hypovolemic shock.

Signs and symptoms

Typically, the patient exhibits signs and symptoms based on the amount and rate of bleeding. With acute GI bleeding and blood loss greater than 30% of the patient's blood volume, the patient exhibits signs and symptoms of hypovolemic shock, including:

- apprehension
- cool, clammy skin

- diaphoresis
- hypotension
- pallor
- restlessness
- syncope
- tachycardia.

What tests tell you
These findings aid in diagnosing acute GI bleeding:
- Upper GI endoscopy reveals the source of esophageal or gastric bleeding.
- CBC reveals the amount of blood loss.
- ABG analysis can indicate metabolic acidosis from hemorrhage and possible hypoxemia.
- Twelve-lead electrocardiogram (ECG) may reveal evidence of cardiac ischemia secondary to hypoperfusion.
- Abdominal X-ray may indicate air under the diaphragm, suggesting ulcer perforation.
- Angiography may aid in visualizing the bleeding site.

How it's treated
Treatment goals include stopping the bleeding and providing fluid replacement while maintaining the patient's function. Treatment may include:
- fluid volume replacement with crystalloid solutions initially, followed by colloids and blood component therapy
- respiratory support
- gastric intubation with gastric lavage (unless the patient has esophageal varices) and gastric pH monitoring
- drug therapy, such as antacids, H_2-receptor antagonists, and proton pump inhibitors
- endoscopic or surgical repair of bleeding sites.

What to do
- Type and cross-match at least 2 units of blood.
- Start at least two large-bore IV lines (16G or 18G preferred). Assess the patient for blood loss and begin fluid replacement therapy as ordered, initially delivering crystalloid solutions such as normal saline or lactated Ringer solution, followed by blood component products.
- Ensure your patient's patent airway. Monitor cardiac and respiratory status and assess LOC at least every 15 minutes until the patient stabilizes and then as indicated by the patient's condition. Assist with insertion of hemodynamic monitoring devices and assess hemodynamic parameters.

Don't forget oxygen

- Administer supplemental oxygen as ordered. Monitor oxygen saturation levels.
- Monitor the patient's skin color and capillary refill for signs of hypovolemic shock.
- Obtain serial hemoglobin and hematocrit levels. Administer albumin or blood as ordered.
- Monitor the patient's intake and output closely, including all losses from the GI tract. Check all stools and gastric drainage for occult blood.
- Assist with or insert an NG tube and perform lavage using room temperature saline to clear blood and clots from the stomach.
- Assess the patient's abdomen for bowel sounds and gastric pH as ordered. Expect to resume enteral or oral feedings after bowel function returns and when there's no evidence of further bleeding.
- Provide appropriate emotional support to the patient.
- Prepare the patient for endoscopic repair or surgery, if indicated. Anticipate transfer of the patient to the critical care unit.

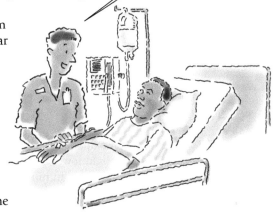

Just a little bit of emotional support can go a long way for a patient who has suffered dramatic blood loss.

Appendicitis

Appendicitis is the most common major surgical emergency. It occurs when the appendix becomes inflamed. More precisely, this disorder is an inflammation of the vermiform appendix, a small, fingerlike projection attached to the cecum just below the ileocecal valve. Although the appendix has no known function, it does regularly fill and empty itself of food.

What causes it

Appendicitis may be due to:
- barium ingestion
- fecal mass (fecalith)
- mucosal ulceration
- stricture
- viral infection.

How it happens

Mucosal ulceration triggers inflammation, which temporarily obstructs the appendix. The obstruction blocks mucus outflow. Pressure in the now-distended appendix increases, and the appendix contracts. Bacteria multiply, and inflammation and pressure continue to increase, restricting blood flow to the organ and causing severe abdominal pain.

Inflammation can lead to infection, clotting, tissue decay, and perforation of the appendix. If the appendix ruptures or perforates, the infected contents spill into the abdominal cavity, causing peritonitis, the most common and most dangerous complication (Martin, 2018).

What to look for

Initially, look for these signs or symptoms:
- abdominal pain, generalized or localized in the right lower abdomen and eventually localizing in the right lower abdomen (McBurney point)
- anorexia
- nausea and vomiting following onset of pain.
  Other signs pointing to location of inflammation of the appendix:
- McBurney point tenderness
- Rovsing sign—on palpation of the left lower abdominal quadrant, pain is felt in the right lower quadrant.
- Psoas sign—on passive right hip extension, pain is felt in the right lower quadrant.
- Obturator sign—on passive flexion of right hip and knee then internal rotation of the right hip, pain is felt in the right lower quadrant.

. . . and then later

Later, look for these signs or symptoms:
- constipation (although diarrhea is also possible)
- fever of 99° to 102° F (37.2° to 38.9° C)
- tachycardia
- increasingly severe abdominal spasms and rebound spasms (rebound tenderness on the opposite side of the abdomen suggests peritoneal inflammation). Then sudden cessation of abdominal pain (indicates perforation or infarction of the appendix).

What tests tell you

These tests help diagnose appendicitis:
- White blood cell (WBC) count is moderately elevated, with increased immature cells.
- Ultrasound of the abdomen and pelvis can be helpful in diagnosing a nonperforated appendix.
- A CT scan is now being used more often than ultrasound in the diagnosis of appendicitis.

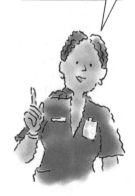

Sometimes, there's only one way to go with treatment. In the case of appendicitis, it's surgical removal.

Teaching the patient with appendicitis

• Explain what happens in appendicitis.
• Help the patient understand the required surgery and its possible complications.
• If time allows, provide preoperative teaching, including coughing and deep breathing exercises and incentive spirometry.
• Discuss postoperative care and activity limitations. Tell the patient to follow the health care provider's orders for driving, returning to work, and resuming physical activity (Gorter et al., 2016).

How it's treated

The current standard of treatment for appendicitis is an appendectomy (Smink & Soybel, 2018). An appendectomy is the only effective treatment for appendicitis. If peritonitis develops, treatment involves GI intubation, parenteral replacement of fluids and electrolytes, and administration of antibiotics.

What to do

If appendicitis is suspected or you're preparing for an appendectomy, follow these steps:

- Administer IV fluids to prevent dehydration. Never administer cathartics or enemas because they may rupture the appendix.
- Maintain the patient on NPO status and administer analgesics judiciously because they may mask symptoms of rupture.
- Place the patient in Fowler position to reduce pain. (This position is also helpful postoperatively.)
- Never apply heat to the lower right abdomen or perform palpation; these actions may cause the appendix to rupture.
- Provide support to the patient and family; prepare them for surgery as indicated.
- Begin educating the patient about his or her condition and care. (See *Teaching the patient with appendicitis*.)

Cholecystitis

Cholecystitis refers to an acute or chronic inflammation of the gallbladder, usually associated with a gallstone impacted in the cystic duct, causing painful gallbladder distention. The acute form is most common during middle age, whereas the chronic form is more common in the elderly. Prognosis is good with treatment.

What causes it

The exact cause of cholecystitis is unknown. However, certain risk factors have been identified, including:

- high-calorie, high-cholesterol diet associated with obesity
- elevated estrogen levels from hormonal contraceptives, postmeno-pausal therapy, pregnancy, or multiparity
- diabetes mellitus, ileal disease, hemolytic disorders, liver disease, or pancreatitis
- genetic factors
- weight reduction diets with severe calorie restriction and rapid weight loss.

How it happens

Certain conditions (such as age, obesity, and estrogen imbalance) cause the liver to secrete bile that's abnormally high in cholesterol or that lacks the proper concentration of bile salts. Excessive water and bile salts are reabsorbed, making the bile less soluble. Cholesterol, calcium, and bilirubin then precipitate into gallstones.

What to look for

In acute cholecystitis, look for:

- classic attack signs and symptoms with severe midepigastric or right upper quadrant pain radiating to the back or referred to the right scapula, commonly after meals rich in fats
- recurring fat intolerance
- belching that leaves a sour taste in the mouth
- flatulence
- indigestion
- diaphoresis
- nausea
- chills and low-grade fever
- possible jaundice and clay-colored stools with common duct obstruction
- local and rebound tenderness.

What tests tell you

These tests help diagnose cholecystitis:

- Ultrasonography reveals calculi in the gallbladder with 96% accuracy. Percutaneous transhepatic cholangiography distinguishes between gallbladder disease and cancer of the pancreatic head in patients with jaundice.
- CT scan may identify ductal stones.
- Endoscopic retrograde cholangiopancreatography (ERCP) visualizes the biliary tree after endoscopic examination of the duodenum, cannulation of the common bile and pancreatic ducts, and injection of a contrast medium.
- Cholescintigraphy detects obstruction of the cystic duct.

Bad to the stone

- If stones are identified in the common bile duct by radiologic examination, a therapeutic ERCP may be performed before cholecystectomy to remove the stones.
- Oral cholecystography shows calculi in the gallbladder and biliary duct obstruction.
- Laboratory tests showing an elevated icteric index and elevated total bilirubin, urine bilirubin, and alkaline phosphatase levels support the diagnosis.
- WBC count is slightly elevated during a cholecystitis attack.
- Serum amylase levels distinguish gallbladder disease from pancreatitis.
- Serial enzyme tests and an ECG should precede other diagnostic tests if heart disease is suspected.

How it's treated

- During an acute attack, treatment may include insertion of an NG tube and IV line as well as antibiotic administration.
- Surgery is the treatment of choice for severe cholecystitis. Cholecystectomy (removal of the gallbladder) restores biliary flow. The surgery may be performed conventionally via a large incision or laparoscopically using a laser. The laparoscopic procedure aids in speeding recovery and reducing the risk of infection and herniation.
- A patient may be discharged home with proper education on preventing a future attack. A low-fat diet is prescribed. Avoiding foods that aggravate the pain and follow-up with a surgeon need to be stressed.
- Ursodiol, a drug that dissolves the solid cholesterol in gallstones, provides an alternative for patients who are poor surgical risks or who refuse surgery. However, use of ursodiol is limited by the need for prolonged treatment (2 years), the incidence of adverse reactions, and the frequency of calculi reformation after treatment.
- Lithotripsy, the ultrasonic breakup of gallstones, is usually unsuccessful, and the rate of recurrence after this treatment is significant. The relative ease, short length of stay, and cost-effectiveness of laparoscopic cholecystectomy have made dissolution and lithotripsy less viable options.

What to do

- Monitor the patient's vital signs and intake and output.
- Insert an NG tube as ordered and attach it to low, intermittent suction.
- Administer medications to control reports of nausea and vomiting.
- Give opioid analgesics for pain.
- Assist in stabilizing the patient's nutritional and fluid balance before surgery.

- Withhold food and fluids by mouth; determine the time when the patient last ate.
- Provide preoperative care including teaching and administration of preoperative medications.
- Ensure that an informed consent form has been signed and is on the patient's chart.

Diverticulitis

Diverticulitis is a form of diverticular disease. In diverticular disease, bulging, pouchlike herniations (diverticula) in the GI wall push the mucosal lining through the surrounding muscle. Diverticula occur most commonly in the sigmoid colon, but they may develop anywhere from the proximal end of the pharynx to the anus. Other typical sites are the duodenum, near the pancreatic border or the ampulla of Vater, and the jejunum.

Diverticula in the stomach are rare and are usually a precursor to peptic or neoplastic disease. Diverticular disease of the ileum (Meckel diverticulum) is the most common congenital anomaly of the GI tract. Diverticular disease has two clinical forms:
1. *diverticulosis*—diverticula that are present but produce no symptoms
2. *diverticulitis*—inflamed diverticula that may cause potentially fatal obstruction, infection, and hemorrhage.

What causes it

The exact cause of diverticular disease is unknown, but it may result from:
- diminished colonic motility and increased intraluminal pressure
- defects in colon wall strength.

How it happens

Diverticula probably result from high intraluminal pressure on an area of weakness in the GI wall where blood vessels enter. Diet may be a contributing factor because insufficient fiber reduces fecal residue, narrows the bowel lumen, and leads to high intra-abdominal pressure during defecation.

Packed in the sac

In diverticulitis, undigested food and bacteria accumulate in the diverticular sac. This accumulation causes the formation of a hard mass that cuts off the blood supply to the thin walls of the sac, making them more susceptible to attack by colonic bacteria. Inflammation follows and may lead to perforation, abscess, peritonitis, obstruction, or hemorrhage. Occasionally, the inflamed colon segment adheres to the bladder or other organs and causes a fistula.

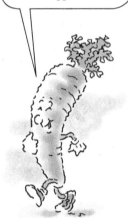

A lack of fiber may contribute to the formation of diverticula, so at the risk of my own safety, I say eat those veggies!

What to look for

- Meckel diverticulum usually produces no symptoms.
- In diverticulosis, recurrent left lower abdominal quadrant pain is relieved by defecation or passage of flatus. Constipation and diarrhea alternate.
- In diverticulitis, the patient may have moderate left lower abdominal quadrant pain, mild nausea, gas, irregular bowel habits, low-grade fever, leukocytosis, rupture of the diverticula (in severe diverticulitis), and fibrosis and adhesions (in chronic diverticulitis).

What tests tell you

These tests aid diagnosis of diverticular disease:

- An upper GI series confirms or rules out diverticulosis of the esophagus and upper bowel.
- Barium enema confirms or rules out diverticulosis of the lower bowel.
- Biopsy rules out cancer; however, a colonoscopic biopsy isn't recommended during acute diverticular disease because of the strenuous bowel preparation it requires.
- Blood studies may show an elevated erythrocyte sedimentation rate in diverticulitis, especially if the diverticula are infected.

How it's treated

Treatment of mild diverticulitis without signs of perforation must prevent constipation and combat infection. It may include bed rest, a liquid diet, stool softeners, a broad-spectrum antibiotic, opioids to control pain and relax smooth muscle, and an antispasmodic, such as dicyclomine (Bentyl), to control muscle spasms (Burchum & Rosenthal, 2019).

What to do

If the patient with a history of diverticulosis comes to the ED, observe the patient's stool carefully for frequency, color, and consistency; monitor pulse and temperature for changes that may signal developing inflammation or complications. Care of the patient with diverticulitis depends on the severity of symptoms:

- In mild disease, administer medications, as ordered. Explain diagnostic tests and preparations for such tests; observe stool carefully; and maintain accurate records of temperature, pulse rate, respiratory rate, and intake and output. Begin patient teaching for discharge. (See *Teaching the patient with diverticulitis*, page 308.)

Severe steps

If the patient's condition is more severe:

- Insert an IV line to administer fluids for rehydration.
- Maintain the patient on NPO status and anticipate insertion of an NG tube to low intermittent suction if the patient experiences persistent vomiting.

Teaching the patient with diverticulitis

• Explain what diverticula are as well as how they form.
• Make sure the patient understands the importance of dietary fiber and the harmful effects of constipation and straining at stool.
• Encourage increased intake of foods high in digestible fiber.
• Advise the patient to relieve constipation with stool softeners or bulk-forming laxatives, but caution against taking bulk-forming laxatives without plenty of water.

• Administer antispasmodic agents to reduce colon spasms; give analgesics to manage pain and antibiotics for infection as ordered.
• Assess the patient for signs and symptoms of peritonitis, such as tachycardia, hypotension, abdominal rigidity, rebound tenderness, and fever.
• Monitor the patient carefully if the patient requires angiography and catheter placement for vasopressin infusion. Inspect the insertion site frequently for bleeding, check pedal pulses frequently, and have the patient avoid flexing at the hips.
• Watch for signs and symptoms of vasopressin-induced fluid retention (apprehension, abdominal cramps, seizures, oliguria, and anuria) and severe hyponatremia (hypotension; rapid, thready pulse; cold, clammy skin; and cyanosis).
• Prepare the patient for surgery as indicated; provide preoperative teaching and support to the patient and family.

Quick quiz

1. A patient with abdominal trauma has purplish discoloration along the flank. How will the nurse document this assessment?
    A. Grey Turner sign.
    B. iliopsoas sign.
    C. obturator sign.
    D. Cullen sign.

Answer: A. Grey Turner sign refers to the purplish discoloration along the patient's flank.

2. The nurse assesses hyperactive bowel sounds when auscultating a patient's abdomen. How will the nurse interpret this assessment data?

    A. turbulent blood flow in the arteries.

    B. inflammation of the peritoneal surface.

    C. increased peristaltic activity.

    D. obstruction in the intestine.

Answer: C. Hyperactive bowel sounds indicate that peristalsis is increased.

3. Which assessment will the nurse anticipate in a patient with acute cholecystitis?

    A. Fever greater than 101.4° F (38.6° C)

    B. Left lower quadrant pain that radiates down the leg

    C. Belching that leaves a sour taste in the mouth

    D. Intolerance to all dairy foods.

Answer: C. With cholecystitis, the patient usually has right upper quadrant pain that radiates to the back or shoulder, a history of fat intolerance (not dairy), and belching that leaves a sour taste in the mouth. The patient may have a fever but it is usually low grade.

4. Which nursing intervention is appropriate for a patient diagnosed with appendicitis?

    A. Maintain NPO status as ordered

    B. Apply a heating pad on the abdomen for pain.

    C. Administer an enema prior to surgery

    D. Give frequent PRN doses of opioid analgesics.

Answer: A. For the patient with appendicitis, the nurse should maintain the patient on NPO status and administer IV fluids. In addition, analgesics are given cautiously because they may mask the signs and symptoms of rupture. Heat and enemas are never used because they could lead to rupture.

Scoring

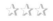 If you answered all four questions correctly, you deserve a gourmet meal! You're a GI genius!

 If you answered three questions correctly, read up and try again! Your hunger for GI information makes it easy to swallow.

 If you answered fewer than three questions correctly, you may be fact-starved. Chew over the chapter and then take the test again.

Selected references

Aggarwal, A., & Bhatt, M. (2014). Commonly used gastrointestinal drugs. *Handbook of Clinical Neurology, 120*, 633–643. doi:10.1016/B978-0-7020-4087-0.00043-7

Burchum, J., & Rosenthal, L. (2019). *Lehne's pharmacology for nursing care* (10th ed.). St. Louis, MO: Elsevier.

Gorter, R., Eker, H., Gorter-Stam, M., et al. (2016). Diagnosis and management of acute appendicitis. EAES consensus development conference 2015. *Surgical Endoscopy, 30*(11), 4668–4690.

Martin, R. F. (2018). *Acute appendicitis in adults: Clinical manifestations and differential diagnosis*. Retrieved from https://www.uptodate.com/contents/acute-appendicitis-in-adults-clinical-manifestations-and-differential-diagnosis

Penner, R., & Fishman, M. (2019). *Evaluation of the adult with abdominal pain*. Retrieved from https://www.uptodate.com/contents/evaluation-of-the-adult-with-abdominal-pain

Smink, D., & Soybel, D. (2018). *Management of acute appendicitis in adults*. Retrieved from https://www.uptodate.com/contents/management-of-acute-appendicitis-in-adults?topicRef=1386&source=see_link

Urden, L., Stacy, K., & Lough, M. (2018). *Critical care nursing: Diagnosis and management* (8th ed.). St. Louis, MO: Elsevier.

Velissaris, D., Karanikolas, M., Pantzaris, N., et al. (2017). Acute abdominal pain in the emergency department: The experience of a Greek university hospital. *Journal of Clinical Medicine Research, 9*(12), 987–993.

Chapter 7

Musculoskeletal emergencies and wound management

Just the facts

In this chapter, you'll learn:

◆ musculoskeletal assessment techniques

◆ tests to diagnose musculoskeletal emergencies

◆ common musculoskeletal emergencies, their causes, and treatments.

Understanding musculoskeletal emergencies

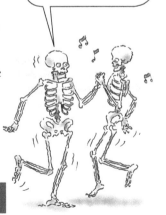

They can be life-threatening, and musculoskeletal emergencies can sure mess up a patient's groove!

Musculoskeletal injuries are common in hospital emergency departments (EDs). They can be life-threatening, and they result in significant pain, long-term disability, and possible disfigurement. These emergencies can involve the entire musculoskeletal system or any part of it. Conditions include strains, sprains, contusions, fractures, or traumatic amputation along with injuries to the muscles, tendons, and ligaments.

Be prepared to call on your full range of nursing skills when providing orthopedic care. Although some musculoskeletal problems are subtle and require comprehensive assessment, others are obvious or even traumatic. Any musculoskeletal concern can affect the patient physically and emotionally. Orthopedic injuries are often distracting in nature because they can be deforming or disfiguring. Don't let them distract you from assessing other possible injuries!

Assessment

Your sharp assessment skills will help you uncover orthopedic abnormalities and evaluate the patient's ability to perform activities of daily living (ADLs). However, because many musculoskeletal injuries are emergencies, you may have to rely on the patient's caregivers for information about his or her history. With any musculoskeletal injury or concern, you must carefully evaluate neurologic and vascular status.

Health history

If possible, question the patient about current and past illnesses and injuries, including allergies, medications, and social history.

Current illness or injury

Ask the patient about the chief concern. Questions about the patient's pain level, factors and events that took place before the illness or injury, and capabilities following the illness or injury will help you decide how to plan care.

Any ouchies?

For example, when a patient comes to the ED with hip pain, ask: When did the pain start? Was there an injury sustained before the pain? If so, what was the injury? Was it blunt trauma (a fall, a motor vehicle collision) or penetrating trauma (stabbing, puncture wound)?

How did it happen? For example, did the patient experience a hip injury after being hit by a car, or did he or she fall from a ladder and land on the coccyx? This information will help guide your assessment and predict other hidden trauma that needs attention.

Out-of-joint, fractured, or all muscle

Patients with joint injuries usually report pain, swelling, or stiffness in the affected area. They may experience decreased range of motion (ROM) or be unable to bear weight. Patients with bone fractures have sharp pain when they move the affected area and will attempt to guard the affected area. Swelling may be present. Patients with muscular injury commonly describe their pain as a burning sensation. Muscular injuries are commonly associated with swelling, bruising, and weakness.

Ask the patient if the ability to carry out ADLs is affected. Has the patient noticed abnormal sounds (grating, crunching, clicking) when moving certain parts of the body? When do these sounds occur (only after exercise, all of the time, upon certain movements, etc.)? Has ice, heat, or other remedies been used to treat the problem? If so, what was the outcome?

Past illness or injury

Inquire whether the patient has ever had gout, arthritis, tuberculosis, or cancer, which may cause bony metastases. Ask about a history of osteoporosis or degenerative joint disease. Also ask whether assistive devices, such as a cane, walker, or brace, are used, and if so, under what circumstances. Some people use these regularly; others only use them periodically or situationally. If the patient does use a device, ask to watch him or her use it and assess for appropriate or compromised movement.

Medications

Question the patient about the medications taken regularly because many drugs can affect the musculoskeletal system. Corticosteroids, for example, can cause muscle weakness, myopathy, osteoporosis, pathologic fractures, and avascular necrosis of the heads of the femur and humerus. Also ask whether the patient uses over-the-counter medications, vitamin or mineral supplements, or cultural remedies.

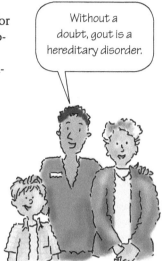

Without a doubt, gout is a hereditary disorder.

Family history

Ask the patient if there is a family history of joint disease. Disorders with a genetic component include:
- gout
- osteoarthritis of the interphalangeal joints
- rheumatoid arthritis
- spondyloarthropathies (such as ankylosing spondylitis, Reiter syndrome, psoriatic arthritis, and enteropathic arthritis).

Social history

Inquire about occupation, hobbies, and personal habits. Knitting or crocheting, playing football or tennis, working at a computer, or doing construction work can all cause repetitive stress injuries or injure the musculoskeletal system in other ways. Even carrying a heavy knapsack or purse can cause injury or increase muscle size.

What goes in

Inquire about the patient's social habits: smoking, drug or alcohol use, and amount of caffeine consumed. (Caffeine can cause demineralization of bones, causing bones to be more brittle.) Most facilities have general questions to ask all patients about safety; these questions screen for potential abuse situations, especially that of intimate partner violence.

Physical assessment

Because the central nervous system and musculoskeletal system are interrelated, assess them together. To assess the musculoskeletal system, use inspection and palpation to test all the major bones, joints, and muscles. Perform a complete examination if the patient has generalized symptoms, such as aching in several joints. Perform an abbreviated examination if pain is reported in only one body area, such as the ankle.

The Six P's of musculoskeletal injury

To swiftly assess a musculoskeletal injury, remember the six P's: pain, paresthesia, pressure, paralysis, pallor, and pulse.

Pain

Ask the patient about pain and assess its location, severity, and quality.

Paresthesia

Assess the patient for loss of sensation by touching the injured area with the tip of an open safety pin. Abnormal sensation or loss of sensation can indicate neurovascular involvement.

Pressure

Assess for areas of pressure, whether by gravity, dressings, or casts.

Paralysis

Assess whether the patient can move the affected area to assess for nerve or tendon damage.

Pallor

Paleness, discoloration, and coolness on the injured side may indicate neurovascular compromise.

Pulse

Check all pulses distal to the injury site. A decreased or absent pulse means reduced blood supply to the area.

Adapted from Ignatavicius, D., Workman, L., & Rebar, C. (2018). *Medical-surgical nursing: Concepts for interprofessional collaborative care* (9th ed.). St. Louis, MO: Elsevier.

First thing's first

Always perform a primary assessment of the patient's airway, breathing, and circulation (ABC), and disability. Base your initial care on that assessment. Then evaluate the neurovascular status of each injured limb. Because any patient experiencing trauma to an extremity risks neurovascular injuries and tissue ischemia, use the "five Ps" to evaluate limb circulation, sensation, and motor function. (See *The Six P's of musculoskeletal injury*.)

After you've established the patient's ABCs, begin your physical assessment. As you do, ask questions that relate to the patient's history and the events leading to the injury.

With feeling

As you palpate, note:
- skin temperature
- pain and the point of tenderness
- bony crepitus
- joint instability
- peripheral nerve function (sensory and motor).

A watchful eye

During inspection, be mindful of:
- color
- disruption of skin integrity
- position of the extremity

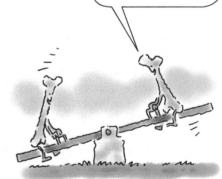

Checking alignment isn't child's play, it's a vital part of musculoskeletal assessment.

- edema, swelling, or ecchymosis
- ROM or lack of ROM
- symmetry, alignment, and deformity.

Assessing the bones and joints

After you finish your head-to-toe evaluation using inspection and palpation, you can perform ROM exercises to determine whether the joints are healthy (Jarvis, 2020). Never force movement; ask the patient to tell you when pain is experienced. Also, watch facial expressions for signs of pain or discomfort.

Head, jaw, and neck

First, inspect the patient's face for swelling, symmetry, and evidence of trauma. The mandible should be in the midline, not shifted to the right or left.

Is the TMJ A-OK?

Next, evaluate ROM in the temporomandibular joint (TMJ). Place the tips of your first two or three fingers in front of the middle of the patient's ear and ask him or her to open and close the mouth. Then place your fingers into the depressed area over the joint, noting the motion of the mandible. The patient should be able to open and close the jaw and protract and retract the mandible easily, without pain or tenderness. If you hear or palpate a click as the patient's mouth opens, suspect an improperly aligned jaw (Jarvis, 2020). TMJ dysfunction may also lead to swelling of the area, crepitus, or pain.

Check the neck

Before performing an examination of the neck, radiologic studies of the cervical spine may be indicated to rule out injury. Spinal cord injury should be suspected whenever there is a history of significant trauma, such as a high-speed motor vehicle collision; fall from higher than 3′ (1 m); significant trauma with loss of consciousness; loss or decrease of movement or sensation in the extremities; significant swelling, pain, or tenderness to the neck; or penetrating trauma to the neck. (See Chapter 3, *Neurologic emergencies*, for more information on spinal cord injury.)

Before cervical spine clearance, the neck should be examined by removing the cervical collar and manually immobilizing the neck. Inspect the front, back, and sides of the patient's neck. Observe for obvious signs of injury to the cervical spine. Also assess the patient's ability to move extremities and feel pain. Palpate the cervical area for pain, tenderness, deformity, and crepitus. *Crepitus* is an abnormal grating sound, not the occasional crack we hear from our joints, and indicates fracture. Be sure to replace the collar when the neck examination is complete.

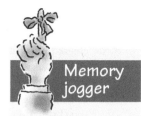

Memory jogger

Here's an easy way to remember adduction and abduction.

Adduction is moving a limb toward the body's midline; think of it as adding two things together.

Abduction is moving a limb away from the body's midline; think of it as taking something away like abducting or kidnapping.

Head circles and chin-ups

When the health care provider states that the cervical spine has been cleared of injury, you can remove the cervical collar. At that time, check ROM in the neck. Ask the patient to try touching the right ear to the right shoulder and the left ear to the left shoulder. The usual ROM is 40 degrees on each side. Next, ask the patient to touch the chin to the chest and then point the chin toward the ceiling. The neck should flex forward 45 degrees and extend backward 55 degrees.

To assess rotation, ask the patient to turn the head to each side without moving the trunk. The chin should be parallel to the shoulders. Lastly, ask the patient to move the head in a circle; normal rotation is 70 degrees.

Spine

Before performing an examination of the spine, radiologic studies may be indicated to rule out injury. As with cervical spine injury, injury to the spinal vertebrae should be suspected when there's significant trauma or clinical signs of injury.

The patient should be immobilized (as indicated in Chapter 3) and log-rolled with the assistance of three people. The remainder of the spine should be examined just as the cervical spine was examined. When the spine has been cleared of injury by the health care provider, immobilization can be discontinued. Observe the spine; it should be in midline position without deviation to either side. Lateral deviation suggests scoliosis.

Spine-tingling procedure

Palpate the spinal processes and the areas lateral to the spine. Have the patient bend at the waist and let the arms hang loosely at the sides; palpate the spine with your fingertips. Repeat the palpation using the side of your hand. Note tenderness, swelling, or spasm.

Shoulders and elbows

Start by observing the patient's shoulders, noting asymmetry, muscle atrophy, or deformity. Swelling or loss of normal, rounded shape could mean that one or more bones is dislocated or out of alignment. Remember, even if the patient seeks care for shoulder pain, the problem may not have started in the shoulder. Shoulder pain may originate from other sources, including a heart attack or ruptured ectopic pregnancy.

Palpate the shoulders with the palmar surfaces of your fingers to locate bony landmarks; note crepitus or tenderness. Using your entire hand, palpate the shoulder muscles for firmness and symmetry. Also palpate the elbow and the ulna for subcutaneous nodules that may signal rheumatoid arthritis.

Lift and rotate

If the patient's shoulders don't seem dislocated, assess rotation. Start with the patient's arm straight at the side—the neutral position. Ask to lift the arm straight up to shoulder level and then to bend the elbow horizontally until the forearm is at a 90-degree angle to the upper arm. The patient's arm should be parallel to the floor, and the fingers should be extended with palms down.

To assess external rotation, have the patient bring the forearm up until the fingers point toward the ceiling. To assess internal rotation, have the patient lower the forearm until the fingers point toward the floor. Normal ROM is 90 degrees in each direction.

Flex and extend

To assess flexion and extension, start with the patient's arm in the neutral position. To assess flexion, ask the patient to move the arm anteriorly over the head, as if reaching for the sky. Full flexion is 180 degrees. To assess extension, have the patient move the arm from the neutral position posteriorly as far as possible. Normal extension ranges from 30 to 50 degrees.

Swing into position

To assess abduction, ask the patient to move the arm from the neutral position laterally as far as possible. Normal ROM is 180 degrees. To assess adduction, have the patient move the arm from the neutral position across the front of the body as far as possible. Normal ROM is 50 degrees.

Up to the elbows

Next, assess the elbows for flexion and extension. Have the patient rest the arm at neutral position. Ask the patient to flex the elbow from this position and then extend it. Normal ROM is 90 degrees for flexion and extension.

To assess supination and pronation of the elbow, have the patient place the side of the hand on a flat surface with the thumb on top. Ask the patient to rotate the palm down toward the table for pronation and upward for supination. The normal angle of elbow rotation is 90 degrees in each direction.

Wrists and hands

Inspect the wrists and hands for contour and compare them for symmetry. Also check for nodules, redness, swelling, deformities, and webbing between fingers. Use your thumb and index finger to palpate both wrists and each finger joint. Note tenderness, nodules, or bogginess. To avoid causing pain, be especially gentle with older adults and those with arthritis.

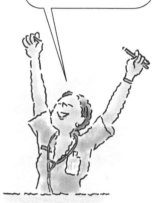

Reach for the sky—a good motto and a great way to check arm flexion!

Rotate and flap

Assess ROM in the wrist. Ask the patient to rotate the wrist by moving his or her entire hand—first to the left and then to the right—as if waxing a car. Normal ROM is 55 degrees laterally and 20 degrees medially. Observe the wrist while the patient extends fingers up toward the ceiling and down toward the floor, as if flapping the hand. The patient should be able to extend the wrist 70 degrees and flex it 90 degrees.

Lift a finger; make a fist

To assess extension and flexion of the metacarpophalangeal joints, ask the patient to keep the wrist still and move only the fingers—first up toward the ceiling and then down toward the floor. Normal extension is 30 degrees; normal flexion is 90 degrees.

Next, ask the patient to touch the thumb to the little finger of the same hand. The patient should be able to fold or flex the thumb across the palm so that it touches or points toward the base of the little finger.

To assess flexion of all of the fingers, ask the patient to form a fist and then spread the fingers apart to demonstrate abduction and draw them back together to demonstrate adduction.

At arm's length

If you think one arm is longer than the other, take measurements. Extend a measuring tape from the acromial process of the shoulder to the tip of the middle finger. Drape the tape over the outer elbow. The difference between the left and right extremities should be no more than ⅜" (1 cm).

Hips and knees

Inspect the hip area for contour and symmetry. Next, inspect knee position, noting whether the patient is bowlegged (having knees that point out) or knock-kneed (having knees that turn in). Then watch the patient walk to assess the gait.

Palpate each hip over the iliac crest and trochanteric area for tenderness or instability. Palpate both knees—they should feel smooth, and the tissues should feel solid. (See *Assessing bulge sign.*)

Hip, hip, hooray!

Assess ROM in the hip; these exercises are typically performed with the patient in a supine position. To assess hip flexion, place your hand under the patient's lower back and have him or her pull one knee as far as possible toward the abdomen and chest. You'll feel the patient's back touch your hand as the normal lumbar lordosis of the

Assessing bulge sign

The bulge sign indicates excess fluid in the joint (Maricar et al., 2016). To assess for this sign, ask the patient to lie down so that you can palpate the knee. Then give the medial side of the knee two to four firm strokes, as shown top right, to displace excess fluid.

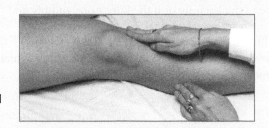

Lateral check

Next, tap the lateral aspect of the knee while checking for a fluid wave on the medial aspect, as shown bottom right.

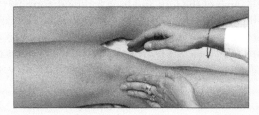

spine flattens. As the patient flexes the knee, the opposite hip and thigh should remain flat on the bed. Repeat on the opposite side.

To assess hip abduction, stand alongside the patient and press down on the superior iliac spine of the opposite hip with one hand to stabilize the pelvis. With your other hand, hold the patient's leg by the ankle and gently abduct the hip until you feel the iliac spine move. That movement indicates the limit of hip abduction. Then, while still stabilizing the pelvis, move the ankle medially across the patient's body to assess hip adduction. Repeat on the other side. Normal ROM is about 45 degrees for abduction and 30 degrees for adduction.

To assess hip extension, have the patient lie prone (facedown) and gently extend the thigh upward. Repeat on the other thigh.

As the hip turns

To assess internal and external rotation of the hip, ask the patient to lift one leg up and, keeping the knee straight, turn the leg and foot medially and laterally. Normal ROM for internal rotation is 40 degrees; for external rotation, 45 degrees.

On bended knees

Assess ROM in the knee. If the patient is standing, ask him or her to bend the knee as if trying to touch the heel to the buttocks. Normal ROM for flexion is 120 to 130 degrees. If the patient is lying down, have him or her draw the knee up to the chest; the calf should touch the thigh.

Knee extension returns the knee to a neutral position of 0 degrees; however, some knees may normally be hyperextended 15 degrees. If the patient can't extend the leg fully or if the knee pops audibly and painfully, consider the response abnormal.

Other abnormalities include pronounced crepitus, which may signal a degenerative disease of the knee, and sudden buckling, which may indicate a ligament injury.

Ankles and feet

Inspect the ankles and feet for swelling, redness, nodules, and other deformities. Check the arch of the foot and look for toe deformities. Also note edema, calluses, bunions, corns, ingrown toenails, plantar warts, trophic ulcers, hair loss, or unusual pigmentation.

Use your fingertips to palpate the bony and muscular structures of the ankles and feet. Palpate each toe joint by compressing it with your thumb and fingers.

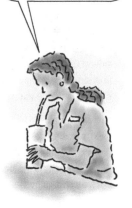

Pop (soda) in a glass? Absolutely! But pop in a knee? Abnormal!

The ankle angle

To examine the ankle, have the patient sit in a chair or on the side of a bed. To test plantar flexion, ask the patient to point toes toward the floor. Test dorsiflexion by asking to point the toes toward the ceiling. Normal ROM for plantar flexion is about 45 degrees; for dorsiflexion, 20 degrees.

Next, assess ROM in the ankle. Ask the patient to demonstrate inversion by turning the feet inward and eversion by turning the feet outward. Normal ROM for inversion is 45 degrees; for eversion, 30 degrees.

To assess the metatarsophalangeal joints, ask the patient to flex and then straighten the toes.

The long and short of it

Take measurements if you think that one leg is longer than the other. Put one end of the tape at the medial malleolus at the ankle and the other end at the anterior iliac spine. Cross the tape over the medial side of the knee. A difference of more than ⅜″ (1 cm) is considered abnormal.

Assessing the muscles

When assessing the muscles, start by inspecting all major muscle groups for tone, strength, and symmetry (Potter et al., 2017). If a muscle appears atrophied or hypertrophied, measure it by wrapping a tape measure around the largest circumference of the muscle on each side of the body and comparing the two numbers.

Other abnormalities of muscle appearance include contracture and abnormal movements, such as spasms, tics, tremors, and fasciculation (fine movements of a small area of muscle).

Grading muscle strength

Grade muscle strength on a scale of 0 to 5:
- **5/5 = Normal**—Patient moves joint through full range of motion (ROM) and against gravity with full resistance.
- **4/5 = Good**—Patient completes ROM against gravity with moderate resistance.
- **3/5 = Fair**—Patient completes ROM against gravity only.
- **2/5 = Poor**—Patient completes full ROM with gravity eliminated (passive motion).
- **1/5 = Trace**—Patient's attempt at muscle contraction is palpable but without joint movement.
- **0/5 = Zero**—There is no evidence of muscle contraction.

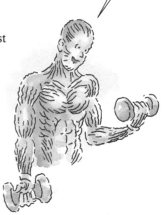

Nurses can't resist me, but I have to resist them pretty often. I tell them it's for the sake of muscle tone.

Tuning in to muscle tone

Muscle tone describes muscular resistance to passive stretching. To test the patient's arm muscle tone, move the shoulder through passive ROM exercises. You should feel a slight resistance. Then let the arm drop. It should fall easily to his or her side.

Test leg muscle tone by putting the patient's hip through passive ROM exercises and then letting the leg fall to the examination table or bed. Like the arm, the leg should fall easily.

Abnormal findings include muscle rigidity and flaccidity. Rigidity indicates increased muscle tone, possibly caused by an upper motor neuron lesion after a stroke. Flaccidity may result from a lower motor neuron lesion.

Wrestling with muscle strength

Observe the patient's gait and movement to gauge general muscle strength. Grade muscle strength on a scale of 0 to 5, with 0 representing no strength and 5 representing maximum strength. Document the results as a fraction, with the score as the numerator and maximum strength as the denominator. (See *Grading muscle strength*.)

To test specific muscle groups, ask the patient to move the muscles while you apply resistance and then compare the contralateral muscle groups. (See *Testing muscle strength*, page 322.)

Shoulder, arm, wrist, and hand strength

Test the strength of the patient's shoulder girdle by asking him or her to extend his or her arms with the palms up and hold this position for 30 seconds. If the patient can't lift both arms equally and keep the palms up, or if one arm drifts down, there may be shoulder girdle weakness on that side. If the patient passes the first part of the test, gauge strength by placing your hands on the arms and applying downward pressure as he or she resists this action.

Testing muscle strength

To test the muscle strength of your patient's arm and ankle muscles, use the techniques shown here.

Biceps strength

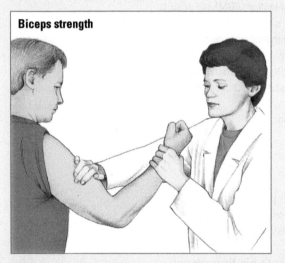

Ankle strength: Plantar flexion

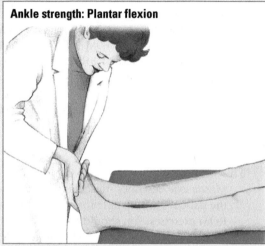

Triceps strength

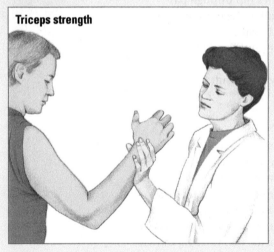

Ankle strength: Dorsiflexion

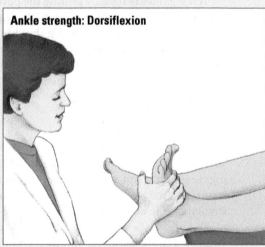

Testing the bi's and tri's

Next, have the patient hold the arm in front with the elbow bent. To test bicep strength, pull down on the flexor surface of the forearm as the patient resists. To test triceps strength, have the patient try to straighten the arm as you push upward against the extensor surface of his or her forearm.

Forcing the hand

Assess the strength of the patient's flexed wrist by pushing against it. Test the strength of the extended wrist by pushing down on it. Test the strength of finger abduction, thumb opposition, and handgrip the same way. (See *Testing handgrip strength*.)

Leg strength

Ask the patient to lie in a supine position on the examining table or bed and lift both legs at the same time. Note whether both legs can be lifted at the same time and to the same distance. To test quadriceps strength, have the patient lower his or her legs and raise them again while you press down on the anterior thighs.

Then ask the patient to flex the knees and put the feet flat on the bed. Assess lower leg strength by pulling the patient's lower leg forward as he or she resists and then pushing it backward as he or she extends the knee.

Lastly, assess ankle strength by having the patient push the foot down against your resistance and then pull the foot up as you try to hold it down.

Testing handgrip strength

When testing handgrip strength, face the patient, extend the first and second fingers of each hand, and ask him or her to grasp your fingers and squeeze. Don't extend fingers with rings on them; a strong handgrip on those fingers can be painful.

Diagnostic tests

Diagnostic tests help confirm the diagnosis and identify the underlying cause of musculoskeletal emergencies. Common procedures include arthrocentesis, computed tomography (CT) scan, magnetic resonance imaging (MRI), and X-ray.

Arthrocentesis

Arthrocentesis is a joint puncture that's used to collect synovial fluid for analysis to identify the cause of pain and swelling, to assess for infection, and to distinguish forms of arthritis, such as pseudogout and infectious arthritis. The health care provider will probably choose the knee for this procedure but may tap synovial fluid from the wrist, ankle, elbow, or first metatarsophalangeal joint.

Telltale findings

In joint infection, synovial fluid looks cloudy and contains more white blood cells (WBCs) and less glucose than normal. When trauma causes bleeding into a joint, synovial fluid contains red blood cells. In specific types of arthritis, crystals can confirm the diagnosis, such as urate crystals indicating gout.

Doing double duty

Arthrocentesis also has therapeutic value. For example, in symptomatic joint effusion, removing excess synovial fluid relieves pain.

Practice pointers

- Describe the procedure to the patient. Explain that he or she will be asked to assume a certain position, depending on the joint being aspirated, and that he or she will need to remain still.
- After the test, the health care provider may ask you to apply ice or cold packs to the joint to reduce pain and swelling.
- If the health care provider removed a large amount of fluid, tell the patient that he or she may need to wear an elastic bandage.

CT scan

A CT scan aids diagnosis of bone tumors and other abnormalities. It helps assess questionable fractures, fracture fragments, bone lesions, and intra-articular loose bodies.

Beam me up

A computerized body scanner directs multiple X-ray beams at the body from different angles. The beams pass through the body and strike radiation detectors, producing electrical impulses. A computer then converts these impulses into digital information, which is displayed as a three-dimensional image on a video monitor.

Practice pointers

- Verify patient allergies and hypersensitivities.
- The patient should be in a hospital gown and instructed to remove all jewelry, hair accessories (e.g., bobby pins), piercings, watches, eyeglasses, hearing aids, and dental appliances.
- Inform the patient that he or she won't be in an enclosed space, that the machine isn't enclosed, and that it's shaped like a doughnut. Teach that there is a low-pitched spinning sound that will be heard during the test.
- Assure the patient that there will be no pain involved.
- Instruct the patient to remain still during the test. Although he or she will be alone in the room, assure the patient that communication can take place through an intercom system with the technician.

MRI

MRI can show irregularities of soft tissue (such as brain tissue), bone, and muscle.

Must be your animal magnetism

The MRI scanner uses a powerful magnetic field and radiofrequency energy to produce images based on the hydrogen content of body tissues. The computer processes signals and displays the resulting high-resolution image on a video monitor. The patient can't feel the magnetic fields, and no harmful effects have been observed.

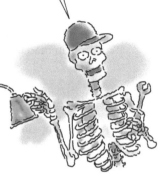

Metal and magnets don't mix! Make sure patients remove all metal objects before entering the MRI.

Practice pointers

- Make sure the patient is in a hospital gown and has removed all metal objects, including jewelry, hair accessories (e.g., bobby pins), piercings, watches, eyeglasses, hearing aids, and dental appliances. Belongings should be secured—including credit, bank, and parking cards—because the scan could erase their magnetic codes.
- Explain to the patient that he or she will be positioned on a narrow bed that slides into a large cylinder housing the MRI magnets. Ask if the patient has ever experienced claustrophobia. If so, sedation may be helpful in tolerating the scan.
- Tell the patient that there will be soft thumping noises heard during the test.
- Instruct the patient to remain still during the test. Although he or she will be alone in the room, assure the patient that communication can take place through an intercom system with the technician.

X-rays

Anteroposterior, posteroanterior, and lateral X-rays allow three-dimensional visualization. They help diagnose:

- fractures and dislocations
- bone disease, including solitary lesions, multiple focal lesions in one bone, or generalized lesions involving all bones
- joint disease (such as arthritis), infection, degenerative changes, synoviosarcoma, osteochondromatosis, avascular necrosis, slipped femoral epiphysis, and inflamed tendons and bursae around a joint
- masses and calcifications.

If the health care provider needs further clarification of standard X-rays, a CT scan or an MRI may be ordered.

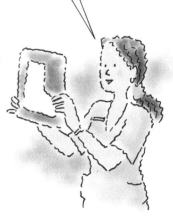

Sure, X-rays help diagnose fractures, but did you know they can also point out joint disease, bone disease, and masses?

Practice pointers
- Explain the procedure to the patient.
- Make sure the patient removes all jewelry from the area to be X-rayed.
- Verify that the X-ray order includes pertinent recent history such as trauma and identifies the point tenderness site. It should also include past fractures, dislocations, or surgery involving the affected area.
- Medicate patients for pain before radiography. Radiography can involve movement of the affected area, increasing the patient's level of discomfort, which can lead to a poor radiography quality and an inaccurate diagnosis.

Treatments

Pain and impaired mobility are good motivators for obtaining medical care. Consequently, most patients with musculoskeletal problems eagerly seek treatment.

Get up and go again

To restore a patient's mobility, several treatments are used alone or in combination:
- drug therapy to control pain, inflammation, or muscle spasticity
- nonsurgical treatments, including closed reduction or immobilization
- surgery with subsequent immobilization in a cast, brace, or other device.

Drug therapy

Nonsteroidal anti-inflammatory drugs are the first line of defense against arthropathies. Other drug therapy includes analgesics, corticosteroids, and skeletal muscle relaxants, depending on the degree of injury and patient presentation.

Nonsurgical treatments

Some patients with musculoskeletal emergencies require nonsurgical treatment. Treatment options include closed reduction of a fracture or immobilization.

Teaching about immobilization devices

When discharging a patient with a musculoskeletal injury who has been prescribed an immobilization device, be sure to include these teaching points:
• Teach to promptly report signs of complications, including increased pain, drainage, or swelling in the involved area.
• Stress the need for strict compliance with activity restrictions while the immobilization device is in place.
• If the patient was given a walker, cane, or crutches to use with a leg or ankle cast, splint, or knee immobilizer, make sure he or she is able to demonstrate correct ambulation using the device.
• If the patient has a removable device, such as a knee immobilizer, teach how to apply it correctly.
• Advise the patient to keep scheduled follow-up appointments to evaluate healing.

Closed reduction

Closed reduction involves external manipulation of fracture fragments or dislocated joints to restore their normal position and alignment. It may be done under conscious sedation or local, regional, or general anesthesia.

Immobilization

Immobilization devices are commonly used to maintain proper alignment, limit movement, and help relieve pain and pressure.

Don't move a muscle!

Immobilization devices include:
- plaster and synthetic casts applied after closed or open reduction of fractures or after other severe injuries
- splints to immobilize fractures, dislocations, or subluxations
- slings to support and immobilize an injured arm, wrist, or hand or to support the weight of a splint or hold dressings in place
- skin or skeletal traction, using a system of weights and pulleys to reduce fractures, treat dislocations, correct deformities, or decrease muscle spasms
- braces to support weakened or deformed joints
- cervical collars to immobilize the cervical spine, decrease muscle spasms and, possibly, relieve pain
- long spine boards with cervical immobilization devices to fully immobilize the entire spine. (See *Teaching about immobilization devices*.)

Casts can be applied after severe injuries or closed or open fracture reductions.

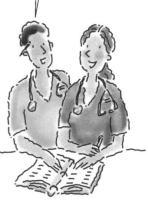

Surgery

Surgical procedures include open reduction and internal fixation. During open reduction, the surgeon restores the normal position and alignment of fracture fragments or dislocated joints and then inserts internal fixation devices—such as pins, screws, wires, nails, rods, or plates—to maintain alignment until healing begins.

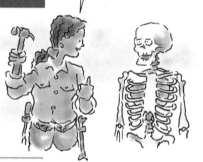

Can you pick up more screws and nails at the store? I need them for home repair, and you need them for bone repair.

Common disorders

In any musculoskeletal emergency, neurologic and vascular status must be evaluated carefully because a patient with a musculoskeletal illness or injury is at risk for potential neurovascular injuries and tissue ischemia. Musculoskeletal emergencies may include amputations (traumatic), compartment syndrome, contusions, dislocations and fractures, puncture wounds, and strains and sprains.

Amputations (traumatic)

Amputation is the removal of a part of the body by traumatic means. Two common types of amputations are the complete (guillotine) or incomplete (crush or tear). A *complete amputation* occurs when the appendage has been completely severed from the body. An *incomplete amputation* occurs when an attachment of the appendage to the body is still present, even if small in size.

What causes it

Amputation that originates from human or mechanical error is accidental and traumatic. Potential for traumatic amputations exists anywhere there are humans working around machinery or hand tools.

How it happens

Complete and incomplete amputations occur with equal frequency. Incomplete amputations acquire greater tissue damage because of the distortion and destruction of the involved and surrounding structures, especially the vasculature. Tissue damage in complete amputations is minor because there's a precise cut between the body and affected part.

What to look for

- Observe the extent and location of the injury. Some amputations will require the patient to go immediately to the operating room.
- Assess what's missing and how much, if any, of the appendage is left intact.

- Determine the amount and color of the blood. Dark blood indicates a venous injury, whereas bright red blood indicates an arterial injury.
- Palpate pulses distal to the injury. If the pulses aren't palpable, immediate intervention is warranted.
- Capillary refill should be less than 2 seconds to indicate adequate perfusion.
- Pain may be present depending on the extent of nerve involvement and damage.
- Determine the underlying physiologic or psychological pathology prompting the injury because this can help you better plan further care. For example, did the patient get dizzy and fall into machinery? Or, was the leg amputated by a train as part of a suicide attempt?

What tests tell you
- X-rays will evaluate the extent to which underlying bony structures are involved or damaged and also determine the level of injury and suitability for replantation.
- Vascular studies, such as arteriograms, determine the extent of vascular compromise caused by the injury.
- Laboratory tests ordered for initial management and preoperative screening may include complete blood count (CBC) with differential, chemistry, type, and screen; prothrombin time; partial thromboplastin time; international normalized ratio level; urine drug screen; and urinalysis. These studies reveal infections and evaluate blood loss, electrolyte balance, and kidney function. Bleeding times and clotting times are important factors for patient management.
- An electrocardiogram evaluates cardiac activity and can identify disease processes that cause complications from fluid resuscitation or anesthesia. These studies can also give clues about the injury's cause—for example, perhaps the patient had a syncopal episode while using the circular saw, which in turn caused the amputation of a finger.

How it's treated
Treatment for amputation may include surgical replantation. Antibiotics are administered before surgery and postoperatively.

What to do
- If available, preserve the amputated part for possible reimplantation by wrapping it in saline-moistened gauze and placing it in a sealed plastic bag. The bag should then be placed in a bath of ice water. Make sure that the part doesn't freeze. Don't allow the part to be submerged directly in the ice.
- Assess the patient's ABCs and manage life-threatening concerns. The patient's ABCs and cervical spine should be cleared before addressing secondary findings.

- Administer oxygen.
- Control bleeding. Current evidence indicates the efficacy of tourniquet use to control life/limb-threatening hemorrhage. If used for the right patient, at the right time, and in the right way, tourniquets are a lifesaving treatment and should be utilized to control life/limb-threatening bleeding (Teixeira et al., 2018).
- Insert two large-bore (18G or larger) intravenous (IV) lines; depending on the site of amputation, you may need a central access device.
- Clean the site using normal saline solution irrigation only; don't scrub or use cleaning solution on the stump.
- Administer tetanus prophylaxis if last booster was greater than 10 years ago (Centers for Disease Control and Prevention, 2018).
- Administer analgesics and antibiotics as ordered.
- Apply sterile dressings.
- Prepare the patient for transfer to an appropriate facility or the operating room.
- Facilitate communication with caregivers.
- Immobilize the limb in its correct anatomic position.

Compartment syndrome

Compartment syndrome is a condition in which increased pressure within a closed-tissue space compromises circulation to the capillaries, muscles, and nerves within that space (American Association of Orthopaedic Surgeons, 2019). It's considered one of the few true orthopedic emergencies that occur in the ED. The key to a favorable patient outcome is early recognition, diagnosis, and intervention. If left untreated, it can be one of the most devastating and debilitating injuries a patient can experience.

What causes it
Compartment syndrome can result from external or internal compression.

External
- Casts
- Tight dressing
- Splints
- Skeletal traction
- Prolonged entrapment of a limb-crush injury

Internal
- Frostbite
- Snakebite

- Fractures or contusions
- Bleeding into a muscle
- IV infiltration or extravasation

How it happens

Compartments are composed of arteries, veins, nerves, muscles, and bones. The compartments most clinically relevant to the ED health care provider are the upper and lower extremities. Compartment syndrome occurs when there's an increase of pressure within the compartment, causing ischemia to its contents. This ischemia causes severe pain, but because the cause isn't readily observed, it will seem out of proportion to the injury. Compartment syndrome can occur immediately or as long as 4 days after the injury.

What to look for

Signs and symptoms of compartment syndrome include:
- swelling
- paresthesia
- pain out of proportion to injury (especially on passive movement)
- diminished pulse (a late sign).

What tests tell you

These tests are used to diagnose compartment syndrome:
- X-rays will help rule out other diagnoses.
- Obtaining a compartment pressure can be accomplished quickly and easily using a commercially available battery-powered monitor.
- Normal pressure is approximately zero but always less than 10 mm Hg.
- Compromise of capillary blood flow occurs at a pressure of 10 to 30 mm Hg; this indicates an immediate risk because muscle and nerve tissue necrosis will occur if pressure isn't alleviated (Stracciolini & Hammerberg, 2018).
- Laboratory studies should include CBC to evaluate hemoglobin level, hematocrit, WBC, and platelet count and chemistry for analysis of metabolic stability and renal function. Myoglobinuria is a common adverse effect; it can develop within 4 hours of the onset of compartment syndrome (Stracciolini & Hammerberg, 2018). Close observation of renal function is imperative for a favorable patient outcome.

How it's treated

- Constant observation, assessment, and reassessment in conjunction with frequent monitoring of compartment pressures is key to management of compartment syndrome.
- Do not apply ice.

- Do not elevate the limb but maintain the limb at the level of the heart.
- Surgical decompression by fasciotomy may be required when compartment pressure exceeds 30 mm Hg (Stracciolini & Hammerberg, 2018).
- Cases that aren't diagnosed expeditiously may require fasciotomy. This procedure involves surgically opening the fascia through the entire length of both compartments of the affected limb. Opening both compartments prevents swelling and ischemia in a lateral area. The surgical site is left open until all the swelling has resolved (approximately 3 to 5 days) and is then closed by skin grafting.

What to do

- Assess the patient's ABCs and manage life-threatening concerns. The patient's ABCs and cervical spine should be cleared before addressing secondary findings.
- Obtain a thorough history of the present illness.
- Remove any constrictive or restrictive clothing, dressings, or devices (especially jewelry).
- Administer analgesia as ordered.
- Obtain IV access.
- Administer tetanus toxoid if last booster was greater than 10 years ago (Centers for Disease Control and Prevention, 2018).

Contusions

A *contusion* is an injury resulting from a direct blow to the affected area.

What causes it

The causes of contusion vary but can include motor vehicle collisions, falls, being struck by a blunt object, or striking an immovable object with a part of the body.

How it happens

A contusion results from minor hemorrhaging underneath unbroken skin. Following the injury, blood extravasates into the surrounding tissue, causing swelling or ecchymosis. This "black-and-blue" mark will change to a yellowish-green color after approximately 2 days as the healing process progresses. The patient may experience minor discomfort from the initial injury, but it will subside as swelling decreases and the blood is reabsorbed by the body.

What to look for

- Report of recent trauma to the area causing discomfort
- Bruising or swelling to the injured area (If the patient reports pain that seems out of proportion to the observed injury, consider the possibility of compartment syndrome.)

What tests tell you

The diagnosis of a contusion is based on clinical findings. Diagnostic tests are performed based on the mechanism of injury only to rule out underlying pathologic conditions such as a fracture.

How it's treated

Treatment is supportive and is based on symptoms:

- Ice helps prevent or decrease swelling and prevent further complications.
- A mild analgesia may be prescribed, if appropriate.
- Observation may be necessary depending on the location and severity of the contusion. If symptoms progress or new ones develop, further evaluation and consultation may be warranted.

What to do

- Assess the patient's ABCs and manage life-threatening concerns. The patient's ABCs and cervical spine should be cleared before addressing secondary findings.
- Obtain a thorough patient history, including mechanism of injury, time, and treatment performed before the patient's arrival at the ED.

History of violence

- Be alert when obtaining the patient's history for any red flags indicating abuse. (See *Abuse alerts*, page 334.)
- Provide physical care, including ice application and, if appropriate, immobilization to decrease pain.
- Mild analgesia, such as acetaminophen (Tylenol) or ibuprofen (Motrin), should be effective; if these drugs provide no decrease in pain, be alert to signs of compartment syndrome.
- Patient education should include trauma prevention and early signs and symptoms of compartment syndrome. The patient should follow up with the primary health care provider or return to the ED if symptoms worsen or the condition doesn't improve.

Stay on the ball

Abuse alerts

Red flags indicating abuse might include:
- multiple bruises in various stages of healing
- impatience with treatment times
- desire to leave by a specific time
- inconsistent reasons given for multiple injuries (e.g., "falling down the stairs," "banged into something")
- lack of direct eye contact when describing what happened
- conflicting stories from patient and significant other.

If the patient arrives with a significant other, observe their interaction. The patient should be interviewed privately and specifically asked about abuse. If the patient reports being a victim of abuse, take appropriate measures to ensure the patient's and the medical staff's safety. Contact security and a social services representative as soon as possible. The social services representative will provide emotional support during hospitalization and assist the patient with legal processes and aftercare.

Dislocations and fractures

A *dislocation* is an injury that occurs at the articulation of two or more bones, causing these bones to move out of their anatomically correct position. Dislocations may also include associative soft tissue and vascular or nerve injury. (See *Types of dislocations.*)

A *fracture* is an interruption in the continuity and stability of the bone. Fractures themselves, although painful and temporarily debilitating, don't cause fatalities. However, complications of fracture can lead to permanent disability and even death if not recognized and treated. Fractures are classified by five characteristics:
1. anatomic location
2. direction of fracture lines
3. relationship of fragments to each other
4. stability
5. associated soft tissue injury.

Trauma and force

Direct trauma describes an injury caused by a force that directly impacted or caused the damage, whereas *indirect trauma* refers to an injury caused by the transmission of force from one area to another.

Types of dislocations

This chart lists the common sites of dislocations, causes, common signs and symptoms, and treatments for each type.

Area of dislocation	Causes	Signs and symptoms	Treatments
Acromioclavicular separation	• Common athletic injury • Fall or direct blow to the point of the shoulder	• Severe pain in the joint area • Inability to raise the arm or adduct the arm across the chest • Deformity • Point tenderness	• Depends on the degree of dislocation • Reduction, which should take place as soon as possible to avoid complications • Postreduction treatment of minor injuries, including splinting in position of comfort with sling and swath, which the patient should maintain for approximately 7 to 10 days • Open reduction or having the patient wear the splint for a longer period for more severe injuries
Shoulder	***Anterior*** • Usually an athletic injury resulting from a fall on an extended arm that is externally rotated and abducted ***Posterior*** • Rare but may be seen when the arm has been forcefully abducted and internally rotated	• Decreased or limited range of motion (ROM) • Decreased function • Deformity	• Closed reduction after associative fracture is ruled out • Reduction, which should occur immediately if neurovascular compromise is present • Operative interventions when indicated, as when there's soft tissue interposition, displaced greater tuberosity fracture, and glenoid rim fracture measuring greater than 5 mm • Surgery, possibly the treatment of choice for athletes
Elbow	• Fall on an extended arm	• Pain that increases with movement • Decreased or limited ROM • Decreased function • Deformity	• Varied, based on direction of dislocation, but usually closed reduction followed by splint application • Surgical repair for a dislocation that's irreducible or one that has associative neurovascular compromise
Wrist	• Fall on an outstretched hand	• Pain, especially with movement • Deformity	• Support in position of comfort • Closed reduction • Surgical intervention

(continued)

Types of dislocations *(continued)*

Area of dislocation	Causes	Signs and symptoms	Treatments
Hand or finger	• Fall on an outstretched hand • Direct blow to the fingertip or a jamming force to the fingertip	• Pain • Swelling • Deformity • Inability to move the joint	• Support in position of comfort • Reduction
Hip	• Major trauma such as frontal motor vehicle collision (foot on brake pedal or knee hits dashboard)	• Hip pain • Knee pain • Pain that may radiate to groin • Hip flexed, adducted, and internally rotated (posterior dislocation) • Hip slightly flexed, abducted, and externally rotated (anterior dislocation [rare]) • Patient reports joint feeling locked • Inability to move the leg	• Support in position of comfort • Surgical reduction • For postsurgical dislocation, closed reduction under moderate sedation or, if unsuccessful, completed under general anesthesia
Knee	• Major trauma • High-speed motor vehicle collision • Sports injury	• Severe pain • Deformity • Gross swelling • Inability to move the joint	• Splint in position of comfort • Immediate reduction (within 24 hours) • Admission or transfer to the operating room
Patella	• History of spontaneous dislocation • Direct trauma • Rotation of a planted foot	• Knee in flexed position • Pain • Loss of function • Swelling • Tenderness	• Possible spontaneous reduction into place • Splint or cast • Crutches
Ankle	• Commonly associated with a motor vehicle collision (foot on pedal) • Commonly associated with a fracture	• Swelling • Deformity • Pain • Inability to move the joint	• Possible surgical reduction • Splint or cast • Crutches

Adapted from Beutler, A. (2018). *General principles of fracture management: Bone healing and fracture description.* Retrieved from https://www.uptodate.com/contents/general-principles-of-fracture-management-bone-healing-and-fracture-description

Location and direction

Anatomic location describes exactly where in the bone the fracture is located. A long bone is divided into sections:

- proximal
- middle or distal
- head, shaft, or base.

Classifying fractures

One of the best-known systems for classifying fractures uses a combination of terms—such as *simple, nondisplaced,* and *oblique*—to describe them.

General classification of fractures
- *Simple (closed)*—Bone fragments don't penetrate the skin.
- *Compound (open)*—Bone fragments penetrate the skin.
- *Incomplete (partial)*—Bone continuity isn't completely interrupted.
- *Complete*—Bone continuity is completely interrupted.

Classification by fragment position
- *Comminuted*—The bone breaks into small pieces.
- *Impacted*—One bone fragment is forced into another.
- *Angulated*—Fragments lie at an angle to each other.
- *Displaced*—Fracture fragments separate and are deformed.
- *Nondisplaced*—The two sections of bone maintain essentially normal alignment.

- *Overriding*—Fragments overlap, shortening the total bone length.
- *Segmental*—Fractures occur in two adjacent areas with an isolated central segment.
- *Avulsed*—Fragments are pulled from normal position by muscle contractions or ligament resistance.

Classification by fracture line
- *Linear*—The fracture line runs parallel to the bone's axis.
- *Longitudinal*—The fracture line extends in a longitudinal (but not parallel) direction along the bone's axis.
- *Oblique*—The fracture line crosses the bone at roughly a 45-degree angle to the bone's axis.
- *Spiral*—The fracture line crosses the bone at an oblique angle, creating a spiral pattern.
- *Transverse*—The fracture line forms a right angle with the bone's axis.

Adapted from Beutler, A. (2018). *General principles of fracture management: Bone healing and fracture description.* Retrieved from https://www.uptodate.com/contents/general-principles-of-fracture-management-bone-healing-and-fracture-description

The *direction* of the fracture line is categorized as:
- *transverse*—when the fracture is perpendicular to the bone
- *oblique*—when the line runs across the bone at a 45- to 60-degree angle
- *spiral*—when the direction of the fracture line looks twisted
- *comminuted*—when the bone is broken into more than two fragments
- *impacted*—when the ends of the fracture are compressed together. (See *Classifying fractures* and *Classification of pediatric fractures,* page 338.)

Transverse, oblique, and comminuted fractures generally occur as a result of direct force. Avulsion, spiral, and stress fractures are typically caused by indirect force.

Relationship and stability

The relationship of the fracture fragments to each other is described by *alignment* and *apposition. Alignment* describes how the bones are positioned or placed. *Apposition* describes the contact between the fracture surfaces.

Stability describes the tendency of a fracture to displace after reduction. A *stable* fracture doesn't displace; an *unstable* fracture does.

Ages and stages

Classification of pediatric fractures

Children's fractures are classified according to where in the epiphyseal growth plate the fracture occurs. The growth plate is located at the ends of bones between the epiphysis and metaphysis. The plate is responsible for longitudinal bone growth, and injury can cause disturbance in growth. The Salter-Harris classification system is used to grade pediatric fractures. Type I carries the lowest risk for growth plate injury, and type V carries the highest. The higher the classification, the greater the potential for interference with bone growth.

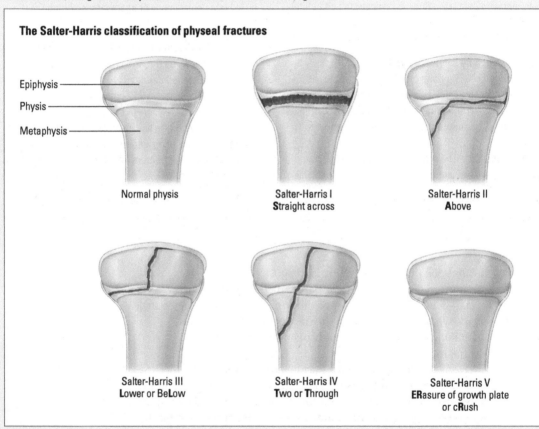

The Salter-Harris classification of physeal fractures

Epiphysis
Physis
Metaphysis

Normal physis

Salter-Harris I
Straight across

Salter-Harris II
Above

Salter-Harris III
Lower or Be**Low**

Salter-Harris IV
Two or **T**hrough

Salter-Harris V
E**R**asure of growth plate
or c**R**ush

Adapted from Mathison, D., & Agrawal, D. (2019). *General principles of fracture management: Fracture patterns and description in children*. Retrieved from https://www.uptodate.com/contents/general-principles-of-fracture-management-fracture-patterns-and -description-in-children

Don't go soft on us now

Associated soft tissue injury is divided into:

- *simple*—when there's no break in the skin
- *compound*—when overlying skin is broken, but there's no direct communication between open skin and the fracture
- *complicated*—when there's associative neurovascular, visceral, ligament, or muscular damage. (Intra-articular fractures are also categorized as complicated.)

What causes it

Most dislocations and fractures are caused by direct or indirect trauma, although some have different causes. Stress fractures result from repetitive use or motion. Pathologic fractures occur in a bone weakened by a preexisting disease. They can be preceded by injury or occur during normal activity. Regardless of underlying disease, the mechanism of injury plays an important role. (See *Understanding fractures*, pages 340 to 343.)

How it happens

The extent and severity of dislocations or fractures depends on extrinsic factors; amount, direction, and duration of force; and the frequency of the injury-causing act.

Dislocation

A dislocation occurs when there's a disruption in the relationship of the bones at their articulation. Reduction of dislocations should be completed as soon as possible to prevent the injury from progressing to adjacent vasculature and nerves.

Fracture

A fracture occurs when the stress applied to the bone exceeds its malleability. The bone's strength is directly related to its density. Factors affecting the osseous structure, such as an underlying disease process, specific medication regimens, and some congenital anomalies, affect its density. Immediately after a fracture occurs, the bone body initiates its own healing process. This process occurs in three phases:

1. inflammatory phase
2. reparative phase
3. remodeling phase.

It's a hematoma!

Because the periosteum is torn, a hematoma forms between the two separated areas of bone. In the *inflammatory phase*, the hematoma begins to clot and deprives the osteocytes at the bones' ends of oxygen and nutrients, which causes them to die. A significant inflammatory response ensues, including vasodilation, causing release of inflammatory cells, leukocytes, and macrophages.

(*Text continues on page 344.*)

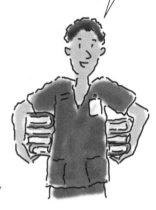

Soft tissue injuries are like good stories; some are simple, and some are complicated.

Understanding fractures

Fractures can occur in almost every part of every limb. Depending on where and how they occur, each has specific complications to monitor for and therapeutic interventions to perform. The chart below describes common fractures, their causes, signs and symptoms, interventions, and the possible complications associated with each type (see chart below).

Fracture	Causes	Signs and symptoms	Interventions	Possible complications
Clavicle	• Most common in pediatric patients • Fall on extended arm or shoulder • Direct blow to shoulder	• Pain in clavicle area • Swelling • Deformity • Bony crepitus • Patient can't or won't raise arm.	• Shoulder immobilization	• Brachial plexus injury • Ligament damage • Malunion • Subclavian vascular injury
Shoulder and humerus	• Fall on outstretched arm • Direct shoulder trauma from a fall or a blunt instrument	• Pain in shoulder area • Point tenderness • Posterior rotation • Inability to move affected arm • Adduction of the humerus • Abduction of humerus • Gross edema and discoloration that can extend to chest wall	• Immobilization of arm in a sling or swath • Surgery if fracture is impacted, comminuted, or displaced	• Laceration of the axillary artery • Brachial plexus injury • Avascular necrosis of the humeral head • Frozen shoulder syndrome • Nonunion
Scapula	• Direct trauma; penetrating or blunt	• Pain on shoulder movement • Point tenderness • Arm held in adduction with resistance to abduction • Ecchymosis • Palpable bony displacement • Swelling	• Immobilization of arm in a sling or swath • Padding the axilla to avoid injury to the brachial plexus and artery	• Injury to the ribs • Pneumothorax • Hemothorax • Compression fractures of the spine
Upper arm	• Fall on arm or direct blow • Twisting or throwing of the arm	• Bony crepitus • Bruising • Inability to move arm • Pain • Point tenderness • Severe deformity • Swelling	• Immobilization of arm in a sling or swath • Surgical intervention (for fracture that extends below the elbow, spiral fractures, or shaft fractures)	• Laceration or stretching of the radial nerve resulting in neuropraxia
Elbow	• Fall on extended arm • Fall on flexed elbow	• Severe pain • Point tenderness • Rapid swelling • Shortening of the arm • Delayed capillary refill	• Splint the arm "as it lies." • Orthopedic consult • Arteriogram to assess for vascular compromise	• Brachial artery laceration • Nerve damage • Volkmann ischemic contracture

Understanding fractures *(continued)*

Fracture	Causes	Signs and symptoms	Interventions	Possible complications
Radius or ulna	• Fall on extended arm • Direct blow such as in "nightstick" fractures • Forced pronation of the forearm	• Pain • Point tenderness • Swelling • Deformity • Angulation • Shortening	• Closed reduction • Casting • Referral to orthopedic surgeon • Open reduction and internal fixation	• Paralysis of the radial nerve • Malunion • Volkmann ischemic contracture
Wrist	• Dorsiflexion, usually following a fall on an extended arm or open hand	• Pain • Snuff box tenderness • Swelling • Deformity • Limited range of motion • Numbness • Weakness	• Closed reduction • Rigid splint or a thumb spica cast • Referral to orthopedic surgeon	• Rare aseptic necrosis
Hand and finger	• Forceful hyperextension • Direct trauma • Crush injury	• Pain • Point tenderness • Severe swelling • Deformity • Inability to use hand	• Closed reduction • Finger traction • Splinting distal phalanges with a padded aluminum guard • Buddy taping an injured finger to an uninjured one • Antibiotics for open fractures	• Malunion • Osteomyelitis • Subungual hematoma
Pelvis	• Motor vehicle collision • Fall from a height • Crush injury • Direct trauma	• Tenderness when iliac wings are compressed • Paraspinous muscle spasms • Sacroiliac joint tenderness • Hematuria • Pelvic ecchymosis • Groin pain • Blood at the urethral meatus • Perineal hematomas • Prostate displacement and loss of sphincter tone	• Aggressive resuscitation (oxygen, crystalloids, blood transfusion) • Immobilization of the spine and legs • Pelvic stabilization (pneumatic antishock garment-abdominal section, pelvic binder, internal or external fixation) • Pelvic computed tomography (CT) scan • Abdominal CT scan • Antibiotics	• Hemorrhage, shock, death • Bladder, genital, or lumbosacral trauma • Ruptured internal organs • Osteomyelitis • Compartment syndrome • Chronic pain • Gastrointestinal (GI) tract injury • Pulmonary or fat emboli

(continued)

Understanding fractures *(continued)*

Fracture	Causes	Signs and symptoms	Interventions	Possible complications
Hip (acetabulum, greater trochanter, femoral head)	• Direct blow or fall • Common injury in older adults • Axial transmission of force from knees as in knee-to-dashboard injuries	• Pain in hip or groin area • Severe pain with movement • Inability to bear weight • External rotation of the affected hip and leg • Shortening of the affected limb	• Immobilization in a comfortable position • Traction • Referral to an orthopedic surgeon • Surgical intervention	• Avascular necrosis of the femoral head • Phlebitis of the femoral vein • Osteoarthritis • Sciatic nerve injury • Hypovolemic shock • Fat embolism syndrome
Femur	• Indirect force upward through a flexed knee • Direct trauma • Falls • Gunshot wounds • Motor vehicle collision (especially vehicle–pedestrian collision)	• Angulation • Shortening of the limb • Severe muscle spasm • Bony crepitus • Severe pain • Swelling of the thigh • Hematoma in the thigh • Inability to bear weight on the affected leg	• Aggressive resuscitation (oxygen, crystalloids, blood transfusion) • Immobilization of the thigh with a traction splint • Referral to an orthopedic surgeon • Open reduction with internal fixation	• Hemorrhage • Severe muscle damage • Knee trauma (commonly overlooked)
Knee	• High-velocity vehicle trauma • Pedestrian trauma (such as from a bumper or fender) • Fall from a height onto a flexed knee • Hyperabduction	• Bony crepitus • Tense swelling in the popliteal area • Hemarthrosis, swelling around the joint • Knee pain and tenderness • Inability to straighten or bend the knee	• Nonweight-bearing cast • Traction • Crutches • Referral to an orthopedic surgeon • Open reduction and internal fixation	• Popliteal nerve or artery injury • Fat emboli • Rotational deformities • Traumatic arthrosis
Patella	• Direct trauma (dashboard impact) or a fall • Indirect trauma (after quadriceps muscle pull or contraction)	• Knee pain • Hemarthrosis • Inability to extend the knee	• Surgery for quadriceps repair	• Avascular necrosis

Understanding fractures *(continued)*

Fracture	Causes	Signs and symptoms	Interventions	Possible complications
Tibia and fibula	• Twisting or rotating forces • Direct trauma • Fall with compression forces • Fall with foot fixed in place such as in a ski injury	• Pain • Point tenderness • Swelling • Deformity • Bony crepitus	• Assessment for puncture wound associated with tibia (open fracture) • Wound debridement and irrigation • Casting • Crutches • Open reduction and internal fixation	• Compartment syndrome • Infection • Osteomyelitis • Nonunion
Ankle	• Direct trauma • Indirect trauma • Torsion, eversion, or inversion	• Popping sound at time of injury (torn ligaments) • Ecchymosis • Bony crepitus • Pain on ambulation or altered gait • Inability to bear weight if injury is unstable	• Closed reduction • Posterior splint • Possible open reduction and internal fixation • Casting • Crutches	• Nonunion • Infection • Posttrauma arthritis
Foot	• Similar to ankle injury • Athletic injuries • Direct trauma	• Deep pain • Point tenderness • Ecchymosis • Swelling • Subungual hematoma • Inability to bear weight • Deformity	• Bulky dressing • Orthopedic shoe • Posterior splint • Cane or crutches	• Avascular necrosis • Malunion • Gait abnormalities
Heel	• Fall from a height	• Increased pain with hyperflexion • Point tenderness • Pain in hindfoot • Soft tissue ecchymosis • Superficial skin blistering • Deformity	• Bulky and compression dressings • Ensuring nonweight bearing or partial weight bearing • Crutches • Surgery (usually not scheduled for 2 days to 2 weeks following injury) • Closed reduction for displaced fractures • Assessment for associated trauma	• Chronic pain • Nerve entrapment
Toe	• Direct trauma (stubbing or kicking) • Crush injuries • Athletic injuries	• Subungual hematoma • Pain • Deformity • Discoloration	• Compression bandage • Buddy taping • Orthopedic shoe • Cane as needed	• None

Organization is key

Next, in the *reparative phase*, cells within the hematoma (mesenchymal cells) organize, localize, and begin to form bone. Osteoblasts move from inside the bone toward the damaged ends and assist in the healing process.

I'm brand new!

New bone is formed from trabeculae organization—causing the reconnection of the previously separated bone edges—in the *remodeling phase* of healing.

What to look for

The most common signs and symptoms of dislocations and fractures include:

- pain
- swelling
- ecchymosis
- point tenderness.

What's more . . .

Deformity may also be present and can be associated with a loss of normal function ranging from minimal to complete, depending on the injury. Associative blood loss shouldn't be overlooked during patient care; blood loss volumes can be minimal to shock inducing. Estimated blood loss can range from 150 (with a radius fracture) to 3,000 mL (in conjunction with a pelvic fracture), leading to hypovolemia and shock.

A pathologic fracture can produce painless swelling and generalized bone pain without swelling.

Signs and symptoms of stress fractures can vary depending on the area of injury. However, the patient's chief concern is of pain that has been getting progressively worse over time during an activity.

What tests tell you

These tests help determine dislocation or fracture:

- Arteriograms are used with dislocations and fractures to assess associative vascular involvement.
- MRIs are most helpful with the diagnosis of tendon, ligament, and soft tissue injuries.
- CT scans can be used to evaluate a bone for a fracture, especially when serial radiography has been negative but the patient complains of persistent pain.
- X-rays provide evidence of most fractures. Some fractures will only show up after an extended time, so follow-up radiography is an important part of fracture management.

How it's treated

Fracture management is based on evaluation of the type and classification of the injury and health care provider preference based on evidence-based practice:

- Pain management is a primary concern for all dislocations and fractures.
- Splinting applied in the ED is the initial treatment for most fractures. Splints are used to prevent further soft tissue injury from fracture fragments, to decrease pain by providing support and position of comfort, and to lower the risk of clinical fat emboli. (See *Common splint types.*)
- General indications for surgical treatment of fractures include displaced intra-articular fractures, associated arterial injury, when closed methods of treatment have failed, fractures through metastatic lesions, or for patients who can't be confined to bed. Postoperatively, a splint or cast is applied to maintain correct alignment.
- Closed reduction should be performed within 6 to 12 hours of the time of injury because swelling makes the procedure difficult.

Inspired casting

- Indications for applying a cast include pain relief, immobilization of a fracture to allow for healing, and stabilization of an unstable fracture. Remember that unstable fractures are treated surgically. Casts are individually molded for the patient using plaster or fiberglass casting material and are generally reserved for application until swelling has resolved—approximately 3 to 5 days after the injury or surgery.
- Pathologic fractures are treated with immobilization and rest as well as pain control.
- Stress fracture treatment varies depending on severity and location and is similar to the treatment of a sprain or strain. The injuring activity is limited or eliminated. Rest is one of the most important interventions for recovery. Treatment for stress fracture in the lower extremity likely involves crutches. The healing timeframe is approximately 4 to 6 weeks. The few cases in which casting treatment is preferred over splinting are usually managed by an orthopedist.

What to do

- Assess the patient's ABCs and ensure that the cervical spine has been cleared before addressing secondary findings.
- Assess for paresthesia.
- Assess the injured area for vascular stability, capillary refill, and pulses distal to the injury.
- Remove jewelry from or distal to the affected area because it can act as a tourniquet if left in place.
- Evaluate the patient's tetanus status. Administer a booster if the patient hasn't had an immunization in the last 10 years (Centers for Disease Control and Prevention, 2018).

Common splint types

Examples of commonly used splints include:

- the Hare traction and Sager splints for reduction and immobilization of femur fractures preoperatively
- prefabricated splints for immobilization and support of the wrist or ankle
- air splints used in the prehospital environment to provide immobilization to extremities
- fiberglass and plaster ready-to-mold splinting material in a variety of widths and lengths.

Don't forget about tetanus! Give your patient a booster if his or her last immunization was more than 10 years ago.

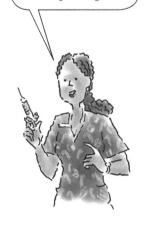

- Apply ice for 20-minute intervals to decrease swelling.
- Assist with splinting as appropriate.
- Cover open fractures with a moist, sterile dressing.
- Administer analgesia as ordered.
- Prepare the patient for admission, if appropriate.
- Prepare the patient for the operating room, if appropriate.

Pelvic plan

If the patient has a suspected pelvic fracture, follow these steps:
- Immobilize by using a long spine board or pneumatic antishock garment.
- If not contraindicated, decrease pain by having the patient flex the knees.
- Monitor vital signs, including neurovascular assessment, every 5 minutes.
- If the pelvic fracture is unstable, initiate open trauma protocol.
- Administer fluids and antibiotics via a large-bore IV line (18G or larger) and administer supplemental oxygen. Prepare the patient for a CT scan or an MRI.
- Prepare the patient for the operating room to receive definitive care.
- Prepare for and assist with procedural sedation, if ordered.
- Administer blood products as ordered.

Puncture wounds

A *puncture wound* is a piercing of the skin by a foreign object, causing a hole in the skin and underlying tissues. Puncture wounds can be superficial and only involve the skin, or can extend through tissue and into the bone, depending on the mechanism of injury.

What causes it

Puncture wounds are caused by direct trauma. The possible mechanisms of injury are endless, but some examples include bites and foreign objects, such as nails, needles, pins, and knives.

What to look for

Assess the wound for signs and symptoms of infection and obvious presence of a retained foreign body.

What tests tell you

X-rays should be completed if the puncture wound is near a joint or bone to rule out underlying fracture and presence of any foreign bodies.

How it's treated

In some cases, cleaning and irrigating the wound is all that's necessary. In other cases, as determined by the health care provider, antibiotics may be prescribed based on the type of injury and potential other exposures (Baddour & Brown, 2018).

What to do

- Assess the patient's ABCs and ensure cervical spine clearance before addressing secondary findings.
- Control bleeding with direct pressure and elevation; note the amount of blood loss from the wound. Notify the health care provider if blood loss is significant or bleeding doesn't stop within 10 minutes of applying pressure.
- Evaluate the patient's tetanus status. Administer a booster if the patient hasn't had an immunization in the last 10 years (Centers for Disease Control and Prevention, 2018).
- Irrigate the wound if it isn't associated with an underlying fracture.
- If the wound contains foreign matter, is associated with a fracture, or is more than 8 hours old, you may need to administer oral or IV antibiotics as ordered.
- Perform wound care and apply necessary dressings or immobilization devices.

Strains and sprains

Strain is the term used to describe a pulling apart of muscle fibers, whereas a *sprain* describes a pulling apart of the fibers within a ligament. Both can result from direct or indirect trauma.

What causes it

The most common cause of strains and sprains is sports-related trauma or falling. Other common causes include motor vehicle collisions.

How it happens

A strain is classified by degree and location of the muscle:

1. A *first-degree* strain is caused by a forceable overstretching of a muscle.
2. A *second-degree* strain is a disruption of more muscle fibers (more forceful contraction or stretch) than a first-degree strain.
3. A *third-degree* strain entails a complete disruption of the muscle fibers and may be accompanied by a rupture of the overlying fascia or an avulsion fracture of the underlying bone.

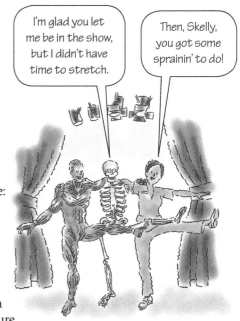

Sprain, sprain, go away!

A sprain is also diagnosed by degree and location but of ligaments (not muscle):

1. In a *first-degree* sprain, the involved ligament stretches without tearing—the joint remains stable and joint function remains normal.
2. A *second-degree* sprain involves stretching and tearing of the involved ligament, causing moderate function loss and mild to moderate joint instability.
3. A *third-degree* sprain is the most painful and physically limiting. It involves a complete disruption of the tendon, causing profound joint instability, moderate to severe loss of function, and an inability to hold an object (if located in the upper extremity) or bear weight (if located in the lower extremity).

What to look for

First- and second-degree strains are similar in presentation; therefore, differentiation is based on the degree of loss of function and level of swelling. Characteristics of first- and second-degree strains include:

*   mild localized swelling
*   ecchymosis
*   mild spasms
*   localized discomfort, possibly aggravated by movement or pressure
*   minimal but transient loss of function and strength.
    Characteristics of a third-degree strain include:
*   moderate to severe swelling with ecchymosis
*   moderate to severe pain
*   muscle spasm
*   moderate to complete loss of function
*   knot-like protrusion on the muscle at the injury site.

Sprain symptoms

Patients with a first-degree sprain demonstrate:

*   minimal swelling
*   little or no joint instability
*   mild discomfort.
    Symptoms of a second-degree sprain are more pronounced. They include:
*   moderate to severe swelling
*   ecchymosis
*   moderate functional loss
*   mild to moderate joint instability.
    A third-degree sprain causes:
*   patient's inability to bear weight or hold an object
*   moderate to severe swelling
*   ecchymosis
*   joint instability.

Any good chef will tell you that presentation is everything. That goes double when you're assessing strains and sprains.

What tests tell you

Just like contusions, strains and sprains are diagnosed by clinical presentation. X-rays will only verify the lack of an underlying fracture. Thus, radiography isn't always needed before diagnosis. For example, if a patient has lower back pain and mild spasms but denies recent trauma such as a fall, then radiography may not be indicated.

How it's treated

Treatment depends on the extent of the injury. All strains and sprains are treated with analgesia, ice, elevation, and immobilization on arrival at the ED. When a differential diagnosis has been made by the health care provider, treatment methods and recovery periods vary:

- *First-degree* strains and sprains are treated with ice and rest over a couple of days. Analgesics may be prescribed. Activity can be gradually resumed as tolerated.
- In addition to analgesia, rest, ice, and elevation, a *second-degree* strain or sprain is immobilized and all patient activity is restricted until swelling and pain subside. Use of immobilizers (for upper extremity injuries) and crutches (for lower extremity injuries) is common. Ice is applied for the first 24 to 48 hours, after which the use of heat is prescribed. Use of the injured muscle is gradual and stopped if pain is experienced. Slow and steady progression is the key to recovery. Returning to normal activity too soon will cause reinjury.
- A *third-degree* strain or sprain is initially treated in the same way as a second-degree strain: with analgesia, ice, elevation, and immobilization. After these interventions, the patient is referred to a specialist for further evaluation and treatment, which may include surgical repair. A more substantial analgesia medication may be required by these patients because of the injury's extent.

What to do

- Assess the patient's ABCs and manage life-threatening concerns. The patient's ABCs and cervical spine should be cleared before addressing secondary findings.
- Immediately apply ice, provide support with a splint or other immobilization device, and elevate the area for comfort.
- Obtain a thorough history of the present illness, including precipitating factors. For example, a patient may have ankle pain as a current concern, but further assessment may reveal that he or she fell down the steps after syncope.
- Remove jewelry from or distal to the affected area because it can act as a tourniquet if left in place.

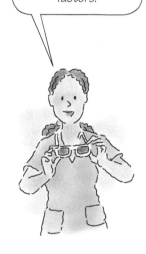

There's often a lot more to a strain or sprain than meets the eye. Be sure to ask about precipitating factors.

Teaching about strains and sprains

Teaching about strains and sprains should include:

• explanation of the diagnosis

• information regarding prescribed medications

• instruction on use of supportive, immobilization, and assistive devices.
   In addition, follow these guidelines:

• The patient should be able to demonstrate understanding of the use of the assistive devices provided.

• Emphasize applying ice and elevating and resting the affected area.

• Stress that use of the affected area shouldn't be initiated until all swelling and pain have subsided. When this occurs, the patient should begin progressively active exercises and perform them to the limit of pain.

• Instruct the patient to follow up with outside resources or return to the emergency department as directed.

• Explain the importance of follow-up care and the risks if follow-up care isn't completed.

• Administer analgesics as ordered.
• Assist the patient into a wheelchair or onto a stretcher, if appropriate, to prevent further injury from weight-bearing activity.
• Provide patient education. (See *Teaching about strains and sprains.*)

Quick quiz

1.   What impairment will the nurse document when a patient cannot move the right arm away from the body?
    A. Supination
    B. Abduction
    C. Eversion
    D. Adduction

Answer: B. Abduction is the ability to move a limb away from the midline. Supination is the rotation of an arm or limb (i.e., rotating the palm of the hand facing outward). Eversion is the action of turning an arm or limb inside out. Adduction is the ability to move a limb toward the midline of the body.

2.   When a patient with a tightly applied arm cast reports a high degree of pain and swelling of the fingers, what condition does the nurse anticipate?

    A.   Sprain

    B.   Strain

    C.   Compression fracture

    D.   Compartment syndrome

Answer: D. Compartment syndrome is characterized by increased pressure within a closed-tissue space compromising circulation to its contents; pain that exceeds normal expectations is often reported. A sprain is the sudden twisting of a joint that causes pain and swelling but does not result in a fracture or dislocation of the joint. A strain is the overstretching of a muscle with results in pain; however, it does not result in swelling. A compression fracture is most commonly found in the vertebrae of the spine. This occurs when one bone is compressed against another bone.

3.   Which condition does the nurse identify that accurately describes an injury that occurs at the articulation of two or more bones and causes the bones involved to be moved out of the anatomically correct position?

    A.   Fracture

    B.   Sprain

    C.   Strain

    D.   Dislocation

Answer: D. A dislocation is defined as an injury that occurs at the articulation of two or more bones, causing the bones involved to be moved out of the anatomically correct position. A fracture is the breaking of a bone. Most commonly, fractures are the result of a traumatic event; however, certain medical conditions such as osteopenia, osteoporosis, or cancer can weaken the bone and result in what is called a pathologic fracture. A sprain is the sudden twisting of a joint that causes pain and swelling but does not result in a fracture or dislocation of the joint. A strain is simply the overstretching of a muscle which causes pain; however, it does not result in swelling.

Scoring

 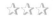 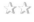   If you answered all three questions correctly, way to go! You're a bred-in-the-bone musculoskeletal maven!

If you answered two questions correctly, impressive! Make no bones about it; you have a mastery of musculoskeletal matters!

If you answered fewer than two questions correctly, don't become unhinged! Just bone up a bit!

Selected references

American Association of Orthopaedic Surgeons. (2019). *Compartment syndrome.* Retrieved from https://orthoinfo.aaos.org/en/diseases--conditions/compartment-syndrome/

Baddour, L., & Brown, A. (2018). *Infectious complications of puncture wounds.* Retrieved from https://www.uptodate.com/contents/infectious-complications-of-puncture-wounds

Beutler, A. (2018). *General principles of fracture management: Bone healing and fracture description.* Retrieved from https://www.uptodate.com/contents/general-principles-of-fracture-management-bone-healing-and-fracture-description

Centers for Disease Control and Prevention. (2018). *Diphtheria, tetanus, and pertussis vaccine recommendations.* Retrieved from https://www.cdc.gov/vaccines/vpd/dtap-tdap-td/hcp/recommendations.html

Ignatavicius, D., Workman, L., & Rebar, C. (2018). *Medical-surgical nursing: Concepts for interprofessional collaborative care* (9th ed.). St. Louis, MO: Elsevier.

Jarvis, C. (2020). *Physical examination and health assessment* (8th ed.). St. Louis, MO: Elsevier.

Maricar, N., Callaghan, M. J., Parkes, M. J., Felson, D. T., O'Neill, T. W. (2016). Clinical assessment of effusion in knee osteoarthritis—A systematic review. *Seminars in Arthritis and Rheumatism, 45*(5), 556–563.

Mathison, D., & Agrawal, D. (2019). *General principles of fracture management: Fracture patterns and description in children.* Retrieved from https://www.uptodate.com/contents/general-principles-of-fracture-management-fracture-patterns-and-description-in-children

Potter, P., Perry, A., Stockert, P., & Hall, A. (2017). *Fundamentals of nursing* (9th ed.). St. Louis, MO: Elsevier.

Stracciolini, A., & Hammerberg, E. M. (2018). *Acute compartment syndrome of the extremities.* Retrieved from https://www.uptodate.com/contents/acute-compartment-syndrome-of-the-extremities

Teixeira, P. G., Brown, C. V., Emigh, B., et al. (2018). Civilian prehospital tourniquet use is associated with improved survival in patients with peripheral vascular injury. *Journal of the American College of Surgeons, 226*(5), e1.769–e1.776.

Chapter 8

Renal, genitourinary, and gynecologic emergencies

Just the facts

In this chapter, you'll learn:

♦ emergency assessment of the genitourinary (GU) and reproductive systems

♦ diagnostic tests and procedures for GU and gynecologic emergencies

♦ GU and gynecologic disorders and their treatments in the emergency department.

Understanding GU and gynecologic emergencies

The genitourinary (GU) and reproductive systems are closely related, and identifying subtle changes within them can mean the difference between effective and ineffective emergency care.

An emergency involving the urinary or reproductive system can have far-reaching consequences. In addition to affecting the system itself, it can trigger problems in other body systems and affect the patient's quality of life, self-esteem, and sense of well-being.

Despite these factors, patients are sometimes reluctant to discuss their problems with a nurse or have intimate areas of their bodies examined. Your challenge is to professionally perform a skilled, sensitive assessment. To do so, you must put the patient at ease; if you appear comfortable discussing the problem, the patient will feel encouraged to talk more openly.

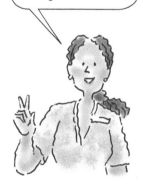

Compassion and comfort are two Cs that will put GU emergency patients right at ease.

Assessment

When your patient comes to the emergency department (ED) with a GU or gynecologic emergency, your assessment can help determine whether the symptoms are related to a current medical problem or indicate a new one. You need to assess the patient thoroughly, always being alert for subtle changes that may indicate a potential change in condition.

Unless the patient requires immediate stabilizing treatment, begin by taking a comprehensive patient history and then conduct a thorough physical examination.

Peruse the record

If you can't interview the patient because of his or her condition, gather information from electronic health records. In some cases, you may need to ask the patient's family or significant other(s) for history. The emergency medical response team that transported the patient to the ED can also provide important information.

Sex-specific

The urinary system consists of the kidneys, ureters, bladder, and urethra. Remember natal sex differences; for the male patient, the urethral meatus is also part of the reproductive system, carrying semen as well as urine. The male reproductive system also includes the penis, scrotum, testicles, epididymis, vas deferens, seminal vesicles, and prostate gland.

For the female patient, the reproductive system consists of the external genitalia (collectively called the *vulva*—mons pubis, labia majora, labia minora, clitoris, opening of the vagina, urethral meatus, and Skene and Bartholin glands) and the internal genitalia (vagina, uterus, ovaries, and fallopian tubes).

Tailor assessment and care of GU and reproductive emergencies from a natal sex perspective. Ensure patient-centered and culturally sensitive care is provided for all patients, especially those who identify as transgender because their natal sex organs may differ from their personal identity. Be certain to ask what name the patient wishes to be addressed by and which pronouns the patient prefers.

Health history

When gathering a health history, focus first on the patient's chief concern and then explore previous health status and a sexual-reproductive history. Ask the patient to describe symptoms in personal words, encouraging free and open speech. As you obtain a history, remember that the patient may feel uncomfortable discussing urinary or reproductive problems. Remain professional and objective, which will help to put the patient more at ease. (See *Putting your patient at ease.*)

Putting your patient at ease

Here are some tips for helping your patient feel more comfortable as you collect the health history:

* Make sure that the room is private and that you won't be interrupted.
* Tell the patient that answers will remain confidential.
* Phrase your questions tactfully.
* Start with less sensitive topic areas and work up to more sensitive areas such as sexual function.
* Don't rush or omit important facts because the patient seems embarrassed. Give the patient time to express thoughts, especially ones that are difficult to discuss.
* When asking questions, keep in mind that the patient may view sexual problems as a sign of diminished masculinity or femininity. Phrase your questions carefully and offer support as needed.
* Consider the patient's educational and cultural background. If slang or euphemisms are used to talk about sexual organs or function, clarify that you're both talking about the same thing by repeating back what the patient has said and asking for confirmation.

Chief concern

Because the locations of the urinary and reproductive systems are so close, you and the patient may have trouble differentiating signs and symptoms. Even if the patient's concern seems minor, investigate it; ask about its onset, duration, characteristics, aggravating versus alleviating factors, severity, and the measures taken to treat it.

The most common concerns associated with GU problems involve output changes, such as polyuria, oliguria, and anuria. Patients commonly report issues related to voiding pattern changes, including:

* hesitancy
* frequency
* urgency
* dysuria
* nocturia
* incontinence
* urine color changes
* pain
* leaking
* blood in urine.

Common concerns associated with male reproductive problems include penile discharge, scrotal or inguinal masses, or pain and tenderness. For women, common reproductive concerns include vaginal discharge, abnormal uterine bleeding, abdominal pain, dyspareunia, and pruritus.

Current health status

Ask the patient about current problems and medications:

- Is there a history of diabetes (which increases the risk of urinary tract infection [UTI]), cardiovascular disease (which can alter kidney perfusion), or hypertension (which can contribute to renal failure and nephropathy)?
- Has the patient noticed a change in the color or odor of urine?
- Is there pain or burning during urination?
- Does the patient have problems with incontinence or frequency?
- Does the patient have allergies? (Allergic reactions can cause tubular damage; a severe anaphylactic reaction can cause temporary renal failure and permanent tubular necrosis.)
- Which prescribed medications and over-the-counter items does the patient take? Be sure to include birth control and hormones, herbal preparations, and vitamins. Some drugs can affect the appearance of urine; nephrotoxic drugs can alter kidney function.

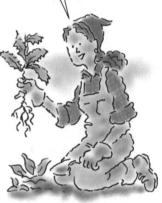

When digging through your patient's health history, pay particular attention to existing health conditions such as diabetes, cardiovascular disease, or hypertension.

Previous health status

Past illnesses and preexisting conditions can affect a patient's GU and reproductive health:

- Has the patient ever had a kidney or bladder infection or an infection of the reproductive system?
- Has the patient ever had kidney or bladder trauma, surgery, congenital problems, cancer, autoimmune disorders, or kidney stones?
- Has he or she ever been catheterized?
- Does the patient have past or current prostate complications?

Also ask about the patient's family history to get information about the risk of developing kidney failure or kidney disease.

Sexual-reproductive history

Some patients feel uncomfortable answering questions about their sexual health or reproductive history. To establish a rapport, begin with less personal questions and then transition to the more personal questions.

Female patients

Start by asking a female patient about her menstrual cycle. How old was she when she began to menstruate? In girls, menses generally starts by age 15. If it hasn't and if no secondary sex characteristics have developed, the patient should be evaluated by a health care provider.

How long does her menses usually last, and how often does it occur? When was her last menstrual period? The normal cycle for menstruation is one menses every 21 to 38 days. The normal duration is 2 to 8 days.

Does she have cramps, spotting, or an unusually heavy or light flow? Does she use pads or tampons? Spotting between menses, or *metrorrhagia*, may be normal in patients taking low-dose hormonal contraceptives or progesterone; otherwise, spotting may indicate infection, cancer, or some other abnormality, so evaluation by a health care provider is warranted.

Comfort zone

When the patient seems comfortable, ask about:
- sexual practices
- sexual orientation
- number of current and past sexual partners
- whether she uses protection (contraception, condoms)
- pain with intercourse (dyspareunia)
- sexually transmitted infection (STI) history and precautions taken to prevent STI contraction
- HIV status
- history of human papilloma virus (HPV) diagnosis
- date of last intercourse
- date and results of last Papanicolaou (Pap) test or vaginal exam
- vaginal discharge
- external lesions
- itching or burning.

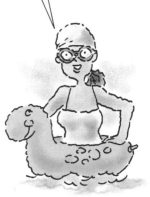

Talking about sexual-reproductive history should go swimmingly after you establish a rapport with your patient.

Pregnancy clues

Ask the patient if she has ever been pregnant. If so:
- How many times has she been pregnant, and how many times did she give birth?
- Has she had any miscarriages or therapeutic abortions?
- Did she have a vaginal or cesarean birth?
- What kind of birth control, if any, does she use?
- Is she possibly pregnant now?

If the patient is sexually active, talk to her about the importance of safer sex and the prevention of and long-term negative effects of untreated STIs.

If your patient is postmenopausal, ask for the date of her last menses. To find out more about her menopausal symptoms, ask if she's having hot flashes, night sweats, mood swings, flushing, or vaginal dryness or itching.

Male patients

As with a female, ask the male patient about his sexual practices and orientation. Also ask about:

- number of current and past sexual partners
- STI history and precautions taken to prevent STI contraction
- HIV status (See *Don't forget to ask the older adult patient.*)
- birth control measures.

Also ask about his sexual health:

- Has he ever experienced trauma to his penis or scrotum?
- Was he ever diagnosed with an undescended testicle?
- Has he had a vasectomy?
- Has he ever been diagnosed with a low sperm count?
- If he participates in sports, how does he protect himself from possible genital injuries?

Physical examination

Physical examination of the GU system usually includes inspection, auscultation, percussion, and palpation. Reproductive system examination involves inspection and palpation.

At ease, please

Before starting, explain the techniques you'll be using and advise the patient that some procedures may be uncomfortable. Perform the examination in a private, quiet, warm, well-lit room.

Renal red flags

Begin the physical examination by assessing your patient's vital signs and mental status. These observations will provide clues about renal dysfunction. For example, a patient's vital signs might reveal hypertension, which can cause renal dysfunction if it isn't controlled.

Behavioral hints

Observing the patient's behavior can give you clues about mental status. Kidney dysfunction can cause symptoms such as trouble concentrating, memory loss, and disorientation. Progressive, chronic kidney failure can cause lethargy, confusion, disorientation, stupor, seizures, and coma.

It's in the skin

Observe the patient's skin. A person with decreased renal function may be pale because of a low hemoglobin level or may even have *uremic frost* (snow-like crystals on the skin that arise from

Ages and stages

Don't forget to ask the older adult patient

Older adults who are sexually active with multiple partners have as high a risk for developing a sexually transmitted disease as younger adults. However, because of decreased immunity, poor hygiene, poor symptom reporting, and, possibly, several concurrent conditions, they may seek treatment for different symptoms.

It is important to gather a thorough understanding of the older adult patient's complete active medication list. These patients often take multiple medications daily (polypharmacy). Decreased ability of organs such as the kidneys to absorb, metabolize, and excrete waste products is common in this population.

metabolic wastes). Also look for signs of fluid imbalance, such as dry mucous membranes, tenting of skin, sunken eyeballs, edema, or ascites.

Inspection

Inspection includes examination of the abdomen and external genitalia.

Leading off: The abdomen and back

Ask the patient to urinate and then help the patient into the supine position with arms at the sides. As you proceed, expose only the areas being examined. Don't forget, collect a clean catch urine specimen at this point.

First, inspect the patient's abdomen. When supine, the abdomen should be symmetrical and smooth, flat, or concave. The skin should be free from lesions, bruises, discolorations, and prominent veins.

Watch for abdominal distention with tight, glistening skin and *striae*—silvery streaks caused by rapidly developing skin tension. These are signs of ascites, which may accompany nephrotic syndrome. This syndrome is characterized by edema, increased urine protein levels, foamy urine, weight gain, and decreased serum albumin levels.

Auscultation

Auscultate the renal arteries in the left and right upper abdominal quadrants by pressing the stethoscope bell lightly against the abdomen and instructing the patient to exhale deeply. Begin auscultating at the midline and work to the left and then return to the midline and work to the right. Listen for systolic bruits or other abnormal sounds, which may indicate a significant problem. For example, a systolic bruit may signal renal artery stenosis or an aortic aneurysm.

Percussion

Kidney percussion, performed by the health care provider, can indicate costovertebral angle tenderness that occurs with inflammation.

Bladder percussion, performed by the health care provider, should sound like tympany. A dull sound signals retained urine.

Palpation

Because the kidneys lie behind other organs and are protected by muscle, they normally aren't palpable unless they're enlarged. However, in very thin patients, you may feel the lower end of the right kidney as a smooth round mass that drops on inspiration. Palpate the inguinal area to identify enlarged lymph nodes or the presence of a hernia. The male scrotum should be assessed for masses or tenderness.

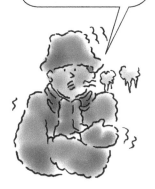

Uremic frost isn't cold, but it sure is frosty! The uremic flakes found on the skin are a positive sign of decreased renal function.

Genitalia concerns

Lastly, inspect the external genitalia for inflammation or discharge from the urethral meatus, skin lesions, drainage from penile or vaginal opening, erythema, edema, and pubic hair distribution. Inspect the location of meatus on the penis for male patients. If uncircumcised, the prepuce (foreskin) should be retracted so the entire glans can be inspected.

Observation of women reporting a previous childbirth should include assessment for vaginal bulging, which could indicate cystocele, rectocele, or vaginal prolapse. Several foreign cultures still perform female genital mutilation even after immigrating to countries where this is not practiced. If noted, inspect for signs or symptoms of infection, bleeding, lacerations, or scarring (World Health Organization, 2018).

Diagnostic tests

Many tests provide information to guide your care of a GU or gynecologic emergency patient. Even if you don't participate in testing, you must know why the test was ordered; what the results mean; and what your nursing responsibilities are before, during, and after the test.

Common diagnostic tests include blood studies, computed tomography (CT) scan, intravenous pyelography (IVP), kidney–ureter–bladder (KUB) radiography, laparoscopy, magnetic resonance imaging (MRI), percutaneous renal biopsy, renal angiography, renal scan, ultrasonography, and urine studies.

Blood studies

Blood studies used to diagnose and evaluate GU function include:
- complete blood count (CBC) to evaluate white blood cell (WBC) count, red blood cell (RBC) count, hemoglobin level, and hematocrit
- blood urea nitrogen (BUN) level
- electrolyte measurements to evaluate calcium, phosphorus, chloride, potassium, and sodium levels
- serum osmolality; creatinine clearance and urea clearance measurements; glomerular filtration rate (GFR); and serum creatinine, serum protein, and uric acid levels. (See *Interpreting blood studies.*)

Interpreting blood studies

Here's how you may interpret the results of blood studies used in diagnosing problems of the genitourinary system.

Complete blood count

An increased white blood cell count may indicate urinary tract infection, peritonitis (in peritoneal dialysis patients), or kidney transplantation infection or rejection.

Red blood cell (RBC) count, hemoglobin level, and hematocrit (HCT) decrease in a patient with chronic renal insufficiency, resulting from decreased erythropoietin production by the kidneys. HCT also provides an indication of fluid balance because it indicates the percentage of RBCs in the blood.

Blood urea nitrogen

Increased blood urea nitrogen (BUN) levels may indicate glomerulonephritis, extensive pyogenic infection, oliguria (from dehydration, mercuric chloride poisoning, or posttraumatic renal insufficiency), tubular obstruction, or other obstructive uropathies. Because nonrenal conditions can also cause BUN levels to increase, interpret BUN levels in conjunction with serum creatinine levels.

Electrolytes

Because the kidneys regulate fluid and electrolyte balance, a critically ill patient with renal disease may experience significant serum electrolyte imbalances. The most commonly measured electrolytes are:

• *calcium and phosphorus*—Calcium and phosphorus levels have an inverse relationship; when one increases, the other decreases. In renal failure, the kidneys aren't able to excrete phosphorus, resulting in hyperphosphatemia and hypocalcemia.

• *chloride*—Chloride levels relate inversely to bicarbonate levels, reflecting acid–base balance. In renal disease, elevated chloride levels suggest metabolic acidosis. Hyperchloremia occurs in renal tubular necrosis, severe dehydration, and complete renal shutdown. Hypochloremia may also occur with pyelonephritis.

• *potassium*—Hyperkalemia occurs with renal insufficiency or acidosis. In renal shutdown, potassium may rapidly increase to life-threatening levels. Hypokalemia may reflect renal tubular disease.

• *sodium*—Sodium helps the kidneys regulate body fluid. Renal disease may result in the loss of sodium through the kidneys.

Serum creatinine

The serum creatinine level reflects the glomerular filtration rate (GFR). Renal damage is indicated more accurately by increases in serum creatinine than by the BUN level. Use in conjunction with the BUN.

Serum osmolality

An increase in serum osmolality with a simultaneous decrease in urine osmolality indicates diminished distal tubule responsiveness to circulating antidiuretic hormone. This provides information regarding the balance between fluid and solutes.

Serum proteins

Levels of the serum protein albumin may decline sharply from its loss in the urine during nephrotic syndrome, inflammation, malnutrition, cirrhosis, and hepatitis. Nephrosis may also cause total serum protein levels to decrease.

Uric acid

Because uric acid clears from the body by glomerular filtration and tubular secretion, elevated levels may indicate impaired renal function; below-normal levels may indicate defective tubular absorption.

Creatinine clearance

Creatinine clearance estimates GFR. Typically, high creatinine clearance rates have little diagnostic value. Low creatinine clearance rates may indicate reduced renal blood flow (associated with shock or renal artery obstruction), acute tubular necrosis, acute or chronic glomerulonephritis, advanced bilateral chronic pyelonephritis, advanced bilateral renal lesions, or nephrosclerosis.

Urea clearance

Although urea clearance is a less reliable measurement of GFR than creatinine clearance, it still provides a good measure of overall renal function. High urea clearance rates rarely have diagnostic value. Low urea clearance rates may reflect decreased renal blood flow, acute or chronic glomerulonephritis, advanced bilateral chronic pyelonephritis, acute tubular necrosis, nephrosclerosis, advanced bilateral renal lesions, bilateral ureteral obstruction, or dehydration.

Practice pointers
- Tell the patient that the test requires a blood sample. Fasting is not necessary.
- Check the patient's active medication list for drugs that might influence test results.

CT scan

CT scan is a diagnostic imaging procedure that uses a combination of X-rays and computer technology to produce horizontal, or axial, images (often called *slices*) of the body. A CT scan, which is more detailed than a standard X-ray, shows detailed images of bones, muscles, fat, and organs.

A CT scan may involve the abdomen or pelvis; in addition, a renal CT scan may be done. In a renal CT scan, the image's density reflects the amount of radiation absorbed by renal tissue, thus permitting identification of masses or other lesions. A CT scan may be done with or without a contrast medium, but use of a contrast medium is preferred unless the patient has an allergy, kidney disease, or an increased BUN or creatinine level.

Practice pointers
- Confirm that the patient is not pregnant prior to CT testing.
- Explain the procedure to the patient and instruct to lie still, relax, and breathe normally during the test.
- Explain the procedure to the patient and confirm that he or she does not have an allergy to iodine or shellfish. A patient with these allergies may have an adverse reaction to the contrast medium. Notify the health care provider.
- If the health care provider has ordered an intravenous (IV) contrast medium (for patients who do not have an allergy to iodine or shellfish), explain that the patient may experience discomfort from the needle puncture and a localized feeling of warmth on injection.
- Ascertain when the patient last ate or drank; restrict food and fluids as soon as possible but continue any drug regimen as ordered.
- If the patient is on nothing-by-mouth status, increase the IV fluid rate as ordered after the procedure to flush contrast medium from the system. Monitor serum creatinine and BUN levels for signs of acute renal failure, which may be caused by the contrast medium.

IVP

After IV administration of a contrast medium, IVP, also known as *excretory urography* or *intravenous urography* (IVU), a diagnostic X-ray of the kidneys, ureters, and bladder, may be performed. This allows visualization of the renal parenchyma, calyces, pelvises, ureters, bladder, and, in some cases, the urethra. In the first minute after injection (the *nephrographic stage*), the contrast medium delineates the kidneys' size and shape. After 3 to 5 minutes (the *pyelographic stage*), the contrast medium moves into the calyces and pelvises, allowing visualization of cysts, tumors, and other obstructions.

Practice pointers

- Explain the procedure to the patient and confirm that he or she does not have an allergy to iodine, iodine-containing foods, or contrast media containing iodine. A patient with these allergies may have an adverse reaction to the contrast medium. Notify the health care provider.
- Ensure the ordering health care provider is aware if the patient is pregnant because IVP is not generally performed on pregnant patients.
- Ensure that the patient is well hydrated.
- Inform the patient that a transient burning sensation and metallic taste when the contrast medium is injected may be experienced.

KUB radiography

A KUB X-ray may be performed to assess the abdominal area. It consists of plain, contrast-free X-rays and shows kidney size, position, and structure. It can also reveal calculi and other lesions. Before performing a renal biopsy, the health care provider may use this test to determine kidney placement.

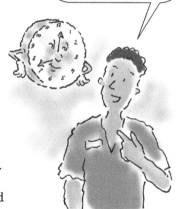

Watch the clock with KUB radiography to identify kidney changes, such as size, position, structure, or the presence of calculi or lesions.

Practice pointers

- KUB radiography requires no special pretest or posttest care. It's commonly a portable X-ray test performed at the bedside.
- Determine the patient's status regarding pregnancy prior to radiographic testing because X-rays are not usually performed on pregnant patients.
- Explain the procedure to the patient.

Laparoscopy

Laparoscopy allows the health care provider to inspect organs in the peritoneal cavity by inserting a *laparoscope* (small fiber-optic telescope) through the anterior abdominal wall. This test is used to:

- detect such abnormalities as cysts, adhesions, fibroids, and infection
- identify the cause of pelvic pain
- diagnose endometriosis, ectopic pregnancy, or pelvic inflammatory disease (PID)
- evaluate pelvic masses or the fallopian tubes of infertile patients
- stage cancer.

This procedure may also be used therapeutically for analysis of adhesions, tubal sterilization, removal of foreign bodies, and fulguration of endometriotic implants.

Practice pointers

- Check the time the patient last ingested food or fluids; if possible, nothing should be taken by mouth (PO) for approximately 8 hours before the test.
- Assure the patient that a general anesthetic will be received. Advise that there may be pain at the puncture site and in the shoulders.
- Check the patient's history to assess for hypersensitivity to the anesthetic. Make sure that all laboratory work is completed and results are reported before the test.
- Provide preoperative care.
- Explain that the patient will probably be transferred to the outpatient care unit after the procedure.

MRI

MRI is a diagnostic procedure that uses a combination of a large magnet, radiofrequencies, and a computer to produce detailed images of organs and structures within the body.

MRI provides tomographic images that reflect the differing hydrogen densities of body tissues. Physical, chemical, and cellular microenvironments modify these densities, as do the fluid characteristics of tissues. MRI can provide precise images of anatomic detail and important biochemical information about the tissue examined and can efficiently visualize and stage kidney, bladder, and prostate tumors.

Practice pointers

- Before the patient enters the MRI chamber, make sure that he or she has removed all metal objects, such as earrings, watches, necklaces, bracelets, and rings. Patients with internal metal objects, such as pacemakers, aneurysm clips, or metal orthopedic fixtures, cannot undergo MRI testing.
- If you're accompanying the patient, be sure to remove metal objects from your pockets, including scissors, forceps, penlights, metal pens, and identification or bank cards containing code strips because the magnetic field will erase the data stored in that area.
- Tell the patient to remain still throughout the test, which takes about 45 minutes, and that there will be a loud thumping noise heard during the test. If the patient reports claustrophobia, reassure and provide emotional support. Be prepared to administer antianxiety or sedative medications if prescribed by the health care provider for claustrophobia.

Percutaneous renal biopsy

A biopsy is a procedure performed to remove tissue or cells from the body for examination under a microscope. Histologic examination can help differentiate glomerular and tubular renal disease, monitor the disorder's progress, and assess the effectiveness of therapy. It can also reveal a malignant tumor such as Wilms tumor.

Histologic studies can help diagnose:
- disseminated lupus erythematosus
- amyloid infiltration
- acute and chronic glomerulonephritis
- renal vein thrombosis
- pyelonephritis. (See *Assisting with percutaneous renal biopsy,* page 366.)

Practice pointers

- Check to ensure that the patient has had nothing by mouth for 8 hours before the test. Inform the patient that a mild sedative will be given before the test to aid relaxation.
- After the test, tell the patient that pressure will be applied to the biopsy site to stop superficial bleeding and then a pressure dressing will be applied.
- Instruct the patient to lie flat on his or her back without moving for at least 6 hours after the biopsy to prevent bleeding.

Assisting with percutaneous renal biopsy

To prepare for percutaneous renal biopsy, position the patient on his or her abdomen. To stabilize the kidneys, place a sandbag or rolled towels beneath the abdomen as shown.

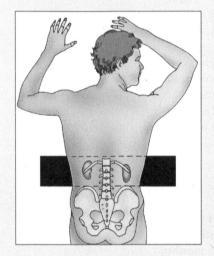

After administering a local anesthetic, the health care provider instructs the patient to hold his or her breath and remain immobile. Then the health care provider inserts a needle with the obturator between the patient's last rib and the iliac crest as shown below. After asking the patient to breathe deeply, the health care provider removes the obturator and inserts cutting prongs, which gather blood and tissue samples. This test is commonly performed in the radiology department so that special radiographic procedures may be used to help guide the needle.

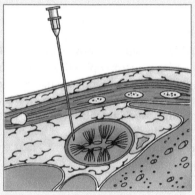

Renal angiography

An angiogram, also called an *arteriogram*, is an X-ray image of the blood vessels. Renal angiography is used to visualize the arterial tree, capillaries, and venous drainage of the kidneys. The test uses a contrast medium injected under fluoroscopy into a catheter in the femoral artery or vein.

On closer inspection

Renal arteriography (angiography of the arteries) may reveal:
- abnormal renal blood flow
- hypervascular renal tumors

- renal cysts
- renal artery stenosis
- renal artery aneurysms and arteriovenous fistulas
- pyelonephritis
- renal abscesses or inflammatory masses
- renal infarction
- renal trauma (Chong et al., 2016).

Practice pointers

- Explain the procedure to the patient and confirm that he or she does not have an allergy to iodine or shellfish. A patient with these allergies may have an adverse reaction to the contrast medium. Notify the health care provider.
- Preprocedural testing should include evaluation of renal function (serum creatinine and BUN levels) and the potential risk of bleeding (prothrombin time, partial thromboplastin time, and platelet count). Notify the health care provider if results are abnormal.
- Report adverse reactions, such as nausea, vomiting, dizziness, headache, and urticaria.
- Depending on the patient's renal status, the health care provider may order increased fluids after the procedure or an increased IV infusion rate to flush the contrast medium out of the patient's system.
- After the procedure, check the patient's serum creatinine and BUN levels to evaluate renal function (because contrast media can cause acute renal failure).

Renal scan

A kidney scan is a specialized radiology procedure used to assess the function and structure of the kidneys as well as the perfusion (blood flow) to the kidney tissue. A radionuclide renal scan, which may be substituted for IVP in patients who are hypersensitive to contrast media, involves IV injection of a radionuclide, followed by scintigraphy. Observation of uptake concentration and radionuclide transit during the procedure allows assessment of renal blood flow, nephron and collecting system function, and renal structure.

Practice pointers

- Inform the patient that injection with a radionuclide will take place and that transient flushing and nausea may be experienced. Emphasize that it's only a small amount of radionuclide and is usually excreted within 24 hours.
- After the test, instruct the patient to flush the toilet immediately upon every urination within the next 24 hours as a radiation precaution.

Ultrasonography

A kidney ultrasound is a noninvasive procedure (in which the skin is not pierced) that uses high-frequency sound waves to reveal internal structures; it can involve the abdomen, pelvis, or specifically the renal structures. This test provides information about internal structures of the abdomen; pelvis; and, more specifically, the kidney's size, shape, and position. It's also used to detect pregnancy.

Practice pointers

- Tell the patient to lie prone (the renal examination position) or supine during the test.
- Explain that a technician will place gel on the skin and then move a probe or transducer against the skin across the area being tested.
- If a pelvic ultrasound is being done, make sure that the patient has a full bladder, which is used as landmark for defining pelvic organs.

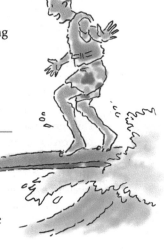

Ride the wave! The wave of high-frequency sound waves that is, of ultrasonography to examine the structure of internal organs.

Urine studies

Urine studies, such as urinalysis (DeMoranville, 2018) and urine osmolality, can indicate acute renal failure, renal trauma, UTI, and other disorders. Urinalysis can indicate renal or systemic disorders, warranting further investigation. A random urine specimen is used. (See *What urinalysis findings mean.*)

Concentrate, concentrate

Urine osmolality is used to evaluate the diluting and concentrating ability of the kidneys and varies greatly with diet and hydration status. The ability to concentrate urine is one of the first functions lost in renal failure.

Practice pointers

- For urinalysis, collect a random urine specimen as a clean-catch specimen or from the indwelling urinary catheter. Send the specimen to the laboratory immediately.
- For urine osmolality testing, collect a random urine sample.

What urinalysis findings mean

Test	Normal values or findings	Abnormal findings	Possible causes of abnormal findings
Color and odor	Straw color	Clear to black	Dietary changes; use of certain drugs (methyldopa, metronidazole, nitrofurantoin, rifampin); dehydration; metabolic, inflammatory, or infectious disease
	Slightly aromatic odor	Fruity or foul odor	Diabetes mellitus, starvation, dehydration or infection
	Clear appearance	Turbid appearance	Renal infection, diet high in purine-rich foods
Specific gravity	1.005 to 1.030, with slight variations from one specimen to the next	Below-normal specific gravity	Diabetes insipidus, glomerulonephritis, pyelonephritis, acute renal failure, alkalosis, diuretic use, adrenal insufficiency, aldosteronism
		Above-normal specific gravity	Dehydration, nephrosis, glycosuria, syndrome of inappropriate antidiuretic hormone, medication use (mannitol)
		Fixed specific gravity	Severe renal damage, intrinsic renal insufficiency
pH	4.6 to 8.0	Alkaline pH (above 8.0)	Fanconi syndrome (chronic renal disease), urinary tract infection (UTI), metabolic or respiratory alkalosis
		Acidic pH (below 4.5)	Renal tuberculosis, phenylketonuria, acidosis
Protein	No protein	Proteinuria	Renal disease (such as glomerulosclerosis, acute or chronic glomerulonephritis, nephrolithiasis, polycystic kidney disease, and acute or chronic renal failure), congestive heart failure; may also be caused acutely by dehydration, emotional stress, exercise, fever
Ketones	No ketones	Ketonuria	Diabetes mellitus, starvation, conditions causing acutely increased metabolic demands and decreased food intake (such as vomiting, diarrhea)
Glucose	No glucose	Glycosuria	Diabetes mellitus, Cushing syndrome, liver and pancreatic disease, Fanconi syndrome
Red blood cells (RBCs)	0 to 2 RBCs/high-power field	Numerous RBCs	UTI, obstruction, inflammation, trauma, or tumor; glomerulonephritis; renal hypertension; lupus nephritis; renal tuberculosis; renal vein thrombosis; hydronephrosis; pyelonephritis; parasitic bladder infection; polyarteritis nodosa; hemorrhagic disorder, Wegener granulomatosis, Goodpasture syndrome, renal infarct, subacute bacterial endocarditis

(continued)

What urinalysis findings mean *(continued)*

Test	Normal values or findings	Abnormal findings	Possible causes of abnormal findings
Epithelial cells	Few epithelial cells	Excessive epithelial cells	Acute tubular necrosis, toxic ingestion (mercury, diethylene glycol, salicylate), cytomegalovirus, viral hepatitis, renal tubular degeneration
White blood cells (WBCs)	0 to 4 WBCs/high-power field	Numerous WBCs	UTI, especially cystitis or pyelonephritis
		Numerous WBCs and WBC casts	Renal infection (such as acute pyelonephritis and glomerulonephritis, nephrotic syndrome, pyogenic infection, and lupus nephritis); poststreptococcal acute glomerulonephritis
Leukocyte esterase	None	Positive	Pyuria, balanitis, urethritis, tuberculosis, bladder tumors, viral infections, nephrolithiasis, foreign bodies, exercise, glomerulonephritis, corticosteroid, and cyclophosphamide
Nitrites	None	Positive	Gram-negative and some gram-positive organisms
Bilirubin	None	Positive	Liver dysfunction, biliary obstruction
Urobilinogen	Small amounts	Large	Hemolysis, hepatocellular disease
Casts	No casts (except occasional hyaline casts)	Excessive casts	Renal disease
		Excessive hyaline casts	Renal parenchymal disease, inflammation, glomerular capillary membrane trauma
		Epithelial casts	Renal tubular damage, nephrosis, eclampsia, chronic lead intoxication
		Waxy casts	Nephrotic syndrome, chronic renal disease, diabetes mellitus
		Fatty casts	High urinary protein nephrotic syndrome
		RBC casts	Renal parenchymal disease (especially glomerulonephritis), renal infarction, subacute bacterial endocarditis, sickle cell anemia, blood dyscrasias, malignant hypertension, collagen disease
Crystals	Some crystals	Numerous calcium oxalate crystals	Hypercalcemia, kidney stones
		Cystine crystals (cystinuria)	Inborn metabolic error, obstructive renal failure
		Triple phosphate crystals	May be normal or associated with alkaline urine and UTI (typically *Proteus*)
Yeast cells	No yeast cells	Yeast cells in sediment	External genitalia contamination, vaginitis, urethritis, prostatovesiculitis
Parasites	No parasites	Parasites in sediment	External genitalia contamination or schistosomiasis related to foreign travel

Adapted from Centers for Disease Control and Prevention. (2018). *Parasites: Schistosomiasis*. Retrieved from https://www.cdc.gov/parasites/schistosomiasis/

Treatments

GU and gynecologic emergencies present many treatment challenges because they stem from various mechanisms occurring separately or simultaneously. Common treatments include drug therapy and non-surgical or surgical procedures.

Drug therapy

Ideally, drug therapy should be effective and not impair urologic function. However, because GU disorders can affect the chemical composition of body fluids and the pharmacokinetic properties of many drugs, standard regimens of some drugs may require adjustment. For example, dosages of drugs that are mainly excreted by the kidneys unchanged or as active metabolites may require adjustment to avoid nephrotoxicity.

Drug therapy for GU disorders can include:
- urinary tract antimicrobials
- bladder control medications (antispasmodics, anticholinergics, cholinergics)
- diuretics
- impotence agents
- benign prostatic hyperplasia medications.

In addition, electrolytes and replacements may be necessary depending on the underlying cause of the GU dysfunction.

Drug therapy for gynecologic disorders commonly includes antibiotics, antifungals, and analgesics for pain.

Nonsurgical procedures

Nonsurgical procedures employed to treat GU emergencies include calculi basketing via uteroscope, lithotripsy (ultrasonic lithotripsy, electrohydraulic lithotripsy, or extracorporeal shock wave lithotripsy [ESWL]), and urinary bladder catheterization.

Calculi basketing

When ureteral calculi are too large for normal elimination, removal with a basketing instrument is the treatment of choice. This helps to relieve pain and prevent infection and renal dysfunction. In this technique, a basketing instrument is inserted through a cystoscope or ureteroscope into the ureter to capture the calculus, which is then withdrawn to remove it.

Calculi basketing may not be fun and games, but it's a total score for the patient to eliminate their pain and improve their kidney health.

Nursing considerations
- Tell the patient that after calculi removal, he or she may have an indwelling urinary catheter inserted for 24 to 28 hours to ensure normal urine drainage.
- The patient may receive a stent during the procedure. Discuss that this is to help ensure the ureter stays open after the procedure as there is the possibility of swelling at the site. The health care provider will schedule a follow-up to have this removed days to weeks after the procedure.
- Tell the patient he or she will receive IV fluids during and immediately after the procedure to maintain urine output and prevent such complications as hydronephrosis and pyelonephritis.
- Administer fluids as ordered, usually to maintain a urine output of 3 to 4 L/day.

Basket boomerang
If the patient returns to the ED after the basketing procedure, follow these steps:
- Observe the color of urine drainage from the indwelling urinary catheter; typically, it's blood tinged at first, with gradual clearing over 24 to 48 hours. Irrigate the catheter as ordered using sterile technique.
- Administer analgesics as ordered.
- Observe for and report signs or symptoms of septicemia, which may result from ureteral perforation during basketing.
- Assess for signs and symptoms of acute ureteral obstruction, such as severe pain and the inability to void.

Extracorporeal shock wave lithotripsy
ESWL is a noninvasive technique for removing obstructive renal calculi. It uses high-energy shock waves to break up calculi and allow their normal passage.

Nursing considerations
- Confirm that the patient is not pregnant prior to ESWL.
- Determine if the patient has a pacemaker, in which case a cardiologist should be present during the procedure.
- Tell the patient he or she may receive a general or epidural anesthetic, depending on the type of lithotriptor and the intensity of shock waves needed.
- Insert an IV line.

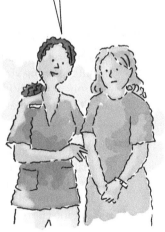

Take time to walk with your patient after ESWL to facilitate the passing of calculi fragments. Drinking extra fluids will help, too!

- Inform the patient that an indwelling urinary catheter will likely be in place after the procedure.
- Explain to the patient that, after the procedure, ambulation will be encouraged as soon as possible and fluids will be increased as ordered to aid the passage of calculi fragments.
- If the patient returns to the ED after the procedure, strain all urine for calculi fragments and send to the laboratory for analysis.
- Monitor urine for frank or persistent bleeding. Keep in mind that slight hematuria usually occurs for several days.
- Assess for severe, unremitting pain; persistent hematuria; inability to void; fever and chills; or recurrent nausea and vomiting.

Urinary catheterization

Catheterization—the insertion of a drainage device into the urinary bladder—may be intermittent or continuous.

Intermittent catheterization drains urine remaining in the bladder after voiding. It's used for patients with urinary incontinence, urinary retention, urethral strictures, cystitis, prostatic obstruction, neurogenic bladder, or other disorders that interfere with bladder emptying. It may also be used postoperatively.

Indwelling urinary catheterization helps relieve bladder distention caused by such conditions as urinary tract obstruction and neurogenic bladder. It allows continuous urine drainage in patients with a urinary meatus swollen from local trauma or childbirth as well as from surgery. Catheterization can also provide accurate monitoring of urine output when normal voiding is impaired.

Nursing considerations

- Thoroughly review the procedure with the patient and provide reassurance that although catheterization may produce slight discomfort, it shouldn't be painful. Explain that you'll stop the procedure if severe discomfort is experienced.
- Obtain a sterile catheterization package.
- Perform the catheterization; document difficulty or ease of insertion, patient discomfort, and the amount and nature of urine drainage.
- During urine drainage, monitor for pallor, diaphoresis, and painful bladder spasms. If these occur, clamp the catheter tubing for 10 to 15 minutes. When symptoms resolve, resume drainage.
- Remove the catheter as soon as possible or as ordered to prevent catheter-associated UTIs.

Fluid watch

- Frequently assess intake and output. Encourage fluid intake to maintain continuous urine flow through the catheter and decrease the risk of infection and clot formation.
- Make sure the collection bag is kept below bladder level to enhance drainage and prevent backflow, which can lead to infection.
- To help prevent infection, avoid separating the catheter and tubing unless absolutely necessary.
- Closely assess for signs and symptoms of UTI and for signs of catheter obstruction.

Surgical procedures

Suprapubic catheterization surgery may be necessary when conservative measures fail to control the patient's problem.

Suprapubic catheterization

Suprapubic catheterization is a type of urinary diversion connected to a closed drainage system that involves transcutaneous insertion of a catheter through the suprapubic area into the bladder. Suprapubic catheterization provides temporary urinary diversion after certain gynecologic procedures, bladder surgery, or prostatectomy and relieves obstruction from calculi, severe urethral strictures, or pelvic trauma. Less commonly, it may be used to create a permanent urinary diversion, thereby relieving obstruction from an inoperable tumor or for patients with neurogenic bladder.

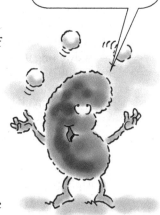

Like most juggling acts, suprapubic catheterization is usually temporary, and their primary purpose is to create a diversion.

Nursing considerations
- Explain that the health care provider will insert a soft plastic tube through the skin of the abdomen and into the bladder and then connect the tube to an external collection bag.
- Explain the procedure is done under local anesthesia, causes little or no discomfort, and takes 15 to 45 minutes.
- Closely assess the insertion site.
- To ensure adequate drainage and tube patency, check the suprapubic catheter at least hourly for the first 24 hours after insertion. Make sure the collection bag is below bladder level to enhance drainage and prevent backflow, which can lead to infection.
- Tape the catheter securely in place on the abdominal skin to reduce tension and prevent dislodgment. To prevent kinks in the tube, curve it gently but don't bend it.
- Assess dressings frequently and change as necessary. Observe the skin around the insertion site for signs of infection and encrustation.

Common disorders

GU and gynecologic disorders commonly encountered in the ED include kidney trauma, ovarian cyst, PID, pyelonephritis, renal calculi, sexual assault, testicular torsion, and UTI.

Kidney trauma

Kidney trauma can involve damage to minor tissues or, possibly, major vascular structures. Trauma to the kidney can be wide ranging, from contusions and subcapsular hematomas to fractured kidney, renal artery thrombosis, or avulsion of the major renal artery or vein. Kidney trauma may be classified by severity using a grading scale of 1 to 5 or using the categories of minor, major, and critical trauma.

The American Association for Surgery of Trauma (AAST) (2018) classifies kidney injury by grade, and type and description of injury. Grade I kidney injury represents a contusion or hematoma, with microscopic or gross hematuria; this injury is subcapsular, and non-expanding without parenchymal laceration (AAST, 2018). Severity of injury increases through Grade V, which represents a laceration with vascular compromise, in which the kidney is shattered and there is avulsion of renal hilum which devascularizes the kidney (AAST, 2018).

What causes it

Kidney trauma is commonly classified as *penetrating* or *blunt*, depending on the type of injury.

Penetrating kidney trauma involves an injury by a foreign object, such as a bullet (or a bullet fragment or effect of the blast) or knife. A gunshot wound involving the kidney typically results in a complex array of injuries.

Blunt kidney trauma is the cause of the majority of all kidney injuries, many of which result from motor vehicle collisions. Other less common causes include sports injuries, occupational injuries, falls, and assaults.

Kidney trauma may also result from iatrogenic causes. These causes may include percutaneous nephrostomy, renal biopsy, and ESWL.

How it happens

Three mechanisms are responsible for causing blunt kidney trauma:
1. direct blow to the flank area
2. laceration of the parenchyma from a fractured rib or vertebra
3. sudden deceleration leading to shearing and subsequent damage.

What to look for

Assessment findings may vary based on the type and extent of kidney trauma. One common finding is hematuria, which may be gross or microscopic. However, the degree of hematuria doesn't correlate with the severity of kidney trauma.

And that's not all

Additional findings may include:
- abdominal or flank pain
- tenderness along the back
- report of colicky pain with the passage of clots in the urine
- hematoma over the flank area, usually in the area of the 11th or 12th rib
- obvious wounds, bruises, or abrasions in the flank area or abdomen
- Grey Turner's sign, which demonstrates bruising of the flanks and blue discoloration; may take 24 to 48 hours to develop
- costovertebral angle pain or tenderness
- palpable mass in the flank or abdominal area
- signs and symptoms of hemorrhage and hypovolemic shock, such as pallor, diaphoresis, hypotension, tachycardia, and changes in mental status
- hematuria.

What tests tell you

Diagnostic testing depends on the patient's condition and extent of injuries. Some diagnostic tests may include:
- KUB radiography to identify the path and appearance of the object causing the penetrating trauma and to determine the outline or fragmentation of the kidney
- IVP to stage the degree of kidney injury
- ultrasound, CT scan, and MRI to evaluate kidney structure and identify hematomas, lacerations, and vascular disruptions
- renal angiography to detect arterial injury.
  Other tests include:
- arterial blood gas analysis to evaluate respiratory and acid–base status secondary to blood loss and shock
- CBC to evaluate the degree of blood loss
- type and screen or type and cross—prepare for possible blood transfusion
- coagulation studies to determine the patient's clotting ability
- serum electrolyte level to determine possible imbalances
- renal panel—BUN and creatinine, GFR, creatinine clearance to determine kidney function.

How it's treated

Treatment of blunt kidney trauma typically focuses on bed rest with frequent assessments and serial specimens for urinalysis. Analgesics are used to manage pain. A penetrating kidney trauma, such as a laceration to the kidney, requires surgical intervention.

Hemodynamics count

A kidney trauma patient who's hemodynamically stable requires close monitoring in the initial period after injury. Surgery is typically performed later, based on the patient's condition.

For a patient who is hemodynamically unstable, has other associated trauma, or exhibits shock, treatment focuses on immediate stabilization, assessing and maintaining airway and circulation as well as breathing (ABCs), assessing level of consciousness (LOC), and preparing the patient for transport or for exploratory laparotomy.

Bed rest is the very best for a kidney after experiencing blunt trauma! But, your job is to check, check, check!

Wound care

If the patient has a wound, treatment may include controlling bleeding—usually by applying firm, direct pressure—and cleaning the wound. Pain medication and antibiotic therapy are instituted as indicated. In addition, IV therapy is started to ensure fluid balance and maintain the patient's hemodynamic status.

What to do

- Assess the patient's ABCs and initiate emergency measures, if necessary.
- Monitor the patient's vital signs and note significant changes.
- Assess oxygen saturation and administer supplemental oxygen, as ordered.
- Assess heart for arrhythmias.
- Assess neurologic status, including LOC and pupillary and motor response.
- Obtain blood studies, including type and cross-match.
- Insert two large-bore IV catheters and infuse fluids as ordered.
- Quickly and carefully assess for other areas of trauma.
- Institute complete bed rest with frequent assessments, such as every 15 to 30 minutes or as indicated by the patient's condition.
- Assess wounds and provide wound care as appropriate. Cover open wounds and control bleeding by applying pressure.

And that's not all

- Assess for increased abdominal distention.
- Administer blood products as appropriate.
- Monitor for signs of hypovolemic shock.
- Provide pain medication, as appropriate.
- Prepare the patient and family for diagnostic testing and possible surgery.
- Provide therapeutic support to the patient and family.

Ovarian cyst

An ovarian cyst refers to the development of a saclike structure on the ovary. The sac can contain fluid, semifluid, or solid material. Cysts may be categorized as *endometrial, follicular,* or *corpus luteal* depending on the underlying mechanism associated with their development.

What causes it

Ovarian cysts vary in size, consistency, and development. The underlying cause of the cyst identifies its type:

- *endometrial cyst*—results from an overgrowth of endometrial tissue such as endometriosis
- *follicular cyst*—results from failed follicular rupture from the ovary at ovulation
- *corpus luteal cyst*—results from the continued presence of a corpus luteum that has failed to atrophy.

How it happens

Within the ovary, the follicle develops because of hormonal influences. At the midpoint of a woman's menstrual cycle, a follicle, now mature, ruptures from the ovary (with follicular cysts, this rupture doesn't occur).

After ovulation, the follicle becomes the corpus luteum and travels to the fallopian tube where it may be fertilized by spermatozoa. If the corpus luteum isn't fertilized, it degenerates. With corpus luteal cysts, this degeneration doesn't occur.

Normally, endometrial tissue is located in the uterine cavity. However, for unknown reasons, the tissue sometimes appears outside of the endometrial cavity, commonly around the ovaries. This tissue responds to estrogen and progesterone secretion and proliferates. Upon menstruation, the tissue bleeds and becomes inflamed, leading to fibrosis.

What to look for

Most patients with ovarian cysts may be asymptomatic. Typically, they experience signs and symptoms when rupture, hemorrhage, or torsion (twisting) of a cyst occurs. Follicular cysts commonly rupture in the first half of the menstrual cycle with strenuous exercise or sexual intercourse, whereas corpus luteal cysts typically rupture in the last half of the cycle, usually in the weeks before the woman's menses.

If the patient is experiencing symptoms, they may include:

- pressure or abdominal pain on the affected side
- dull ache in the lower back and thighs
- abnormal or prolonged menstruation
- mittelschmerz pain (pain with ovulation) with rupture of the cyst
- nausea and vomiting may be present with torsion of an ovary.

Pelvic examination may reveal ovarian tenderness and enlargement. With rupture, the patient may exhibit signs and symptoms of hypovolemic shock, especially with rupture of a blood-filled cyst such as a mature corpus luteal cyst. These symptoms may range from mild to severe, depending on the extent of blood loss.

What tests tell you

There's no specific test used to identify ovarian cysts. Usually, ultrasound is used to rule out other conditions, such as appendicitis, ectopic pregnancy, and intraperitoneal bleeding, which demonstrate similar symptoms. In addition, a pregnancy test is performed to rule out pregnancy. Routine diagnostic tests, such as CBC and urinalysis, are done to establish a baseline and rule out other possible disorders.

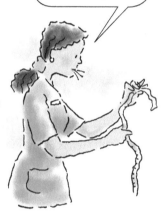

Ruling out other conditions with similar symptoms is the primary way of diagnosing an ovarian cyst.

How it's treated

Treatment for an unruptured cyst includes analgesics for pain management and support for the patient. In most cases, nonopioids, such as nonsteroidal anti-inflammatory drugs (NSAIDs), are used. If necessary, opioids may be given for a short term, although this is not the preferred method of treatment.

Additional treatment may include:

- surgical excision of the endometrial cyst
- low-dose hormonal contraceptives may be considered to slow the development of new cysts (Office on Women's Health, 2019a)
- pelvic rest if the patient is having moderate to severe pain.

Poly problems

If the patient has polycystic ovarian syndrome or PCOS (multiple follicular cysts on both ovaries), clomiphene citrate or metformin may be used to induce ovulation; alternatively, a wedge resection of the ovary may be performed (National Institutes of Health, 2018).

Typically, surgery isn't done unless the patient exhibits signs and symptoms of hypovolemic shock. Then treatment focuses on stabilizing the patient and preparing her for surgery as quickly as possible.

What to do

- Assess vital signs and be alert for signs and symptoms of hemorrhage (hypovolemic shock).
- Administer analgesics as ordered for pain management.
- Provide support to the patient; explain that small cysts usually reabsorb on their own.
- Review the treatment plan for the patient, including drug therapy if ordered.
- Teach the patient about signs and symptoms of possible torsion.
- Prepare the patient for surgery if indicated.
  If the patient develops hypovolemic shock:
- Monitor and maintain ABCs.
- Start IV line if one isn't already in place and administer fluids as ordered.
- Obtain a specimen for blood typing and cross-matching.

Pelvic inflammatory disease

PID refers to an infectious and inflammatory disorder of the upper female genital tract (Centers for Disease Control and Prevention, 2015). It is an acute, subacute, recurrent, or chronic infection of the oviducts and ovaries, with adjacent tissue involvement. It includes inflammation of the cervix (cervicitis), uterus (endometritis), fallopian tubes (salpingitis), and ovaries (oophoritis), which can extend to the connective tissue lying between the broad ligaments (parametritis). (See *Three types of PID.*)

Early diagnosis and treatment prevent damage to the reproductive system. Complications of PID include infertility and potentially fatal septicemia, pulmonary emboli, and shock.

What causes it

PID can result from infection with aerobic or anaerobic organisms. The organisms that cause gonorrhea and chlamydia are common in up to 50% of the cases of PID (Centers for Disease Control and Prevention, 2017). Overgrowth of one or more of the common bacterial species found in cervical mucus, including staphylococci, streptococci, diphtheroids, *Gardnerella vaginalis*, *Haemophilus influenzae*, and such coliforms as *Pseudomonas* and *Escherichia coli*, may be implicated. PID also results from infection with *Neisseria gonorrhoeae*. Finally, multiplication of typically nonpathogenic bacteria in an altered endometrial environment can cause PID. This multiplication occurs most commonly during parturition.

Three types of PID

This chart lists the types of pelvic inflammatory disease (PID), their signs and symptoms, and diagnostic test findings.

Type and signs and symptoms	Diagnostic test findings
Cervicitis	
• *Acute*: purulent, foul-smelling vaginal discharge; vulvovaginitis with itching or burning; red, edematous cervix; pelvic discomfort; sexual dysfunction; metrorrhagia; infertility; spontaneous abortion • *Chronic*: cervical dystocia, laceration or eversion of the cervix, ulcerative vesicular lesion (when cervicitis results from herpes simplex virus type 2)	• Cultures for *Neisseria gonorrhoeae* or *Chlamydia trachomatis* are positive; with chronic cervicitis, causative organisms are usually *Staphylococcus* or *Streptococcus*. • Cytologic smears may reveal severe inflammation. • If cervicitis isn't complicated by salpingitis, white blood cell (WBC) count is normal or slightly elevated; erythrocyte sedimentation rate (ESR) is elevated. • With acute cervicitis, cervical palpation reveals tenderness.
Endometritis (usually postpartum or postabortion)	
• *Acute*: mucopurulent or purulent vaginal discharge oozing from cervix; edematous, hyperemic endometrium, possibly leading to ulceration and necrosis (with virulent organisms); lower abdominal pain and tenderness; fever; rebound pain; abdominal muscle spasm; thrombophlebitis of uterine and pelvic vessels • *Chronic*: recurring acute episodes (usually from having multiple sexual partners and sexually transmitted infections)	• With severe infection, palpation may reveal boggy uterus. • Uterine and blood samples are positive for causative organism, usually *Staphylococcus*. • WBC count and ESR are elevated.
Salpingo-oophoritis	
• *Acute*: sudden onset of lower abdominal and pelvic pain, usually after menses; increased vaginal discharge; fever; malaise; lower abdominal pressure and tenderness; tachycardia; pelvic peritonitis • *Chronic*: recurring acute episodes	• WBC count is elevated or normal. • X-ray may show ileus. • Pelvic examination reveals extreme tenderness. • Smear of cervical or periurethral gland exudate shows gram-negative intracellular diplococci.

Upping the ante

These factors increase the patient's chances of developing PID:
- history of STIs
- multiple sexual partners
- history of sexual abuse
- intrauterine contraceptive devices within the first 3 weeks
- conditions (such as uterine infection) or procedures (such as conization or cauterization of the cervix) that alter or destroy cervical mucus, allowing bacteria to ascend into the uterine cavity

- procedures that risk transfer of contaminated cervical mucus into the endometrial cavity by instrumentation, such as use of a biopsy curet or an irrigation catheter, tubal insufflation, abortion, or pelvic surgery
- infection during or after pregnancy
- infectious focus within the body, such as drainage from a chronically infected fallopian tube, a pelvic abscess, a ruptured appendix, or diverticulitis of the sigmoid colon.

How it happens

Various conditions, procedures, or instruments can alter or destroy the cervical mucus, which usually serves as a protective barrier. As a result, bacteria enter the uterine cavity, causing inflammation of various structures.

Your chances of ending up in the bed because of PID greatly increase if you've had an intrauterine infection or procedure.

What to look for

Signs and symptoms vary with the affected area and include:

- profuse, purulent vaginal discharge in most of cases
- unanticipated vaginal bleeding, often postcoital in more than one-third of the cases (Murano & Della Fave, 2018)
- low-grade fever and malaise (especially if *N. gonorrhoeae* is the cause)
- lower abdominal pain in up to 90% of cases (Murano & Della Fave, 2018)—dull, aching or crampy, bilateral, and constant
- extreme pain on movement of the cervix or palpation of the adnexa.

What tests tell you

- Endometrial biopsy if evidence of endometritis is present
- Laparoscopy to identify salpingitis and determine bacteriologic presence
- Gram stain of secretions on wet mount from the vaginal, endocervix, or cul-de-sac areas help identify the infecting organism.
- Culture and sensitivity testing aid selection of the appropriate antibiotic. Urethral and rectal secretions may also be cultured.
- Testing for STIs with presentation of PID is standard, including gonorrhea, chlamydia, and HIV.
- Transvaginal sonography or MRI determines changes such as thickened, fluid-filled tubes. Free pelvic fluid and/or tubo-ovarian complex may also be identified.
- Doppler studies may identify tubal hyperemia.
- Culdocentesis obtains peritoneal fluid or pus for culture and sensitivity testing.

How it's treated

Effective management eradicates the infection, relieves symptoms, and leaves the reproductive system intact. It includes:

- aggressive therapy with appropriate antibiotics beginning immediately after culture specimens are obtained
- reevaluation of therapy as soon as laboratory results (culture and sensitivity) are available (usually after 24 to 48 hours)
- supplemental treatment, including bed rest, analgesics, and IV therapy
- adequate drainage if a pelvic abscess develops
- NSAIDs for pain relief (preferred treatment); opioids if necessary.

Additional considerations

Treatment for patients suffering from PID may include the following:

- IV antibiotic regimens may be administered as prescribed; these often include cefotetan or cefoxitin plus doxycycline, or clindamycin plus gentamycin.
- An alternative IV regimen with limited but positive results is ampicillin/sulbactam and doxycycline.
- If the patient is expected to be discharged, regimens may include ceftriaxone, cefoxitin, or a third-generation cephalosporin intramuscularly (IM) or IV with additional PO doxycycline.
- Regimens routinely include metronidazole to treat anaerobes.
- If an allergy to cephalosporins is present and the risk of gonorrhea is low, treatment with fluoroquinolones is acceptable until cultures are returned. Otherwise, infectious disease will need to be consulted.
- If isolated, treatment of gonorrhea includes ceftriaxone IM and azithromycin PO.

A total abdominal hysterectomy with bilateral salpingo-oophorectomy may be recommended for patients suffering from a ruptured pelvic abscess (a life-threatening complication).

What to do

- Institute aggressive antibiotic therapy as ordered.
- Position the patient with the head of the bed elevated approximately 30 to 45 degrees—this helps keep secretions pooled in the lower pelvic area.
- Administer analgesics as ordered for pain.
- Monitor vital signs for changes, especially temperature.
- Assess the abdomen for rigidity and distention, which are possible signs of developing peritonitis.
- Provide frequent perineal care if vaginal drainage occurs.
- Support the patient and her family.

PID teaching tips

If your patient has pelvic inflammatory disease (PID), cover these important points:
• To prevent recurrence, encourage adherence with the treatment regimen and explain the nature and seriousness of PID.
• Teach the importance of avoiding sexual activity during treatment and until symptoms have resolved.
• Stress the need for the any sexual partners within the last 60 days to be examined and treated for infection. If no partners exist, the most recent partner outside of 60 days should undergo treatment. Social services may need to assist with referrals and treatment. As a last resort, expedited partner therapy or EPT may be used in some states to deliver the medications to partners.
• To prevent infection after minor gynecologic procedures, such as dilation and curettage, teach to immediately report fever, increased vaginal discharge, or pain. After such procedures, instruct her to avoid douching and intercourse for at least 7 days.

- Prepare the patient for possible surgery if a ruptured abscess is suspected.
- If the patient will be discharged, review the medication therapy regimen for outpatient therapy. Provide education related to recurrence prevention. (See *PID teaching tips*.)

Severe situation

If the patient's PID is considered severe, expect her to be admitted for IV antibiotic administration. Criteria for possible hospitalization include:
- child or adolescent age
- pregnancy or HIV infection
- suspected or positive evidence of a pelvic abscess or peritonitis
- temperature greater than 104° F (40° C)
- inability to eat or drink
- failed response to outpatient therapy
- decreased resistance to infection because of her condition
- inability to confirm diagnosis
- lack of available follow-up
- nonadherence to outpatient treatment plan.

Understanding chronic pyelonephritis

Chronic pyelonephritis, or persistent inflammation of the kidneys, can scar the kidneys and may lead to chronic renal failure. Its cause may be bacterial, metastatic, or urogenous. This disease occurs most commonly in patients who are predisposed to recurrent acute pyelonephritis such as those with urinary obstructions or vesicoureteral reflux.

Signs and symptoms
Patients with chronic pyelonephritis may have a childhood history of unexplained fevers or bed-wetting. Signs and symptoms include flank pain, anemia, low urine specific gravity, proteinuria, leukocytes in urine, and, especially in late stages, hypertension. Uremia rarely develops from chronic pyelonephritis unless structural abnormalities exist in the urinary system. Bacteriuria may be intermittent. When no bacteria are found in the urine, diagnosis depends on excretory urography (where the renal pelvis may appear small and flattened) and renal biopsy.

Treatment
Treatment requires control of hypertension, elimination of the existing obstruction (when possible), and long-term antimicrobial therapy.

Pyelonephritis

One of the most common renal diseases, acute pyelonephritis is a sudden bacterial inflammation. It primarily affects the interstitial area, the renal pelvis, and, less commonly, the renal tubules. With treatment and continued follow-up care, the prognosis is good; extensive permanent damage is rare. (See *Understanding chronic pyelonephritis*.)

What causes it

The two causes of pyelonephritis are:
1. bacterial infection
2. hematogenous or lymphatic pathogen dissemination.

Risk factors include:
- use of diagnostic and therapeutic instruments, such as those used in catheterization, cystoscopy, or urologic surgery
- inability to empty the bladder
- urinary stasis
- urinary obstruction
- sexual activity (in women)
- use of diaphragms and condoms with spermicidal gel
- pregnancy

- diabetes
- other renal diseases
- UTI.

How it happens

Typically, the infection spreads from the bladder to the ureters and then to the kidneys. Bacteria refluxed to intrarenal tissues may create colonies of infection within 24 to 48 hours. However, pathogens may be carried to one or both kidneys via the blood or lymphatic systems.

What to look for

Signs and symptoms of pyelonephritis include:
- fever
- flank pain, including on palpation (costovertebral tenderness)
- nausea and/or vomiting
- urinary urgency, frequency, burning, pain
- pain over one or both kidneys
- nocturia, hematuria
- cloudy urine with an ammonia or fish odor
- shaking chills
- anorexia
- general fatigue (NIDDK, 2017a).
  See *Additional symptoms in the older adult.*

What tests tell you

- Urinalysis reveals pyuria and, possibly, a few RBCs; low specific gravity and osmolality; slightly alkaline pH; and, possibly, proteinuria, glycosuria, and ketonuria.
- Urine culture reveals more than 100,000 organisms/mL of urine.
- Blood culture is positive for bacteria.
- KUB radiography may reveal calculi, tumors, or cysts in the kidneys and the urinary tract.
- Excretory urography may show asymmetrical kidneys.
- Renal CT scan can show calculi, fluid collections (abscess), and pathology.

How it's treated

Therapy centers on antibiotic therapy appropriate to the specific infecting organism after it has been identified by urine culture and sensitivity studies. When the infecting organism can't be identified, therapy usually consists of a broad-spectrum antibiotic. If the patient is pregnant, antibiotics must be prescribed cautiously. Urinary analgesics are also appropriate.

Antibiotic aid

Symptoms may disappear after several days of antibiotic therapy. Although urine usually becomes sterile within 48 to 72 hours, the

Ages and stages

Additional symptoms in the older adult

Older adults with acute pyelonephritis may exhibit other symptoms such as mental status changes and decompensation in another organ system.

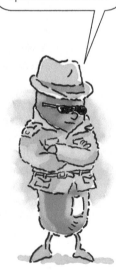

The pyelonephritis perpetrator may remain undercover, but it usually can't hide from a broad-spectrum antibiotic.

course of such therapy is 10 to 14 days. Follow-up treatment includes reculturing urine 1 week after drug therapy stops and then periodically for the next year to detect residual or recurring infection. Most patients with uncomplicated infections respond well to therapy and don't suffer reinfection.

Infection from obstruction or vesicoureteral reflux may be less responsive to antibiotics. Treatment may then necessitate surgery to relieve the obstruction or correct the anomaly. Patients at high risk for recurring UTIs and kidney infections, such as those using an indwelling urinary catheter for a prolonged period and those on maintenance antibiotic therapy, require long-term follow-up care.

What to do

- Obtain a clean-catch urine specimen for culture and sensitivity.
- Monitor the patient's vital signs, especially temperature, and administer antipyretics for fever.
- Ensure pain management is implemented.
- Ensure adequate hydration with fluids. Encourage increased fluid intake to achieve a urine output of more than 2,000 mL/day. Don't encourage intake of more than 2 to 3 qt (2 to 3 L) because this amount of fluid intake may decrease the effectiveness of antibiotics. If the patient has difficulty with oral fluid intake, expect to administer IV fluids.
- Prepare the patient for discharge. Review the medication therapy regimen and teach recurrence prevention measures. (See *Acute pyelonephritis teaching tips*, page 388.)

Renal calculi

Renal calculi may form anywhere in the urinary tract but usually develop in the renal pelvis or calyces. Such formation follows precipitation of substances normally dissolved in urine (calcium oxalate, calcium phosphate, magnesium ammonium phosphate, or, occasionally, urate or cystine). Renal calculi vary in size and may be solitary or multiple. They may remain in the renal pelvis or enter the ureter and may damage renal parenchyma. Large calculi cause pressure necrosis. In certain locations, calculi cause obstruction (with resultant hydronephrosis) and tend to recur. (See *A close look at renal calculi*, page 389.)

What causes it

Renal calculi may result from:
- dehydration, as decreased urine production concentrates calculus-forming substances
- decreased urine production/flow (for reasons other than dehydration)

Education edge

Acute pyelonephritis teaching tips

• Teach measures to reduce and avoid bacterial contamination, including using proper hygienic toileting practices such as wiping the perineum from front to back after bowel elimination.

• Teach the proper technique for collecting a clean-catch urine specimen and instruct to refrigerate a urine specimen within 30 minutes of collection to prevent overgrowth of bacteria.

• Stress the need to complete the entire prescribed antibiotic therapy even after symptoms subside.

• Advise routine checkups for a patient with chronic urinary tract infections.

• Teach signs and symptoms of infection, such as cloudy urine, burning on urination, and urinary urgency and frequency, especially when accompanied by a low-grade fever.

• Encourage long-term follow-up care for high-risk patients.

Adapted from Johnson, J. R., & Russo, T. A. (2018). Acute pyelonephritis in adults. *The New England Journal of Medicine, 378*(1), 48–59. doi:10.1056/NEJMcp1702758

- elevated urinary levels of calcium, oxalate, and uric acid and citrate levels
- infection. Infected, damaged tissue serves as a site for calculus development. Infected calculi (usually magnesium ammonium phosphate or staghorn calculi) may develop if bacteria serve as the nucleus in calculus formation. Such infections may promote destruction of renal parenchyma.
- changes in urine pH. Consistently acidic or alkaline urine provides a favorable medium for calculus formation.
- obstruction. Urinary stasis (such as in immobility from spinal cord injury) allows calculus constituents to collect and adhere, forming calculi. Obstruction also promotes infection that, in turn, compounds the obstruction.
- diet. Increased intake of calcium or oxalate-rich foods encourages calculus formation.
- immobilization. Immobility from spinal cord injury or other disorders allows calcium to be released into the circulation and eventually filtered by the kidneys.
- metabolic factors. Hyperparathyroidism; renal tubular acidosis; elevated uric acid levels (usually with gout); defective metabolism of oxalate; genetically defective metabolism of cystine; and excessive intake of vitamin D, protein, or dietary calcium may predispose a patient to renal calculi.

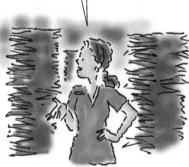

A person's chances of developing renal calculi can really stack up when you consider all of these potential causes.

A close look at renal calculi

Renal calculi vary in size and type. Small calculi may remain in the renal pelvis or pass down the ureter as shown below left. A staghorn calculus, shown below right, is a cast in the innermost part of the kidney—the calyx and renal pelvis. A staghorn calculus may develop from a calculus that stays in the kidney.

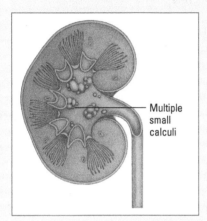 Multiple small calculi

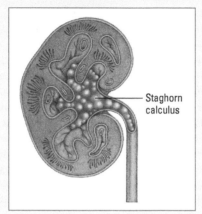 Staghorn calculus

How it happens

Calculi form when substances that normally dissolve in urine, such as calcium oxalate and calcium phosphate, precipitate. Large, rough calculi may occlude the opening to the ureteropelvic junction. The frequency and force of peristaltic contractions increase, causing pain.

What to look for

Clinical effects vary with size, location, and cause of the calculus. Pain is the key symptom. The pain of classic renal colic travels from the costovertebral angle to the flank, the suprapubic region, and the external genitalia. The pain fluctuates in intensity and may be excruciating at its peak. If calculi are in the renal pelvis and calyces, pain may be more constant and dull. Back pain occurs from calculi that produce an obstruction within a kidney. Nausea and vomiting usually accompany severe pain.

Other symptoms include:
- abdominal distention
- fever and chills
- hematuria, pyuria, and, rarely, anuria
- restlessness
- inability to lie in a supine position.

What tests tell you

- KUB radiography reveals most renal calculi.
- Renal CT scan detects localized renal calculi.
- Calculus analysis shows mineral content.
- Excretory urography confirms the diagnosis and determines the size and location of calculi.
- Renal ultrasonography may detect obstructive changes such as hydronephrosis.
- Urine culture of a midstream specimen may indicate UTI.
- Urinalysis results may be normal or may show increased specific gravity and acid or alkaline pH suitable for different types of calculus formation. Other urinalysis findings include hematuria (gross or microscopic), crystals (urate, calcium, or cystine), casts, and pyuria with or without bacteria and WBCs. A 24-hour urine collection is evaluated for calcium oxalate, phosphorus, and uric acid excretion levels.
- Other laboratory results support the diagnosis. Serial blood calcium and phosphorus levels detect hyperparathyroidism and show increased calcium levels in proportion to normal serum protein levels. Blood protein levels determine free calcium unbound to protein. Blood chloride and bicarbonate levels may show renal tubular acidosis. Increased blood uric acid levels may indicate gout as the cause.

> Look at all this water! Increasing fluids, either by mouth or parenteral, will help flush out renal calculi while decreasing resistance.

How it's treated

Because most renal calculi are smaller than 5 mm in diameter, treatment usually consists of measures to promote their natural passage. Along with vigorous hydration, treatment includes:

- antimicrobial therapy with struvite stones (varying with the cultured organism) for infection
- diuretics to prevent urinary stasis and further calculus formation (thiazide diuretics decrease calcium excretion into the urine, which reduces calculus formation)
- allopurinol (Aloprim) to reduce uric acid
- Tiopronin (Thiola) for cystine stones
- potassium citrate increases urine pH
- analgesics, such as ketorolac for pain (if available) (U.S. Food and Drug Administration, 2018).

Calculus formation prevention measures include increasing fluid intake, which increases urine output; a low-calcium diet for absorptive hypercalciuria; avoiding excessive salt and protein intake; parathyroidectomy for hyperparathyroidism; allopurinol for uric acid calculi; and daily administration of ascorbic acid (vitamin C) by mouth to acidify the urine. A calculus that's too large for natural passage may require surgical removal, percutaneous ultrasonic lithotripsy and ESWL, or chemolysis.

What to do
- Promote sufficient intake of fluids to maintain a urine output of greater than 2 L/day (urine should be very dilute and colorless). If the patient can't drink the required amount of fluid, supplemental IV fluids may be given.
- Strain all urine through a strainer and save the solid material recovered for analysis.
- Administer analgesics as ordered.
- Encourage ambulation, if appropriate, to aid in spontaneous passage of stones.
- Record intake, output, and weight to assess fluid status and renal function.
- If surgery is necessary, support the patient by supplementing and reinforcing what the surgeon has disclosed about the procedure. Explain preoperative and postoperative care.
- Prepare the patient for discharge, if appropriate. Assist in arranging a follow-up visit with a urologist in 2 to 3 days. Provide discharge teaching and review at-home procedures, including how to strain urine for stones, and signs and symptoms that should be reported to the health care provider. (See *Renal calculi teaching tips*.)

Sexual assault

Sexual assault, which includes *rape*, refers to actual or attempted sexual contact without the person's consent. It includes many behaviors—including physical and psychological coercion and force—that result in varying degrees of physical and psychological trauma.

Most information related to sexual assault is derived from statistics involving adult women who have been sexually assaulted. However, men and children can also be victims.

What's in a name?

Persons who have experienced sexual assault may be referred to as *survivors* or *victims*. Some people use the term *survivor* because it's empowering and positive. Some use the term *victim* because it underscores the event's overwhelming severity and devastation. Others feel that the term *victim* denotes hopelessness and helplessness. In this chapter, the term *survivor* is used most frequently.

Rape-trauma syndrome

Persons who have been sexually assaulted or have experienced an attempted sexual assault may develop rape-trauma syndrome. This syndrome involves the survivor's short- and long-term reactions to the trauma and the methods used to cope with it. With support and counseling to help the patient deal with feelings, the prognosis is favorable.

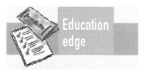

Renal calculi teaching tips

- Before discharge, teach the patient and family the importance of following the prescribed dietary and medication regimens to prevent recurrence of calculi.
- Encourage increased fluid intake.
- Instruct to immediately report symptoms of acute obstruction (such as pain and inability to void).
- Advise to return to the health care facility right away if experiencing fever, uncontrolled pain, or vomiting.

What causes it

Sexual assault is the result of a crime involving power, anger, and control enacted by the perpetrator. It isn't the result of the survivor wearing suggestive clothing or a specific sexual orientation.

How it happens

The person committing the assault uses sex as a means to control and humiliate the victim. In this situation, all options for consent are removed from the victim. Subsequently, the attacker uses sexual contact forcibly and degradingly.

What to look for

Sexual assault is commonly characterized by:

- signs of physical trauma, including bruising, lacerations, abrasions, and avulsions
- clothing that is ripped, stained, or cut
- tearfulness, crying, and shaking
- withdrawal
- anxiety.

What tests tell you

Typically, several tests rule out possible STIs and pregnancy. Other tests may be done depending on the extent of the patient's injuries; for example, X-rays may be done to rule out fractures.

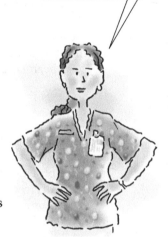

There is not a standard presentation for sexual assault survivors. Some may demonstrate fear, anxiety, or be completely withdrawn, whereas others are able to discuss the attack openly.

How it's treated

Treatment focuses on proper evidence collection, immediate care of apparent or life-threatening wounds or injuries, and medication therapy to prevent STIs and pregnancy. Nurses must follow local laws in determining their role during the examination of a sexual assault survivor (Delgadillo, 2017).

Each institution or agency has a specific protocol for specimen collection in cases involving sexual assault. Specimens can be collected from many sources. Typically, they include blood, hair, nails, tissues, and body fluids, such as urine, semen, saliva, and vaginal secretions. Evidence can also be obtained via diagnostic tests, such as CT scan and radiography. Regardless of the protocol or specimen source, accurate and precise specimen collection is essential in conjunction with thorough, objective documentation because, in many cases, this information will be used as evidence in legal proceedings.

In good hands

Many institutions have a sexual assault response team and may also have a sexual assault nurse examiner (SANE) available to care for survivors. SANEs are skilled professionals who provide comprehensive care to sexual assault survivors, collect specimens, and sometimes testify in legal proceedings.

What to do

When caring for the survivor of a sexual assault, follow these steps:
- Develop a therapeutic relationship with the patient.
- Stay with the patient at all times; offer comfort and support.
- Ask about calling a person for the patient who can also provide support, such as a friend, family member, or counselor.
- Assure that informed consent for testing that may be performed has been obtained.
- Inform and assure the patient's understanding of the facility's responsibility in reporting the assault.
- Arrange for an advocate to talk with the patient about choices and decision making.
- Assist with history taking and physical examination; obtain the following key information: date and time of the assault; where it occurred and the surroundings; injuries occurred; areas penetrated, including the use of foreign objects; and other sexual acts.
- Ask actions the survivor has taken after the assault, such as showering, urinating, douching, or changing clothing; recent gynecologic treatment or surgery; and history of sexual intercourse (other than the rape) within the past 72 hours.

Collecting evidence

- Explain which specimens are being taken and why; guide the patient through each step of the process.
- Assist with evidence collection. (See *Collecting evidence in a sexual assault*, page 394.)
- Make sure that the chain of custody for all evidence collected is maintained and logged according to the facility's protocol. Document all information completely, including the date and time that evidence was given to law enforcement officers. Include the names of the individuals receiving the evidence in the patient's medical record.
- After the examination and evidence collection are completed, assist the patient with showering and donning clean clothing.

Medication and follow-up

- Administer medications as ordered to prevent STIs and pregnancy (if "morning after" pill has been accepted by the patient).
- Review instructions about medications and follow-up and what to expect physically and psychologically.
- Encourage that a support person accompany the survivor to a safe place and stay with him or her.
- Ensure that the patient has a follow-up appointment in 10 to 14 days with a health care provider or clinic and has the name and contact number of a rape crisis counselor.

Collecting evidence in a sexual assault

Accurate, precise specimen collection for evidence of a sexual assault is essential. Thorough, objective documentation with proper evidence collection is crucial because, in most cases, this information will be used as evidence in legal proceedings.

Although specific protocols and policies may vary among facilities, some general guidelines are listed here.

Patient preparation

• Assess the patient's ability to undergo the specimen collection procedure.
• Explain the procedures that the patient will undergo and what specimens will be collected and from where and provide emotional support throughout.
• Obtain consent from the patient for specimens to be obtained.
• Ask the patient if someone—such as a family member, friend, or other person—is desired to stay during the specimen collection.
• Ensure the patient's privacy throughout the collection procedure.

Guidelines for specimen collection

If you're responsible for collecting specimens in a sexual assault, follow these important guidelines:
• Be knowledgeable about your institution's policy and procedures for specimen collection in sexual assault cases.
• Obtain a special sexual assault evidence collection kit, which contains all the necessary items for specimen collection based on the evidence required by the local crime laboratory. The kit also contains a form for the examiner to complete, sign, and date.
• When obtaining specimens, be sure to collect them from the survivor and, if possible, the suspect.
• When collecting specimens for moist secretions, typically a one-swab technique is used; if secretions are dry, then a two-swab technique is used.
• Check with local law enforcement agencies regarding additional specimens that may be needed—for example, trace evidence, such as soot, grass, gravel, glass, or other debris.

• Wear gloves and change them frequently, washing hands in between; use disposable equipment and instruments if possible.
• Avoid coughing, sneezing, or talking over specimens or touching your face, nose, or mouth when collecting specimens.
• Include the survivor's clothing as part of the collection procedure.
• Place all items collected in separate paper bags.
• Never allow a specimen or item considered as evidence to be left unattended.
• Document each item or specimen collected; have another nurse witness each collection and document it.
• If the patient consents, obtain photographs of all injuries for inclusion in documentation in the electronic health record (Delgadillo, 2017). Comply with Health Insurance Portability and Accountability Act (HIPAA) laws.
• Include written documentation of the survivor's physical and psychological condition on the first encounter, throughout specimen collection, afterward, and at time of discharge.

Clothing for specimen collection

• Ask the patient to stand on a clean piece of examination paper, if possible. If the patient can't stand, then have him or her remain on the examination table or bed.
• Have the patient remove each article of clothing, one at a time, and place each article in a separate, clean paper bag.
• Fold the examination paper onto itself and place it into a clean paper bag.
• Fold over, seal, label, and initial each bag.

Anal secretion collection

• *Note*: The forensic pelvic examination must be performed by a health care provider (Delgadillo, 2017). The nurse supports the provider and the patient by keeping the patient informed of each step of the examination, providing materials for the collection of evidence as requested by the provider, and documenting the examination as performed.

Collecting evidence in a sexual assault *(continued)*

• Collect these swabs first due to contamination of the area.

• If rectal penetration is suspected, obtain rectal and anal swabs.

• Insert the swab gently into the patient's rectum approximately 1" to 1¼" (2 to 3 cm).

• Rotate the swab gently and then remove it.

• Allow the swabs to air dry and then place them in an envelope.

• Seal and label the envelope appropriately.

Vaginal or cervical secretion collection

• *Note*: The forensic pelvic examination must be performed by a health care provider (Delgadillo, 2017). The nurse supports the provider and the patient by keeping the patient informed of each step of the examination, providing materials for the collection of evidence as requested by the provider, and documenting the examination as performed.

• Swab the vaginal area thoroughly with the swabs provided; next, swab the cervical area, being sure to keep the vaginal swabs separate from the cervical swabs.

• Allow the swabs to air dry; do not apply heat to speed drying.

• Place the vaginal swabs in the swab container and close; repeat for the cervical swabs.

• Place the swab container into the prelabeled envelope and seal the envelope securely.

Complete the information on the front of the envelope; if vaginal and cervical swabs are obtained, use a separate envelope for each.

Penile secretion collection

• *Note*: The forensic pelvic examination must be performed by a health care provider (Delgadillo, 2017). The nurse supports the provider and the patient by keeping the patient informed of each step of the examination, providing materials for the collection of evidence as requested by the provider, and documenting the examination as performed.

• Swab the entire external surface of the penis. Repeat this at least one more time (so that at least two swabs are obtained). Allow the swab to air dry and then place it in an envelope.

• Swab the scrotum (Riviello & Rozzi, 2016). Repeat this at least one more time (so that at least two swabs are obtained). Allow the swab to air dry and then place it in an envelope.

• Seal and label the envelope appropriately.

Pubic hair collection

• Use the comb provided in the kit and comb through the pubic hair.

• Collect approximately 20 to 30 pubic hairs and place them in the envelope.

• Alternatively, obtain 20 to 30 plucked hairs from the patient; allow the patient the option of plucking pubic hair.

Testicular torsion

Testicular torsion is the abnormal twisting of the spermatic cord that results from rotation of a testis or the *mesorchium*, a membrane that supports the testis. It causes strangulation and, if untreated, eventual infarction of the testis.

This condition is almost always unilateral. Although it's most common between ages 12 and 18, it may occur at any age. The prognosis is favorable with early detection and prompt treatment.

What causes it

Testicular torsion is caused in part by abnormalities inside or outside the *tunica vaginalis,* the serous membrane covering the internal scrotal cavity. Normally, the tunica vaginalis envelops the testis and attaches to the epididymis and spermatic cord. Testicular torsion can be intravaginal or extravaginal.

Intra vs. extra

Intravaginal torsion is caused by:
- abnormality of the tunica vaginalis and the position of the testis
- incomplete attachment of the testis and spermatic fascia to the scrotal wall, leaving the testis free to rotate around its vascular pedicle
- increased weight of testicle after puberty
- sudden forceful contraction of the cremaster muscle due to physical exertion or irritation of the muscle.
  Extravaginal torsion (more common in neonates) is caused by:
- loose attachment of the tunica vaginalis to the scrotal lining, causing spermatic cord rotation above the testis.

How it happens

In testicular torsion, the testis rotates on its vascular pedicle and twists the arteries and vein in the spermatic cord. This twisting interrupts blood flow to the testis, resulting in vascular engorgement, ischemia, and scrotal swelling.

What to look for

Torsion produces excruciating pain in the affected testis or iliac fossa. Physical examination reveals tense, tender swelling in the scrotum or inguinal canal and hyperemia of the overlying skin. Scrotal swelling is unrelieved by rest or elevation of the scrotum.

What tests tell you

Doppler ultrasonography helps distinguish testicular torsion from strangulated hernia, undescended testes, or epididymitis.

How it's treated

If manual reduction or detorsion is unsuccessful, torsion must be surgically corrected within 6 hours after the onset of symptoms to preserve testicular function. Treatment consists of immediate surgical repair by *orchiopexy* (fixation of a viable testis to the scrotum) or *orchiectomy* (excision of a nonviable testis). Without treatment, the testis begins to experience ischemic damage after just 4 to 8 hours (Kostakis et al., 2017).

What to do

- Administer analgesics as ordered to aid pain relief.
- Assess vital signs and prepare the patient for surgery.
- Perform preoperative teaching.
- Provide emotional support to the patient and family.
- Inform the patient and family about transfer to the patient care unit after surgery.

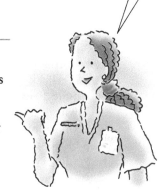

Sexually active teenage females have a significantly increased risk of developing a UTI.

Urinary tract infection

UTI typically refers to infection of the lower urinary tract. Lower UTIs commonly respond readily to treatment, but recurrence and resistant bacterial flare-up during therapy are possible. Lower UTIs are much more common in women than in men. Lower UTIs also occur in relatively large percentages in sexually active teenage girls. Lower UTIs fall into two types:

- *cystitis*, which is an inflammation of the bladder that usually results from an ascending infection
- *urethritis*, which is an inflammation of the urethra.

What causes it

UTI may be caused by (Office on Women's Health, 2019b):

- infection by gram-negative enteric bacteria, such as *E. coli*, *Klebsiella*, *Proteus*, *Enterobacter*, *Pseudomonas*, or *Serratia*
- simultaneous infection with multiple pathogens in a patient with neurogenic bladder
- indwelling urinary catheters
- fistula between the intestine and the bladder
- use of a diaphragm or spermicide
- being sexually active or pregnant
- a diagnosis of diabetes.

How it happens

Recent studies suggest that infection results from a breakdown in local defense mechanisms in the bladder that allows bacteria to invade the bladder mucosa and multiply. These bacteria can't be readily eliminated by normal micturition.

What to look for

Characteristic signs and symptoms include:

- urinary urgency and frequency
- dysuria
- bladder cramps or spasms
- itching
- feeling of warmth during urination

- nocturia
- possible hematuria
- fever
- urethral discharge in males.

Other common features include lower back pain, malaise, confusion, nausea, vomiting, abdominal pain or tenderness over the bladder, chills, and flank pain.

What tests tell you

- A clean-catch urinalysis reveals a bacteria count of 100,000/mL, confirming UTI. Lower counts don't necessarily rule out infection, especially if the patient is urinating frequently, because bacteria require 30 to 45 minutes to reproduce in urine. Culture and sensitivity testing determine the exact organism and the appropriate antimicrobial drug.
- A blood test or stained smear rules out STI.
- Voiding cystourethrography or excretory urography may detect congenital anomalies.

How it's treated

A 7- to 10-day course of an appropriate antibiotic is usually the treatment of choice for an initial lower UTI. After 3 days of antibiotic therapy, a urine culture should show no organisms. If the urine isn't sterile, bacterial resistance has probably occurred, making the use of a different antimicrobial necessary. Single-dose antibiotic therapy with amoxicillin or sulfamethoxazole trimethoprim (Bactrim DS) may be effective in women with acute uncomplicated UTI. A urine culture taken 1 to 2 weeks later indicates whether the infection has been eradicated.

Recurrent infections caused by renal calculi, chronic prostatitis, or a structural abnormality may require surgery. If there are no predisposing conditions, long-term, low-dose antibiotic therapy is preferred.

What to do

- Assess the patient's vital signs and obtain a clean-catch urine specimen for urinalysis and culture and sensitivity.
- Encourage fluid intake; if necessary, administer IV fluids.
- Initiate antimicrobial therapy as ordered.
- Provide comfort measures, such as a warm sitz bath and warm compresses.
- Prepare the patient for discharge. Teach medication regimen and measures to promote infection resolution and prevent recurrence. (See *UTI teaching tips.*)

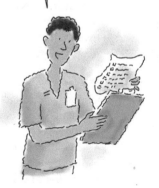

When E. coli, Klebsiella, Proteus, Enterobacter, Pseudomonas, *or* Serratia *grow to numbers over 100,000, the patient has a UTI.*

Education edge

UTI teaching tips

Follow these guidelines below when teaching your patient with a urinary tract infection (UTI):

• Explain the nature and purpose of antimicrobial therapy. Emphasize the importance of completing the prescribed course of therapy and, with long-term prophylaxis, of adhering strictly to the ordered dosage.

• Encourage intake of plenty of water (at least eight glasses per day). Teach to avoid alcohol while taking antibiotics. Fruit juices, especially cranberry juice, and oral doses of vitamin C may help acidify urine and enhance the action of the medication.

• If therapy includes a urinary analgesic, teach that this drug may turn urine red orange.

• Teach the patient about general perineal hygiene measures; females should be taught to wipe from front to back, avoid bubble baths and douching, and wear cotton-lined underwear.

Quick quiz

1.   When assessing for costovertebral angle tenderness during a physical assessment, where does the nurse place the ball of his or her nondominant hand?

    A.   On the back at the level of the 12th rib
    B.   On the abdomen just below the rib cage
    C.   At the symphysis pubis
    D.   At the midclavicular line on each side of the abdomen

Answer: A. When checking costovertebral angle tenderness, the nurse will place the ball of the nondominant hand on the back at the costovertebral angle of the 12th rib.

2.   When assessing a patient for PID, which assessment finding does the nurse anticipate?

    A.   Upper abdominal pain
    B.   Lack of vaginal discharge
    C.   Fever greater than 104° F (40° C)
    D.   Absence of pain upon palpation of the adnexa

Answer: C. A patient with PID typically has a fever with malaise, profuse purulent vaginal discharge, pain on palpation of the adnexa, and lower abdominal pain.

3. Which condition does the nurse teach a patient that contributes to the development of renal calculi?
    A. Heart failure
    B. Hypocalcemia
    C. Hypothyroidism
    D. High calcium diet

Answer: D. A diet high in calcium or the presence of hyperparathyroidism (not hypothyroidism) may contribute to the development of renal calculi. Heart failure and hypocalcemia are not associated with increased renal calculi formation.

4. When collecting evidence in a sexual assault, which nursing action would be most appropriate?
    A. Instruct to void before obtaining specimens.
    B. Collect secretion specimens only from the vagina.
    C. Place each item of evidence in a separate paper bag.
    D. Place all articles of clothing in one plastic, sealable bag.

Answer: C. When evidence is collected from a survivor of sexual assault, it's important to place each item of evidence, including clothing, in a separate paper bag. Using plastic bags can promote faster deterioration of body fluids and other trace evidence. It is important to collect secretion specimens from the vagina and other areas. The patient should not void until secretion specimens are obtained.

Scoring

☆☆☆ If you answered all four questions correctly, get up and cheer! You're a GU and gynecologic genius!

☆☆ If you answered three questions correctly, pat yourself on the back! You're gearing up for GU success.

☆ If you answered fewer than three questions correctly, don't be sad. Just review the chapter and give it another go.

Selected references

Centers for Disease Control and Prevention. (2015). *Pelvic inflammatory disease (PID)*. Retrieved from https://www.cdc.gov/std/tg2015/pid.htm

Centers for Disease Control and Prevention. (2017). *2015 Sexually transmitted diseases treatment guidelines*. Retrieved from https://www.cdc.gov/std/tg2015/default.htm

Centers for Disease Control and Prevention. (2018). *Parasites: Schistosomiasis*. Retrieved from https://www.cdc.gov/parasites/schistosomiasis/

Chong, S. T., Cherry-Bukowiec, J., Willatt, J. M., et al. (2016). Renal trauma: Imaging evaluation and implications for clinical management. *Abdominal Radiology (New York)*, *41*(8), 1565–1579. doi:10.1007/s00261-016-0731-x

Delgadillo, D. C. (2017). When there is no sexual assault nurse examiner: Emergency nursing care for female adult sexual assault patients. *Journal of Emergency Nursing, 43*(4), 308–315. doi:10.1016/j.jen.2016.11.006

DeMoranville, V. E. (2018). Urinalysis. In J. L. Longe (Ed.), *The Gale encyclopedia of nursing and allied health* (4th ed.). Detroit, MI: Gale.

Johnson, J. R., & Russo, T. A. (2018). Acute pyelonephritis in adults. *The New England Journal of Medicine, 378*(1), 48–59. doi:10.1056/NEJMcp1702758

Kostakis, I. D., Zavras, N., Damaskos, C., et al. (2017). Erythropoietin and sildenafil protect against ischemia/reperfusion injury following testicular torsion in adult rats. *Experimental and Therapeutic Medicine, 13*(6), 3341–3347. doi:10.3892/etm.2017.4441

Murano, T., & Della Fave, A. (2018). Pelvic inflammatory disease. *Emergency Medicine Reports, 39*(14). Retrieved from https://www.proquest.com/

National Institute of Diabetes and Digestive and Kidney Diseases. (2017a). *Symptoms & causes of kidney infection (pyelonephritis)*. Retrieved from https://www.niddk.nih.gov/health-information/urologic-diseases/kidney-infection-pyelonephritis/symptoms-causes

National Institutes of Health. (2018). *Treatments for infertility resulting from PCOS*. Retrieved from https://www.nichd.nih.gov/health/topics/pcos/conditioninfo/treatments/infertility

Office on Women's Health. (2019a). *Ovarian cysts*. Retrieved from https://www.womenshealth.gov/a-z-topics/ovarian-cysts

Office on Women's Health. (2019b). *Urinary tract infections*. Retrieved from https://www.womenshealth.gov/a-z-topics/urinary-tract-infections

Riviello, R., & Rozzi, H. (2016). *How to conduct a sexual assault examination and collect evidence*. Retrieved from https://www.acepnow.com/article/conduct-sexual-assault-examination-collect-evidence/?singlepage=1&theme=print-friendly

The American Association for the Surgery of Trauma. (2018). *Injury scoring scale*. Retrieved from http://www.aast.org/library/traumatools/injuryscoringscales.aspx#kidney

U.S. Food and Drug Administration. (2018). *FDA drug shortages. Current and resolved drug shortages and discontinuations reported to FDA*. Retrieved from https://www.accessdata.fda.gov/scripts/drugshortages/dsp_ActiveIngredientDetails.cfm?AI=Ketorolac+Tromethamine+Injection&st=c&tab=tabs-4&panels=1

World Health Organization. (2018). *Female genital mutilation*. Retrieved from http://www.who.int/news-room/fact-sheets/detail/female-genital-mutilation

Chapter 9

Obstetric emergencies

Just the facts

In this chapter, you'll learn about emergency management of:

♦ neonates with meconium-stained amniotic fluid

♦ neonates with shoulder dystocia

♦ neonates with prolapsed umbilical cord

♦ maternal patients with a ruptured uterus

♦ maternal patients with amniotic fluid embolism.

Understanding obstetric emergencies

Emergency departments are frequented by pregnant women for urgent needs even though they may have routine access to obstetric health care and resources (Kilfoyle et al., 2016). Pregnancy-type problems are the fifth most common reason patients visit the emergency room. The occurrence of an urgent obstetric emergency does not occur frequently; however, these types of emergencies can lead to maternal and fetal mortality (Janicki et al., 2016).

Emergency departments are most effective when they work with ancillary obstetric units and collaborate on the structure and triage guidelines used when evaluating pregnant patients through this environment of care (ACOG, 2016). These guidelines may vary from facility to facility. Keep in mind that the patient may come in through the emergency department and the emergency nurse will begin care; yet, the obstetric team may take over at any time depending on the facility protocols and availability of the specialized teams. This short chapter gives you the most important interventions that you need to know to undertake in the emergency department as you await transfer to the health care provider and obstetric team.

There are five common obstetric emergencies that are most commonly seen in the emergency department. These emergencies occur as delivery of the fetus is imminent and rapid assessment of the mother and neonate must occur. There should always be a team on hand to care for the mother and a separate team to care for the neonate immediately upon its delivery.

Meconium–stained amniotic fluid

The first obstetric emergency is that of meconium-stained amniotic fluid. The amniotic fluid is contained within the amniotic sac in which the fetus is protected in utero. Normal amniotic fluid is clear or pale yellow. When the amniotic fluid is stained, it is an indication that the fetus has passed the first meconium (stool) prior to delivery. Meconium is green and is typically documented as thin or thick in consistency.

There are three main reasons that the fluid may become stained with meconium. The first is the natural process of maturity of the infant after the 38th week of gestation. The second is that some type of hypoxic event may have occurred, which stimulated the function of peristalsis in the fetus. The third reason is that the umbilical cord may be compressed, which can stimulate the occurrence of this process in the fetus.

The highest risk associated with this obstetric emergency is that of meconium aspiration syndrome in the neonate during delivery. This type of aspiration can cause pneumonia in the neonate. Immediate postbirth care is dependent on the presentation of the infant. If the infant is vigorous (active), demonstrates good respiratory effort, and has good muscle tone, the initial steps of routine infant care can be done while the infant is placed on the mother (American College of Obstetricians and Gynecologists [ACOG], 2017). A bulb syringe can be used to gently clear meconium from the mouth and nose, if necessary. If the infant has inadequate breathing effort and poor muscle tone, the initial resuscitation is to be completed under a radiant warmer (ACOG, 2017). If the airway is obstructed, suction and intubation may be necessary.

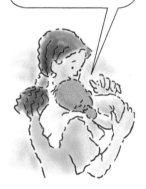

If I am active, breathing well, and have good muscle tone, I can stay with my mom.

Emergency nursing management of meconium-stained amniotic fluid

Prior to delivery, assess the amniotic fluid once the membranes are ruptured. If the fluid is positive for the meconium stain, gather neonatal resuscitation supplies and activate the neonatal advanced life support team, a team of credentialed individuals who have full resuscitation and endotracheal intubation skills.

Immediately after delivery, assess the neonate's respiratory effort, heart rate, and tone. Follow the Neonatal Resuscitation Program (NRP), an evidence-based interprofessional approach to newborn care at birth (American Academy of Pediatrics, 2018). Suction the neonate's mouth first and then the nose, with the bulb syringe. If respiratory depression is noted, NRP guidelines should be followed.

Shoulder dystocia

During a vaginal delivery, shoulder dystocia occurs if the infant's head is delivered first and there is a complication in the anterior shoulder passing under the pubic arch. This may occur if the fetal size is different than the opening between the fetal shoulders and the pelvic inlet. This is not common, but occurrences are happening more frequently due to women giving birth to larger babies. (See *Shoulder dystocia.*)

Shoulder dystocia can cause trauma to the fetus during delivery and also asphyxia due to the prolonged delivery. A fractured clavicle, brachial plexus injury, and fractured humerus are among the common injuries that may occur.

Emergency nursing management of shoulder dystocia

Before delivery:
- Assess the stage of labor. In the presence of shoulder dystocia, there is a slowing of progress in the second stage of labor.
- Assess for caput succedaneum (swelling of the baby's scalp) that gets larger.
- Assess for fetal head retraction against the perineum.
- Stay calm and call for assistance.

Shoulder dystocia

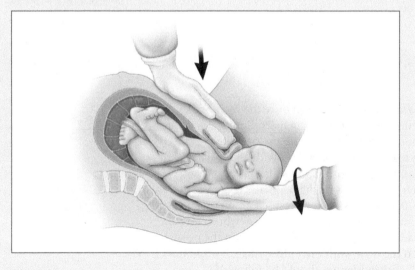

- Assist with positioning.
- Monitor the mother and fetus while the health care provider implements the McRoberts maneuver and applies suprapubic pressure to attempt to dislodge the shoulder.
  Immediately after delivery:
- Assess the neonate for trauma or injury.
- Assess the mother's vagina, perineum, and rectum for signs of trauma and bleeding.

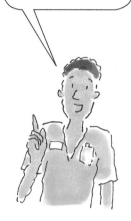

An important part of caring for a patient experiencing an obstetric emergency is staying calm and calling for assistance.

Prolapsed umbilical cord

A prolapsed umbilical cord can happen when the umbilical cord locates itself beneath the presenting part of the fetus. (See *Prolapsed umbilical cord*.) In this condition, the cord may not be visible at any

Prolapsed umbilical cord

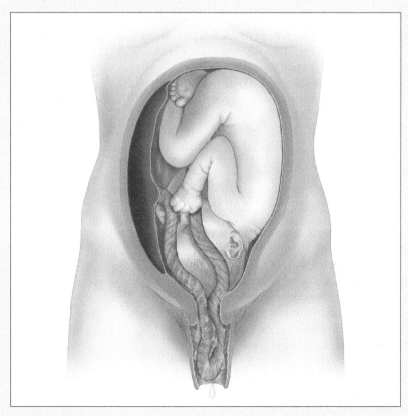

Transverse lie

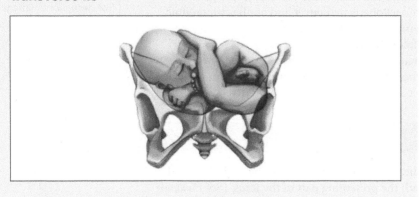

point during labor, even if the rupture of membranes has occurred. The most common presentation is visualization of the cord once the membranes have ruptured.

Risks for this condition include transverse lie or breech position of the fetus, a long cord, prematurity, delivery of multiples (e.g., twins or triplets), excessive amniotic fluid, and lack of engagement of the presenting part of the fetus. (See *Transverse lie*.)

One of the most critical risks associated with a prolapsed umbilical cord is fetal hypoxia because of cord compression. Other risks also include damage to the central nervous system or even fetal death.

Emergency nursing management of prolapsed umbilical cord

Before delivery:
- Monitor fetal heart rates and patterns for variable/prolonged decelerations during contractions.
- Assess whether the mother has felt the cord outside of her body after the membranes are ruptured or whether the cord is visible.
- Call immediately for assistance and do not leave the patient alone.
- Position the patient in a modified Sims or Trendelenburg position to use gravity to decrease the pressure on the cord.
- Wrap the prolapsed cord in a sterile towel.
- Place the mother on oxygen, 8 to 10 L/minute, until the fetus is delivered.
- Begin or increase intravenous fluids as ordered.
- Monitor fetal and maternal heart rates and patterns.

When caring for a patient experiencing a prolapsed umbilical cord, wrap the cord in a sterile towel, place the mother in modified Sims or Trendelenburg position, apply oxygen to the mother, and call for help. Do not leave the patient alone!

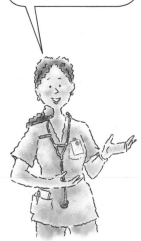

- Prepare for a cesarean section delivery.
- Recognize that the health care provider may place a gloved hand inside the vagina to hold the presenting part up and off of the umbilical cord.
  Immediately after delivery:
- Assess the neonate for trauma or injury.
- Support the mother and family with communication.
- Assist the health care provider as needed.

Rupture of the maternal uterus

Rupture of the maternal uterus is due to the disruption and separation of the layers of the uterus. When the disruption occurs, all or some of the fetal parts can be ejected into the peritoneal cavity. The risk of this condition is low; however, it is considered an emergency for both the mother and the fetus if it occurs. Uterine rupture can lead to excessive bleeding of the mother and severe hypoxia for the fetus. This can happen if the uterus has scar tissue from previous deliveries or surgeries. Prevention is the most important method of avoiding uterine rupture; this is accomplished by not allowing the mother to labor through a vaginal delivery if she has risk factors. (See *Uterine rupture.*)

Uterine rupture

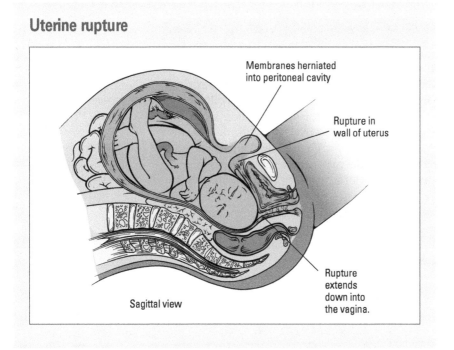

Membranes herniated into peritoneal cavity

Rupture in wall of uterus

Rupture extends down into the vagina.

Sagittal view

Emergency nursing management of rupture of the maternal uterus

Before delivery:
- Monitor the maternal and fetal heart rates and patterns for abnormality, an abrupt decrease in fetal heart rate, variable/prolonged decelerations, and/or absent baseline variability.
- Monitor the mother closely if she is on oxytocin or prostaglandin.
- Assess carefully for bright red vaginal bleeding and signs of shock if the mother reports sharp shoulder pain or ripping or tearing sensation (in addition to the contractions that are occurring).
- Place mother on oxygen 8 to 10 L/minute until the fetus is delivered.
- Begin or increase intravenous fluids as ordered.
- Continue monitoring maternal and fetal heart rates and patterns.
- Prepare for a cesarean section delivery.
  Immediately after delivery:
- Assess the neonate for trauma or injury.
- Prepare the mother for possible laceration repair or surgery for hysterectomy.
- Prepare for blood transfusion to the mother.
- Administer oxygen to the mother if needed.
- Support the mother and family with communication.

Amniotic fluid embolus

Amniotic fluid embolus is not common; yet, it can be devastating if this complication occurs (Perry et al., 2018). With this condition, there is a sudden onset of hypoxia, hypotension, cardiovascular collapse, and coagulopathy as a foreign substance enters the mother's circulatory system. The foreign substance is most likely amniotic fluid that has entered the mother's circulation; yet, it could also be fetal debris. This can be caused by a defect in the maternal membranes. This complication can occur during labor, during delivery, or approximately 30 minutes after delivery. The risks for this condition include an unusually fast labor, meconium-stained fluid, older age of the mother, post-term delivery, eclampsia, having a cesarean section birth, having an assisted vaginal birth, or having placenta abruption or placenta previa. (See *Amniotic fluid embolus*.)

Amniotic fluid embolus

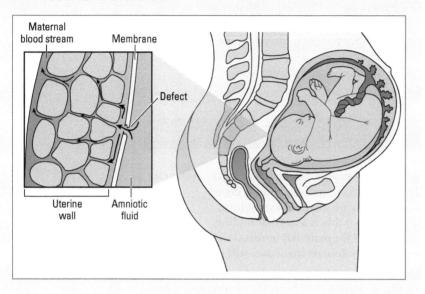

Maternal blood stream
Membrane
Defect
Uterine wall
Amniotic fluid

Emergency nursing management of amniotic fluid embolus

Before delivery:
- Assess for signs and symptoms of maternal respiratory distress (e.g., cyanosis, dyspnea, restlessness, pulmonary edema, respiratory arrest).
- Assess for signs and symptoms of maternal circulatory collapse (e.g., hypotension, tachycardia, shock, cardiac arrest).
- Assess for maternal hemorrhage (bleeding from incisions or intravenous sites, petechiae, ecchymosis, purpura).
- Assess for maternal uterine atony (a condition in which the uterus fails to contract, which can lead to postpartum hemorrhage).
- Position the mother on her side.
- Administer oxygen as ordered.
- Replace fluid loss as ordered.
- Assist with or perform cardiopulmonary resuscitation (CPR) if needed.
- Be prepared for intubation.
- Prepare for blood transfusion to the mother.
- Continue to monitor maternal and fetal heart tones.
- Prepare for a cesarean delivery once stable.
- Support the mother and family with communication.

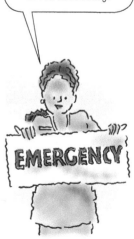

An amniotic fluid embolus is a medical emergency. Be prepared to perform CPR if necessary.

EMERGENCY

Immediately after delivery:
- Assess the neonate for trauma or injury.
- Prepare for maternal transport to the intensive care unit.
- Administer blood, oxygen, and fluids to the mother as ordered.
- Monitor closely if the mother has been placed on mechanical ventilation.
- Continue supporting the mother and family with communication.

Quick quiz

1. What nursing action is appropriate upon finding that a pregnant patient's membranes have ruptured and the fluid is green?
   A. Prepare to suction the neonate for meconium.
   B. Ensure the patient that this is a normal finding.
   C. Type and cross blood for maternal transfusion.
   D. Anticipate that the McRoberts maneuver will be needed.

Answer: A. Meconium is green, and it is not considered a normal finding in fluid. If the nurse assesses that the fluid contains meconium, preparation should be made to suction the neonate with a bulb syringe. Further interventions will be dependent on the presentation of the neonate at birth. The nurse does not need to obtain blood for a type and cross. The McRoberts maneuver is used in the presence of shoulder dystocia.

2. What nursing action is appropriate when a laboring patient reports sudden, sharp shoulder pain?
   A. Massage the affected shoulder.
   B. Reassure that this is likely a gas sensation.
   C. Place into lithotomy position to begin pushing.
   D. Prepare for emergency cesarean delivery.

Answer: D. Sudden, sharp shoulder pain in a laboring patient can be indicative of uterine rupture so the nurse will prepare for an emergency cesarean delivery, not a vaginal delivery (which requires lithotomy position). The shoulder should not be massaged. Although some postsurgical gas pain presents in the shoulder, this is not expected in a laboring patient; therefore, rupture of the uterus should be considered.

3. When caring for four patients, which does the nurse recognize is least likely to experience an amniotic fluid embolus?
    A. The 24-year-old patient in early stages of labor
    B. The 29-year-old patient who is actively pushing
    C. The 31-year-old patient who delivered 15 minutes ago
    D. The 34-year-old patient whose newborn is 2 days old

Answer: D. Amniotic fluid embolisms can occur during any stage of labor and delivery, up to 30 minutes past delivery. The patient whose newborn is 2 days old is the least likely to experience this condition.

4. Which nursing action is appropriate when caring for a pregnant patient who came to the emergency department with the umbilical cord prolapsed?
    A. Cut the cord and anticipate a quick delivery.
    B. Wrap the prolapsed cord in a sterile towel.
    C. Leave the cord as is and have patient lie down.
    D. Seat mother in a wheelchair and call the health care provider.

Answer: B. The cord should be wrapped in a sterile towel for infection control purposes and to preserve its function as much as possible while the nurse immediately calls for emergent assistance. Having the patient lie down does not preserve the cord's integrity. Seating the patient places more pressure on the cord, increasing the risk of hypoxia to the fetus. Cutting the cord dangerously compromises the fetus.

Scoring

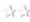 If you answered all four questions correctly, get up and cheer! You're an obstetric emergency genius!

 If you answered three questions correctly, pat yourself on the back! You're gearing up for obstetric success.

If you answered fewer than three questions correctly, don't be sad. Just review the chapter and give it another go.

Selected references

American Academy of Pediatrics. (2018). *Neonatal Resuscitation Program.* Retrieved from https://www.aap.org/en-us/continuing-medical-education/life-support/NRP/Pages/NRP.aspx

American College of Obstetricians and Gynecologists. (2016). *Committee Opinion Number 667. Hospital-based triage of obstetric patients.* Retrieved from https://www.acog.org/Clinical-Guidance-and-Publications/Committee-Opinions/Committee-on-Obstetric-Practice/Hospital-Based-Triage-of-Obstetric-Patients

American College of Obstetricians and Gynecologists. (2017). *Delivery of a newborn with meconium-stained amniotic fluid.* Retrieved from https://www.acog.org/Clinical-Guidance-and-Publications/Committee-Opinions/Committee-on-Obstetric-Practice/Delivery-of-a-Newborn-With-Meconium-Stained-Amniotic-Fluid?IsMobileSet=false

Janicki, A. J., MacKuen, C., Hauspurg, A., et al. (2016). Obstetric training in emergency medicine: A needs assessment. *Medical Education Online, 21*, 28930. doi:10.3402/meo.v21.28930

Kilfoyle, K. A., Vrees, R., Raker, C. A., et al. (2016). Nonurgent and urgent emergency department use during pregnancy: An observational study. *American Journal of Obstetrics and Gynecology, 216*(2), 181.e1–181.e7. doi:10.1016/j.ajog.2016.10.013

Perry, S. E., Hockenberry, M., Lowdermilk, D., et al. (2018). *Maternal child nursing care* (6th ed.). St. Louis, MO: Mosby.

Chapter 10

Maxillofacial and ocular emergencies

Just the facts

In this chapter, you'll learn:

♦ emergency assessment of the face and associated structures of the eyes, ears, nose, and mouth

♦ diagnostic tests and procedures for maxillofacial and ocular emergencies

♦ maxillofacial and ocular disorders in the emergency department and their treatments.

Understanding maxillofacial and ocular emergencies

The face consists of various structures that are closely related, and as such, an injury in one area can affect surrounding areas as well. Numerous bones and the organs of sight, hearing, taste, and smell are located on the face. In addition, the facial nerve (cranial nerve VII), its branches, and several other cranial nerves provide motor and sensory function for the face.

Maxillofacial and ocular emergencies typically involve some discomfort and pain. In addition, they may affect the patient's functional ability and physical appearance. Moreover, because of the proximity of the patient's airway to the structures of the face, the potential for the patient's airway to be compromised in some way, from edema or due to an extension of the injury, is always present (Jose et al., 2016).

Quickness counts

When faced with a maxillofacial or an ocular emergency, you must assess the patient thoroughly and quickly, always staying alert for subtle changes that might indicate a potential deterioration in the patient's condition. A thorough assessment forms the basis for your interventions, which must be instituted quickly to minimize potentially life-threatening risks to the patient. As with any emergency, the patient's airway, breathing, circulation, disability, and exposure and environment (ABCDE) are priorities. (See *Primary assessment of the trauma patient* in Chapter 1.)

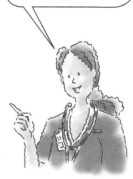

Maxillofacial and ocular emergencies can affect a patient's physical appearance as well as functional ability.

Assessment

Assessment of a patient's face and associated structures includes a health history and physical examination. If the patient's condition does not allow for an interview, you may gather information from the patient's medical record. In some cases, you may need to ask a family member or the emergency medical response team that transported the patient to the emergency department (ED) for information.

Health history

To obtain a health history, begin by introducing yourself and explaining what happens during the health history and physical examination. Use a systematic approach, focusing on one area of the face and then proceeding to another to gather information on the patient's chief concern, past health status, family history, and cultural factors that may influence your assessment.

Chief concern

When obtaining the patient's history, adapt the questions to the patient's specific concerns. Focus your questions on the onset, location, duration, and characteristics of the symptom as well as what aggravates or relieves it. Be sure to question the patient's reports of pain or changes or loss of function in the area as well as the use of medications such as eye drops.

> Frequent headaches can be symptoms of larger problems, so be sure to ask about them.

Eye spy

Key questions related to the eye should address:
- routine problems with the eyes
- use of glasses or contact lenses and why
- problems with blurred vision or changes in the visual field
- history of eye surgery or injury, glaucoma, or cataracts
- medications to treat eye problems.

Earmark past problems

Key questions related to the ears, nose, and throat should address:
- changes in hearing, smell, or the ability to taste or swallow
- reports of frequent headaches, nasal discharge, or postnasal drainage
- history of ear infections, sinus infections, or nosebleeds.

Personal and family health and lifestyle

Next, question the patient about possible familial disorders related to the eyes, ears, nose, and throat. Also explore the patient's daily habits that might affect these structures. Appropriate questions may include:

- Does your occupation require intensive use of your eyes or require you to be exposed to loud noises or chemicals?
- Does the air where you work or live contain anything that causes you problems?
- Do you wear safety equipment, such as goggles and ear protection?

Physical examination

Maxillofacial and ocular emergencies affect people of all ages and can take many forms. To best identify abnormalities, use a consistent, methodical approach to the physical examination. Because of the emergency nature of the patient's condition, remember that you may need to limit your examination to specific problem areas or stop it entirely to intervene should the patient exhibit signs and symptoms of a deteriorating condition.

Examination of extraocular structures

Start by observing the patient's face. With the scalp line as the starting point, check that the patient's eyes are in a normal position—about one-third of the way down the face and about one eye's width apart from each other. Then assess the eyelid, conjunctiva, cornea, anterior chamber, iris, and pupil.

Looking at lids

To examine the eyelid, follow these steps:

- Inspect the eyelids; each upper eyelid should cover the top quarter of the iris, so the eyes look alike.
- Check for an excessive amount of visible sclera above the limbus (corneoscleral junction).
- Ask the patient to open and close their eyes to see if they close completely.
- If the downward movement of the upper eyelid in down gaze is delayed, the patient has a condition known as *lid lag*, which is a common sign of hyperthyroidism.
- Assess the lids for redness, edema, inflammation, or lesions.
- Check for a stye, or hordeolum, a common eyelid lesion. Check for a chalazion, which is a cyst in the eyelid that is caused by inflammation of a blocked meibomian gland. Also check for excessive tearing or dryness.
- The eyelid margins should be pink, and the eyelashes should turn outward.
- Observe whether the lower eyelids turn inward toward the eyeball (called *entropion*) or outward (called *ectropion*).

- Examine the eyelids for lumps.
- Put on examination gloves and gently palpate the *nasolacrimal sac*, the area below the inner canthus. Note any tenderness, swelling, or discharge through the lacrimal point, which could indicate blockage of the nasolacrimal duct.

Conjunctiva

Next, inspect the conjunctiva. To inspect the *bulbar conjunctiva* (the delicate mucous membrane that covers the exposed surface of the sclera), ask the patient to look up and gently pull the lower eyelid down. The bulbar conjunctiva should be clear and shiny; note excessive redness or exudate.

With the lid still secured, inspect the bulbar conjunctiva for color changes, foreign bodies, and edema. Also observe the sclera's color, which should be white. In a black patient, you may see flecks of tan. A bluish discoloration may indicate scleral thinning.

To examine the *palpebral conjunctiva* (the membrane that lines the eyelids), ask the patient to look down. Then lift the upper lid, holding the upper lashes against the eyebrow with your finger. The palpebral conjunctiva should be uniformly pink. In the patient with a history of allergies, the palpebral conjunctiva may have a cobblestone appearance.

Corneal matters

Examine the cornea by shining a penlight from both sides and then from straight ahead. The cornea should be clear without lesions. Test corneal sensitivity by lightly touching the cornea with a wisp of cotton. (See *Tips for assessing corneal sensitivity.*)

Observe the iris, which should appear flat, and the cornea, which should appear convex. The irises should be the same size, color, and shape.

Pupil examination

Each pupil should be round, equal in size, and about one-fourth the size of the iris in average room lighting. About one person in four has asymmetrical pupils without disease. Unequal pupils may indicate neurologic damage, iritis, glaucoma, or therapy with certain drugs. A fixed pupil that doesn't react to light can be an ominous neurologic sign.

Testing

Test the pupils for direct and consensual response. In a slightly darkened room, hold a penlight about 20″ (51 cm) from the patient's eyes and direct the light at the eye from the side. Note the reaction of the pupil you're testing (direct response) and the opposite pupil (consensual response). They should both react the same way. Also, note sluggishness or inequality in the response. Repeat the test with the

Tips for assessing corneal sensitivity

To test corneal sensitivity, touch a wisp of cotton from a cotton ball to the cornea, as shown below.

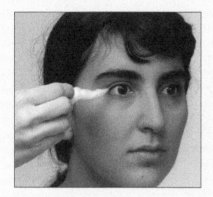

The patient should be able to blink. If the patient is unable to blink, the patient may have suffered damage to the sensory fibers of cranial nerve V or to the motor fibers controlled by cranial nerve VI.

Keep in mind that people who wear contact lenses may have reduced sensitivity because they're accustomed to having foreign objects in their eyes.

Just a wisp
Remember that a wisp of cotton is the only safe object to use for this test. Even though a 4" × 4" gauze pad or tissue is soft, it can cause corneal abrasions and irritation.

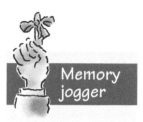

Memory jogger

To make sure that your pupil assessment is complete, think of the acronym PERRLA.

Pupils

Equal

Round

Reactive

Light-reacting

Accommodative-reacting

other pupil. *Note:* If you shine the light in a blind eye, neither pupil will respond. If you shine the light in a seeing eye, the pupils will respond consensually.

To test the pupils for accommodation, place your finger approximately 4" (10 cm) from the bridge of the patient's nose. Ask the patient to look at a fixed object in the distance and then at your finger. The pupils should constrict and the eyes converge as the patient focuses on your finger.

Assessment of ocular muscle function

Evaluation of ocular muscle function involves assessing the corneal light reflex and the cardinal positions of gaze.

To assess the corneal light reflex, ask the patient to look straight ahead and then shine a penlight on the bridge of the nose from about 12" to 15" (30.5 to 38 cm) away. The light should fall at the same spot on each cornea. If it doesn't, the eyes aren't being held in the same plane by the extraocular muscles. This inequality commonly occurs in a patient who lacks muscle coordination, a condition called *strabismus* (cross-eye) (Bagheri & Wajda, 2016).

Cardinal concerns

Cardinal positions of gaze evaluate the oculomotor, trigeminal, and abducens nerves as well as the extraocular muscles. To perform this test, ask the patient to remain still while you hold a pencil or other small object directly in front of the patient's nose at a distance of

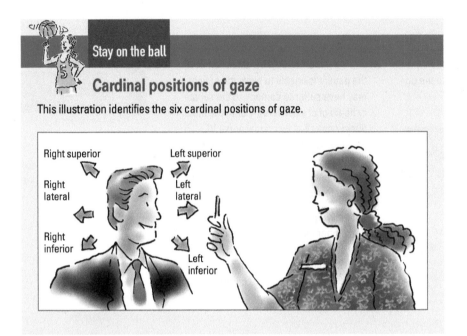

Cardinal positions of gaze

This illustration identifies the six cardinal positions of gaze.

Right superior

Left superior

Right lateral

Left lateral

Right inferior

Left inferior

about 18″ (46 cm). Ask the patient to follow the object with their eyes without moving the head. Then move the object to each of the six cardinal positions, returning to the midpoint after each movement. The patient's eyes should remain parallel as they move. Note abnormal findings, such as nystagmus. (See *Cardinal positions of gaze*.)

Testing

If time and the patient's condition allow, you may perform the cover–uncover test. This test usually isn't done unless you detect an abnormality when assessing the corneal light reflex and cardinal positions of gaze.

Ask the patient to stare at a wall on the other side of the room. Cover one eye and watch for movement in the uncovered eye. Remove the eye cover and watch for movement again. Repeat the test with the other eye.

Eye movement while covering or uncovering the eye is considered abnormal. It may result from weak or paralyzed extraocular muscles, which may be caused by cranial nerve impairment.

Visual acuity testing

Visual acuity testing is performed on the patient with an ocular emergency or who reports eye or vision problems. In most cases, it's the first test performed; however, if the patient has experienced chemical exposure to the eyes, it follows eye irrigation.

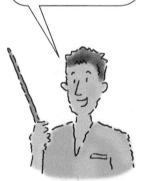

When testing with cardinal positions of gaze, make sure that the patient's head stays still.

A very telling Snellen

To test your patient's far and near vision, use a Snellen chart and a near-vision chart (Jarvis, 2020). To test peripheral vision, use confrontation. Before each test, ask the patient to remove corrective lenses if corrective lenses are worn.

Have the patient sit or stand 20′ (6.1 m) from the chart and then cover the left eye with an opaque object. Ask the patient to read the letters on one line of the chart and then to move downward to increasingly smaller lines until the patient is no longer able to discern all of the letters. Have the patient repeat the test covering the right eye. Lastly, ask the patient to read the smallest line possible with both eyes uncovered to test binocular vision.

If the patient wears corrective lenses, have the patient repeat the test wearing them. Record the vision with and without correction.

If a Snellen chart is unavailable, you can use other methods to assess the patient's visual acuity, including:
- using a pocket vision screener held 14″ (35.6 cm) from the patient's nose
- having the patient read newsprint
- asking the patient to identify the number of fingers being held up
- having the patient identify hand motion if he or she unable to discern the number of fingers being held up.

With these methods, be sure to document the distance at which the patient identified or perceived it (Bagheri & Wajda, 2016).

E for everyone else

Use the Snellen E chart to test visual acuity in a young child and a patient who can't read. Cover the patient's left eye to check the right eye; point to an E on the chart and ask the patient to indicate which way the letter faces. Repeat the test on the other side. (See *Visual acuity charts*, page 420.)

If the test values between the two eyes differ by two lines—for example, 20/30 in one eye and 20/50 in the other—suspect an abnormality, such as amblyopia (the failure of one eye to follow an object, also called lazy eye), especially in children.

To test near vision, cover one of the patient's eyes with an opaque object and hold a Rosenbaum near-vision card 14″ (35 cm) from the patient's eyes. Have the patient read the line with the smallest letters he or she can distinguish. Repeat the test with the other eye. If the patient wears corrective lenses, have the patient repeat the test with glasses on or contacts in. Record the visual acuity with and without lenses.

To assess peripheral vision, use a method known as *confrontation*. (See *Using confrontation*, page 421.)

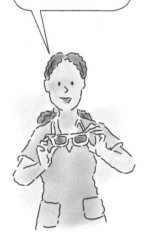

If the patient wears corrective lenses, have him or her repeat the Snellen test without them and record the difference.

Visual acuity charts

The most commonly used charts for testing vision are the Snellen alphabet chart (left) and the Snellen E chart (right), which are used for young children and adults who can't read. Both charts are used to test distance vision and measure visual acuity. The patient reads each chart at a distance of 20' (6.1 m).

Recording results

Visual acuity is recorded as a fraction. The top number (20) is the distance between the patient and the chart. The bottom number is the distance from which a person with normal vision could read the line. The larger the bottom number, the poorer the patient's vision.

Age differences

In adults and children aged 6 and older, normal vision is measured as 20/20. For children aged 3 and younger, normal vision is 20/50; for children aged 4, 20/40; and for children aged 5, 20/30 (Bagheri & Wajda, 2016).

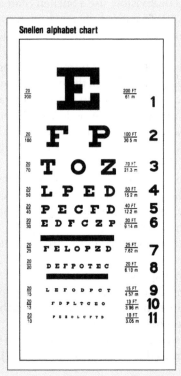

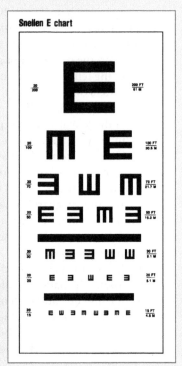

Hearing acuity testing

Test your patient's gross hearing acuity. Ask the patient to occlude one ear or occlude it for the patient. Then stand at a distance of 1' to 2' (30.5 to 61 cm) away, exhale fully, and whisper softly toward the unoccluded ear. Choose numbers or words that have two syllables that are equally accented such as "nine-four" or "baseball." If you note diminished hearing, perform tuning fork tests, such as the Weber and Rinne tests (Wahid & Attia, 2019).

Examination of the nose and sinuses

Begin by observing the patient's nose for position, symmetry, and color. Note such variations as discoloration, swelling, and deformity. Variations in size and shape are largely caused by differences in cartilage and in the amount of fibroadipose tissue.

Using confrontation

Follow these steps to assess peripheral vision with confrontation:
- Sit directly across from the patient and ask them to focus their gaze on your eyes.
- Place your hands on either side of the patient's head at ear level so that they're about 2' (61 cm) apart (as shown).
- Tell the patient to focus their gaze on you as you gradually bring your wiggling fingers into their visual field.
- Instruct the patient to tell you as soon as they can see your wiggling fingers; they should see them at the same time you do.
- Repeat the procedure while holding your hands at the superior and inferior positions.

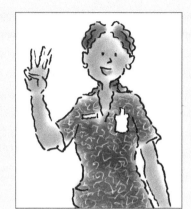

Observe for nasal discharge or flaring. If discharge is present, note the color, quantity, and consistency; if you notice flaring, observe for other signs of respiratory distress.

Test nasal patency and olfactory nerve (cranial nerve I) function. Ask the patient to block one nostril and inhale a familiar aromatic substance through the other nostril. Possible substances include soap, coffee, citrus, tobacco, or nutmeg. Ask the patient to identify the aroma and then repeat the process with the other nostril using a different aroma.

Now, inspect the nasal cavity. Ask the patient to tilt the head back slightly and then push the tip of the nose up. Use the light from the otoscope to illuminate the nasal cavities. Check for severe deviation or perforation of the nasal septum. Examine the vestibule and turbinates for redness, softness, swelling, and discharge.

When life gives you lemons, use them to test cranial nerve I!

Upon closer inspection

Examine the nostrils by direct inspection, using a nasal speculum, a penlight or small flashlight, or an otoscope with a short, wide-tip attachment. Have the patient sit in front of you with the head tilted back. Put on gloves and insert the tip of the closed nasal speculum into one nostril to the point where the blade widens. Slowly open the speculum as wide as possible without causing discomfort. Shine the flashlight in the nostril to illuminate the area.

Inspecting the nostrils

This illustration shows the proper placement of the nasal speculum during direct inspection and the structures you should be able to see during this examination.

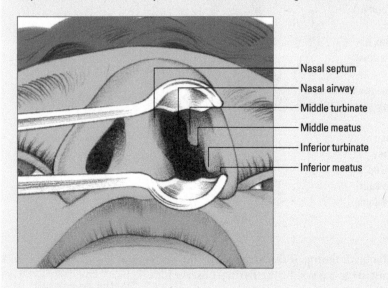

- Nasal septum
- Nasal airway
- Middle turbinate
- Middle meatus
- Inferior turbinate
- Inferior meatus

Observe the color and patency of the nostril and check for exudate. The mucosa should be moist, pink to light red, and free from lesions and polyps. After inspecting one nostril, close the speculum, remove it, and inspect the other nostril. (See *Inspecting the nostrils.*)

Lastly, palpate the patient's nose and surrounding soft tissue with your thumb and forefinger, assessing for pain, tenderness, swelling, and deformity.

Face and sinuses

Next, examine the facial structures using both hands and simultaneously palpating for irregularities and crepitus. Palpate in an upward fashion and then laterally. Observe the patient's face using a downward approach from the eyebrows to the chin. Then observe in the opposite manner to identify deformities.

Examine the sinuses. Remember, only the frontal and maxillary sinuses are accessible; you won't be able to palpate the ethmoidal and sphenoidal sinuses. Begin by checking for swelling around the eyes, especially over the sinus area. Then palpate the sinuses, checking for tenderness. To palpate the frontal sinuses, place your thumbs above the patient's eyes just under the bony ridges of the upper orbits, and place your fingertips on the patient's forehead. Apply gentle pressure. Next, palpate the maxillary sinuses.

Stay on the ball

Transilluminating the sinuses

Transillumination of the sinuses helps demonstrate opacity and requires only a penlight (Patel & Hwang, 2018). Before you start, darken the room and have the patient close both eyes.

Frontal sinuses
Place the penlight on the supraorbital ring and direct the light upward to illuminate the frontal sinuses just above the eyebrow, as shown here.

Maxillary sinuses
Place the penlight on the patient's cheekbone just below one eye and ask them to open their mouth, as shown here. The light should transilluminate easily and equally.

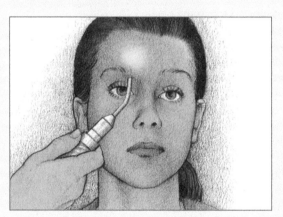

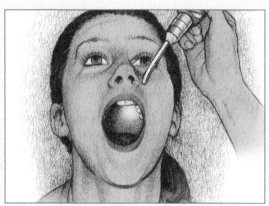

If the patient reports tenderness during palpation, use transillumination to see if the sinuses are filled with fluid or pus. Transillumination can also help reveal tumors and obstructions. (See *Transilluminating the sinuses*.)

Examination of the mouth and throat
First, inspect the patient's lips. They should be pink, moist, symmetrical, and without lesions. A bluish hue or flecked pigmentation is common in patients with dark skin.

Use a tongue blade and a bright light to inspect the oral mucosa. Have the patient open their mouth and then place the tongue blade on top of the tongue. The oral mucosa should be pink, smooth, moist, and free from lesions and unusual odors. Increased pigmentation is seen in patients with dark skin.

Gums . . .

Next, observe the gingivae, or gums; they should be pink, moist, and have clearly defined margins at each tooth. They shouldn't be retracted.

Inspect the teeth, noting their number, condition, and whether any are missing or crowded. If the patient is wearing dentures, ask the patient to remove them, so you can inspect the gums underneath. Ask the patient to open their jaw and palpate the interior of the mouth while wearing gloves.

. . . and tongues

Lastly, inspect the tongue. It should be midline, moist, pink, and free from lesions. The posterior surface should be smooth, and the anterior surface should be slightly rough with small fissures. The tongue should move easily in all directions, and it should lie straight to the front at rest.

Ask the patient to raise the tip of their tongue and touch the palate directly behind the front teeth. Inspect the ventral surface of the tongue and the floor of the mouth. Next, wrap a piece of gauze around the tip of the tongue and move the tongue first to one side then the other to inspect the lateral borders. They should be smooth and even-textured.

Gag order

Inspect the patient's oropharynx by asking them to open their mouth while you shine the penlight on the uvula and palate. You may need to insert a tongue blade into the mouth and depress the tongue. Place the tongue blade slightly off center to avoid eliciting the gag reflex. The uvula and oropharynx should be pink and moist, without inflammation or exudate. The tonsils should be pink and shouldn't be hypertrophied. Ask the patient to say "Ahhh." Observe for movement of the soft palate and uvula.

Lastly, palpate the lips, tongue, and oropharynx. Note lumps, lesions, ulcers, or edema of the lips or tongue. Assess the patient's gag reflex by gently touching the back of the pharynx with a cotton-tipped applicator or the tongue blade. This should produce a bilateral response.

Diagnostic tests

Diagnostic tests include computed tomography (CT) scan, facial X-rays, fluorescein angiography, fluorescein staining, and ultrasonography.

CT scan

A CT scan aids in diagnosing complex facial fractures. It's considered the standard for assessing soft tissue injury and provides useful information in identifying soft tissue injury involving the optic nerve. It also confirms the diagnosis of cervical spine injury, which may be present in a patient with maxillofacial or ocular injuries.

It's orbital

Performed specifically for an ocular emergency, an orbital CT scan allows visualization of abnormalities not readily seen on standard X-rays, such as size and position delineation, and relationship to adjoining structures. Contrast media may be used in orbital CT scanning to define ocular tissues and help confirm a suspected circulatory disorder or hemangioma.

The application of CT scanning to ophthalmology extends beyond the evaluation of the orbital and adjoining structures; it also permits precise diagnosis of many intracranial lesions that affect vision.

Orbital CT scan reveals ocular abnormalities that standard X-rays can't such as a hemangioma!

Practice pointers

- Check the patient's history for hypersensitivity reactions to iodine, shellfish, or radiographic dyes.
- Tell the patient that they will be positioned on a CT scan table and that the table's head will be moved into the scanner, which will rotate around their head.
- If a contrast medium will be used, tell the patient that they may feel flushed and warm and may experience a metallic taste and nausea or vomiting after injection of the medium. Reassure the patient that these reactions are typical.

Facial X-rays

Various types of X-rays may be used to determine maxillofacial injuries. These include:

- *posteroanterior (Waters) view*, considered the most useful X-ray in helping to identify problems in the orbital rim and floor
- *Towne view*, which detects problems in the mandibular condyles
- *anterior, posterior, and lateral views*, which provide information about the skull, sinuses, and roof of the orbit
- *submental vertex*, which provides information about the zygomatic arch and base of the skull
- *anteroposterior and lateral oblique views* to detect injuries to the condylar and coronoid processes and the symphysis (of the mandible).

Practice pointers

- Prepare the patient for the X-ray to be performed; inform the patient of the reason for the X-ray.
- Verify that the X-ray order includes a pertinent history, such as trauma, and identifies the site of tenderness or pain.
- Make sure that the patient removes all jewelry from the head and neck area.

Fluorescein angiography

Fluorescein angiography records the appearance of blood vessels inside the eye through rapid sequence photographs of the fundus (posterior inner part of the eye) (Rebar, 2018). The photographs, which are taken with a special camera, follow the intravenous (IV) injection of sodium fluorescein. This contrast medium enhances the visibility of microvascular structures of the retina and choroid, allowing evaluation of the entire retinal vascular bed, including retinal circulation.

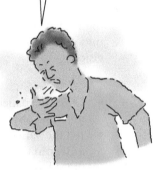

Gesundheit! Sudden sneezing after contrast dye injection could mean hypersensitivity.

Practice pointers

- Check the patient's history for an intraocular lens implant, glaucoma, and hypersensitivity reactions, especially reactions to contrast media and dilating eye drops.
- If mydriatic eye drops are ordered, ask the patient with glaucoma if they have used eye drops that day.
- Observe the patient for hypersensitivity reactions to the dye, such as vomiting, dry mouth, metallic taste, sudden increased salivation, sneezing, light-headedness, fainting, and hives. Rarely, anaphylactic shock may result.
- Explain that eye drops will be instilled to dilate the pupils and that a dye will be injected into their arm. Remind the patient to maintain their position and fixation as the dye is injected. Tell the patient that they may briefly experience nausea and a feeling of warmth.
- Remind the patient that their skin and urine will be a yellow color for 24 to 48 hours after the test and that their near vision will be blurred for up to 12 hours.

Fluorescein staining

Fluorescein staining is used to evaluate ocular structures, specifically the cornea. It uses a stain that, when applied to the conjunctival sac, is distributed over the cornea. The cornea is then examined using a cobalt blue light; colors denote corneal irregularities. For example, corneal abrasions appear bright yellow like a highlighter, and loss of the protective conjunctiva appears as orange-yellow. Foreign bodies can vary in color depending on their material.

Colorful AND informative! Fluorescein staining uses stain and a cobalt blue light to reveal corneal irregularities.

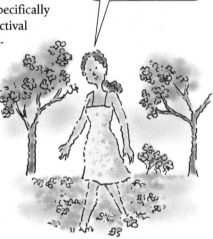

Practice pointers

- Explain the procedure and the reason for its use to the patient; make sure that they have removed contact lenses if worn.
- Put on gloves and remove the strip from the package, being sure to keep the strip sterile.

Technique for fluorescein staining

When performing fluorescein staining, be sure to touch the dampened edge of the fluorescein strip to the conjunctiva at the inner canthus of the lower eyelid.

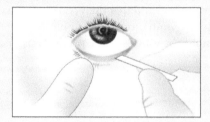

- Moisten the strip with normal saline solution (or an anesthetizing agent if ordered).
- Using your nondominant hand, gently pull down the eye's lower lid.
- Touch the tip of the fluorescein strip to the inner canthus of the lower lid. (See *Technique for fluorescein staining.*)
- Have the patient blink several times so that tears can help transport the stain throughout the eye.
- Examine the patient's eye under cobalt blue light, looking for colored areas or spots.
- After completion, flush the patient's eye with normal saline solution to remove the stain.
- Instruct the patient to wait at least 1 hour before inserting contact lenses.

Ultrasonography

Ultrasonography involves the transmission of high-frequency sound waves. For ocular emergencies, the transmission of high-frequency sound waves through the eye is measured based on their reflection from ocular structures.

Illustrating the eyes' structures through ultrasound especially helps to evaluate a fundus clouded by an opaque medium, such as a cataract, or changes in density due to fractures. This test can identify pathologies that are normally undetectable through ophthalmoscopy. Ocular ultrasonography may also be performed before such surgeries as cataract removal with intraocular lens implantation.

Practice pointers
- Tell the patient that a small transducer will be placed on the closed eyelid and will transmit high-frequency sound waves that are reflected by the structures in the eye.
- Tell the patient that they may be asked to move the eyes or change gaze during the procedure and that their cooperation is required to ensure accurate determination of test results.
- After the test, remove the water-soluble gel that was placed on the patient's eyelids.

Treatments

Treatments vary depending on the specific maxillofacial or ocular emergency. Common treatment measures include drug therapy, ophthalmic agents, and surgery.

Drug therapy

Various drugs may be used in maxillofacial and ocular emergencies. Topical and systemic medications, including analgesic, antibiotic, and anti-inflammatory agents, are commonly employed.

Ophthalmic agents

Ophthalmic agents are usually administered in drop form but may also come in ointment form. Generally, ophthalmic agents fall into one of two groups:
1. miotics
2. mydriatics.

   Miotics constrict the pupil; mydriatics dilate the pupil. In most cases, mydriatics are anticholinergic agents that also paralyze the muscle of accommodation (termed *cycloplegics*). (See *Examples of miotics and mydriatics*.)

Examples of miotics and mydriatics

Commonly used miotics include:
- acetylcholine (Miochol-E)
- carbachol (Miostat)
- pilocarpine (Isopto Carpine).

Commonly used mydriatics include:
- atropine (Isopto Atropine)
- cyclopentolate (Cyclogyl)
- epinephrine
- homatropine (Isopto Homatropine)
- scopolamine (Hyoscine)
- tropicamide (Mydriacyl).

Memory jogger

Generally, the caps are color coded by the effect of the medication on the pupil. Mydriatics have a red cap, and miotics have a green cap.

Instilling eye ointment and eye drops

To teach about instilling eye ointment, instruct the patient to:

• Hold the tube for several minutes to warm the ointment.

• Squeeze a small amount of ointment—¼" to ½" (0.6 to 1.3 cm)—inside the lower lid.

• Gently close the eye and roll the eyeball in all directions with the eye closed.

• Wait 10 minutes before instilling other ointments.

• If eye drops are also ordered, administer eye drops first and wait 5 minutes before instilling the eye ointment (National Institutes of Health Clinical Center, 2018).

To teach about instilling eye drops, instruct the patient to:

• Tilt the head back and pull down on the lower lid.

• Drop the medication into the conjunctival sac.

• Apply pressure to the inner canthus for 1 minute after administration.

• Wait 5 minutes before instilling a second drop or other eye solutions (National Institutes of Health Clinical Center, 2018).

Nursing considerations

- Administer the agent as ordered, making sure that the proper form, such as solution or ointment, is used.
- Instill topical agents appropriately, making sure you keep the tip of the applicator (eye drop bottle or ointment tip) sterile.
- Provide patient teaching about the proper method for instilling eye ointment and eye drops, especially if the patient is to continue the medication at home. (See *Instilling eye ointment and eye drops*.)

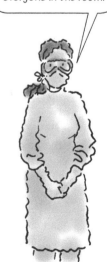

Safety first; laser surgery requires using lots of precautions—including eye protection—for everyone in the room.

Surgery

Surgery, such as laser surgery or scleral buckling, may be performed for ocular emergencies.

Laser surgery

Laser surgery is often the treatment of choice for many ophthalmic disorders because it's relatively painless and especially useful for elderly patients, who may be at poor risks for conventional surgery. Depending on the type of laser, the finely focused, high-energy beam shines at a specific wavelength and color to produce various effects. Laser surgery can be used to treat such ocular emergencies as retinal tears.

Scleral buckling for retinal detachment

In scleral buckling, cryotherapy (cold therapy), photocoagulation (laser therapy), or diathermy (heat therapy) creates a sterile inflammatory reaction that seals the retinal hole and causes the retina to re-adhere to the choroid. The surgeon then places a silicone plate or sponge—called an *explant*—over the site of reattachment and holds it in place with a silicone band. The pressure exerted on the explant indents (buckles) the eyeball and gently pushes the choroid and retina closer together.

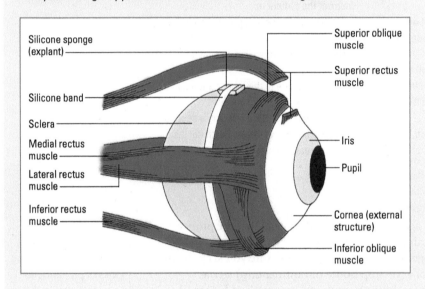

Nursing considerations

- Be aware that laser surgery requires safety precautions, including the use of eye protection for everyone in the room. Reflection of the laser beam from a smooth surface, such as a refractor, to a surface, such as a disposable drape, can start a fire.
- Advise the patient that eye pain may be experienced after the surgery. Encourage the use of ice packs as needed to help decrease the pain.

Scleral buckling

Used to repair retinal detachment, scleral buckling involves applying external pressure to the separated retinal layers, bringing the choroid into contact with the retina. Buckling (or *indenting*) brings the layers together so that an adhesion can form. It also prevents vitreous fluid from seeping between the detached layers of the retina and leading to further detachment and possible blindness. (See *Scleral buckling for retinal detachment*.)

Another method of reattaching the retina is pneumatic retinopexy. This procedure involves sealing the tear or hole with cryotherapy and introducing gas to provide a tamponade of the retina.

Nursing considerations

- Prepare the patient for surgery; depending on the patient's age and the surgeon's preference, advise the patient whether local or general anesthetic will be administered.
- Instruct the patient to report fever or eye pain that's sharp, sudden, or severe.

Common disorders

Common maxillofacial and ocular emergencies you're likely to "face" include:

- chemical burns to the eye
- corneal abrasion
- epistaxis
- facial fractures
- foreign body in the ear
- orbital fracture
- retinal detachment
- soft tissue facial injuries.

Regardless of the disorder, the priorities are always to ensure vital functioning (the ABCDEs).

Chemical burns to the eye

Chemical burns to the eye can cause serious eye injury. These injuries may be work related or may occur while using common household products.

What causes it

Chemical injury to the eye involves splashing or spraying hazardous materials into the eyes. It may also result from exposure to fumes or aerosols. Chemical burns may be caused by an acidic or alkaline substance or an irritant:

- Alkaline substances have a high pH and tend to cause the most severe ocular damage. Examples include lye, cement, lime, and ammonia.
- Acidic substances have a low pH and tend to cause less severe damage. (Even so, hydrofluoric acid, found in rust removers, aluminum brighteners, and heavy-duty cleaners, is an exception and causes severe burns.) An automobile battery explosion, causing a sulfuric acid burn, is the most common injury to the eye involving an acidic substance. Other common acids that can cause chemical burns include sulfurous acid, hydrochloric acid, nitric acid, acetic acid, and chromic acid.
- Irritant substances have a neutral pH and tend to cause discomfort rather than ocular damage. Examples of irritants include pepper spray and many household detergents.

How it happens

The severity of chemical injury to the eye depends on the chemical's pH, the duration of contact with the chemical, the amount of chemical, and the chemical's ability to penetrate the eye.

Alkaline substances can penetrate the surface of the eye into the anterior chamber within 5 to 15 minutes, causing damage to such internal structures as the iris, ciliary body, lens, and trabecular network.

Acidic substances can't penetrate the corneal epithelial layer of the eye, which limits injury to superficial, nonprogressive damage. However, because hydrofluoric acid has properties similar to alkaline substances, it can cause more progressive and severe damage.

Household cleaning solutions carry with them a risk of eye irritation.

What to look for

- Obtain the patient's history; ask about a chemical spraying or splashing in the face or exposure to fumes or aerosols. Also ask about the use of cleaning solutions, solvents, or lawn and garden chemicals.
- Ask the patient about pain, irritation, inability to keep the eyes open, blurred vision, and a sensation of having something in the eye.
- Note patient reports of severe pain and burning; observe for extreme redness, irritation, and excessive tearing.

What tests tell you

Chemical burns to the eye are an immediate threat to the patient's vision and are considered the most urgent of all ocular emergencies. Typically, no diagnostic tests are initially performed because eye irrigation takes priority.

How it's treated

The patient's eye is irrigated continuously with copious amounts of normal saline solution. Irrigation continues for at least 30 minutes and until the ocular pH reaches the desired level. Topical antibiotics, cycloplegic agents, and corticosteroids are ordered; opioid analgesia may also be ordered. Follow-up care with an ophthalmologist is essential.

What to do

- Assess the patient's eye pH before irrigating the eye with sterile normal saline solution. Assessing the patient's visual acuity can be delayed until after irrigation.
- Flush the patient's eyes with copious amounts of sterile isotonic saline solution for at least 30 minutes. Intermittently check the pH of the eye (because ocular pH may be increased if the offending

Eye irrigation for chemical burns

The patient's eye may be irrigated using a Morgan lens or an intravenous (IV) tube.

Morgan lens

Connected to irrigation tubing, a Morgan lens permits continuous lavage and also delivers medication to the eye. Use an adapter to connect the lens to the IV tubing and the solution container. Begin the irrigation at the prescribed flow rate. To insert the device, ask the patient to look down as you insert the lens under the upper eyelid (as shown). Then have the patient look up as you retract and release the lower eyelid over the lens.

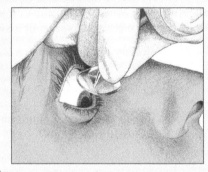

IV tube

If a Morgan lens isn't available, set up an IV bag and tubing without a needle. Direct a constant, gentle stream at the inner canthus so that the solution flows across the cornea to the outer canthus (as shown). Flush the eye for at least 15 minutes (Stevens, 2016).

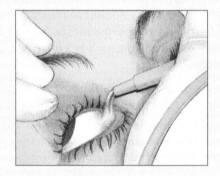

chemical is alkaline, decreased if it's acidic, or neutral if it's an irritant). Continue to irrigate until the pH returns to a normal level (6.5 to 7.6). (See *Eye irrigation for chemical burns*.)

- After irrigation, inspect for conjunctival and scleral redness and tearing and corneal opacification.
- Prepare the patient for an ophthalmic examination.
- Provide analgesics as needed for pain.
- Administer other medications—topical or oral antibiotics, cycloplegics to prevent ciliary spasms and reduce inflammation, and topical lubricants—as ordered.
- Be prepared to administer beta-adrenergic blockers to lower intraocular pressure (IOP) if secondary glaucoma develops.
- If the patient has face burns from an alkaline substance, assess the patient for tracheal or esophageal burns; these burns can cause life-threatening injuries.

- Because burns resulting from hydrofluoric acid may cause severe hypocalcemia, monitor serum calcium levels as ordered.
- Apply eye dressings or patches as needed to reduce eye movement.
- Teach the patient how to apply ophthalmic medications as necessary.
- Strongly advise patients to wear protective goggles or eyewear when working with toxic substances and to keep all toxic home products out of children's reach.

Corneal abrasion

A corneal abrasion is a scratch on the surface epithelium of the cornea. With treatment, prognosis is usually good.

What causes it

A corneal abrasion usually results from a foreign body—such as a cinder or a piece of dust, dirt, or grit—becoming embedded under the eyelid (Ignatavicius et al., 2018). Additional causes include small pieces of metal; improperly fitted contact lenses or falling asleep wearing hard contact lenses; or other items, such as a fingernail, piece of paper, or other organic substance.

How it happens

Small pieces of metal that get in the eyes of workers who don't wear protective glasses quickly form a rust ring on the cornea and cause corneal abrasion. Such abrasions are also common in the eyes of people who fall asleep wearing hard contact lenses or whose lenses aren't fitted properly. A corneal scratch caused by a fingernail, a piece of paper, or other organic substance may cause a persistent lesion. The epithelium doesn't always heal properly, possibly resulting in recurrent corneal erosion with delayed effects more severe than the original injury.

What to look for

- Reports of eye trauma or wearing contact lenses for a prolonged period
- Reports of a sensation of something in the eye, sensitivity to light, decreased visual acuity (if the abrasion occurs in the pupillary region), and pain
- Redness, increased tearing
- Evidence of a foreign body on the cornea or eyelid

What tests tell you

Fluorescein staining confirms the diagnosis. The health care provider uses a cobalt blue light and slit-lamp examination. The injured area appears yellow like a highlighter when examined.

How it's treated

If a foreign body is identified, the eye is irrigated and a topical anesthetic eye drop is used. The health care provider uses a foreign body spud to remove a superficial foreign body. If the foreign body is a rust ring, it must be removed by the health care provider using an ophthalmic burr. When only partial removal is possible, reepithelialization lifts what remains of the ring to the surface so that removal can be completed the next day.

What to do

- Assist with the eye examination. Check visual acuity before beginning treatment.
- If a foreign body is visible, carefully irrigate the eye with normal saline solution.
- Instill topical anesthetic eye drops in the affected eye before assisting the health care provider with removal.
- Instill broad-spectrum antibiotic eye drops in the affected eye every 3 to 4 hours.
- Reassure the patient that the corneal epithelium usually heals in 24 to 48 hours.
- Provide tetanus prophylaxis.

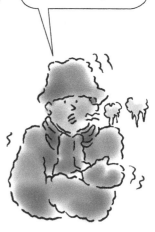

Brrr is for the cold, but a burr is for removing a rust ring from the eye.

To patch or not to patch

- If a patch is ordered, tell the patient to leave it in place for 6 to 12 hours. Warn the patient that a patch alters depth perception and advise caution in performing daily activities, such as climbing stairs or stepping off a curb. (Patching is no longer routinely recommended in the treatment of corneal abrasions.)
- Stress the importance of instilling antibiotic eye drops as ordered because an untreated corneal abrasion, if infected, can lead to a corneal ulcer and permanent vision loss. Teach the patient the proper way to instill eye medications. (See *Corneal ulceration*, page 436.)
- Advise the patient who wears contact lenses to abstain from wearing them until the corneal abrasion heals.
- Urge the patient to wear safety glasses to protect the eyes from flying fragments.
- Review instructions for wearing and caring for contact lenses to prevent further trauma.

Epistaxis

Epistaxis refers to a nosebleed. Such bleeding in children generally originates in the anterior nasal septum and tends to be mild. In adults, such bleeding most likely originates in the posterior septum and can be severe.

Corneal ulceration

A major cause of blindness worldwide, corneal ulcers result in corneal scarring or perforation. They occur in the central or marginal areas of the cornea, vary in shape and size, and may be singular or multiple. Prompt treatment (within hours of onset) can prevent vision impairment.

Corneal ulcers generally result from bacterial, protozoan, viral, or fungal infections, but other causes may include ocular trauma, exposure, toxins, and allergens (McCance & Huether, 2019).

Signs and symptoms

Typically, corneal ulceration begins with pain (aggravated by blinking) and photophobia, followed by increased tearing. Eventually, central corneal ulceration produces pronounced visual blurring. The eye may appear red. Purulent discharge is possible if a bacterial ulcer is present.

Treatment

Prompt treatment is essential for all forms of corneal ulcer to prevent complications and permanent vision impairment. Treatment aims to eliminate the underlying cause of the ulcer and relieve pain.

A corneal ulcer should never be patched because patching creates the dark, warm, moist environment ideal for bacterial growth. However, it should be protected with a perforated shield. Antibiotics, antivirals, or antifungals are prescribed based on culture and sensitivity findings. Artificial tears and lubricating ointments may be prescribed as needed.

Nursing considerations

- Because corneal ulcers are quite painful, give analgesics as needed.
- Watch for signs of secondary glaucoma (transient vision loss and halos around lights).
- The patient may be more comfortable in a darkened room or when wearing dark glasses.

What causes it

Epistaxis may be a primary disorder or may occur secondary to another condition. It usually follows trauma from external or internal causes, such as a blow to the nose, nose picking, or insertion of a foreign body. Less commonly, it results from polyps; inhalation of chemicals that irritate the nasal mucosa; vascular abnormalities; or acute or chronic infections, such as sinusitis or rhinitis, that cause congestion and eventual bleeding from capillary blood vessels. Epistaxis may also follow sudden mechanical decompression (caisson disease) and strenuous exercise.

How it happens

A rich supply of fragile blood vessels makes the nose particularly vulnerable to bleeding. Air moving through the nose can dry and irritate the mucous membranes, forming crusts that bleed when they're removed.

Dry mucous membranes are also more susceptible to infections, which can lead to epistaxis as well. In addition, trauma to the mucous membranes leads to bleeding.

What to look for

The patient with epistaxis commonly comes to the ED holding bloody tissues, towels, or cloths. Bleeding from one or both nostrils is visible and may range from a slow trickle to a profuse continuous flow. Unilateral bleeding is typical; bilateral bleeding suggests a blood dyscrasia or severe trauma.

Bright red blood oozing from the nostrils suggests anterior bleeding. Blood visible in the back of the throat originates in the posterior area and may be dark or bright red. It's commonly mistaken for hemoptysis because of expectoration.

The patient's history may reveal trauma to the nose or evidence of a predisposing factor, such as anticoagulant therapy, hypertension, chronic aspirin use, high altitudes and dry climate, sclerotic vessel disease, Hodgkin disease, vitamin K deficiency, or blood dyscrasias.

Life at a high altitude can predispose you to epistaxis.

What tests tell you

Diagnosis is determined by assessment findings. Facial X-rays may be done to determine if a fracture is present. If the patient's bleeding is severe, complete blood count and coagulation studies may be done to evaluate the patient's status. In addition, blood typing and cross-matching is done if the patient requires a transfusion because of blood loss.

How it's treated

The nose is cleared of blood clots by having the patient blow their nose or with suctioning via an 8 or 10 French Frazier catheter. If the bleeding is anterior, treatment typically includes stopping the bleeding with topical vasoconstrictors, direct pressure for 5 to 10 minutes, cautery (chemical or electrical), and packing if needed. Nasal packing, which is coated with an antibiotic ointment before insertion, can be in the form of petroleum iodoform gauze, which requires removal in 24 to 72 hours, or commercial packing products that dissolve and don't require removal.

Posterior bleeding is treated with nasal packing in the form of nasal sponges, special epistaxis balloon devices, or a 12 to 16 French urinary catheter (with the distal tip removed). This type of packing is usually removed in 2 to 3 days. Drug therapy to treat an underlying condition, such as hypertension, is ordered. If bleeding doesn't respond to treatment, surgery involving ligation or embolization may be necessary.

What to do

- Assess the patient's ABCs. If bleeding is severe or if there's associated trauma, institute emergency interventions as necessary, such as suctioning, oxygen saturation monitoring and oxygen therapy, IV therapy, and cardiac monitoring.
- Determine the location of the bleeding (anterior or posterior) and whether epistaxis is unilateral or bilateral. Inspect for blood seeping behind the nasal septum, in the middle ear, and in the corners of the eyes.
- Apply direct pressure to the soft portion of the nostrils against the septum continuously for 5 to 10 minutes. Maintain the patient in an upright position with the head tilted slightly downward as you compress the nostrils.
- Apply an ice collar or cold compresses to the nose. Bleeding should stop after 10 minutes.
- Assist with treatment for anterior bleeding, including the application of external pressure and a topical vasoconstrictor (such as a cotton ball saturated with 4% topical cocaine solution or a solution of 4% lidocaine and topical epinephrine at 1:10,000) to the bleeding site, followed by cauterization with electrocautery or a silver nitrate stick. If these measures don't control bleeding, petroleum gauze nasal packing may be needed. (See *Types of nasal packing.*)

Pack it up

- Assist with treatment for posterior bleeding, including the use of a nasal balloon catheter to control bleeding effectively, gauze packing inserted through the nose, or postnasal packing inserted through the mouth, depending on the bleeding site.
- If local measures fail to control bleeding, assist with additional treatment, which may include supplemental vitamin K and, for severe bleeding, blood transfusions and surgical ligation or embolization of a bleeding artery.
- Monitor the patient's vital signs and skin color; record blood loss.
- Assess oxygen saturation levels via pulse oximetry and administer oxygen as needed.
- Tell the patient to breathe through the mouth and not to swallow blood, talk, or blow their nose.
- Keep vasoconstrictors, such as phenylephrine (Neo-Synephrine) nasal spray, on hand.
- Reassure the patient and family that epistaxis usually looks worse than it is.
- Administer antibiotics as ordered if packing must remain in place for longer than 24 hours.
- If the bleeding is controlled effectively, prepare the patient for discharge; if the patient required posterior nasal packing, prepare the patient for admission. (See *Teaching tips to prevent epistaxis*, page 440.)

Types of nasal packing

Nosebleeds may be controlled with anterior or posterior nasal packing.

Anterior nasal packing

The health care provider may treat an anterior nosebleed by packing the anterior nasal cavity with an antibiotic-impregnated petroleum gauze strip (shown at right) or with a nasal tampon.

A nasal tampon is made of tightly compressed absorbent material with or without a central breathing tube. The health care provider inserts a lubricated tampon along the floor of the nose and, with the patient's head tilted backward, instills 5 to 10 mL of antibiotic or normal saline solution. This solution causes the tampon to expand, stopping the bleeding. The tampon should be moistened periodically, and the central breathing tube should be suctioned regularly.

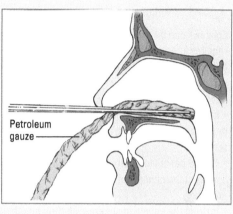

In a patient with blood dyscrasias, the health care provider may fashion an absorbable pack by moistening a gauzelike, regenerated cellulose material with a vasoconstrictor. Applied to a visible bleeding point, this substance will swell to form a clot. The packing is absorbable and doesn't need removal.

Posterior nasal packing

Posterior packing consists of a gauze roll shaped and secured by three sutures (one suture at each end and one in the middle) or a balloon-type catheter. To insert the packing, the health care provider advances one or two soft catheters into the patient's nostrils (shown at right). When the catheter tips appear in the nasopharynx, the health care provider grasps them with a Kelly clamp or bayonet forceps and pulls them forward through the mouth. He secures the two end sutures to the catheter tip and draws the catheter back through the nostrils.

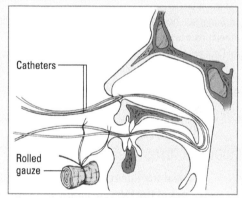

This step brings the packing into place with the end sutures hanging from the patient's nostril. (The middle suture emerges from the patient's mouth to free the packing, when needed.)

The health care provider may weigh the nose sutures with a clamp. Then the packing is pulled securely into place behind the soft palate and against the posterior end of the septum (nasal choana).

After the health care provider examines the patient's throat (to ensure that the uvula hasn't been forced under the packing), the anterior packing is inserted and secured by tying the posterior pack strings around rolled gauze or a dental roll at the nostrils (shown at right).

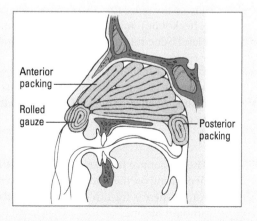

Teaching tips to prevent epistaxis

Epistaxis can be a frightening experience for a patient, especially if the patient requires interventions other than just applying pressure to the nostril area. Therefore, educating the patient in measures to prevent epistaxis can help to alleviate anxiety and decrease the risk of a recurrent episode. Be sure to include the following information in your discharge teaching:

• If anterior packing is required, instruct the patient to return to the emergency department (ED) or make an appointment with the health care provider for packing removal.

• Tell the patient to return to the ED if bleeding recurs or if packing becomes dislodged.

• Instruct the patient not to insert foreign objects into the nose and to avoid bending and lifting.

• Instruct the patient to sneeze with their mouth open.

• Emphasize the need for follow-up examinations and periodic blood studies after an episode of epistaxis. Advise the patient to seek prompt treatment for nasal infection or irritation.

• Suggest a humidifier if the patient lives in a dry climate or at a high elevation or if their home is heated with circulating hot air.

• Caution the patient against inserting cotton or tissues into the nose because these objects are difficult to remove and may further irritate nasal mucosa (Morgan & Kellerman, 2014).

Facial fractures

A facial fracture refers to an injury that results in a broken bone or bones of the face. Facial fractures may involve damage to almost any of the bone structures of the face, including the nose, zygoma (cheekbone), mandible, frontal region, maxilla, and supraorbital rim. Nasal bone fractures are the most common type of facial fracture.

What causes it

Many facial fractures result from sports-related injuries. Other mechanisms of injury may include motor vehicle accidents, manual blows to the face, and falls.

How it happens

The amount of force necessary to fracture bones of the face varies depending on the bone. Nasal fractures require the least amount of force, whereas fractures of the supraorbital rim require the greatest amount of force.

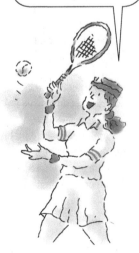

Watch that return! Sports-related injuries are a main facial fracture culprit.

What to look for
General findings related to facial fractures include:
- swelling
- displacement
- ecchymosis
- pain
- possible loss of function.

Specific signs and symptoms vary depending on the areas and structures involved. (See *Assessing facial fractures,* page 442.)

What tests tell you
Typically, facial X-rays reveal the type of fracture and its location. CT scan may be used to determine the injury's extent.

How it's treated
Treatment of facial fractures involves stabilizing the patient's airway, including frequent suctioning if bleeding and secretions are profuse, and ruling out cervical spine injury. Orotracheal intubation is preferred for airway maintenance. Oxygen therapy and assisted ventilation are used as necessary. Hemorrhage is treated with direct pressure, ice packs, or an external compression dressing. Nasal fractures require splinting and setting of the bone. Surgery with open reduction and internal fixation or wiring is used to treat mandibular fractures.

What to do
- Because facial fractures typically involve structures located near the airway, immediately assess ABCs. If the patient has sustained severe facial trauma, oral airway insertion or endotracheal intubation and mechanical ventilation may be necessary.
- Immobilize the cervical spine until spinal injury is ruled out. Because of the force needed to cause a facial fracture, cervical spine injury may be present in 1% to 4% of those with facial fractures.
- Obtain facial X-rays and a CT scan of the face as ordered to locate the fracture and determine the level of severity.
- Initiate measures to reduce swelling and control bleeding (which may include elevating the patient's head if cervical spine injury has been ruled out); apply ice to the area.
- Administer analgesics and other medications as ordered, including tetanus prophylaxis.
- Prepare the patient for surgery as indicated.

Assessing facial fractures

When a patient experiences a facial fracture, signs and symptoms vary based on the area of injury. This chart highlights some of the common assessment and diagnostic test findings associated with various facial fracture areas.

Fracture area	Assessment findings	Diagnostic test findings
Nasal	• Pain • Changes in vision • Edema of the periorbital area and upper face • Ecchymosis • Epistaxis • Crepitus • Possible intracranial injuries	Facial computed tomography (CT) scan or nasal bone X-ray revealing disruption of the bone
Zygomatic arch	• Pain in the lateral cheek • Difficulty closing the jaw • Swelling and crepitus • Visible asymmetry	Facial X-ray or facial CT scan showing depressed arch
Mandibular	• Point tenderness • Crepitus • Trismus (tonic contracture of chewing muscles) • Asymmetrical facial appearance • Swelling • Ecchymosis • Malocclusion • Possible lower lip and chin paresthesia • Inability to grasp a tongue blade between the teeth	Facial X-ray or CT scan revealing displacement at the site of fracture (most commonly mandibular angle, condyle, molar, and mental areas)
Maxillary	• Severe facial pain • Lack of sensation or paresthesia of the upper lip • Vision changes • Severe facial edema and ecchymosis • Elongated facial appearance • Periorbital or orbital edema • Subconjunctival hemorrhage • Facial asymmetry • Malocclusion • Rhinorrhea • Moveable maxilla	Facial X-ray revealing displacement and site of fracture; CT scan identifying the extent and severity of the fracture

Foreign body in the ear

Foreign body in the ear, as the name suggests, refers to any object in the ear canal that causes some obstruction. This problem is most commonly associated with children ages 9 months to 4 years.

What causes it

The most common cause of a foreign body in the ear is cerumen, commonly as a result of inserting cotton swabs into the ear and pushing cerumen further into the ear canal. Cerumen impaction is another cause, most commonly seen in the older adult. Other causes include insects and such objects as beads, small stones, beans, corn, and dry cereal.

How it happens

The object becomes lodged in the ear canal. Cerumen blocks the transmission of sound to the eardrum. Other objects, such as beans or insects, become lodged in the canal, leading to inflammation, pain, and possible infection.

What to look for

Typically, the patient reports a change in hearing. The patient may report ear pain or feelings of fullness. Signs and symptoms of ear infection or purulent foul-smelling drainage may be seen. If an insect is the cause, the patient commonly reports a feeling of buzzing or something moving in the ear.

What tests tell you

Gross hearing screening may be done to estimate the degree of hearing loss. Otoscopic examination reveals evidence of an obstruction.

How it's treated

Removal of the foreign body is key. This removal may be achieved with suctioning, irrigation, or special tools while directly visualizing the ear canal. These tools may include an ear curette, right-angle hook, Frazier suction catheter, funnel-tipped flexible catheter, or alligator forceps. Eardrops may be used to help soften impacted cerumen. If a patient has a live insect in their ear, mineral oil or 2% lidocaine may be used to kill the insect before its removal.

What to do

- Assess the patient's gross hearing acuity and determine evidence of obstruction.
- Prepare the patient for ear irrigation; provide comfort to the patient and family.

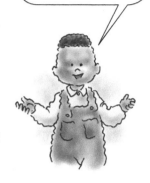

Little hands, big trouble! Children ages 9 months to 4 years are the usual suspects when it comes to foreign bodies in the ear.

• Explain procedures and treatments to the patient and family to help alleviate anxiety.
• If ordered, administer eardrops to soften cerumen or insert mineral oil or 2% lidocaine to kill a live insect.
• Assist with the instrument removal of a foreign object.
• Irrigate the ear as ordered using warm tap water or a solution of 1:1 hydrogen peroxide and warm water; make sure that the solution is warmed to body temperature to prevent stimulating the inner ear, which could lead to dizziness, nausea, and vomiting (Hayter, 2016). (See *Contraindications for irrigation*.)

Orbital fracture

Orbital fracture refers to a break in the orbital floor and rim. This type of fracture is a serious condition and can lead to vision impairment or injury to the globe.

What causes it
Orbital fracture is usually caused by direct blunt trauma to the eye, such as from a motor vehicle collision, assault, or fall. A blowout fracture occurs when the direct injury causes such a significant increase in IOP that the floor of the orbit breaks.

How it happens
The direct force of the blunt trauma causes disruption to the orbital floor and rim. Fracture of the floor occurs when orbital pressure rises significantly. Subsequently, the contents of the orbit can herniate into the maxillary and ethmoid sinuses. The inferior rectus muscle may also become trapped in the area.

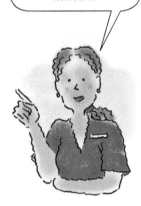

Eyelid ecchymosis, swelling, pain, and difficulty blinking all point to orbital fracture.

What to look for

The patient with an orbital fracture typically reports some type of blunt trauma. Signs and symptoms may include:

- ecchymosis of the eyelid
- swelling
- pain
- difficulty blinking.
    If the patient has a blowout fracture, the following may be present:
- periorbital ecchymosis
- sunken eye
- upward gazing
- diplopia.
    Because of the close proximity of other facial structures and the location on the skull, there may be evidence of facial fractures or head trauma.

What tests tell you

Facial X-rays are used to determine the extent of the fracture and aid in the diagnosis of an orbital blowout fracture. CT scan helps to confirm entrapment of the inferior rectus and oblique extraocular muscles.

How it's treated

Treatment of an orbital fracture is conservative. If globe injury or muscle involvement hasn't occurred, the patient is referred to an ophthalmologist. If there's an associated nasal fracture, antibiotics are most likely ordered. Surgery for globe injury is typically postponed for approximately 2 weeks while swelling diminishes.

What to do

- Evaluate the patient's ABCs and intervene as necessary.
- Assess for evidence of associated trauma, including facial fractures and head trauma.
- Determine the type of injury, including the mechanism, time, force, and object causing the trauma.
- Assess visual acuity and perform an ophthalmic examination.
- Apply ice and elevate the patient's head.
- Provide reassurance to help alleviate anxiety.
- Refer the patient to an ophthalmologist as indicated.
- Advise the patient to avoid Valsalva maneuver, coughing, and nose blowing; these activities can increase IOP, possibly leading to a blowout fracture.

Retinal detachment

Retinal detachment occurs when the outer retinal pigment epithelium splits from the neural retina, creating a subretinal space (Arroyo, 2018). This space then fills with fluid called *subretinal fluid*.

Retinal detachment usually involves only one eye but may later involve the other eye. Surgical reattachment is typically successful. However, the prognosis for good vision depends on which area of the retina has been affected.

What causes it

Predisposing factors include high myopia and cataract surgery. The most common causes are degenerative changes in the retina or vitreous humor. Other causes include:

- trauma or inflammation
- systemic diseases such as diabetes mellitus.

Retinal detachment is rare in children. However, it occasionally develops as a result of retinopathy of prematurity, tumors (retinoblastomas), trauma, or myopia, which tends to run in families.

How it happens

A retinal tear or hole allows the vitreous humor to seep between the retinal layers, separating the retina from its choroidal blood supply. Retinal detachment may also result from seepage of fluid into the subretinal space or from traction placed on the retina by vitreous bands or membranes. (See *Understanding retinal detachment.*)

What to look for

Signs and symptoms of retinal detachment include:

- floaters
- light flashes
- sudden, painless vision loss that may be described as a curtain that eliminates a portion of the visual field
- wavy or watery vision.

What tests tell you

Ophthalmoscopic examination through a well-dilated pupil confirms the diagnosis. It shows the usually transparent retina as gray and opaque; in severe detachment, it reveals folds in the retina and ballooning out of the area. Indirect ophthalmoscopy is also used to search the retina for tears and holes. Ocular ultrasonography may be necessary if the lens is opaque or if the vitreous humor is cloudy.

How it's treated

Treatment depends on the location and severity of the detachment:

- Eye movements are restricted through bed rest and sedation. If the patient's macula is threatened, the head may be positioned so the tear or hole is below the rest of the eye before surgical intervention.
- Bed rest is typically ordered with bilateral eye patching.
- A hole in the peripheral retina can be treated with cryotherapy; a hole in the posterior portion, with laser therapy.
- Retinal detachment rarely heals spontaneously. Surgery— including scleral buckling, pneumatic retinopexy, or vitrectomy (or a combination of these procedures)—can reattach the retina.

Understanding retinal detachment

Traumatic injury or degenerative changes cause retinal detachment by allowing the retina's sensory tissue layers to separate from the retinal pigment epithelium. This permits fluid—for example, from the vitreous humor—to seep into the space between the retinal pigment epithelium and the rods and cones of the tissue layers.

The pressure that results from the fluid entering the space balloons the retina into the vitreous cavity away from choroidal circulation. Separated from its blood supply, the retina can't function. Without prompt repair, the detached retina can cause permanent vision loss.

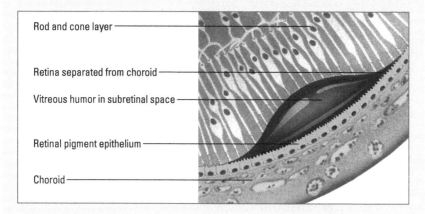

Rod and cone layer

Retina separated from choroid

Vitreous humor in subretinal space

Retinal pigment epithelium

Choroid

What to do

- Provide emotional support because the patient may be distraught about vision loss.
- Maintain complete bed rest and instruct the patient to restrict eye movements until surgical reattachment is performed.
- To avoid pressure to the globe of the eye, which could cause further extrusion of intraocular contents into the subretinal space, apply goggles or a metallic eye shield.
- Urge the patient to avoid activities in bed that could increase IOP, such as straining at stool, bending down, forceful coughing, sneezing, or vomiting.
- Prepare the patient for surgery; if indicated, wash the patient's face with no-tears shampoo. Give antibiotics and cycloplegic–mydriatic eye drops.
- Provide preoperative and postoperative teaching, including care measures to avoid increased IOP. (See *Teaching tips for the patient with retinal detachment*, page 448.)

Teaching tips for the patient with retinal detachment

• Explain to the patient undergoing laser surgery that he may have blurred vision for several days afterward.
• Show the patient having scleral buckling how to instill eye drops properly. Remind the patient to lie in the position recommended by the health care provider after surgery.
• Reinforce the need to rest and avoid driving, bending, heavy lifting, and other activities that affect intraocular pressure for several days after eye surgery. Discourage activities that could cause the patient to bump the eye.
• Review early symptoms of retinal detachment and emphasize the need for immediate treatment.

Soft tissue facial injuries

Soft tissue facial injuries include contusions, lacerations, abrasions, and friction injuries. These injuries are problematic because they can cause considerable upset or changes in physical appearance. Therefore, facial lacerations are typically repaired as soon as possible.

What causes it

Soft tissue facial injuries can be the result of numerous causes; motor vehicle collisions are a common one. Air bag deployment commonly causes minor abrasions of the face, neck, and upper chest.

Lacerations and contusions may result from blunt or penetrating trauma. Animal or human bites are a common cause of lacerations. Friction injuries, commonly called *road rash,* may be the result of a vehicle collision or, possibly, gunpowder fragments.

How it happens

During the trauma, the skin of the face comes in contact with the offending cause. For example, in the case of a bite, the animal's teeth penetrate the outer layer of the skin, causing damage to the underlying tissue. Contact of skin with asphalt leads to shearing of the outer surface and abrasion.

What to look for

Signs and symptoms associated with soft tissue facial injuries may include:
• superficial to deep lacerations on any area of the face
• evidence of skin opening or revealing teeth marks

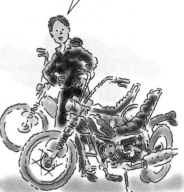

Skin plus asphalt equals shearing and abrasion. Wearing protective clothing and a helmet protects me from injury.

- epidermal staining (friction injuries)
- intraoral deformities, including lacerations and bleeding.
  If the patient sustains deep lacerations of the cheek, you may note:
- forehead asymmetry due to damage of the temporal branch of the facial nerve
- inability to close the eye on the affected side due to damage of the temporal or zygomatic branch of the facial nerve
- inability to purse lips due to damage to the buccal branch of the facial nerve
- elevation of the lower lip at rest with an inability to lower the lower lip from damage to the mandibular branch.

What tests tell you
Facial X-rays, CT scan, and magnetic resonance imaging aid in diagnosing the extent of injury and ruling out fractures.

How it's treated
Treatment of soft tissue facial injuries varies, depending on the type of injury and its severity. Regardless, bleeding is controlled and the wound area is cleaned and irrigated if necessary. In addition:
- Superficial lacerations are sutured as soon as possible to minimize cosmetic disfigurement.
- Lacerations due to bites are thoroughly cleaned and irrigated; consultation with a plastic surgeon is recommended for the decision to close the wounds to minimize possible disfigurement. Animal bites require rabies evaluation and tetanus prophylaxis.
- Friction injuries are vigorously scrubbed with mild soap; dermabrasion may be needed.
- Surgical exploration and repair is conducted for large or deep lacerations.
- Debridement is conducted for wounds that are extensively contaminated.
- Antibiotic therapy is instituted to prevent and treat infection (Mayersak, 2018).

What to do
- Assess the patient's ABCDE and intervene as necessary to stabilize the patient's condition.
- Apply direct pressure to any openly bleeding wounds.
- Clean all wounds and irrigate as ordered; apply sterile dressings as appropriate.
- If the patient sustained an animal bite, question the patient about the animal and possible rabies.
- Prepare the patient for cleaning, debridement, suturing, or surgical exploration as appropriate.
- Provide comfort measures and support; patients may be anxious about how they may look after treatment.

Quick quiz

1. The nurse is caring for a patient who reports a foreign body sensation in the eye. For which procedure will the nurse prepare the patient?

    A. Fluorescein staining
    B. Scleral buckling
    C. Posterior nasal packing
    D. Laser surgery

Answer: A. The fluorescein staining is the diagnostic test used to confirm corneal abrasions.

2. What will the nurse use to assess a patient's corneal sensitivity?

    A. A wisp of cotton
    B. A tissue
    C. A gauze pad
    D. Ophthalmoscopy

Answer: A. A wisp of cotton is the only safe object to use for assessing corneal sensitivity. Even though a gauze pad or tissue is soft, it can cause corneal abrasions and irritation.

3. A patient has experienced a soft tissue injury of the face. Which cranial nerve will the nurse anticipate that may be affected?

    A. I
    B. II
    C. VII
    D. IX

Answer: C. With a soft tissue facial injury, the most commonly affected cranial nerve would be cranial nerve VII, the facial nerve, because its branches are responsible for sensory and motor function of various facial structures.

4. The nurse has received a prescription to administer a mydriatic agent. Which will the nurse prepare to give?

    A. Pilocarpine
    B. Epinephrine
    C. Carbachol
    D. Acetylcholine

Answer: B. Epinephrine is a mydriatic agent. Pilocarpine, carbachol, and acetylcholine are miotic agents.

Scoring

☆☆☆ If you answered all four questions correctly, give a big grin! You're tops when it comes to maxillofacial and ocular emergencies.

☆☆ If you answered three questions correctly, say "Tell yourself, "eye" will keep reading to learn more!" You're ahead of the competition in this emergency category.

☆ If you answered two or less questions correctly, don't frown. Keep your eyes on the prize as you look through the chapter again.

Selected references

Arroyo, J. (2018). *Retinal detachment.* Retrieved from https://www.uptodate.com/contents/retinal-detachment

Bagheri, N., & Wajda, B. N. (Eds.). (2016). *The wills eye manual: Office and emergency room diagnosis and treatment of eye disease* (7th ed.). Philadelphia, PA: Wolters Kluwer.

Hayter, K. (2016). Listen up for safe ear irrigation. *Nursing, 46*(6), 62–65. doi:10.1097/01.NURSE.0000481437.02178.3b

Ignatavicius, D., Workman, L., & Rebar, C. (2018). *Medical-surgical nursing: Concepts for interprofessional collaborative care* (9th ed.). St. Louis, MO: Elsevier.

Jarvis, C. (2020). *Physical examination and health assessment* (8th ed.). St. Louis, MO: Elsevier.

Jose, A., Nagori, S. A., Agarwal, B., et al. (2016). Management of maxillofacial trauma in emergency: An update of challenges and controversies. *Journal of Emergencies Trauma and Shock, 9*(2), 73–80.

Mayersak, R. J. (2018). *Facial trauma in adults.* Retrieved from https://www.uptodate.com/contents/facial-trauma-in-adults

McCance, K., & Huether, S. (2019). *Pathophysiology: The biologic basis for disease in adults and children* (8th ed.). St. Louis, MO: Elsevier.

Morgan, D. J., & Kellerman, R. (2014). Epistaxis: Evaluation and treatment. *Primary Care, 41*(1), 63–73.

National Institutes of Health Clinical Center. (2018). *How to apply eye drops.* Retrieved from https://www.cc.nih.gov/ccc/patient_education/pepubs/eyedrops.pdf

Patel, Z., & Hwang, P. (2018). *Acute sinusitis and rhinosinusitis in adults: Clinical manifestations and diagnosis.* Retrieved from https://www.uptodate.com/contents/acute-sinusitis-and-rhinosinusitis-in-adults-clinical-manifestations-and-diagnosis

Rebar, C. (2018). Sensory system. In L. Willis (Ed.), *Professional guide to pathophysiology* (4th ed., pp. 550–564). Philadelphia, PA: Wolters Kluwer.

Stevens, S. (2016). How to irrigate the eye. *Community Eye Health, 29*(95), 56.

Wahid, N. W. B., & Attia, M. (2019). *Weber test.* Retrieved from https://www.ncbi.nlm.nih.gov/books/NBK526135/

Chapter 11

Psychiatric emergencies

Just the facts

In this chapter, you'll learn:

◆ psychiatric emergencies commonly found in the emergency department setting

◆ key areas to assess when caring for patients with psychiatric emergencies

◆ appropriate nursing interventions in related psychiatric emergencies

◆ use of the interprofessional team in emergent psychiatric situations.

A psychiatric emergency is a disturbance of thoughts, perceptions, feelings, and behaviors that require immediate treatment. The emergency is a threat that if not quickly addressed may result in harm to a patient's existence or to others in the patient's environment. At times, the patient recognizes there is a concern and requests treatment. Sometimes, the patient, because of illness or extreme stress, is unable to voluntarily seek care. In either case, the nurse plays a key role in helping to maintain safety for the patient, family members, and others with whom the patient is in contact.

Understanding psychiatric emergencies

There are various types of psychiatric emergencies. Some arise from organic health conditions, others are situational in nature, and sometimes criminal concerns can accompany these circumstances. Types of psychiatric emergencies include:

- acute psychosis
- violent, disruptive, aggressive, or excited behaviors
- suicide ideation or attempt
- acute anxiety or panic
- organic confused states
- intoxication stupor from alcohol, stimulants, and opioids
- situations of abuse—child, older adult, or domestic violence
- iatrogenic emergencies.

Medical versus psychiatric?

Patients who come to the emergency department (ED) must be assessed holistically. There are often physical, psychological, and sociocultural concerns that exist together. Before initiating a full psychiatric assessment of the patient in the ED, an evaluation of potential medical conditions must be addressed. Listening closely to the chief concern and presenting symptoms will help you determine if the patient's priority problem is medical or psychiatric in nature. Sometimes, you may not know if the problem is medical or psychiatric. Therefore, the health care provider may order laboratory and diagnostic studies to rule out health conditions that may mimic psychiatric problems. Examples of those conditions include glucose abnormalities, endocrine disorders, substance-induced psychosis, and fluid–electrolyte imbalances. Once the patient is medically stable, a thorough mental health screening and assessment can begin.

Specialized members of the psychiatric health care team

Mental health professionals work in an interprofessional environment. Common behavioral health specialists who may participate in the evaluation and care of a patient experiencing psychiatric emergencies include the:

- Psychiatrist, who is a licensed physician who has completed at least a 4-year specialized residency in psychiatry, after which the psychiatrist tests for board certification in psychiatry. Psychiatrists evaluate patients, prescribe medications, and conduct psychotherapy.
- Psychiatric mental health nurse practitioner (PMHNP), who is an advanced practice registered nurse, prepared at the master's or doctoral level to diagnose and treat psychiatric disorders and provide psychotherapy in most states. The PMHNP must pass a national specialized certification exam and be licensed by the state.
- Licensed clinical social worker (LCSW), who has completed a master's degree in social work and additional requirements, such as postgraduate supervision and national testing, in order to be licensed by the state. The LCSW can assess and evaluate a patient's mental health and diagnose mental conditions. The LCSW can provide psychotherapy directly with patients and their families.
- Licensed mental health counselor, who has completed at least a master's degree in professional counseling, a supervised clinical internship, and 3,000 hours of postgraduate supervised clinical practice and passed a national examination. The licensed mental health counselor can assist patients in personal and relationship issues, work stress, and other life issues.

- Psychologist, who has completed a doctorate in psychology and is licensed by the state. The psychologist can engage patients in psychotherapy, conduct psychological research, and provide psychological testing.
- Registered nurse, who may be the first to encounter a patient experiencing a psychiatric disturbance. In the emergency setting, the registered nurse is vital to accurate assessment and effective and timely intervention for the patient with a psychiatric problem.

Using the nursing process

The Joint Commission's (TJC) National Patient Safety Goal (NPSG) for hospitals, goal 15, states, "The hospital identifies safety risks inherent in its patient population" (TJC, 2019, p. 13). Included in this NPSG is identifying patients at risk for suicide. This means you will use the nursing process to screen all patients for suicide risk. The nursing process of assessment, planning, implementation, and evaluation helps the nurse to logically and critically think through essential aspects of care needed to keep the patient safe and to implement appropriate treatment. The principles of applying the nursing process remain consistent through different types of psychiatric emergencies. Remember to respect the patient's autonomy and freedom to be involved in the patient's care to the extent possible. An important goal of the treatment process is to build rapport and trust reflecting that you are there to help. Ensure adequate visual and auditory privacy during the assessment for the patient to share personal matters without embarrassment and to maintain confidentiality.

Assessment

The process of obtaining a detailed assessment begins when the patient enters the ED. Individuals who bring a patient into the emergency setting can be a vital source of information for understanding the current crisis. During the assessment, the nurse will obtain information in a structured and deliberate manner using observation, interview, and direct examination. There may be times when the patient is unable to participate in the initial interview.

History and physical assessment

As the nurse, you will collect key patient information prior to performing an objective hands-on assessment. Areas for assessment as well as key nursing questions are included in the *Patient history guide*.

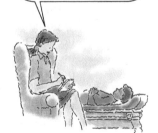

Building trust with patients is important in ensuring patient safety.

Patient history guide

Area for assessment	Key nursing questions
Primary concern	• What are the symptoms and focus of the concern from the patient's perspective?
History of presenting illness	• When did the onset of symptoms begin? • What events or situations had led up to the concerns of today?
Immediate safety concerns	• Does the patient have easy or immediate access to an item that could be used to harm self or others (e.g., drugs, medication, firearms, knives)? • Is the patient at risk for elopement, aggressive behavior, or suicide?
Previous psychiatric or mental health history	• Has the patient received previous ED, inpatient, and/or outpatient treatment for psychiatric care? • Is the patient under the care of a psychiatric health care professional for mediation treatment and/or psychotherapy?
Medical/surgical history	• What medical and/or surgical history does the patient have? • What comorbid conditions may be present? (For example, weight gain, metabolic syndrome, hyperglycemia, hyperlipidemia, and diabetes are common when taken with second-generation antipsychotics; other conditions such as headaches and back pain are common comorbid conditions seen in patients with mental health disorders.)
Social history, including use of substances	• What is the patient's living situation? • What is the patient's occupation? • What is the patient's educational background? • Who does the patient consider to be a support system? • Does the patient perceive interpersonal relationships to be fulfilling or difficult? • Has the patient experienced physical, emotional, or sexual abuse at any time? • Does the patient use alcohol, opiates, cocaine, amphetamines, hallucinogens, prescription and over-the-counter drugs, or tobacco? (Include type, frequency, amount, and any history of withdrawal.)
Family history	• Is there a family history of mental illness and/or suicide?
Medication allergies	• What allergies to medications does the patient have?
Medications taken	• What current medications does the patient take? (Include type, dose, and frequency.) • What former psychiatric medications has the patient taken? (Include response to these drugs.) • What vitamin, mineral, and/or herbal supplements does the patient take? (Include type, amount, and frequency.)
Review of systems for psychiatric disorders	• Does the patient currently have, or has the patient experienced in the past: a. anxiety symptoms b. depressive symptoms c. eating disorders d. mania e. obsessive-compulsive behaviors f. panic g. posttraumatic stress symptoms h. psychotic symptoms i. trauma/abuse?

After performing the patient history assessment, a mental status examination will be conducted. Characteristics of the mental status examination along with nursing areas of assessment can be found in the *Mental status examination*.

Mental status examination

Characteristic	Areas for the nurse to assess	
Appearance	Objectively assess the patient for: • dress (appropriate seasonally and to the occasion) • eye contact or lack thereof	• facial expressions made • grooming and hygiene • posture.
Attitude	Is the patient: • attentive • cooperative • defensive • evasive • friendly	• hostile • indifferent • ingratiating • seductive?
Behavior and activity	Does the patient display: • agitation • combativeness • coordination • gait appropriateness or difficulty • gesturing	• grimaces • restlessness • unusual movements or psychomotor activity?
Speech	Evaluate the patient's speech by: • rate • tone	• type (halting, pressured, spontaneous, talkative, tangential [off topic]) • volume.
Affect	Are the patient's facial expressions: • appropriate • blunted (displays little emotion) • constricted (mildly restricted) • depressed • flat (displays no emotion)	• labile (excessive displays of emotion or expresses emotions inappropriate to the context of the situation) • tearful?
Mood	Determine whether the patient's mood is: • ambivalent (seemingly doesn't care) • anxious • depressed • dysthymic (somewhat depressed) • elevated	• euphoric • euthymic (a normal, peaceful state) • grandiose (excessive elated) • grief stricken • irritable.

Mental status examination *(continued)*

Characteristic	Areas for the nurse to assess	
Thought processes	Can the patient think with: • abstractness • concreteness • goal directedness • logic • organization?	Does the patient exhibit: • blocking (avoidance) • disorganized thinking • flight of ideas (moving from one topic to another, without context) • paranoia • rumination (fixation) • tangential thinking (wanders off topic)?
Thought content	Does the patient exhibit: • compulsions • delusions • obsessions?	• phobias • poverty of thought (very brief or unelaborated answers)
Perceptions	Does the patient experience or exhibit signs of experiencing: • auditory or visual hallucinations • depersonalization (the feeling of being removed from one's body)? • distortions	
Threat of harm to self or others	Does the patient exhibit signs of being: • homicidal • suicidal • violent? If yes, does the patient have a plan, intent, and/or means to carry out homicide, suicide, and/or violence?	
Orientation	Is the patient oriented to: • person • place • time?	
Memory and cognition	Does the patient exhibit the ability to: • concentrate and maintain attention • recall recent and remote memories?	
Insight/judgment	Is the patient's current ability to demonstrate insight/judgment: • adequate • fair • poor?	

Common problems for patients with psychiatric concerns

Self-care problems
- Hygiene
- Personal grooming

Physiologic problems
- Confusion
- Fatigue
- Insomnia
- Ineffective sleep schedule
- Memory alterations
- Nightmares
- Nutritional deficit

Safety problems
- Self-mutilation
- Suicidal ideation
- Violence
- Wandering

Behavior problems
- Aggression
- Escalating behavior

- Lack of impulse control
- Nonadherence to treatment
- Violence

Relational problems
- Altered relational interaction
- Ineffective communication
- Loneliness
- Role conflict

Emotional problems
- Anxiety
- Decisional difficulty
- Denial
- Fear
- Grieving
- Hopelessness
- Impaired self-esteem
- Rape or trauma
- Spiritual conflict
- Stress

Planning

Based on the findings of the assessment, the nurse will create an individualized plan of care for the patient. This requires the nurse to consider the patient's psychological and physiologic needs and set realistic patient goals. The plan must remain flexible to changes in the patient's condition. While planning for the patient's care, think about how to effectively address common problems experienced by patients with psychiatric needs. (See *Common problems for patients with psychiatric concerns.*)

Implementation

Specific interventions for psychiatric emergencies will address existing and potential patient problems. While each patient is unique, there are some interventions that are common to all psychiatric emergencies.

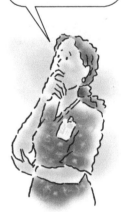

The plan of care will be modified as the patient's condition changes.

Common nursing interventions

- Provide a safe, protective, and calming environment.

  If the patient is threatening harm, has attempted suicide, or demonstrated risk of suicide, it is important to readily identify objects that could be used for self-harm within the room. Clear the room of all sharp objects as well as medical supplies. Remove items from the room that contain cords. Although it is important to respect the patient, it may not be possible to provide total privacy in order to keep the patient safe. Dim the lights and try to decrease ambient noise and adjust the room to a comfortable temperature. Decreasing environmental stimuli can be helpful in the provision of rest.

  Offer self, staying with the patient, when possible. Avoid judgment in the provision of care and listen to the patient. Patients experiencing a psychiatric emergency are often very fearful of judgment as well as fearful of the potential diagnosis. Empathize with and be open with the patient and the patient's family.
- Demonstrate therapeutic nursing care.
- Involve the family in discussions about dealing with patient's behaviors.
- Educate patient about purpose of medication, at the level appropriate to patient's condition.
- Administer medications as prescribed, and monitor for therapeutic effect and adverse side effects.
- Reinforce the need for medication adherence on discharge.
- Engage in timely documentation when possible because circumstances can change quickly. When documenting, stick to objective facts and the patient's words whenever possible to assist in describing behavior.

Evaluation

Ongoing evaluation of the patient's responses to intervention helps demonstrate progress toward patient goals.

Common disorders

Psychiatric disorders commonly encountered in the ED include acute psychosis; violent, disruptive, aggressive, or excited behaviors; suicidal ideation or attempt; acute anxiety and panic; delirium and dementia; intoxication stupor; situations of abuse; and iatrogenic emergencies.

Acute psychosis

Psychosis represents a cluster of symptoms that reflect a severe mental illness. Patients may exhibit psychosis from an acute onset of a new psychiatric disorder, or it may be a relapse of a preexisting chronic psychiatric disorder. During a psychotic episode, an individual's capacity to meet the demands of everyday life is severely impaired and the ability to distinguish reality is affected. Psychosis can occur with brain injuries or diseases (tumors, dementias, neurologic diseases, stroke), schizophrenia and schizoaffective disorder, bipolar disorders, and severe cases of depression, including postpartum depression. Alcohol, illicit drugs, stimulants, steroids, and prescription drugs can also cause substance-induced psychosis. (See *Psychosis is different from delirium*.)

Signs and symptoms of acute psychosis

- Hallucinations—sensory experiences of seeing (visual), hearing (auditory), smelling (olfactory), tasting (gustatory), or feeling (tactile) things that are not real. Most common are auditory hallucinations that convey a hurtful or negative message.
- Delusions—fixed, false beliefs of reasoning and thought, despite evidence to the contrary. Such beliefs may be delusions of grandeur (believing one has a special power) or paranoia (suspiciousness of persons or organizations plotting to cause harm to the individual).
- Mania—a heightened and abnormal state of arousal where a person exhibits hyperactivity, pressured speech, grandiose thoughts, euphoria or irritability, and insomnia
- Catatonia—mute, in a catatonic stupor, unresponsive to external stimuli
- Disorganized thinking—racing thoughts, jumbled speech, inability to form coherent thoughts, flight of ideas (leap from one topic to another), clang association (verbal linking of words with similar sounds)
- Personality changes—becoming socially withdrawn, little display of emotions, avoiding eye contact, loss of interest, lack of spontaneity, distressed, agitated without cause
- Behavior changes—irritability, difficulty engaging in social interactions and conforming to social norms, difficulty performing activities of daily living, may forget to care for personal hygiene

Nursing interventions for patients with psychotic behavior

In addition to the nursing interventions discussed earlier in this chapter for all patients experiencing any psychiatric disorder, the following

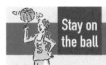

Stay on the ball

Psychosis is different from delirium

Delirium develops over a short period of time, usually hours to days. It causes a disturbance in the level of awareness and consciousness. The causative factor is physiologic in nature. For example, a high fever can cause delirium, which is reversible when the fever is treated.

De-escalation strategies

• Respect personal space by maintaining at least two arm's length distance from the patient.
• Do not be provocative or challenge the patient. Use open body language and a calm demeanor. Maintain a calm but assured tone. Answer the patient honestly.
• Establish verbal contact by introducing yourself and your role. Call the patient by name.
• Communicate concisely by using simple vocabulary with short sentences. Use repetition because the patient may not be able to process information quickly.
• Listen closely to what the patient is saying. Help the patient to identify, reflect, and clarify wants and feelings. Redirect the patient when the conversation is unhelpful.
• Find a way to agree with the patient, or agree to disagree. It can be helpful to find something about patient's situation that you can agree with. For example, if the patient is experiencing a delusion you may say, "I have never experienced that but I believe that you are."
• Set limits with the patient in a respectful manner. Clearly define expected behavior and the need to remain in control.
• Debrief with the patient and staff; offer opportunity to teach the patient alternative ways of expressing intense feelings
• If there is imminent violence:
  – Firmly tell the patient that violence is not acceptable. Try to engage the patient in a dialogue and suggest potential resolutions.
  – Offer pharmacologic treatment to help calm the patient.
  – Firmly explain that physical restraint will be used if necessary to maintain safety of the patient and the staff (Richmond et al., 2012; Vieta et al., 2017).

interventions can also be used when caring for a patient with psychotic behaviors:

• Address the patient by name to facilitate patient orientation to reality.
• Use a larger room, if possible, to prevent feelings of being trapped.
• Use techniques to de-escalate patient, if necessary. (See *De-escalation strategies.*)
• Orient patient to the ED and the staff providing care. Provide consistent caregivers whenever possible.
• Use simple, direct statements when providing directions and explanations.
• Monitor for triggers that escalate patient symptoms.
• Provide adequate personal space between you and patient.
• Explain actions in advance, especially if you need to touch the patient.
• Provide information to help the patient understand the diagnosis and treatment plan.
• Encourage the patient to express feelings and concerns.

Medication management in psychosis

Medications can be used to manage psychotic episodes. When medications are used, consideration is given to previous medications that the patient has tried successfully and unsuccessfully, allergies, current medications, comorbidities, renal and hepatic function, and potential medication interactions that may decrease or increase drug levels. Medication dosages should begin low and slowly increase to decrease the potential for adverse effects. The goal is to calm the patient and reduce symptoms, not to completely sedate the patient. If the patient is cooperative, giving oral medications is preferred over intramuscular (IM) or intravenous (IV) routes. (See *Drugs used to treat or manage psychosis*.)

Violent, disruptive, aggressive, or excited behaviors

Patients exhibiting disruptive, agitated, and violent behaviors are not new to the emergency setting. Previous approaches, such as restraints and chemical sedation, for addressing these behaviors have given way to education of the emergency team members in verbal de-escalation of the agitated or combative patient (Gottlieb et al., 2018). The goal is to help the patient regain control of his or her behavior while avoiding the use of restraints and coercive interventions that increase the patient's agitation. The most important thing is to maintain safety for everyone within the area, including the patient, while avoiding physical confrontation.

After establishing safety, work to triage and obtain a brief history, vital signs, oxygen levels, and blood glucose levels, if possible. Immediate evaluation by a health care provider should occur when the following symptoms are present: abnormal vital signs, slurred speech, unequal dilated pupils, seizures, lack of coordination, overt trauma, hemiparesis, extreme muscle stiffness or weakness, difficulty breathing, disorientation, or loss of memory. The purpose of the initial evaluation is to determine the most likely cause of the behavior, assess safety issues, and develop an initial treatment plan.

It may be necessary to use antipsychotic drugs or sedatives to reduce hallucinations and/or delusions for the patient experiencing agitation. Lorazepam (Ativan) is the most commonly used benzodiazepine for short-term calming and sedation for agitation.

Maintaining safety with the agitated patient

As with all patients experiencing a psychiatric disorder, modify the physical space for patient safety. Remove items from the room that could be used as weapons or for self or staff harm. It is important to know who is educated within the department to manage behavioral emergencies. Verbal de-escalation is a team effort, requiring several

Drugs used to treat or manage psychosis

Drugs	Common side effects
Antipsychotics	
First generation	Extrapyramidal symptoms (abnormal postures, muscle spasms, restlessness, parkinsonism tremors, or muscle rigidity)
Haloperidol (Haldol)	
Risperidone (Risperdal)	
Second generation	Weight gain risk for metabolic syndrome
Olanzapine (Zyprexa)	
Quetiapine (Seroquel)	
Mood stabilizers	
Carbamazepine (Tegretol)	Nausea, vomiting, dizziness, poor concentration, weight gain
Lithium (Eskalith)	
Valproic acid (Depakote)	Lithium only: increased thirst and urination
Antidepressants	
Selective serotonin reuptake inhibitors	Nausea, dry mouth, dizziness, headache, decreased libido
Citalopram (Celexa)	
Escitalopram (Lexapro)	
Fluoxetine (Prozac)	
Fluvoxamine (Luvox)	
Paroxetine (Paxil)	
Sertraline (Zoloft)	
Serotonin norepinephrine reuptake inhibitors	Nausea, dry mouth, dizziness, headache
Desvenlafaxine (Pristiq)	
Duloxetine (Cymbalta)	
Venlafaxine (Effexor)	
Other	
Bupropion (Wellbutrin)	Nausea, vomiting, headache, dry mouth, insomnia
Mirtazapine (Remeron)	Increased appetite, weight gain, dizziness, drowsiness, weakness
Trazodone (Desyrel)	Dizziness, drowsiness, bizarre dreams
Vilazodone (Viibryd)	Nausea, anxiety, irritability, headaches

Adapted from Stahl, S. (2017). *Prescriber's guide: Stahl's essential psychopharmacology* (6th ed.). Cambridge, United Kingdom: Cambridge University Press.

members of the interprofessional health care team. This may include nurses, health care providers, security, and social workers. Using de-escalation strategies can help the patient regain control of his or her own behavior as well as decrease the need for sedation or restraint (Richmond et al., 2012). Verbal de-escalation is also useful in establishing a therapeutic relationship with clear boundaries (Vieta et al., 2017). (See *De-escalation strategies*, page 461.)

Seclusion and restraint in the ED for aggressive or agitated behavior

The Centers for Medicare & Medicaid Services has stipulated that patients have a right to be free from restraint or seclusion as a coercive measure (U.S. Department of Health and Human Services, 2006). "Restraint or seclusion may only be imposed to ensure the immediate physical safety of the patient, a staff member, or others" (Office of the Federal Register National Archives and Records Administration, 2018, §482.13(e)). The hectic pace of an ED, the diminished opportunity to develop rapport over a period of time with patients, and the intensity of ED acuity at times can produce challenges in preventing or de-escalating situations when seclusion and/or restraint is used. However, having a thoughtful and procedural approach to determining how to use the least restrictive intervention can produce great benefits for patients and staff. Knox and Holloman (2012) developed an algorithm for decision making that, together with verbal de-escalation techniques and medication (where appropriate), allows patients to more quickly regain control and be a part of their care. (See *Algorithm for decision making*.) Promoting ongoing staff education on how to work with a patient who is agitated, debriefing after incidents, and continually looking for ways to prevent or de-escalate situations will help make these difficult situations as therapeutic as possible.

Suicidal ideation or attempt

The statistics for suicide in the United States are alarming and reflect overall increases of nearly 30% over the past 17 years (1999–2016) (Centers for Disease Control and Prevention [CDC], 2018b). Further concerning data reflects the following:

- Suicide is the 10th leading cause of death in the United States (CDC, 2019b).
- Suicide is the 2nd leading cause of death within ages 10 to 34 (CDC, 2017b).
- Suicide is the 4th leading cause of death in ages 35 to 54 (CDC, 2017b).
- Males with no known mental health condition are more likely to complete suicide and use a firearm (CDC, 2018b).
- The highest suicide rates for rural areas include American Indians and Alaska native non-Hispanics (CDC, 2018a).
- Lesbian, gay, bisexual, and transgender individuals are statistically more likely to attempt suicide than cisgender (straight) individuals (American Foundation for Suicide Prevention, 2017).
- The most common methods of suicide worldwide are pesticide ingestion, hanging, and the use of firearms (World Health Organization, 2014).
- Prevalence of suicidal ideation is highest among adults ages 18 to 25 (Piscopo, 2017).

Algorithm for decision making

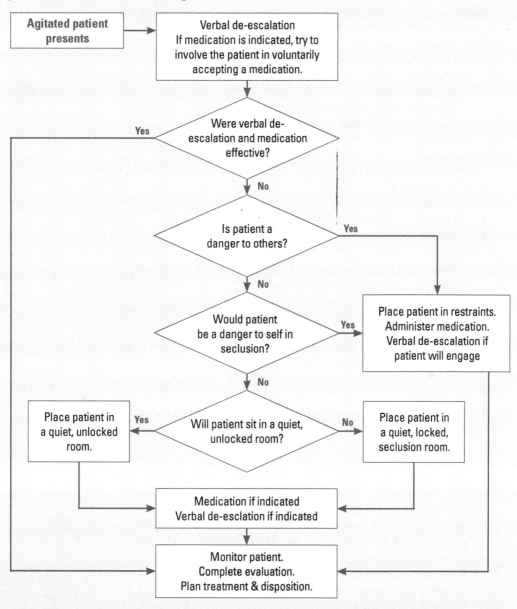

From Knox, D., & Holloman, G. H., Jr. (2012). Use and avoidance of seclusion and restraint: Consensus statement of the American Association for Emergency Psychiatry project BETA Seclusion and Restraint Workgroup. *The Western Journal of Emergency Medicine, 13*(1), 35–40. doi:10.5811/westjem.2011.9.6867; and Stowell, K. R., Florence, P., Harman, H. J., et al. (2012). Psychiatric evaluation of the agitated patient: Consensus statement of the American Association for Emergency Psychiatry project BETA Psychiatric Evaluation Workgroup. *The Western Journal of Emergency Medicine, 13*(1), 11–16. doi:10.5811/westjem.2011.9.6868

Suicide and depression

Not all people who are depressed are suicidal. However, most individuals experiencing suicidal ideation are depressed. The signs and symptoms of depression include the following:

- Thoughts
  - Perception of being a burden to family and friends
  - Pessimism
  - Rigid thinking
  - Slowed thinking; indecisiveness
  - Trouble concentrating
- Emotions
  - Anxiety
  - Excessive sadness or crying
  - Helplessness
  - Hopelessness
  - Loneliness or feelings of isolation
  - Persistent low mood
- Behaviors
  - Anhedonia (loss of interest in formerly pleasurable activities)
  - Changes in attention to appearance
  - Changes in weight or appetite
  - Decrease in sexual drive
  - Fatigue or loss of energy
  - Pulling away from friends, family, social groups
  - Sleep disturbances (too much or too little)

Warning signs of suicide

As an emergency room nurse, be aware of statements or behaviors that are considered warning signs that a patient may attempt suicide in the near future. (See *Warning signs of suicide.*) Remember, this may not be the patient who presents with suicidal ideation. In fact, 54% those who die by suicide do not have a previously diagnosed mental health condition (CDC, 2018c; Stone et al., 2018).

A patient who states he or she has made a decision to commit suicide and has voiced having a concrete plan of action is at significant risk and needs to be in a protective setting. Although all verbalizations of suicidal intent are to be taken seriously, these behaviors or statements warrant immediate attention and intervention by the nurse to protect the patient's safety.

Circumstances that place the patient at even higher risk for a suicide attempt in the presence of these behaviors and statements include:

- the absence of strong support system
- the absence of stable living conditions
- the presence of psychosis or a major psychiatric disorder
- the presence of serious medical condition.

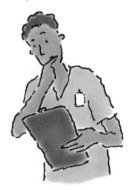

Be aware! According to CDC, 54% of people who die by suicide do not have a previously diagnosed mental health condition!

Warning signs of suicide

Behaviors	Statements
Starting or increasing use of alcohol or drugs	Talking about death and dying, expressing a strong wish to die or "wanting the pain to end"
Engaging in aggressive, impulsive, reckless, or disruptive behavior	Saying goodbye to family and friends
Purchasing a firearm or other means of killing oneself or having easy access to a mode of self-harm	Stating regret for surviving an active suicide attempt
Giving away personal belongings	Admits to visualizing suicide or rehearsing the plan
Putting personal affairs in order	Voices details about a specific plan for suicide with high lethality
Carrying out a serious, near-lethal, or premeditated attempt to self-harm (presently or in the past)	

Caring for patients with suicide risk

Although the ED environment is often fast paced, this does not mean that you cannot establish a therapeutic relationship. It is important to create a calm, empathic, and nonjudgmental environment. Sit down, even if for a short time, make eye contact, and listen to the patient. The Suicide Prevention Resource Center (2015) recommends conducting a brief universal screening of all patients for suicide risk and a more comprehensive assessment of individuals to confirm suspected suicide risk. When conducting the inquiry about suicidal ideation, the Suicide Prevention Resource Center offers a decision support tool to help confirm the risk of suicide and how to rate the responses. (See *Decision support tool*, pages 468 and 469.)

Suicide Assessment Five-Step Evaluation and Triage

The Suicide Assessment Five-Step Evaluation and Triage (SAFE-T) protocol was designed to help identify suicide risk. This protocol supports TJC's NPSGs specific to suicide and is supported by the American Psychiatric Association (Jacobs, 2007). (See *Suicide Assessment Five-Step Evaluation and Triage protocol (SAFE-T)*, page 470.)

Keeping the patient safe

When a patient is identified as a risk for suicide, it is important to take additional steps in the ED to keep the patient safe. Most EDs will have a specific area that is designated for patients at high risk of suicide. The rooms have modifications eliminating materials that could be of harm. If this type of room is not available, staff will need to evaluate the room for means of injury. (See *Common sources of injury*, page 471.)

Decision support tool

Transition question: confirm suicidal ideation Have you had recent thoughts of killing yourself? Is there other evidence of suicidal thoughts, such as reports from family or friends? ***Not part of scoring.***	**Y**	
1. Thoughts of carrying out a plan Recently, have you been thinking about how you might kill yourself? ***If yes, consider the immediate safety needs of the patient.***	**Y**	**N**
2. Suicide intent Do you have any intention of killing yourself?	**Y**	**N**
3. Past suicide attempt Have you ever tried to kill yourself?	**Y**	**N**
4. Significant mental health condition Have you had treatment for mental health problems? Do you have a mental health issue that affects your ability to do things in life?	**Y**	**N**
5. Substance use disorder Have you had four or more (female) or five or more (male) drinks on one occassion in the past month or have you used drugs or medication for non-medical reasons in the past month? Has drinking or drug use been a problem for you?	**Y**	**N**
6. Irritability/agitation/aggression Recently, have you been feeling very anxious or agitated? Have you been having conflicts or getting into fights? Is there direct evidence of irritability, aggitation, or aggression?	**Y**	**N**

Step 1: Inform the patient

Tell your patient that you will be asking a few questions to help you consider next steps.

Step 2: Review the patient's suicidal ideation

If this is your first interaction with the patient, begin by confirming that he or she has suicidal ideation. Ask the patient directly or state your understanding of the nature of his or her suicide risk. This will facilitate a smooth transition to item number 1 (plan).

Step 3: Ask questions for items 1 through 6

The tool includes example questions to ask. Use open, nonjudgmental style to overcome social response bias and encourage honest answers.

Step 4: Review other available information

Use available data (e.g., patient observation, medical records) and consult with available collaterals (e.g., friends, family members, and outpatient providers) to corroborate the patient's report. Let the patient know you would like

to contact his or her collaterals, and that the visit may be delayed while you are awaiting corroborating information.

Can ED providers share patient health information with others?

Yes. For patients with concerning risk factors who minimize or deny suicide risk, it may be life-saving to contact collaterals for corroborating information. First request the patient's permission to contact friends, family, or outpatient treatment providers. If the patient declines to consent after reasonable attempts have been made to obtain permission, there are circumstances in which collaterals may be contacted without the patient's permission. HIPAA permits such contacts when the clinician, in good faith, believes that the patient may be a danger to self or others.

Step 5: Check the score

A "yes" response is equal to 1. Total the number of "yes" responses on items 1 to 6.

Decision support tool *(continued)*

Score 0. If the response to every item (1–6) is "no," discharge may be appropriate following the provision of one or more ED-based brief suicide prevention interventions.
Score ≥1. If the responses to the transition question (i.e., suicidal ideation) *and* any item 1 to 6 are "yes," consider consulting a mental health specialist during the ED visit for further evaluation, including a comprehensive suicide risk assessment. Consider the immediate safety needs of the patient as you determine next steps.

Step 6: Tell the patient what happens next
Explain next steps. For example:
Score 0. Say that you are considering discharging him or her to an outpatient care setting and would first like to provide a brief intervention. Describe the intervention you

plan to use. Ask for the patient's feedback on this plan and discuss any reservations he or she may have about it.
Score ≥1. Say that you would like him or her to see a specialist for further evaluation as part of the ED visit. Explain that the specialist may repeat some of the questions that you've already aksed. Be familiar with the type of suicide risk assessment used in the mental health specialist's evaluation.

Involve the patient in the decision-making process. Research suggests that shared decision making lowers patient stress, gives patients a sense of control, and leads to better outcomes. Patients with suicide risk report higher satisfaction when they are involved in decisions about their care.

Provide a wait time estimate. If wait times are significant, ask what will increase the patient's comfort.

Source: Suicide Prevention Resource Center. (2015). *Caring for adult patients with suicide risk: A consensus guide for emergency departments*. Waltham, MA: Education Development Center. Retrieved from http://www.sprc.org/sites/default/files/EDGuide_full.pdf

Depending on the degree of risk, it may not be possible to leave the patient unsupervised. Safety observations and checks may be implemented every 15 minutes or every 30 minutes according to agency policy. Patients may need to be supervised at all times, even when using the bathroom. Be careful of items that visitors may bring in, such as earbuds or a sweatshirt with a string tie, because these items could be a source of injury.

Acute anxiety states and panic

Patients commonly seek treatment in the ED for acute anxiety attacks. In some cases, acute anxiety and panic bring patients to the ED due to fears of experiencing a potentially life-threatening event. Anxiety attacks can feel very scary and illicit physiologic symptoms. Obtaining a thorough history and conducting a focused physical assessment including vital signs will help to rule out acute medical conditions (i.e., cardiac arrhythmias, endocrine problems).

Suicide Assessment Five-Step Evaluation and Triage protocol (SAFE-T)

The five steps of the protocol (Substance Abuse and Mental Health Services Administration, 2009) include the following:

Step 1: Identify risk factors.	• Demographics • Suicidal thinking and behavior • Previous self-harming behaviors • Psychiatric disorders and comorbidity, especially mood disorders, psychotic disorders, posttraumatic stress disorder, cluster B personality disorders (antisocial, borderline, histrionic, narcissistic) • Family history • Personality disorder/traits	• Substance use/abuse • Life stressors, especially loss of significant other • Suicidal behavior • Recent discharge from inpatient psychiatric facility • History of or exposure to trauma, military, combat, or traumatic emergencies • Access to weapons
Step 2: Identify protective factors.	• Sense of responsibility to family • Pregnancy • Strong ethnic or cultural ties • Religious beliefs that discourage suicide	• Adaptive coping skills • Positive support system • Positive therapeutic relationship • Resiliency and optimism
Step 3: Conduct suicide inquiry.	• Thoughts • Intent • Behavior	• Plans • Frequency and intensity of suicidal thinking within past 48 hours
Step 4: Determine risk level/interventions to reduce risk.	• Acute and chronic stressors • Triggering events • Beliefs about death and suicide	• Quality of relationships • Potentially lethal attempt or intent
Step 5: Document the ED visit.	• How the patient arrived • Specific reason for visit (include patient quotes) • Communication attempts with family • Risk level, as determined by health care provider • Rationale for risk level • Plan for reducing risk • Protective factors • Communication with interprofessional health care team • Interventions provided	• Challenges arising during the ED visit • Patient's preferences regarding treatment • Assessment of patient's access to firearms or other lethal means • Patient safety plan—developed in collaboration with the patient and is based on strengths and supports available to the patient • Educational and crisis center resources provided to patient • Referrals provided, including provider contact information

Common sources of injury

Things ingestible
- Hand foam or soap
- Liquids in room

Things used as ligatures
- Bags or purses with straps
- Belts
- Blinds
- Clothing with strings
- Curtains
- Earbuds with cords
- Linens

Things used as weapons
- Curtain rods
- Sharps containers

Things used for cutting
- Eating utensils
- Razors
- Sharps
- Windows (glass)

Things used to suffocate
- Trash can liners

Symptoms of acute anxiety and panic disorder

Patients with acute anxiety and panic disorder may exhibit symptoms such as:

- chest pain, racing heart, or palpitations
- chills or hot flashes
- dizziness, light-headedness, feeling faint
- numbness or tingling sensations
- profuse sweating
- shortness of breath
- sudden onset of intense anxiety or fear
- trembling or shaking.

Treatment approaches and nursing interventions

Patients experiencing anxiety or panic need reassurance that health care professionals are present and attentive to their needs. Having a calming environment and involving the patient in the unfolding plan of care can help decrease symptoms.

For extreme anxiety, use of fast-acting benzodiazepines as prescribed can be helpful in reducing symptoms.

A panic attack generally lasts 10 to 15 minutes. The patient often feels better within an hour but afterward may feel exhausted. Reassure the patient that this is a normal response. If panic becomes chronic, a patient may have "anxiety about anxiety" or anticipatory panic (Musey et al., 2018). Breaking the cycle of panic is important to restore the patient's sense of well-being. Facilitating long-term treatment with outpatient resources, with referral to the patient's primary care provider or a mental health provider, is appropriate.

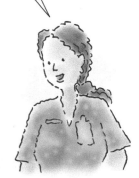

Pounding heart, light-headedness, sweating, and fear of dying are just four symptoms that patients with acute anxiety and panic disorder can experience.

Delirium and dementia

Delirium

Delirium is an acute change in cognition (American Psychiatric Association, 2013). It occurs over hours or days and is reversible. Recognizing delirium in the older adult can be a challenge within the ED setting. Delirium can lead to functional decline, a loss of independent living, emotional stress, and increased mortality. Factors precipitating delirium include:

- comorbidities, such as dementia, chronic kidney disease, liver failure, head trauma, infection, terminal illness, depression
- alcohol or other substance use
- immobility
- sensory impairment
- dehydration
- pain
- urine retention
- constipation
- polypharmacy
- medications with anticholinergic properties, benzodiazepines, and narcotics.
  - ○ Anticholinergics
    - – Antihistamines
    - – Antispasmodics
    - – Antiemetics
    - – Antiparkinsonian drugs
    - – Antipsychotics
  - ○ Psychoactive medications
    - – Benzodiazepines
    - – Anticonvulsants
    - – Narcotic pain medications, especially meperidine
  - ○ Other medications
    - – Digoxin
    - – Beta blockers
    - – Corticosteroids
    - – Nonsteroidal anti-inflammatory drugs
    - – Antibiotics

Screening for delirium

One of the most widely used screening assessment tools for delirium is the Confusion Assessment Method (CAM) (Inouye et al., 1990). This tool is validated for use in the ED. However, it takes 10 minutes to administer. The 3D-CAM is a 3-minute delirium assessment based on CAM that is practical for use in the emergency setting (Marcantonio et al., 2014).

The four elements evaluated in the 3D-CAM screening tool are:
1. altered mental status/fluctuating course
2. inattention
3. altered level of consciousness
4. disorganized thinking.

3D-CAM has been shown to have high sensitivity and specificity relative to a reference standard and to be a key tool for delirium recognition (Marcantonio et al., 2014).

Nursing interventions

While the health care provider is seeking the root cause of delirium, nursing interventions center around keeping the patient safe and treating the root cause of the delirium once diagnosed. In addition to the nursing interventions discussed earlier in the chapter for all patients experiencing any psychiatric disorder, the following interventions can also be used when caring for a patient with delirium:

- Keep consistent personnel, when possible.
- Orient and reorient patient to day, time, and location.
- Describe procedures and interventions that are implemented.
- Keep instructions short and simple; repeat as needed.
- Enlist family/friends to help calm and support patient.
- Use nightlights to help decrease visual disturbances.
- Minimize disruptions in sleep/wake cycles.
- Avoid restraints, which is associated with increased delirium.
- Use intermittent straight catheterization (vs. indwelling catheter, if possible) due to less infection risk.
- Use Beers criteria to avoid medications inappropriate for administering to older adults (especially anticholinergics).
- Administer medications as prescribed, which may include:
  - benzodiazepines (only if delirium is due to alcohol withdrawal)
  - quetiapine (used for sedation)
  - risperidone (can cause prolonged QT interval)
  - haloperidol (used for sedation; increases risk for extrapyramidal symptoms and prolonged QT interval).

Dementia

According to the CDC (2018c), dementia affects 5 million Americans. The fast-paced nature of the ED creates challenges in managing the care of individuals that struggle on a daily basis to understand their environment. Patients may come to the ED for a trauma-associated injury, an acute illness, pain, or complications associated with dementia.

Dementia differs from delirium in that it is a slow progression of cognitive decline caused by a chronic brain disorder that is permanent. Types of dementia include Alzheimer disease, Lewy body

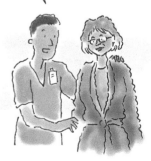

Dementia rarely occurs among persons younger than 50 years, and the incidence increases with age.

dementia, vascular dementia, frontotemporal dementia, mixed dementia, and Creutzfeldt-Jakob disease.

Parkinson disease, Huntington disease, Wernicke-Korsakoff syndrome, and normal pressure hydrocephalus are conditions in which patients often develop dementia.

Dementia is a syndrome—a group of symptoms—that affects attention, orientation, judgment, abstract thinking, and personality. It occurs rarely among persons younger than 50, and the incidence increases with age. Diagnosis is made by symptoms of memory loss (especially for recent events) plus one or more of the following: language problems (aphasia), organizational problems (apraxia), inability to recognize or tell the purpose of objects, and disturbances in executive function.

Nursing interventions

In addition to the nursing interventions discussed earlier in the chapter for all patients experiencing any psychiatric disorder, interventions for a patient with dementia are similar to those for patients with delirium. Patients with dementia may also need assistance with everyday activities depending on their level of impairment. Assess patients individually to determine what level of intervention is needed to accomplish activities of daily living.

Intoxication and overdose of alcohol

Substance use is an increasing public health concern. Patients who use substances often present to the ED due to intoxication, which can be a potentially life-threatening event.

Alcohol

Alcohol intoxication is a clinically harmful condition resulting from an excessive amount of alcohol (or products containing alcohol) consumed over a short period of time. Drinking to excess is called *alcohol overdose*, sometimes known as *alcohol poisoning*. The focus of care is on stabilizing the patient and directing the patient to personalized treatment.

- Men are more likely than women to drink excessively and experience more alcohol-related deaths and hospitalizations (CDC, 2016a).
- Women have a more rapid increase in blood alcohol levels than men and can experience toxic effects of alcohol with less consumption (CDC, 2016b).

Individuals with patterns of ED encounters for alcohol intoxication have higher rates of medical comorbidities including liver disease, chronic kidney disease, ischemic vascular disease, dementia, chronic obstructive pulmonary disease, and history of traumatic brain injury. Alcohol intoxication may be a symptom of other underlying disorders. It is important to conduct a thorough assessment to be able to consider appropriate immediate and follow-up care.

Legal limits

In the United States, the national legal limit for blood alcohol concentration level is 0.08 or above, or 80 mg/dL. It is difficult to give *precise* information about how much alcohol it takes to become acutely intoxicated due to many contributing factors. These factors include alcohol tolerance, age, gender, metabolism, fat/muscle content, hydration, presence or absence of food in the stomach, the strength of alcohol, and time over which the alcohol is consumed. As the individual's blood alcohol level increases, the degree of impairment also increases.

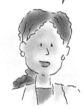

As the blood alcohol level increases, impairment also increases.

- A standard drink is equal to 0.6 oz of pure alcohol. This amount of pure alcohol is found in a 12-oz beer containing 5% alcohol, 5 oz of wine with 12% alcohol, or 1.5 oz (shot) of 80 proof distilled spirits or liquor. The *Blood alcohol concentration* correlates the blood alcohol content with generalizations in effect. Remember, there are many factors that affect the way an individual metabolizes and responds to alcohol.

The intoxicating effects of alcohol

Alcohol consumption affects the entire brain. Effects of intoxication range from slightly impaired judgment, thinking, and decision making to inhibition of behaviors, poor impulse control, and lack of coordination.

Alcohol overdose is a life-threatening condition. This occurs when there is so much alcohol in the bloodstream that the brain cannot control life-support functions such as breathing, heart rate, and temperature (National Institute on Alcohol Abuse and Alcoholism, 2018). Individuals who take opioids, sedative-hypnotic, anxiolytic, and/or antihistamine medications are at particularly high risk for alcohol overdose. (See *Physical signs and symptoms of alcohol intoxication and alcohol overdose*, page 477.)

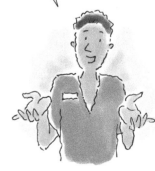

SBIRT stands for screening, brief intervention, and referral to treatment.

Nursing care of the patient with alcohol intoxication or alcohol overdose

Alcohol is metabolized quickly, yet effects can take days to resolve. During this time, care is symptomatic and supportive in the case of the patient with alcohol intoxication. While in the ED:
- Ensure the patient has a patent airway.
- Take measure to prevent aspiration.
- Check vital signs often per orders or agency policy.
- Assess oxygen saturation frequently.

Blood alcohol concentration

As blood alcohol concentration (BAC) increases, so does impairment.

	BAC Level
Life threatening • Loss of consciousness • Danger of life-threatening alcohol overdose • Significant risk of death in most drinkers due to suppression of vital life functions	0.31% to 0.45%
Severe impairment • Speech, memory, coordination, attention, reaction time, balance significantly impaired • All driving-related skills dangerously impaired • Judgment and decision-making dangerously impaired • Blackouts (amnesia) • Vomiting and other signs of alcohol overdose common • Loss of consciouness	0.16% to 0.30%
Increased impairment • Perceived benefical effects of alcohol, such as relaxation, give way to increasing intoxication • Increased risk of aggression in some people • Speech, memory, attention, coordination, balance further impaired • Significant impairments in all driving skills • Increased risk of injury to self and others • Moderate memory impairments	0.06% to 0.15%
Mild impairment • Mild speech, memory, attention, coordination, balance impairments • Perceived beneficial effects, such as relaxation • Sleepiness can begin	0% to 0.05%

Source: National Institute on Alcohol Abuse and Alcoholism. (2018). *Understanding the dangers of alcohol overdose*. Retrieved from https://www.niaaa.nih.gov/publications/brochures-and-fact-sheets/understanding-dangers-of-alcohol-overdose

Physical signs and symptoms of alcohol intoxication and alcohol overdose

It is important to differentiate between signs and symptoms associated with alcohol intoxication versus alcohol overdose. In coordination with early involvement by the health care provider, you could save a life!

Body system	Alcohol intoxication	Alcohol overdose
Neurologic	• Blackouts or seizures • Slurred speech • Loss of balance • Inability to walk straight or stand still	• Seizures • Mental confusion • Difficulty remaining conscious • Depressed or absent gag reflex
Sensory	• Enlarged pupils • Rapid eye movements • Breath that smells of alcohol	• Difficulty opening eyes
Cardiac	• Tachycardia • Cardiac arrhythmias	• Bradycardia
Respiratory	• Decreased respirations	• Difficulty breathing
Gastrointestinal	• Nausea and vomiting	• Vomiting
Integumentary	• Flushed skin	• Clammy skin
Vital signs	• Slightly increased temperature	• Extremely low body temperature

- Monitor laboratory and diagnostic data.
- Administer medications and IV fluids as prescribed.
- Ensure patient safety and comfort. Physical restraints should be considered only in extreme situations and after all other methods of diversion are exhausted.

Prime opportunities exist within the ED setting to provide screening, brief intervention, and referral to treatment (SBIRT) to patients with alcohol intoxication after they have recovered. SBIRT is a clinical model that screens for abuse, uses motivational interviewing skills to help assess willingness for change, focuses on risk reduction and consequences of use, and provides patients with information about referral for treatment.

The patient with alcohol overdose may need intensive care following care provided in the ED. Indications for intensive care unit (ICU) care include vital signs abnormalities, hypoxia, hypoglycemia, and the need for parenteral sedation (Cowan & Su, 2018). ED care focuses on stabilization until transport for admission into the ICU. The priority of care is maintaining the patient's airway. Breathing support may be required, with administration of oxygen or an endotracheal tube and ventilation.

Intoxication and overdose of stimulants or opioids

The number of patients brought to the ED due to intoxication of substance continues to increase. Intoxication can be a potentially life-threatening event. In this section, most frequent intoxicants and nursing roles and interventions are covered.

Stimulants

Stimulants are drugs that stimulate the central nervous system that can produce euphoria and hallucination. Although useful clinically to treat attention deficit hyperactivity disorder and short-term treatment of obesity, recreational use of stimulants is a public health crisis.

Stimulants can be made by combining chemicals with over-the-counter cold medicines containing ephedrine and pseudoephedrine. They can be orally ingested, injected intravenously, or inhaled. The most commonly abused stimulants include cocaine and amphetamines.

- Cocaine comes from the leaves of the coca plant cultivated in South America. Cocaine is highly addictive. Cocaine is street available as:
  o a hydrochloride salt in the form of a water-soluble white crystalline powder. When dissolved, it is either inhaled through the nose or injected into the veins.
  o a freebase cocaine that is smoked, resulting in a quick high felt within seconds of inhaling. "Crack" cocaine is a type of freebase cocaine that is in the form of small crystals. When it is smoked, it makes a distinctive crackling noise.
- Amphetamines are central nervous system stimulants used to treat select medical conditions. Amphetamines increase the activity of neurotransmitters in the brain, particularly norepinephrine and dopamine. These drugs can be prescribed to treat attention deficit hyperactivity disorder and narcolepsy and as a weight loss aid. Examples of common amphetamines include dextroamphetamine/amphetamine combination (Adderall), methylphenidate (Ritalin), and dextroamphetamine (Dexedrine). As a recreational drug, stimulant use increases wakefulness, reduces fatigue, and induces euphoria. When used at higher doses and in routes not prescribed, overuse and repeated abuse can result.
- Methylenedioxymethamphetamine (MDMA), known as *ecstasy* or *molly*, and bath salts are recreational "designer drugs," which can cause similar symptoms as stimulant overdose when taken in toxic amounts. These substances can be injected, snorted, or smoked and are accessible and inexpensive. A single exposure can be very serious and potentially life-threatening, depending on the nature and amount of the substance consumed.

Signs and symptoms of stimulant overdose

Neurologic
- Coma
- Confusion
- Hyperthermia
- Overactive reflexes
- Seizures
- Tremors
- Weakness

Sensory
- Rhinitis

Cardiac
- Blood pressure variability
- Cardiac arrhythmias
- Circulation failure
- Diaphoresis

Respiratory
- Tachypnea

Gastrointestinal
- Nausea and vomiting

Renal
- Acute renal failure

Psychiatric
- Aggression
- Anxiety
- Hallucinations
- Impulsivity
- Insomnia
- Irritability
- Panic
- Paranoia

Musculoskeletal
- Muscle pain
- Rhabdomyolysis

Patients who have chronically abused stimulants may have effects to many body systems. Visible, characteristic symptoms include persistent rhinitis, perforated nasal septum, nasal and gingival ulceration, dental decay, periodontal disease, and dry mouth (xerostomia). (See *Signs and symptoms of stimulant overdose.*)

Nursing care of the patient with stimulant overdose

The management of patients with stimulant overdose is primarily supportive and based on the presenting symptoms. In addition to the nursing interventions discussed earlier in the chapter for all patients experiencing any psychiatric disorder, interventions for a patient with stimulant overdose include:
- providing a quiet environment to avoid added stimulation
- ensuring patient is protected if aggressive, confused, or combative
- administering medications and IV fluids as prescribed
- monitoring blood glucose levels
- ensuring the patient has a patent airway (Mechanical ventilation may be required.)
- checking vital signs often per orders or agency policy
- assessing oxygen saturation frequently
- monitoring laboratory and diagnostic data
- providing external cooling if hyperthermic to prevent rhabdomyolysis and multiorgan failure.

Categories of opioids

Opioids can be divided into categories.

Opioid type	Example	Legal or illegal?	Notes
Prescription opioids	Oxycodone (OxyContin) Hydrocodone (Vicodin) Morphine (MS Contin) Methadone (Methadose)	Legally prescribed	
Fentanyl	Fentanyl (Duragesic)	Legally prescribed, often for cancer pain	50 to 100 times more potent than morphine
		Illegally manufactured	When illegally manufactured, is often mixed with heroin or cocaine
Carfentanil (Carfentanyl)	Not approved for human use	Illegal (for human use)	Has a quantitative potency approximately 10,000 times that of morphine and 100 times that of fentanyl
	Marketed by trade name Wildnil for use as a tranquilizing agent for very large animals	Illegally manufactured	Has been mixed with heroin and cocaine
Heroin		Illegal	
Kratom*	A tree that grows in areas of Southeast Asia whose leaves contain compounds that produce mind-altering effects.	Legal in some of the United States; illegal in other states	

*Although not an opioid by structure, the U.S. Food and Drug Administration (2019) considers kratom to be in the category of drugs that affect the same opioid brain receptors as morphine, which exposes users to risks of addiction, abuse, and dependence.

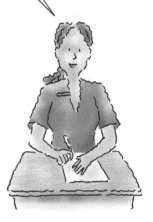

Prevention of addiction is critical. Teach your patients the risks of opioid use!

Opioids

Opioids include prescription pain relievers, heroin, and synthetic preparations such as fentanyl (CDC, 2017a). (See *Categories of opioids.*) Addiction often begins with the patient receiving and using a prescription opioid. It is estimated that between 21% and 29% of patients who are prescribed an opioid for chronic pain misuse the drug and

An extra word about fentanyl

Fentanyl can be potentially hazardous upon exposure to first responders (e.g., police, paramedics, and emergency medical technicians) and health care workers. Highly potent forms of fentanyl acquired through inhalation, mucous membrane contact, ingestion, or needle stick injury can cause the rapid onset of life-threatening respiratory depression. Inhalation is the most common form of exposure.

For personal protection and the safety of the work place, it is necessary for health care workers to recognize the signs and symptoms of secondary opioid exposure. People who have a low tolerance for opioids can have a fast and potentially life-threatening response to accidental exposure. The onset of symptoms, which mirror those associated with direct exposure, can be immediate or delayed and is affected by the strength, purity, and method of exposure.

Best practices for self-protection include not eating, drinking, or using a restroom near where fentanyl is suspected; not touching eyes, nose, or mouth if exposure is anticipated or suspected; frequently changing gloves; and washing hands with soap and water immediately following potential exposure. All personnel who may come in contact with fentanyl should be educated in the use of personal protective equipment according to agency policy.

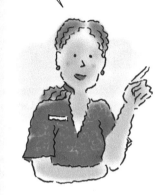

If I suspect that my patient used fentanyl, I use PPE!!

between 8% and 12% of those individuals develop an opioid use disorder (National Institute on Drug Abuse, 2019). Over time, dependence can develop. Approximately 4% to 6% of individuals who misuse opioids transition to use of heroin (National Institute on Drug Abuse, 2019).

Every day in the United States, more than 130 people die from opioid overdose (National Institute on Drug Abuse, 2019). The "opioid crisis" costs the United States $75.8 billion dollars per year to cover the burden of health care costs, lost productivity, treatment for addiction, and issues that must be resolved through the criminal justice system (National Institute on Drug Abuse, 2019). (See *An extra word about fentanyl*.)

Prevention of addiction is critical. Health care providers have been called on to closely monitor use of opioids and judiciously prescribe them only as needed in the lowest dose possible, for the least amount of time possible. Electronic prescription monitoring systems have made it easier to identify patients at high risk for opioid misuse and/or overdose.

Nurses teach patients the risks of opioid use and can engage patients through use of motivational interviewing to explore motivations for change, how to prepare to change, and how to access to follow up resources.

Signs and symptoms of opioid overdose

Common symptoms of opioid overdose result from suppressed respiratory function and breathing because opioids affect the part of the brain that regulates breathing. Even when taken at prescribed doses, opioids can cause respiratory depression when mixed with other substances such as alcohol.

Body system	Symptom of opioid overdose
Neurologic	Confusion Difficulty in awakening or arousing (even with loud stimulus or vigorous sternal rub) Limpness
Sensory	Blue lips Pinpoint pupils
Cardiac	Hypotension Slowed (or stopped) heart rate
Respiratory	Slowed breathing
Gastrointestinal	Vomiting
Integumentary	Blue nail beds Clammy Pale

Nursing care of the patient with opioid overdose

Aggressive airway control is the priority of care when caring for a patient with opioid overdose. (See *Signs and symptoms of opioid overdose.*) While in the ED, you will:

- ensure the patient has a patent airway
- provide supplemental oxygen as prescribed
- perform rescue breathing if indicated
- prepare for potential endotracheal intubation.

Reversing the effects of the opioids can be facilitated by administration of a short-acting opioid antagonist such as naloxone (Narcan). Naloxone is administered nasally, subcutaneously, intramuscularly, or intravenously. In the ED setting, IV administration of naloxone provides the most rapid onset, efficacious, and predictable dosing, but immediate administration of IM naloxone is sometimes essential when IV access is not yet established.

Multiple administrations of naloxone may be required, depending on the duration of action of the opioid within the patient's body. If a patient is addicted to opioids, naloxone can precipitate symptoms of withdrawal, such as nausea and vomiting, agitation, cardiovascular instability, and pulmonary edema. Therefore, the

Abuse by the numbers

- One in 4 children experience some form of abuse or neglect (CDC, 2019a).
- One in 10 adults older than the age of 60 experience emotional, physical, or sexual abuse or neglect within their lifetime. Estimates as high as 5 million older adults are abused each year (National Council on Aging, n.d.).
- One in 3 women and 1 in 6 men have experienced sexual violence during their lifetime (Smith et al., 2017).
- One in 5 women have experienced attempted or completed rape in their lifetime (Smith et al., 2017).
- One in 6 women and 1 in 14 men have experienced intimate partner violence in their lifetime (Smith et al., 2017).
- There are 40.3 million victims of human trafficking globally (International Labour Organization, 2017)
- In the United States, over 8 in 10 suspected incidents of human trafficking involve sex trafficking, and more than half of sex-trafficking victims are younger than the age of 17 (Development Services Group, 2014).

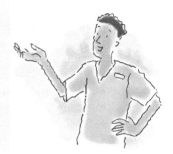

health care provider will usually prescribe the lowest effective dose to minimize these risks.

Be certain to report even the smallest changes in the patient's condition to assure that appropriate medical interventions are made in a timely fashion during the acute treatment phase. If the patient's condition allows, SBIRT can also be used as a brief intervention model to address the abuse of drugs.

Situations of abuse—older adult, child, intimate partner, or human trafficking

Abuse or mistreatment are actions of intent that create a situation of harm or risk to another individual. (See *Abuse by the numbers*.) Abuse or mistreatment can also result from neglect or the failure of a caregiver to meet basic needs or protect the person from harm. Abuse may take the form of physical abuse, sexual abuse, emotional abuse, neglect, and/or financial exploitation. Populations that are particularly vulnerable include children, older adults, and women.

Older adult abuse/neglect

Older adult abuse or neglect, sometimes called *elder abuse*, is abuse of an adult older than the age of 60. Although it is common to think of abuse in terms of physical abuse, older adult abuse includes physical, emotional, sexual, and financial abuse as well as neglect. Signs of abuse include:

Physical abuse
- A caregiver refusing to leave the room
- Abrasions
- Broken bones
- Bruises
- Burns
- Dislocations
- Pressure marks
- Signs of being restrained
- Unexplained injuries.

Emotional abuse
- Forced isolation by caregiver so others are unable to see the abuse
- Humiliation and ridicule
- Nervous or fearful behavior
- Strained relationship between caregiver and the older adult
- Withdrawal and apathy

Sexual abuse
- Bruises around breasts
- Bruises around genital area
- Depressed or withdrawn behavior
- Flirtation by the caregiver
- Sexually transmitted infection
- Vaginal or rectal bleeding

Neglect
- Delay in seeking needed care
- Dirty surroundings
- Lack of bathing, cleanliness
- Lack of hearing aids, glasses, cane
- Lack of suitable clothing for weather
- Pressure injuries
- Unexplained weight loss
- Wearing soiled clothing
- Wet, soiled briefs

Financial abuse
- Adding new persons to accounts
- Bills not being paid
- Forging the older adult's signature
- Identity theft

- Money disappearing
- Suspicious changes to financial and legal documents
- Unusual purchases

Child abuse/neglect

Child abuse can be physical, emotional, or sexual. Child neglect is a form of child abuse where inaction by a parent or caregiver is harmful. Recognizing the signs of child maltreatment is a critical part of helping a child who is a victim of abuse. The child who is a victim of abuse often presents to the ED with an unexplained or poorly explained injury. For example, a child may present to the ED with burns, bruises, abrasions, or broken bones in various stages of healing. The child, as well as the caregiver, may provide inconsistent explanations or an explanation that does not match the degree of injury. In the event of child abuse, the caregiver may be unduly protective or refuse to leave the child alone.

Behavioral abnormalities can also be an indicator of abuse. The child may seem withdrawn, overly compliant, fearful, anxious, depressed, or aggressive.

Other signs of abuse or neglect in children include (Child Welfare Information Gateway, 2019):
- regressive behaviors such as bedwetting, thumb sucking, or fear of dark
- failure to thrive
- apprehension or fear of going home
- weight gain or loss
- changes in sleeping patterns or school performance
- disheveled appearance
- inappropriate sexual behaviors or use of sexual language.

Intimate partner violence

Intimate partner violence can be emotional, physical, sexual, or a combination. Intimate partner violence can occur between spouses, partners, boyfriend, girlfriend, or estranged partners (Videbeck, 2017). Victims of intimate partner violence may present with unexplained injuries or multiple injuries in different states of healing. The partner may accompany the victim, refuse to leave, or try to speak for the victim. Other signs of intimate partner violence include:
- injuries from items that leave patterns such as shoes or belts
- injuries in areas that are hidden by clothing
- history of depression, anxiety, suicide attempts, alcohol and drug abuse
- frequent visits for somatic concerns.

Human trafficking

Human trafficking is the act of force, coercion, or fraud to obtain people (children or adults) for labor or sex (Homeland Security, n.d.). Human trafficking can occur in any community, and traffickers look for individuals who may be vulnerable. Recognizing the signs of human trafficking is a critical skill for all health care providers and especially those who work in the ED. Signs of victimization by human trafficking may include (Polaris, 2019):

- fearful, anxious, or tense behavior
- poor hygiene or malnourished appearance
- signs of physical and/or sexual abuse or restraint
- lack of personal possessions
- lack of own identification documents
- reluctance to speak for self
- minimizing abuse
- inconsistent story regarding injury or reason for ED visit.

Nursing care for victims of abuse

Although it may be difficult to hear about experiences with abuse, the nurse is in a primary position to facilitate the beginning of safety and recovery for the victim of human trafficking (Breuer & Daiber, 2019). There are interventions common to all victims of abuse, as well as specialized interventions for specific populations.

Interventions common to all victims of abuse

- Screen for abuse in a safe, private setting.
- Attempt to meet with the patient privately without others present.
- Take time to build a rapport and gain the patient's trust.
- Maintain eye contact.
- Express a sincere desire to help the patient.
- Ask questions and response to the patient in a calm, respectful, nonthreatening, and nonjudgmental way.
- Contact an interpreter if the patient primarily speaks a different language.
- Validate the patient's feelings and his or her decision to share his or her story.
- Gain specific training in procedures and processes for handling evidence in cases of abuse and/or assault.
- Know agency protocols and legal requirements of local, state, and federal laws for reporting abuse, assault, and violence.
- Maximize abilities of the interprofessional team to aid in the evaluation and care of the patient.

- Be aware of your own feelings and biases about abuse so that these do not adversely affect your ability to intervene in supporting the patient.
- Document using the patient's own words in the electronic health record.

Additional interventions for

The child who is a victim of abuse

- Recognize normal growth and anatomy development for the patient's age and growth pattern.
- Recognize expected developmental milestones for the patient's age and maturity level.
- Use screening tools specific to this population, such as the Escape instrument (Dinpanah & Akbarzadeh Pasha, 2017).
- Use age-appropriate language.

The older adult who is a victim of abuse

- Recognize that self-abuse (the state that occurs when a vulnerable adult is unable or unwilling to adequately and safely care for themselves and refuse assistance to do so) is also considered a type of abuse (Stark, 2012).
- Recognize different types of abuse exclusive to the older adult population, such as financial abuse.
- Recognize caregiver burnout, which can accompany abuse of older adults.
- Use screening tools specific to this population, such as the Elder Abuse Suspicion Index© (Yaffe et al., 2008).
- Listen carefully to interactions between the older adult and caregiver; these dynamics can provide meaningful information from which to continue assessing for abuse.

The individual who is a victim of intimate partner abuse

- Recognize that the patient's partner (who performs the abuse) may often attempt to stay with the patient and answer for the patient. Offer to escort the patient's partner to another area of the hospital while assessing the patient in a private environment.
- Recognize that males, as well as females, can be victims of intimate partner violence.
- Use screening tools specific to intimate partner violence via physical abuse, such as the Universal Violence Prevention Screening Protocol (Dutton et al., 1996) or the Interpersonal Violence New Tool for Identification in Health Care Settings (Family Violence Prevention Fund, 2003).
- Use screening tools specific to intimate partner violence via physical and sexual abuse, such as the Two-Question Screening Tool (McFarlane et al., 1995).

The individual who is a victim of human trafficking
- Recognize that children and vulnerable adults are at risk to be victims of human trafficking.
- Use screening tools specific to human trafficking such as the Human Trafficking Screening Tool (Dank et al., as cited in Mostajabian et al., 2019)
- Involve experts such as the forensic nurse immediately upon recognition of signs of human trafficking (Scannell et al., 2018).

Iatrogenic emergencies

Iatrogenic emergencies are conditions induced by medications or a health care provider. This is an important reason why individuals receiving psychiatric care need to be seen regularly by their prescriber. Three iatrogenic medication-induced emergencies include serotonin syndrome, neuroleptic malignant syndrome (NMS), and medication-induced acute dystonia.

Serotonin syndrome

Serotonin syndrome is a rare condition caused by taking a combination of drugs that results in a potentially lethal amount of serotonin released into the brain. Serotonin is found in the central nervous system, platelets, and gastrointestinal tract. A number of drugs (prescribed as well as illicit) and supplements can cause increases in serotonin levels when taken in combination, including (Volpi-Abadie et al., 2013):
- amphetamines
- antidepressants
- antiemetics
- antimigraine medications (triptans)
- antipsychotics
- anxiolytics
- dietary supplements (e.g., L-tryptophan)
- drugs of abuse (e.g., cocaine, MDMA—"ecstasy" or "molly")
- herbal supplements (e.g., St. John's wort)
- monoamine oxidase inhibitors (MAOIs)
- opiates (meperidine, oxycodone, tramadol).

The most common drugs that cause serotonin syndrome are antidepressants, including MAOIs and selective serotonin reuptake inhibitors. Serotonin syndrome is highly preventable with proper prescribing and taking of serotonergic medications.

Symptoms associated with serotonin syndrome occur rapidly. (See *Signs and symptoms of serotonin syndrome*.)

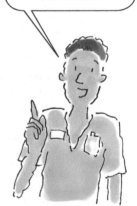

Serotonin syndrome is a rare condition caused from a combination of drugs that results in a potentially lethal amount of serotonin in the brain.

Signs and symptoms of serotonin syndrome

Neurologic
- Confusion
- Headache
- Restlessness
- Seizures (when condition is severe)
- Unconsciousness (when condition is severe)

Sensory
- Dilated pupils

Cardiovascular
- Cardiac arrhythmias (when condition is severe)
- Hypertension
- Hyperthermia (high, when condition is severe)

Musculoskeletal
- Akinesia (loss of voluntary muscle movement)
- Hyperreflexivity

Gastrointestinal
- Diarrhea

Integumentary
- Piloerection (the erection of hairs on the skin; commonly referred to as *goose bumps*)

Psychiatric
- Hallucinations

General
- Shivering

Nursing interventions for the patient with serotonin syndrome

In the mild form of this condition, serotonin syndrome can be resolved by discontinuing medications that contribute to excessive levels of serotonin. In more severe cases, patients need careful observation and supportive hospital treatment.

You will administer IV fluids, muscle relaxants, serotonin-blocking medications ($5\text{-}HT_3$ receptor antagonists such as chlorpromazine), cardiac medications, and oxygen as prescribed. Carefully monitor oxygen saturation and breathing patterns. The patient may need mechanical ventilation until proper breathing can be restored.

Neuroleptic malignant syndrome

NMS is a neurologic emergency caused by a reaction to an antipsychotic or neuroleptic drug (Simon & Callahan, 2018). This is very rare; however, it can be life-threatening. NMS is most commonly associated with first-generation antipsychotic medications. However, it can occur with every class of antipsychotic drugs as well as antiemetics (Wijdicks, 2019).

There are four typical symptoms that are present in almost all cases of NMS. These symptoms include:
- cognitive changes that can include confusion and mutism, with fluctuations between agitation and stupor
- muscular rigidity that is severe and characterized by "lead-pipe rigidity" (Wijdicks, 2019)

- hyperthermia with profuse sweating
- autonomic instability that can present as tachycardia, labile blood pressure, and tachypnea.

Most cases of NMS occur within the first week of taking the drug. Treatment involves recognizing the condition, stopping the medication, and aggressive supportive care. Early detection and supportive care, sometimes within an intensive care setting for close monitoring, has helped to reduce mortality rates. With appropriate care, most cases resolve within 2 weeks.

Medication-induced acute dystonia

Symptoms of medication-induced acute dystonia generally occur after weeks or years of exposure to certain drugs. Severity of symptoms range from mild to severe. Muscle spasms may occur in the neck, trunk, or arms. Tremors may be noticed. More severe dyskinesias include tongue protrusion, lip smacking, mouth puckering, and eye blinking. The patient may experience sustained contracture of the neck (torticollis) or the head (retrocollis), limbs, or trunk. Patients may also experience trouble breathing and/or talking, sweat profusely, and become cyanotic.

Emergency management of medication-induced acute dystonia involves pharmacologic treatment with anticholinergic agents such as benztropine mesylate (Cogentin). Diphenhydramine (Benadryl) can also be beneficial. Patients may need to be placed on a maintenance dose of an anticholinergic drug or changed from the medication that is causing the reaction.

Quick quiz

1. Which term will the nurse document when the patient reports "hearing voices"?
    A. Mania
    B. Delusions
    C. Catatonia
    D. Hallucinations

Answer: D. *Hallucinations* is a term used to describe the sensory experiences of seeing (visual), hearing (auditory), smelling (olfactory), tasting (gustatory), or feeling (tactile) things that are not real. Most common are auditory hallucinations that convey a hurtful or negative message.

2.   Which priority nursing action should be taken in the ED for a patient with suspected opioid overdose?
   A.   Open airway.
   B.   Initiate an IV as prescribed.
   C.   Administer naloxone as prescribed.
   D.   Comfort family members.

Answer: A. Basic airway control is the required treatment for opioid overdose. The nurse should ensure a patent airway, provide supplemental oxygen, initiate rescue breathing as needed, and prepare for endotracheal intubation if needed. Initiating an IV is a prescribed action needed to maintain an open line for fluids. Administering naloxone as prescribed is an action to reverse the opioid effects. Comforting family members is an important nursing action; however, emergency patient care is a priority.

3.   Which prescribed medication will the nurse expect to administer as ordered for a patient with schizophrenia who is exhibiting agitation?
   A.   Sertraline
   B.   Wellbutrin
   C.   Lorazepam
   D.   Citalopram

Answer: C. In patients experiencing agitation due to schizophrenia or bipolar disorder, it is necessary to use appropriate antipsychotic medications to ameliorate hallucinations and/or delusions, not only sedatives. Lorazepam (Ativan) is the most commonly used benzodiazepine for short-term calming and sedation for agitation.

Scoring

 If you answered all three questions correctly, way to go! You're ahead of the game!

 If you answered two questions correctly, impressive! Make no mistake about it, you have a mastery of mental health matters!

If you answered fewer than two questions correctly, don't be depressed. Just gain control and study a bit more!

Selected references

American Foundation for Suicide Prevention. (2017). *Talking about suicide and LGBT populations*. Retrieved from http://afsp.org/wp-content/uploads/2016/01 /talking-about-suicide-and-lgbt-populations-2nd-edition.pdf

American Psychiatric Association. (2013). *Diagnostic and statistical manual of mental disorders* (5th ed.). Arlington, VA: Author.

Breuer, G., & Daiber, D. (2019). Human trafficking awareness in the emergency care setting. *Journal of Emergency Nursing, 45*(1), 67–75.

Centers for Disease Control and Prevention. (2016a). *Fact sheets—Excessive alcohol use and risks to men's health.* Retrieved from https://www.cdc.gov/alcohol/fact-sheets/mens-health.htm

Centers for Disease Control and Prevention. (2016b). *Fact sheets—Excessive alcohol use and risks to women's health.* Retrieved from https://www.cdc.gov/alcohol/fact-sheets/womens-health.htm

Centers for Disease Control and Prevention. (2017a). *Opioid overdose.* Retrieved from https://www.cdc.gov/drugoverdose/opioids/index.html

Centers for Disease Control and Prevention. (2017b). *Leading causes of death reports,* 1981-2017. Retrieved from https://webappa.cdc.gov/sasweb/ncipc/leadcause.html

Centers for Disease Control and Prevention. (2018a). *Suicide in rural America.* Retrieved from https://www.cdc.gov/ruralhealth/Suicide.html

Centers for Disease Control and Prevention. (2018b). *Suicide rising across the US. More than a mental health concern.* Retrieved from https://www.cdc.gov/vitalsigns/pdf/vs-0618-suicide-H.pdf

Centers for Disease Control and Prevention. (2018c). *U.S. burden of Alzheimer's disease, related dementias to double by 2060.* Retrieved from https://www.cdc.gov/media/releases/2018/p0920-alzheimers-burden-double-2060.html

Centers for Disease Control and Prevention. (2019a). *Child abuse prevention.* Retrieved from https://www.cdc.gov/features/healthychildren/index.html

Centers for Disease Control and Prevention. (2019b). *Welcome to WISQARS™.* Atlanta, GA: National Center for Injury Prevention and Control. Retrieved from http://www.cdc.gov/injury/wisqars/index.html

Child Welfare Information Gateway. (2019). *What is child abuse and neglect? Recognizing the signs and symptoms.* Washington, DC: Children's Bureau, U.S. Department of Health and Human Services. Retrieved from https://www.childwelfare.gov/pubpdfs/whatiscan.pdf

Cowan, E., & Su, M. (2018). *Ethanol intoxication in adults.* Retrieved from https://www.uptodate.com/contents/ethanol-intoxication-in-adults

Development Services Group. (2014). *Commercial sexual exploitation of children and sex trafficking. Literature review.* Washington, DC: Office of Juvenile Justice and Delinquency Prevention. Retrieved from https://www.ojjdp.gov/mpg/litreviews/CSECSexTrafficking.pdf

Dinpanah, H., & Akbarzadeh Pasha, A. (2017). Potential child abuse screening in emergency department; a diagnostic accuracy study. *Emergency (Tehran, Iran),* 5(1), e8.

*Dutton, M., Mitchell, B., & Haywood, Y. (1996). The emergency department as a violence prevention center. *Journal of the American Medical Women's Association (1972),* 51, 92–95, 117.

Family Violence Prevention Fund. (2003). Interpersonal violence new tool for identification in health care settings. *Health Alert,* 9, 8–9.

Gottlieb, M., Long, B., & Koyfman, A. (2018). Approach to the agitated emergency department patient. *The Journal of Emergency Medicine,* 54(4), 447–457. doi:10.1016/j.jemermed.2017.12.049

Homeland Security. (n.d.). *What is human trafficking.* Retrieved from https://www.dhs.gov/blue-campaign/what-human-trafficking

Inouye, S., van Dyck, C., Alessi, C., et al. (1990). Clarifying confusion: The confusion assessment method. A new method for detection of delirium. *Annals of Internal Medicine, 113*(12), 941–948.

International Labour Organization. (2017). *Global estimates of modern slavery: Forced labour and forced marriage.* Retrieved from http://www.ilo.org/wcmsp5/groups /public/–dgreports/–dcomm/documents/publication/wcms_575479.pdf

Jacobs, D. (2007). *A resource guide for implementing. The Joint Commission 2007 patient safety goals on suicide: Featuring the Suicide Assessment Five-step Evaluation and Triage (SAFE-T).* Retrieved from http://stopasuicide.org/assets/docs/JCAHO.pdf

Knox, D. K., & Holloman, G. H., Jr., (2012). Use and avoidance of seclusion and restraint: Consensus statement of the American Association for Emergency Psychiatry project BETA Seclusion and Restraint Workgroup. *The Western Journal of Emergency Medicine, 13*(1), 35–40. doi:10.5811/westjem.2011.9.6867

Marcantonio, E., Ngo, L. H., O'Connor, M., et al. (2014). 3D-CAM: Derivation and validation of a 3-minute diagnostic interview for CAM-defined delirium: A cross-sectional diagnostic test study. *Annals of Internal Medicine, 161*(8), 554–561.

*McFarlane, J., Greenberg, L., Weltge, A., et al. (1995). Identification of abuse in emergency departments: Effectiveness of a two-question screening tool. *Journal of Emergency Nursing, 21,* 391–394.

Mostajabian, S., Santa Maria, D., Wiemann, C., et al. (2019). Identifying sexual and labor exploitation among sheltered youth experiencing homelessness: A comparison of screening methods. *International Journal of Environmental Research and Public Health, 16,* E363.

Musey, P. I., Jr., Lee, J. A., Hall, C. A., et al. (2018). Anxiety about anxiety: A survey of emergency department provider beliefs and practices regarding anxiety-associated low risk chest pain. *BMC Emergency Medicine, 18*(1), 10. doi:10.1186/s12873-018-0161-x

National Council on Aging. (n.d.). *Elder abuse facts.* Retrieved from https://www.ncoa .org/public-policy-action/elder-justice/elder-abuse-facts/

National Institute on Alcohol Abuse and Alcoholism. (2018). *Understanding the dangers of alcohol overdose.* Retrieved from https://www.niaaa.nih.gov/publications /brochures-and-fact-sheets/understanding-dangers-of-alcohol-overdose

National Institute on Drug Abuse. (2019). *Opioid overdose crisis.* Retrieved from https:// www.drugabuse.gov/drugs-abuse/opioids/opioid-overdose-crisis#two

Office of the Federal Register National Archives and Records Administration. (2018). *Title 42—Public health.* Retrieved from https://www.govinfo.gov/content/pkg /CFR-2018-title42-vol5/xml/CFR-2018-title42-vol5-sec482-13.xml

Piscopo, K. (2017). *Suicidality and death by suicide among middle-aged adults in the United States.* Retrieved from https://www.samhsa.gov/data/sites/default/files/report _3370/ShortReport-3370.html

Polaris. (2019). *Recognizing the signs.* Retrieved from https://polarisproject.org/human -trafficking/recognize-signs

Richmond, J. S., Berlin, J. S., Fishkind, A. B., et al. (2012). Verbal de-escalation of the agitated patient: Consensus statement of the American Association for Emergency Psychiatry Project BETA De-escalation Workgroup. *Western Journal of Emergency Medicine, 13*(1), 17–25. doi:10.5811/westjem.2011.9.6864

Scannell, M., MacDonald, A. E., Berger, A., et al. (2018). Human trafficking: How nurses can make a difference. *Journal of Forensic Nursing, 14*(2), 117–121.

Simon, L. V., & Callahan, A. L. (2018). *Neuroleptic malignant syndrome.* Retrieved from https://www.ncbi.nlm.nih.gov/pubmed/29489248

Smith, S. G., Chen, J., Basile, K. C., et al. (2017). *The National Intimate Partner and Sexual Violence Survey (NISVS): 2010-2012 State report.* Retrieved from https://www.cdc.gov/violenceprevention/pdf/NISVS-StateReportBook.pdf

Stahl, S. (2017). *Prescriber's guide: Stahl's essential psychopharmacology* (6th ed.). Cambridge, United Kingdom: Cambridge University Press.

*Stark, S. (2012). Elder abuse: Screening, intervention, and prevention. *Nursing, 42*(10), 24–29.

Stone, D. M., Simon, T. R., Fowler, K. A., et al. (2018). Vital signs: Trends in state suicide rates—United States, 1999–2016 and circumstances contributing to suicide—27 states, 2015. *Morbidity and Mortality Weekly Report, 67*, 617–624. doi:10.15585/mmwr.mm6722a1

Stowell, K. R., Florence, P., Harman, H. J., et al. (2012). Psychiatric evaluation of the agitated patient: Consensus statement of the American Association for Emergency Psychiatry project BETA Psychiatric Evaluation Workgroup. *The Western Journal of Emergency Medicine, 13*(1), 11–16. doi:10.5811/westjem.2011.9.6868

Substance Abuse and Mental Health Services Administration. (2009). *SAFE-T: Suicide Assessment Five-Step Evaluation and Triage.* Rockville, MD: U.S. Department of Health and Human Services.

Suicide Prevention Resource Center. (2015). *Caring for adult patients with suicide risk: A consensus guide for emergency departments.* Waltham, MA: Education Development Center. Retrieved from http://www.sprc.org/sites/default/files/EDGuide_full.pdf

The Joint Commission. (2019). *National patient safety goals effective January 2019: Hospital accreditation program.* Retrieved from https://www.jointcommission.org/assets/1/6/NPSG_Chapter_HAP_Jan2019.pdf

U.S. Department of Health and Human Services. (2006). Medicare and Medicaid Programs; hospital conditions of participation: Patients' rights. *Federal Register, 71*(236), 71426–71428.

U.S. Food and Drug Administration. (2019). *FDA and kratom.* Retrieved from https://www.fda.gov/news-events/public-health-focus/fda-and-kratom

Videbeck, S. (2017). *Psychiatric–mental health nursing* (7th ed.). Philadelphia, PA: Wolters Kluwer.

Vieta, E., Garriga, M., Cardete, L., et al. (2017). Protocol for the management of psychiatric patients with psychomotor agitation. *BMC Psychiatry, 17*, 328. doi:10.1186/s12888-017-1490-0

Volpi-Abadie, J., Kaye, A., & Kaye, A. (2013). Serotonin syndrome. *The Ochsner Journal, 13*(4), 533–540.

Wijdicks, E. (2019). *Neuroleptic malignant syndrome.* Retrieved from https://www.uptodate.com/contents/neuroleptic-malignant-syndrome

World Health Organization. (2014). *Preventing suicide: A global imperative.* Geneva, Switzerland: Author. Retrieved from https://www.who.int/mental_health/suicide-prevention/world_report_2014/en/

*Yaffe, M., Wolfson, C., Lithwick, M., et al. (2008). Development and validation of a tool to improve physician identification of elder abuse: The Elder Abuse Suspicion Index (EASI). *Journal of Elder Abuse & Neglect, 20*(3), 276–300.

*Classic reference

Chapter 12

Environmental emergencies

Just the facts

In this chapter, you'll learn:

♦ types of environmental emergencies

♦ assessment methods for environmental emergencies

♦ treatment for hyperthermia

♦ treatment for hypothermia

♦ treatment for frostbite

♦ treatment for bites of animals, spiders, snakes, and humans.

Insects and lightning and fire—oh my! Environmental emergencies give new meaning to "the great outdoors"!

Understanding environmental emergencies

Environmental emergencies are emergencies that occur because of exposure to, or contact with, the environment. Environmental emergencies include injuries from fire, electricity, lightning, chemicals, water, animals, insects, other humans, cold, and heat.

Assessment

Your environmental emergency assessment will depend on the type of injury and its location. First and foremost, assess the patient's airway, breathing, circulation, disability, and exposure (ABCDE). (See *Primary survey*, page 496.)

Diagnostic tests

Diagnostic tests used to help assess environmental emergencies will also depend on the type and location of the injury and the emergency. They may include arterial blood gas (ABG) analysis to assess oxygenation and ventilation; electrocardiogram to assess for possible cardiac arrhythmias; blood tests such as complete blood count (CBC), platelet count, clotting studies, and liver function studies; and electrolyte, blood urea nitrogen (BUN), glucose, and creatinine levels. Bronchoscopy may be performed to visualize the condition of the trachea and bronchi in burn patients.

Primary survey

The primary survey consists of airway, breathing, circulation, disability (level of consciousness), and exposure (an assessment of the possible cause of condition) (ABCDE).

A is for airway

Remember as you assess the airway of an environmental emergency patient to ensure cervical spine immobilization, any patient who has sustained a major trauma must be assumed to have a cervical spine injury until proven otherwise. The best way to achieve this is through the application of a cervical collar.

B is for breathing

The major trauma patient requires high-flow oxygen. If the patient doesn't have spontaneous respirations or has ineffective respirations, ventilate him or her using a bag valve mask device until you can achieve intubation.

C is for circulation

All major trauma patients need two large-bore intravenous (IV) lines. Because these patients may require large amounts of fluids and blood, use a fluid warmer if possible. If external bleeding is present, apply direct pressure over the site.

If the patient has no pulse, cardiopulmonary resuscitation must be started. If there is a suspected injury to the heart (such as a gunshot or knife wound), the health care provider may elect to perform an emergency thoracotomy in the emergency department in an effort to repair the wound.

D is for disability

Assess the patient using the mnemonic AVPU:
- A stands for alert and oriented.
- V stands for responds to voice.
- P stands for responds to pain.
- U stands for unresponsive.

E is for exposure

Exposure involves assessing for the possible cause of the patient's condition and to determine body temperature. You may need to remove the patient's clothing to perform a full assessment that looks for signs such as bleeding, trauma, skin reactions or rashes, needle marks, burns, or other possible causative agents. Do this in a respectful manner to preserve the dignity of the patient.

If the patient isn't alert and oriented, conduct further assessments during the secondary survey.

Remember that ABCDE is a rapid assessment designed to identify life-threatening emergencies. Treat any life-threatening emergencies before continuing your assessment.

Practice pointers
- A health care provider, respiratory therapist, or specially trained emergency nurse draws samples for ABG analysis, usually from an arterial line if one is present.
- After obtaining an ABG sample, apply pressure to the puncture site for 5 minutes and tape a gauze pad firmly in place. Regularly monitor the site for bleeding and check the arm for signs of complications such as swelling, discoloration, pain, numbness, and tingling.
- Monitor cardiac status frequently for changes in heart rate or rhythm. Report tachycardia or evidence of an arrhythmia.
- After bronchoscopy, the patient is positioned on his or her side. The head of the bed may be elevated 30 degrees until the gag reflex returns. Assess respiratory status and monitor vital signs,

oxygen saturation levels, and heart rhythm. Report signs and symptoms of respiratory distress, such as dyspnea, laryngospasm, or hypoxemia.

- If the patient isn't intubated, assess for return of the gag, cough, and swallow reflexes after bronchoscopy.

Treatments

Treatment for environmental emergencies may include cold application, a hypothermia–hyperthermia blanket, gastric lavage, or hemodialysis. Treatment method depends on the type and mechanism of injury.

Temperature related

Temperature-related treatments for environmental emergencies may include cold application and/or use of a hyperthermia–hypothermia blanket.

Cold application

The application of cold constricts blood vessels; inhibits local circulation, suppuration, and tissue metabolism; relieves vascular congestion; slows bacterial activity in infections; reduces body temperature; and may act as a temporary anesthetic during brief, painful procedures.

Cold may be applied in dry or moist forms, but ice shouldn't be placed directly on a patient's skin because it compromises tissue integrity. Moist application is more penetrating than dry because moisture facilitates conduction. Devices for applying cold include an ice bag or collar, K-Pad (which can produce cold or heat), and chemical cold packs and ice packs. Devices for applying moist cold include cold compresses for small body areas and cold packs for large areas.

Nursing considerations
- Observe the site frequently for signs of tissue intolerance, such as blanching, mottling, cyanosis, maceration, and/or blisters.
- Stay alert for shivering or reports of burning or numbness. If these signs or symptoms develop, discontinue treatment and notify the health care provider.
- Refill or replace the cold device as necessary to maintain the correct temperature. Change the protective cover if it becomes wet.
- Apply cold treatments cautiously on patients with impaired circulation, children, elderly patients, or patients with arthritis because of the risk of ischemic tissue damage.

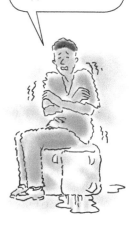

I don't think that this is what cold application is supposed to mean!

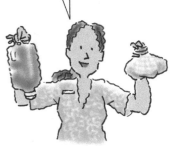

Be careful when you use cold treatments on children, older adults, or patients with arthritis. They run a high risk of ischemic tissue damage.

Hyperthermia–hypothermia blanket

The hyperthermia–hypothermia blanket—which is actually a blanket-sized Aquamatic K-Pad—raises, lowers, or maintains body temperature through conductive heat or cold transfer between the blanket and the patient. It can be operated manually or automatically.

The blanket is used most commonly to reduce high fever when more conservative measures (such as baths, ice packs, and antipyretics) are unsuccessful. Other uses include:

- maintaining normal temperature during surgery or shock
- inducing hypothermia during surgery to decrease metabolic activity and thereby reduce oxygen requirements
- reducing intracranial pressure
- controlling bleeding and intractable pain in patients with amputations, burns, or cancer
- providing warmth in cases of severe hypothermia.

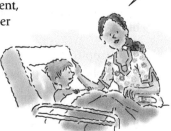

If a patient shivers during hypothermic treatment, banish the blanket! The now-increasing metabolism will elevate body temperature without it.

Nursing considerations

- If the patient shivers excessively during hypothermia treatment, discontinue the procedure and notify the health care provider immediately; by increasing metabolism, shivering elevates body temperature.
- Avoid lowering the temperature more than 1 degree every 15 minutes to prevent premature ventricular contractions.
- Don't use pins to secure catheters, tubes, or blanket covers because an accidental puncture can result in fluid leakage and burns.

Other treatments

Other treatments for environmental emergencies include gastric lavage and hemodialysis.

Gastric lavage

After poisoning or a drug overdose, especially in patients who have central nervous system (CNS) depression or an inadequate gag reflex, gastric lavage flushes the stomach and removes ingested substances through a gastric lavage tube. Gastric lavage can be continuous or intermittent. Typically, this procedure is performed in the emergency department (ED) or intensive care unit by a health care provider, gastroenterologist, or nurse; a wide-bore lavage tube is almost always inserted by a gastroenterologist.

Gastric lavage is contraindicated after ingestion of a corrosive substance (such as lye, petroleum distillates, ammonia, alkalis, or mineral acids) because the lavage tube may perforate the already compromised esophagus.

Correct lavage tube placement is essential for patient safety because accidental misplacement (e.g., in the lungs) followed by lavage can be fatal. Other complications of gastric lavage include bradyarrhythmias and aspiration of gastric fluids.

Nursing considerations

- Never leave a patient alone during gastric lavage. Observe continuously for any changes in level of consciousness (LOC) and monitor vital signs frequently because the natural vagal response to intubation can depress the heart rate.
- If you need to restrain the patient, secure restraints on the same side of the bed or stretcher so you can free them quickly without moving to the other side of the bed. Be sure to obtain proper orders and follow agency policy regarding restraints.

Suck it up

- Remember to keep tracheal suctioning equipment nearby and watch closely for airway obstruction caused by vomiting or excess oral secretions. Throughout gastric lavage, you may need to suction the oral cavity frequently to ensure an open airway and prevent aspiration. For the same reasons, and if the patient doesn't exhibit an adequate gag reflex, an endotracheal (ET) tube may be required before the procedure.
- When aspirating the stomach for ingested poisons or drugs, save the contents in a labeled container to send to the laboratory for analysis along with a laboratory request form. If ordered after lavage to remove poisons or drugs, mix charcoal tablets with the irrigation liquid (water or normal saline solution) and administer the mixture through the nasogastric (NG) tube. The charcoal will absorb remaining toxic substances. The tube may be clamped temporarily, allowed to drain via gravity, attached to intermittent suction, or removed.

Hemodialysis

The underlying mechanism in hemodialysis is differential diffusion across a semipermeable membrane. This diffusion extracts the by-products of protein metabolism (such as urea and uric acid) as well as creatinine and excess body water. This process restores or maintains the balance of the body's buffer system and electrolyte level. It's used in cases of acute poisoning, such as an overdose of barbiturates or analgesics.

Nursing considerations

- Throughout hemodialysis, carefully monitor the patient's vital signs. Measure blood pressure at least hourly or as often as every 15 minutes if necessary.

- Perform periodic tests for clotting time on the patient's blood samples and on samples from the dialyzer.
- Continue necessary drug administration during dialysis unless the dialysate would remove the drug; if so, administer the drug after dialysis.

Common disorders

Common environmental emergencies include burns; caustic substance ingestion; hyperthermia; hypothermia; frostbite; animal, spider, snake, or human bites; and poisoning.

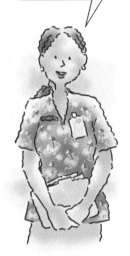

Thermal burn causes range from residential fires to kitchen accidents.

Burns

A burn is a tissue injury resulting from contact with fire, a thermal chemical, or an electrical source. It can cause cellular skin damage and a systemic response that leads to altered body function.

What causes it

Thermal burns, the most common type of burn, typically result from residential fires, automobile collisions, playing with matches, improper handling of firecrackers, scalding and kitchen accidents (such as a child climbing on top of a stove or grabbing a hot iron), abuse (in children and elderly patients), and clothes catching on fire.

It's electric

Electrical burns result from contact with faulty electrical wiring or high-voltage power lines.

Scorching brews

Chemical burns result from contact, ingestion, inhalation, or injection of acids, alkalis, or vesicants.

How it happens

Specific pathophysiology depends on the cause and classification of the burn. (See *Visualizing burn depth.*) The injuring agent modifies the molecular structure of cellular proteins. Some cells die because of traumatic or ischemic necrosis. Loss of collagen cross-linking also occurs that moves intravascular fluid into interstitial spaces. Cellular injury triggers the release of mediators of inflammation, contributing to local and—in the case of major burns—systemic increases in capillary permeability.

Visualizing burn depth

Burn severity is determined by how much of body surface area is involved and the depth of the burn (Ignatavicius et al., 2018). Another system categorizes burns by degree. It is important to remember that most burns involve tissue damage of multiple degrees and thicknesses. This illustration may help you visualize burn damage at the various degrees.

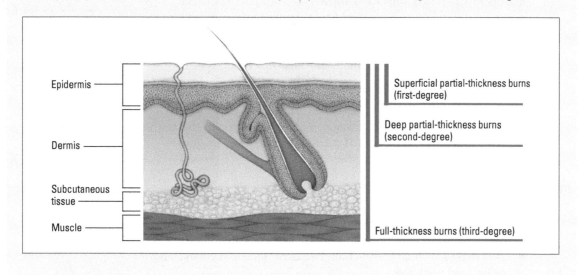

Epidermis

Dermis

Subcutaneous tissue

Muscle

Superficial partial-thickness burns (first-degree)

Deep partial-thickness burns (second-degree)

Full-thickness burns (third-degree)

Not just a matter of degrees anymore

In the past, burns were gauged only by degree. Today, however, assessment of depth of tissue damage is used to describe a burn.

For your epidermis only

Superficial thickness wounds are limited to the epidermis; these burns cause localized injury or destruction to the skin by direct or indirect contact. The barrier function of the skin remains intact.

Two thicknesses

Superficial partial-thickness wounds involve destruction of the upper third of the epidermis. Blood supply to the area remains intact. Pain and tactile responses remain, as nerve endings are exposed, causing treatments to be very painful. The barrier function of the skin is lost. Blistering is common within a 24-hour period following the injury.

In deep partial-thickness wounds, damage extends deeper into the dermis. There is moderate edema, and the wound usually appears wet, waxy, and bright red or white. Pain is often absent because nerve endings are destroyed. Blistering does not occur with this type of wound.

Full-thickness wounds destroy the entire epidermis and dermis; involve muscle, bone, and interstitial tissue; and usually require skin grafting. Within hours following the burn, fluids and protein shift from capillary to interstitial spaces, causing severe edema. These burns are dry and leathery and do not blanch with pressure. They are painless because nerve endings are destroyed. The dead dermis, called *eschar, must slough off or be removed from the wound before healing can occur.* Eschar often sticks to the lower tissue layers, making removal difficult. A full-thickness burn may be waxy white, deep red, yellow, brown, or black. Thrombosed and heat-coagulated blood vessels may be seen beneath the surface of the burn.

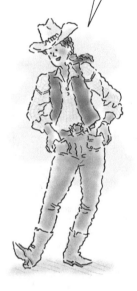

Regardless of color, full-thickness burns tend to look as leathery as my boots.

What to look for

Determine the depth of tissue damage; a partial-thickness burn damages the epidermis and part of the dermis, whereas a full-thickness burn also affects subcutaneous tissue.

Tracking burn traits

Signs and symptoms depend on the type of burn:

- *superficial burn*—localized pain and erythema, usually without blistering
- *more severe superficial burn*—chills, headache, localized edema, and nausea and vomiting
- *superficial partial-thickness burn*—thin-walled, fluid-filled blisters appear within 24 hours of the injury, with mild to moderate edema and pain
- *deep partial-thickness burn*—bright red or white, waxy, wet appearance to damaged area
- *full-thickness burn*—waxy white, deep red, yellow, brown, or black leathery tissue and visible thrombosed vessels due to destruction of skin elasticity but without blisters
- *electrical burn*—silver-colored, raised or charred area, usually at the site of electrical contact.

Configure this

Assess the burn's location and the extent of injury. Note its configuration:

- If the patient has a circumferential burn on an extremity, there is a risk of edema occluding its circulation.
- If the patient has burns on the neck, face, and/or chest, airway obstruction is possible.
- Burns on the patient's chest can lead to restricted respiratory excursion.

More than just skin deep

Inspect the patient for other injuries that may complicate recovery, such as signs of pulmonary damage from smoke inhalation—singed nasal hairs, mucosal burns, voice changes, coughing, wheezing, soot in the mouth or nose, and darkened sputum.

What tests tell you

An assessment method that can be used to determine the size of a burn is the rule of nines chart, which determines the percentage of body surface area (BSA) covered by the burn. (See *Estimating burn size*, page 504.)

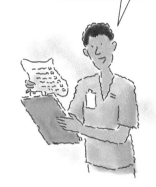

BSA coverage is one way to determine burn category.

Paging severe burns

Severe burns include:
- full-thickness burns on more than 10% of BSA
- partial-thickness burns on more than 25% of BSA in adults and more than 20% in children
- burns on the hands, face, feet, eyes, ears, or genitalia
- burns complicated by fractures or respiratory damage
- all electrical and inhalation burns
- any burn in a poor-risk patient (children younger than 5, adults older than 60, patients with preexisting conditions).

Everything in moderation

Moderate burns include:
- full-thickness burns on 2% to 10% of BSA
- partial-thickness burns on 15% to 25% of BSA in adults and 10% to 20% of BSA in children.

Minor but still important

Minor burns include:
- full-thickness burns on less than 2% of BSA
- partial-thickness burns on less than 15% of BSA in adults and less than 10% of BSA in children.

Meanwhile, back in the lab

Here are some additional diagnostic test results regarding burns:
- ABG levels may be normal in the early stages but reveal hypoxemia and metabolic acidosis later.
- Carboxyhemoglobin level may reveal the extent of smoke inhalation due to carbon monoxide presence.
- CBC may reveal a decreased hemoglobin level due to hemolysis, increased hematocrit (HCT) secondary to hemoconcentration, and leukocytosis resulting from a systemic inflammatory response or the possible development of sepsis.

Estimating burn size

Because body surface area (BSA) varies with age, two different methods are used to estimate burn size in adult and pediatric patients.

Rule of nines

You can quickly estimate the extent of an adult patient's burn by using the rule of nines. This method quantifies BSA in multiples of nine (thus, the name). To use this method, mentally transfer the burns on your patient to the body charts below. Add the corresponding percentages for each body section burned. Use the total—a rough estimate of burn extent—to calculate initial fluid replacement needs.

Lund-Browder classification

The rule of nines isn't accurate for infants or children because their body shapes, and therefore BSA, differ from those of adults. For example, an infant's head accounts for about 17% of total BSA, compared with 7% for an adult. Instead, use the Lund-Browder classification to determine burn size for infants and children.

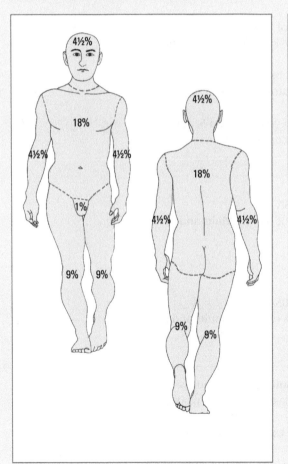

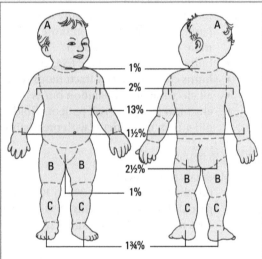

Percentage of burned body surfaced by age

At birth	0 to 1 year	1 to 4 years	5 to 9 years	10 to 15 years	Adult
A: Half of head					
9½%	8½%	6½%	5½%	4½%	3½%
B. Half of one thigh					
2¾%	3¼%	4%	4¼%	4½%	4¾%
C. Half of one leg					
2½%	2½%	2¾%	3%	3¼%	3½%

- Electrolyte levels may show hyponatremia from massive fluid shifting and hyperkalemia from fluid shifting and cell lysis. Other laboratory tests may reveal elevated BUN level secondary to fluid loss or increased protein breakdown and decreased total protein and albumin levels resulting from plasma proteins leaking into the interstitial spaces.
- Creatine kinase (CK) and myoglobin levels may be elevated. Keep in mind that CK and myoglobin are helpful indicators of muscle damage; the higher the CK or myoglobin level, the more extensive the muscle damage. The presence of myoglobin in urine may lead to acute tubular necrosis.

How it's treated

Keep in mind that some EDs aren't equipped to handle full-thickness burns. In cases like these, the patient will be transported to a burn center.

Initial burn treatments are based on the type of burn and may include:

- removing the source of the burn and items that retain heat, such as clothing and jewelry
- maintaining an open airway; assessing airway, breathing, circulation (ABCs)
- preparing for ET intubation if the airway is compromised
- administering supplemental humidified oxygen
- controlling active bleeding
- preventing further contamination of the burns by using sterile gloves
- covering deep partial-thickness burns that are over 30% of BSA or full-thickness burns that are over 5% of BSA with clean, dry, sterile bed sheets (because of the drastic reduction in body temperature, don't cover large burns with saline-soaked dressings)
- fluid replacement (See *A closer look at fluid replacement,* page 506.)

> All jewelry must be removed from patients with burns because it retains heat.

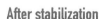

After stabilization

- antimicrobial therapy (for all patients with major burns)
- pain medication as needed
- anti-inflammatory medications
- laboratory tests such as CBC; electrolyte, glucose, BUN, and serum creatinine levels; ABG analysis; type and cross-match; and urinalysis for myoglobinuria and hemoglobinuria
- close monitoring of intake, output, and vital signs
- electrolyte replacement as indicated by laboratory values
- surgical intervention, including skin grafts and thorough surgical debridement for major burns
- tetanus prophylaxis as ordered
- nutritional therapy.

A closer look at fluid replacement

Fluid replacement is essential for the patient with burns because of the massive fluid shifts that occur. However, you must use extreme caution because of the risk of overreplacement.

How much?

Various formulas may be used to determine the amount of fluid replacement to be administered during the first 24 hours after a burn injury. Typically, these formulas use body weight and the percentage of body surface area (BSA) burned. One of the most common formulas used is the Parkland formula shown here:

2 to 4 mL of lactated Ringer's solution/kg

Percentage of BSA burned

Over how long?

Typically, one-half of the calculated amount is administered during the first 8 hours after the injury. (Note that the time of injury—not the time of the patient's arrival in the emergency department—is used as the initial start time of the 8-hour duration.) The remaining one-half of the amount is then administered over the next 16 hours.

Which fluids?

During the first 24 hours, crystalloid solutions are commonly used because capillary permeability is greatly increased, allowing proteins to leak into the interstitial tissues. After the first 24 hours, colloid solutions can be included. Giving colloids before the initial 24-hour period would supply additional protein that could leak into the interstitial tissue.

Too much or too little?

During fluid replacement, always stay alert for indications of overreplacement and underreplacement. Signs and symptoms of heart failure and pulmonary edema suggest overreplacement. Assessment findings of hypovolemic shock suggest underreplacement.

What to do

- Immediately assess the patient's ABCDEs. Institute emergency resuscitative measures as necessary. Monitor arterial oxygen saturation and serial ABG values and anticipate the need for ET intubation and mechanical ventilation if the patient's respiratory status deteriorates, especially with facial or neck burns.

Listen to the lungs

- Auscultate lung sounds for crackles, rhonchi, or stridor. Observe for signs of laryngeal edema or tracheal obstruction, including labored breathing, severe hoarseness, and dyspnea.
- Administer supplemental humidified oxygen as ordered.
- Perform oropharyngeal or tracheal suctioning as indicated by the patient's inability to clear the airway or evidence of abnormal breath sounds.

Electrical burn care

Keep these tips in mind when caring for a patient with an electrical burn:
• Stay alert for ventricular fibrillation as well as cardiac and respiratory arrest caused by the electrical shock; begin cardiopulmonary resuscitation immediately.
• Get an estimate of the voltage that caused the injury.
• Tissue damage from an electrical burn is difficult to assess because internal destruction along the conduction pathway is usually greater than the surface burn would indicate.
• An electrical burn that ignites clothing may also cause thermal burns.

• Initiate continuous cardiac monitoring and monitor cardiac and respiratory status closely—at least every 15 minutes or more frequently depending on condition. Be vigilant for patient for cardiac arrhythmias. Assess LOC for changes, such as increasing confusion, restlessness, or decreased responsiveness. (See *Electrical burn care*.)

Minor burns
• Immerse the burned area in cool water (55° F [12.8° C]) or apply cool compresses.
• Cover the area with an antimicrobial agent and a nonstick bulky dressing after debridement.
• Administer a prophylactic tetanus injection as needed.

Moderate or major burns
• Provide 100% oxygen and prepare for intubation and mechanical ventilation if necessary.
• If the patient has facial or neck burns, anticipate the need for early intubation to reduce the risk of airway obstruction.

Breathing room
• Place in semi-Fowler position to maximize chest expansion.
• Control active bleeding.
• Cover partial-thickness burns over 30% of BSA or full-thickness burns over 5% of BSA with a clean, dry, sterile bed sheet.
• Because of the drastic reduction in body temperature, don't cover large burns with saline-soaked dressings.
• Remove smoldering clothing (first soaking it in saline solution if clothing is stuck to the skin), jewelry, and other constricting items.
• Prepare for emergency escharotomy of the chest and neck for deep burns or circumferential injuries to promote lung expansion.
• Assist with central venous or pulmonary artery catheter placement as needed.

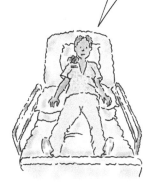

A dry, sterile bed sheet is the best thing to cover full- or partial-thickness burns.

In and out

- Insert an indwelling urinary catheter; monitor intake and output.
- Insert an NG tube to decompress the stomach and prevent aspiration of stomach contents.
- Maintain nothing-by-mouth (NPO) status.
- Watch for signs and symptoms of infection.
- For chemical burns, provide frequent wound irrigation with copious amounts of normal saline solution.
- Prepare for surgical intervention, including skin grafts and more thorough surgical debridement for major burns.

Administration station

Expect to administer:
- pain medication and anti-inflammatories as needed
- analgesics intravenous (IV), rather than intramuscular (IM), because tissue damage associated with the burn injury may impair absorption of the drug if given IM
- lactated Ringer's solution or a fluid replacement formula to prevent hypovolemic shock and maintain cardiac output
- antimicrobial therapy
- bronchodilators and mucolytics to aid in the removal of secretions.

Caustic substance ingestion

Caustic substances can be strong acids or strong bases. The most damaging substances are industrial products because they are highly concentrated. However, some common household products, including toilet bowl and drain cleaners, as well as some dishwasher detergents, contain damaging caustic substances such as sodium hydroxide and sulfuric acid.

Caustic substances are available as solids and liquids. The fact that solids stick to a moist surface (such as the lips) may prevent a person from consuming a large amount of the product. Because liquids don't stick, it's easier to consume more of the product and possibly damage the entire esophagus.

Regular offenders

Common acid-containing sources include:
- toilet bowl–cleaning products
- automotive battery liquid
- rust-removing products
- metal-cleaning products
- cement-cleaning products
- drain-cleaning products
- soldering flux containing zinc chloride.

Common alkaline-containing sources include:
- drain-cleaning products
- ammonia-containing products
- oven-cleaning products
- swimming pool–cleaning products
- automatic dishwasher detergent
- hair relaxers
- Clinitest tablets
- bleaches
- cement.

What causes it

Ingestion of a caustic substance can be accidental, such as ingestion by a young child, or deliberate, as in an attempted suicide.

How it happens

The extent of the injury is determined by the amount of the ingested material, its concentration and form, and whether the patient has vomited or aspirated.
- After ingestion, an extreme inflammatory reaction occurs that results in erythema and edema of the superficial layers.
- Ingestion of caustic substances can cause esophageal stricture and laryngeal stenosis and can increase the risk of esophageal cancer.
- Alkaline cleaners, such as drain cleaner, are generally tasteless and odorless, allowing larger amounts to be ingested. These substances tend to cause injury to the mucosa and submucosa of the esophagus. Alkaline substances cause liquefaction necrosis, a process in which necrosis continues from the superficial layers into the deeper tissues.
- Acidic cleaners, such as chlorinated household cleaners, undergo oxygenation reactions and form hydrochloric acid, which causes gastric injury if ingested. These agents cause coagulation necrosis, a process in which a protective layer forms at the site of the injury and limits its depth.

Less odor equals more danger; because they're generally tasteless and odorless, alkaline cleaners can be ingested in large amounts.

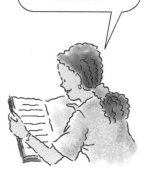

What to look for
- Abdominal pain or guarding
- Airway obstruction
- Altered mental status
- Burns around the mouth
- Diarrhea
- Drooling
- History of ingesting poisons
- Nausea and vomiting
- Odd breath odors (See *Identifying breath odor*, page 510.)
- Respiratory distress
- Saliva or foaming at the mouth
- Unresponsiveness

Identifying breath odor

The patient's breath odor may help determine what has been ingested, especially if unconscious.

Breath odor	Possible substance
Alcohol	• Chloral hydrate • Ethanol • Phenols
Acetone	• Acetone • Isopropyl alcohol • Salicylates
Bitter almond	• Cyanide
Coal gas	• Carbon monoxide
Garlic	• Arsenic • Organophosphates • Phosphorus
Nonspecific	• Possible inhalant use
Wintergreen	• Methyl salicylates

What tests tell you

- pH testing of saliva determines whether the substance is an acid or a base; however, a neutral pH can't rule out ingestion of a caustic substance. A pH of less than 2.0 (acidic substance) or greater than 12.5 (alkaline substance) indicates the potential for severe tissue damage.
- CBC and electrolyte, BUN, creatinine, and ABG levels evaluate the patient's renal status and acid–base balance as well as the blood oxygen ventilation status.
- Urinalysis can evaluate the patient's renal status because many toxic and caustic substances can be excreted through the kidneys.
- Ethanol and toxicologic screens rule out or confirm cases of suspected intentional ingestion by evaluating the levels of these substances in the blood.
- Chest X-ray may reveal mediastinitis, pleural effusions, pneumoperitoneum, and aspiration pneumonitis.
- Abdominal X-ray may reveal pneumoperitoneum or ascites.

What to do

- Provide supplemental oxygen and prepare the patient for emergency ET intubation, cricothyroidotomy, or tracheostomy and mechanical ventilation if necessary.
- Initiate suicide precautions if appropriate.

- Initiate NPO status.
- Obtain a history, including the substance and the amount ingested.
- Assess LOC; airway; and rate, depth, and pattern of respirations.
- Auscultate the lung and heart sounds.
- Obtain vital signs, noting hypotension and fever.
- Observe the electrocardiogram tracing for arrhythmias.
- Don't induce emesis or perform gastric intubation and lavage, which may induce emesis; inducing emesis can reintroduce the caustic substances to the upper gastrointestinal tract.

Call the pros

- Contact Poison Control or a toxicology center to get quick, accurate information, suggestions, and recommendations for treatment.
- Wash the mouth and face to remove any particles of the ingested substance.
- Anticipate administering broad-spectrum antibiotics, antireflux medication, or sucralfate as ordered.

Look, listen, and ask

- Observe for drooling and dysphagia.
- Inspect the oropharyngeal cavity for burns and injury.
- Listen to the patient's voice to detect laryngitis, hoarseness, and dysphagia.
- Assess for chest pain.
- Observe for stridor.
- Ask about vomiting.
- Auscultate bowel sounds.
- Assess for abdominal pain; a boardlike, rigid abdomen; and other signs of peritonitis.
- Signs and symptoms of peritonitis, fever, chest pain, and hypotension suggest a full-thickness gastric injury or perforation, which requires immediate surgical intervention.
- Monitor serum electrolyte levels.
- Contact Child Protective Services or Adult Protective Services if abuse or neglect is suspected of a child or older adult.

Careful preparation

Prepare the patient for:
- flexible nasopharyngoscopy, laryngoscopy, or endoscopy to visualize the injuries
- chest X-ray to check the mediastinal width and detect free air in the mediastinum or abdomen
- neck X-ray if stridor is present
- surgical intervention, such as exploratory laparotomy or thoracotomy with possible esophagectomy, esophagogastrectomy, or gastrectomy for a full-thickness injury

- periodic esophagography with water-soluble contrast and possible esophageal stenting or dilatation with contrast to detect and correct dysphagia.

Hyperthermia

Hyperthermia, also known as *heat syndrome*, refers to an elevation in body temperature to more than 99° F (37.2° C). It may result from environmental or internal conditions that increase heat production or impair heat dissipation.

What causes it

Hyperthermia may result from excessive exercise, infection, or use of drugs such as amphetamines. It may also result from an impaired ability to dissipate heat. (See *Heatstroke in older adults*.) Factors that impair heat dissipation include:
- high temperatures or humidity
- lack of acclimatization
- excess clothing
- cardiovascular disease
- obesity
- dehydration
- sweat gland dysfunction
- drugs, such as amphetamines
- drug and alcohol withdrawal
- prolonged exertion
- the aging process.

Ages and stages

Heatstroke in older adults

As an individual ages, the thirst mechanism and ability to sweat decreases. These factors put the older adult at risk for heatstroke, especially during hot summer days. Heatstroke must be treated rapidly to prevent serious complications or death. To help prevent heatstroke, teach older adult patients to follow these instructions:
- Reduce activity in hot weather, especially outdoor activity.
- Wear lightweight, loose-fitting clothing during hot weather; when outdoors, wear a hat and sunglasses and avoid wearing dark colors that absorb sunlight.

- Drink plenty of fluids, especially water, and avoid tea, coffee, and alcohol because they can cause dehydration.
- Use air conditioning or open windows (making sure that a secure screen is in place) and use a fan to help circulate air. If the patient doesn't have air conditioning at home, during periods of excessive heat, suggest attending community resources that have air conditioning, such as senior centers, libraries, and churches. Some community centers may even provide transportation.

How it happens

Humans normally adjust to excessive temperatures with complex cardiovascular and neurologic changes that are coordinated by the hypothalamus. Heat loss offsets heat production to regulate body temperature. The body loses heat by the process of evaporation or vasodilation, which cools the body's surface by radiation, conduction, and convection. However, when heat loss mechanisms fail to offset heat production, the body retains heat.

- The process of hypothermia begins with dehydration and electrolyte abnormalities and progresses to thermoregulatory dysfunction and ultimately multisystem organ failure. (Saqe-Rockoff et al., 2018).
- As the temperature rises, oxygen consumption and metabolic rate also increase.
- Essential enzymes cease to function above 108° F (42° C), and cellular needs can no longer be met.
- For every 1.8° F (1° C) increase in body temperature, body metabolic rate increases by 13% impairing the ability of the CNS, cells, and cardiac system to function properly.
- At body temperature of 104° F (40° C), the body has a 39% increase in metabolism, and at 107.6° F (42° C), the body's cellular needs cannot be met because of insufficient oxygen.

Feeling hot, hot, hot

Hyperthermia occurs in varying degrees:
- Mild hyperthermia (heat cramps or heat rash) occurs with excessive perspiration and loss of salt from the body.
- Moderate hyperthermia (heat exhaustion) occurs when the body is subjected to high temperatures and blood accumulates in the skin in an attempt to decrease the body's temperature. This accumulation causes a decrease in circulating blood volume, which decreases cerebral blood flow. Heat syncope then occurs (Centers for Disease Control and Prevention, 2018f).
- Critical hyperthermia (heatstroke) occurs when the body's temperature continues to rise and internal organs become damaged, which can eventually result in death.

What to look for

Assessment findings vary with the degree of hyperthermia. (See *Hyperthermia signs and symptoms*, page 514.) Assess older adults who present with altered mental status and are exposed to hot climates. Inadequate fluid intake and dehydration can quickly lead to urinary tract infections.

Hyperthermia signs and symptoms

Hyperthermia may be classified as mild (heat cramps and heat rash), moderate (heat exhaustion and heat syncope), or critical (heatstroke) (Centers for Disease Control and Prevention, 2018a, 2018b, 2018c, 2018d, 2018e, 2018f). This table highlights the major assessment findings associated with each classification.

Classification	Assessment findings
Mild hyperthermia (heat cramps and heat rash)	• Temperature ranging from 99° to 102° F (37.2° to 38.9° C) • Mild agitation (central nervous system findings otherwise normal) • Mild hypertension • Moist, cool skin and muscle tenderness; involved muscle groups possibly hard and lumpy • Muscle twitching and spasms (heat cramps) • Nausea, abdominal cramps (heat cramps) • Report of prolonged activity in a very warm or hot environment without adequate salt intake • Skin irritation from excessive sweating (heat rash) • Tachycardia
Moderate hyperthermia (heat exhaustion and heat syncope)	• Temperature elevated up to 104° F (40° C) • Dizziness • Headache • Hypotension • Muscle cramping • Nausea and vomiting • Oliguria • Pale, moist skin • Rapid, thready pulse • Syncope or confusion (heat syncope) • Thirst • Weakness
Critical hyperthermia (heatstroke)	• Temperature greater than 106° F (41.1° C) • Atrial or ventricular tachycardia • Confusion, combativeness, delirium • Fixed, dilated pupils • Hot, dry, reddened skin • Loss of consciousness • Seizures • Tachypnea

What tests tell you

No single diagnostic test confirms hyperthermia, but these test results may help support the diagnosis:

- ABG results may reveal respiratory alkalosis and hypoxemia.
- Alanine transaminase levels will be elevated (in heatstroke).
- CBC may reveal leukocytosis and increased HCT secondary to hemoconcentration.
- Electrolyte levels may show hypokalemia and hyponatremia.

- Other blood studies may reveal elevated BUN level, increased bleeding and clotting times, and fibrinolysis.
- Urinalysis may show concentrated urine with elevated protein levels, tubular casts, and myoglobinuria and increased specific gravity.

How it's treated

Mild or moderate hyperthermia is treated by allowing the patient to rest in a cool environment. Oral or IV fluid and electrolyte replacement is administered if needed and as ordered.

Critical measures

Measures for treating critical hyperthermia include:

- removing the patient's clothing and applying cool water to the skin and then fanning the patient with cool air
- administering medications that may be ordered, such as to control shivering and urine output
- applying hypothermia blankets and ice packs to the groin and axillae if necessary
- continuing treatment until the patient's body temperature drops to 101° F (38.3° C). Do not allow temperature to drop any further, as hypothermia may develop.

> We could probably all use some rest in a cool environment, but for patients with hyperthermia, it is of the utmost importance.

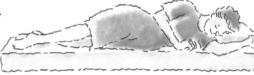

In addition to the cooldown

Supportive measures for hyperthermia include:

- oxygen therapy
- central venous pressure and pulmonary artery wedge pressure monitoring
- rehydration
- ET intubation, if necessary.

What to do

- Assess ABCDEs and initiate emergency resuscitative measures as indicated.
- Remove as much of the patient's clothing as possible.
- Assess oxygen saturation and administer supplemental oxygen as indicated and ordered. Monitor the patient's pulmonary status closely, including respiratory rate and depth and lung sounds; anticipate the need for ET intubation and mechanical ventilation if respiratory status deteriorates.
- Assess neurologic and cardiac status closely, including heart rate and rhythm. Institute continuous cardiac monitoring to evaluate for arrhythmias secondary to electrolyte imbalances. Monitor hemodynamic parameters; assess peripheral circulation, including skin color, peripheral pulses, and capillary refill.

- Monitor vital signs continuously, especially core body temperature. Although the goal is to reduce the patient's temperature rapidly, too rapid a reduction can lead to vasoconstriction, which can cause shivering. Shivering increases metabolic demand and oxygen consumption and should be prevented if possible.
- Establish IV access for hydration and medications as needed.
- Employ external cooling measures, such as cool, wet sheets; tepid baths with a cooling fan to blow over the skin; and cooling blankets.
- Place an indwelling urinary catheter, if ordered, to monitor urine output in patients with heatstroke.
- Monitor fluid and electrolyte balance and laboratory test results. Assess renal function studies to evaluate for rhabdomyolysis.

Hypothermia

Hypothermia is defined as a core body temperature 95° F (35° C) (Zafren & Crawford Mechem, 2018). It may be classified as:
- *mild*—90° to 95° F (32° to 35° C)
- *moderate*—82° to 90° F (28° to 32° C)
- *severe*—below 82° F (below 28° C), which can be fatal.

What causes it

Hypothermia commonly results from drowning in cold water, prolonged exposure to cold temperatures, disease or debility that alters homeostasis, or administration of large amounts of cold solutions or blood products.

Likely candidates

The risk of serious cold injury, especially hypothermia, is higher in patients who are:
- very young
- older than 65 (older adults)
- lacking in insulating body fat
- wearing wet or inadequate clothing
- using drugs or alcohol or smoking
- suffering from cardiac disease
- fatigued
- malnourished with a depletion of caloric reserve.

How it happens

In hypothermia, metabolic changes slow the functions of most major organ systems, resulting in decreased renal blood flow and decreased glomerular filtration. Vital organs are physiologically affected. Severe hypothermia results in depression of cerebral blood flow, diminished oxygen requirements, reduced cardiac output, and decreased arterial pressure.

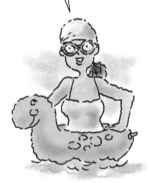

Hypothermia can result from drowning in cold water.

What to look for

Obtaining the history of a patient with a cold injury may reveal:
- cause of hypothermia
- temperature to which the patient was exposed
- length of exposure.

Temperature dependent

Assessment findings in a patient with hypothermia vary with the patient's body temperature:
- **Mild hypothermia (90° to 95° F [32° to 35° C]):** Symptoms may include early tachycardia followed by bradycardia, tachypnea, slurred speech, or impaired judgment.
- **Moderate hypothermia (82° to 90° F [28° to 32° C]):** Symptoms may include unresponsiveness, peripheral cyanosis, and muscle rigidity or atrial arrhythmias. Patients who are improperly rewarmed may show signs of shock.
- **Severe hypothermia below 82° F (below 28° C):** Symptoms may include an absence of palpable pulses, no audible heart sounds, nonreactive or dilated pupils, and a rigor mortis–like state. Ventricular fibrillation and a loss of deep tendon reflexes are common.

How it's treated

Treatment for hypothermia consists of supportive measures and specific rewarming techniques, including:
- passive rewarming (when the patient rewarms on his or her own, without other intervention other than possibly drinking a warm nonalcoholic liquid that is high in carbohydrates; Ignatavicius et al., 2018)
- active external rewarming with heating blankets, warm water immersion, heated objects such as water bottles, and radiant heat
- active core rewarming with warmed IV fluids; warm humidified oxygen; genitourinary tract irrigation; extracorporeal rewarming; hemodialysis; and peritoneal, gastric, and mediastinal lavage.

Cardiac concerns

Arrhythmias that develop usually convert to normal sinus rhythm with rewarming. If the patient has no pulse or respirations, cardiopulmonary resuscitation (CPR) is needed until rewarming raises the core temperature to at least 89.6° F (32° C).

Monitoring dependent

The administration of oxygen, ET intubation, controlled ventilation, IV fluids, and treatment for metabolic acidosis depend on test results and careful patient monitoring.

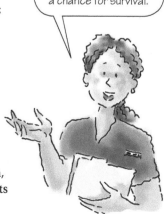

CPR is OK for hypothermia victims. Even when they've been unresponsive for a while, their lack of brain anoxia provides a chance for survival.

What to do

- Assess the patient's ABCDEs.
- Initiate CPR if patient does not have spontaneous circulation (Ignatavicius et al., 2018). Keep in mind that hypothermia helps protect the brain from anoxia, which normally accompanies prolonged cardiopulmonary arrest. Therefore, even if the patient has been unresponsive for a long time, CPR may be resuscitative, especially after a cold water drowning.
- Administer supplemental oxygen and prepare for ET intubation and mechanical ventilation if necessary.
- Initiate continuous cardiac monitoring.
- Assist with rewarming techniques as necessary. (In cases of moderate to severe hypothermia, only experienced personnel should attempt aggressive rewarming.)
- During rewarming, provide supportive measures as ordered, including mechanical ventilation and heated, humidified therapy to maintain tissue oxygenation, and IV fluids that have been warmed with a warming coil to correct hypotension and maintain urine output.
- Continuously monitor the patient's core body temperature and other vital signs during and after initial rewarming. Continuously monitor cardiac status, including continuous cardiac monitoring, for evidence of arrhythmias.
- If using a hyperthermia blanket, discontinue the warming when core body temperature is within 1° to 2° F (0.6° to 1.1° C) of the desired temperature. The patient's temperature will continue to rise even when the device is turned off.

As time goes by

- If the patient has been hypothermic for longer than 45 to 60 minutes, administer additional fluids as ordered to compensate for the expansion of the vascular space that occurs during vasodilation in rewarming. Monitor heart rate and hemodynamic parameters closely to evaluate fluid needs and response to treatment.
- Monitor hourly output, fluid balance, and serum electrolyte levels, especially potassium. Stay alert for signs and symptoms of hyperkalemia. If hyperkalemia occurs, administer calcium chloride, sodium bicarbonate, glucose, and insulin as ordered. Anticipate the need for sodium polystyrene sulfonate (Kayexalate) enemas. If the potassium level is extremely elevated, prepare the patient for dialysis.

Frostbite

Frostbite is a cold-related injury that results in tissue damage due to cold temperature exposure. The extent of damage to the skin and surrounding tissues ranges from first degree (redness, edema, and cold to touch) to fourth degree (full-thickness necrosis that extends into the muscle and bone) (Ignatavicius et al., 2018). The initial assessment and history should include:

- environmental temperature
- duration of exposure
- humidity
- wet or dry conditions
- first aid and rewarming efforts
- ambulation attempts before and after rewarming
- previous frostbite injuries.

What causes it

Tissue damage occurs when ice crystals form within the cells or outside the cells causing intracellular dehydration through osmosis. It also occurs in venous stasis and thrombosis leading to hypoxia and then vasospasm, ischemia, and tissue necrosis. Tissue damage may not be evident until after reperfusion when swelling leads to thrombus formation, inflammatory leukocyte infiltration, and then necrosis. The extent of the damage, which may include gangrene, may evolve over weeks to months. Feet, hands, earlobes, nose, cheeks, and chin are the most frequently affected areas of the body.

Likely candidates

Risk increases in persons who:

- work outdoors
- are homeless
- exhibit poor self-care, intoxication, altered mental status, or immobility
- are athletes engaging in cold weather sports
- are winter outdoor enthusiasts, such as skiers, snowshoers, and mountain climbers.

Various medical conditions increase the risk for frostbite including:

- diabetes
- peripheral vascular disease
- cardiovascular disease
- Raynaud phenomena
- previous history of frostbite.

Stages of frostbite

First-degree frostbite: The skin is hyperemic. Edema forms around the affected area.

Second-degree frostbite: Large blisters filled with milky or clear fluid develop, and partial-thickness necrosis is present.

Third-degree frostbite: Small blisters with dark fluid are present. The affected area is cool, numb, nonblanchable, and either blue or red. The injury requires debridement.

Fourth-degree frostbite: Blistering and edema are absent. Full-thickness necrosis extends to the muscle and bone, and the body part is cold, numb, and devoid of circulation. Gangrene can follow (Ignatavicius et al., 2018).

What tests tell you

Lab tests

- In first-degree frostbite cases, no lab tests are indicated.
- For second-, third-, and fourth-degree frostbite, a CBC, electrolytes, BUN, creatinine, glucose, and a urinalysis for evidence of myoglobinuria may be considered.

Imaging

- Technetium 99m bone scanning is helpful in determining tissue and bone viability and assists in making amputation decisions within 2 to 7 days after cold injury.
- Angiography is helpful in assessing tissue before and after thrombolysis.

How it's treated

Treatment modalities are based on the age of the injury and may require rewarming the affected part, analgesia, administration of fluids to enhance blood flow and tissue perfusion, blister debridement or aspiration, tetanus and antibacterial prophylaxis, and application of topical medications. Rewarming helps to reduce the amount of tissue loss.

What to do

- Remove constrictive clothing or jewelry.
- If injury is less than 24 hours old, rewarm the affected part in warm water (99° to 102° F [37° to 39° C]; Freer et al., 2016) by swirling while avoiding touching the side of the container (Ignatavicius et al., 2018). Avoid dry heat. Stop rewarming when the part is warm, red, and pliable.
- **Do not** remove blood-filled blisters. This exposes deeper underlying structures to dehydration and infection.
- Place sterile gauze between the affected fingers or toes to prevent maceration.

- Wrap affected part in a loose bandage or sterile sheet.
- Splint and elevate the affected part.
- Administer analgesics for pain control and antibiotics to treat infection.
- Administer tetanus prophylaxis if vaccination status is not current or unknown.
- Reassess for soft tissue injury, dehydration, mental status changes, or respiratory difficulty.
- Hypovolemia and hypokalemia may need correction.
- Teach that the full extent of tissue damage may not be evident for 1 to 3 months.
- Instruct to avoid tobacco, alcohol, and caffeine due to their vasoconstrictive effects, thus reducing the blood supply to the affected part.

Animal and human bites

Because many animal and human bites go unreported, it is difficult to estimate the incidence of bite wounds; however, the Centers for Disease Control and Prevention (2018g) states that one in five people bitten by dogs requires medical attention. Other common sources of bites include cats, rats, humans, and, to a lesser extent, exotic animals.

The initial history and assessment should include:

- time and location of the incident
- type of animal and its status (health, vaccination history, behavior, current location, ownership)
- circumstances surrounding the bite (provoked, defensive vs. un-provoked)
- location of the bite
- full description of the bite
- first aid and prehospital treatment
- medical history, including tetanus and rabies vaccination history, and conditions compromising immune function.

What causes it

Most cat and dog bites are inflicted by provoked animals that belong to family or friends. Rat bites occur more commonly among laboratory personnel and children of lower socioeconomic status. Human bites are more frequently associated with rapes, sexual assaults, and other forms of battery.

- Large dogs can inflict the most serious wounds. An adult dog can exert greater than 200 lb (90.7 kg) of pressure, resulting in a crush wound causing damage to vessels, tendons, muscles, nerves, and bones. Most fatalities in children are caused by bites to the face and neck.

- Cat bites place individuals at high risk for infection due to puncture wounds caused by sharp pointed teeth pushing bacteria deep into the tissue. Infection usually appears in less than 24 hours.
- Occlusal human bites frequently cause lacerations or crush injuries. Clenched fist injuries occur when a fist strikes the teeth and mouth of another individual. These appear as several small wounds over the metacarpophalangeal joints in the dominant hand (referred to as *fight bites*). These are serious injuries with high risk of infection. When the hand unclenches, bacteria are trapped in puncture wounds within joints. Most human bites occur in the upper extremities.
- Hand bites have the highest rate of infection due to the relatively poor blood supply of many structures in the hand. Anatomically, it is more difficult to thoroughly irrigate and cleanse hand wounds.
- Local infections and cellulitis are the leading cause of morbidity from bite wounds and can potentially lead to sepsis, particularly in immunocompromised individuals.
- Bites from wild or sick-appearing animals (dogs, cats, skunks, bats, and raccoons) raise concern for rabies exposure.

What to look for

Inspect the wound for bleeding, crush injury, deep penetrating injury, lacerations, and devitalized tissue. Note any signs of infection, redness, drainage, swelling, and pain. Note range of motion of the affected area and any additional injuries. Assess for any numbness, tingling, or loss of sensation distal to the wound. Observe for signs of systemic infection such as fever, tachycardia, hypotension, rashes, or elevated white blood cell count. Assess for fractures and head or neck injuries.

What tests tell you

Lab tests
- Aerobic and anaerobic cultures are taken from infected wounds. Cultures are usually not taken if there are no signs of infection.
- CBC is taken if there are signs of infection.

Imaging
- Plain radiographs are taken when fracture, foreign body, or infection are suspected near a joint space.
- Plain films and computed tomography scans are taken in children who have been bitten in the head.
- Cervical spine films are taken in children who have been shaken.

How it's treated

Treatment modalities are based on the location, age, and severity of the injury. Provide for initial stabilization of homeostasis. Control bleeding. Observe and ensure adequate airway when the bite is located on the head or neck. Treatment may include IV fluids, wound irrigation, debridement, wound closure, administration of antibiotics, analgesics, and tetanus prophylaxis.

Rabies immunoprophylaxis

- Is not required if rabies is not known or suspected
- May be warranted if the bite is from a skunk, raccoon, bat, or fox
- May be warranted if the dog or cat who bit is from a rabies-known area and cannot be quarantined for 10 days
- May be warranted if a previously healthy dog or cat becomes ill while quarantined and awaiting results of rabies fluorescent antibody test

What to do

- Remove constrictive clothing or jewelry.
- Inspect the wound for pus, erythema, or necrosis and culture for abscess, severe cellulitis, devitalized tissue, or signs of sepsis.
- Prepare for wound to be anesthetized prior to a thorough medical evaluation, cleaning, and debridement.
- Photograph the wound per hospital policy for evidence in criminal and legal proceedings.
- Irrigate the wound with copious amounts of saline or prescribed solution.
- Bite wounds that cannot be thoroughly cleansed, like cat bites or other puncture wounds, will usually be left open to avoid trapping bacteria in the wound. Teach to watch for signs of infection.
- Bite wounds to the hands and lower extremities more than 8 to 12 hours old or in an immunocompromised patient may be left open due to the high risk of infection.
- Apply a bulky dressing or splint to limit use and promote elevation of a hand injury.
- Administer analgesics for pain control, antibiotics to treat infection, and tetanus prophylaxis per recommendations in "Rabies immunoprophylaxis."
- Initiate rabies treatment protocol when appropriate. Explain the process and follow-up procedures.
- Instruct proper wound care and to watch for and report signs of infection.

Poisoning

Poisoning refers to inhalation, ingestion, and injection of, or skin contamination from, any harmful substance. It is a common environmental emergency. The prognosis depends on the amount of poison absorbed, its toxicity, and the time interval between poisoning and treatment. (See *Poisoning facts.*)

What causes it

Because of their curiosity and ignorance, children are the most common poison victims. Accidental poisoning (usually from the ingestion of salicylates [aspirin], cleaning agents, insecticides, paints, cosmetics, and plants) is a leading cause of death in children.

In adults, poisoning is common among chemical company employees—particularly those in companies that use chlorine, carbon dioxide, hydrogen sulfide, nitrogen dioxide, and ammonia—and in companies that ignore safety standards. Other causes of poisoning in adults include improper cooking, canning, and storage of food; ingestion of or skin contamination from plants (e.g., dieffenbachia, mistletoe, azalea, and philodendron); and accidental or intentional drug overdose or chemical ingestion.

How it happens

The pathophysiology of poisons depends on the substance that is inhaled or ingested. The extent of damage depends on the pH of the substance, the amount ingested, its form (solid or liquid), and the length of exposure to it.

Substances with an alkaline pH cause tissue damage by liquefaction necrosis, which softens the tissue. Acids produce coagulation necrosis. Coagulation necrosis denatures (changes the molecular composition of) proteins when the substance contacts tissue. This limits the extent of the injury by preventing penetration of the acid into the tissue.

The mechanism of action for inhalants is unknown, but they're believed to act on the CNS similarly to a very potent anesthetic. Hydrocarbons sensitize the myocardial tissue and allow it to be sensitive to catecholamines, resulting in arrhythmias.

What to look for

The patient's history should reveal the poison's source and form of exposure (ingestion, inhalation, injection, or skin contact). Assessment findings vary with the poison. (See *Pinpointing poison's effects.*)

Ages and stages

Poisoning facts

Older adults who accidentally overdose do so usually because of polypharmacy, improper use of their prescribed medication, improper storage of the medication (not in its original container), or mistaking the identity of the medication.

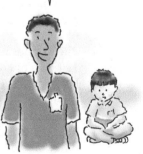

Household plant ingestion is one of the most common poisoning sources in children.

Pinpointing poison's effects

Review the assessment findings and possible toxins listed below to help determine what type of poison is causing your patient's signs and symptoms.

Agitation, delirium
Alcohol, amphetamines, atropine, barbiturates, neostigmine, scopolamine

Coma
Atropine, barbiturates, bromide, carbon monoxide, chloral hydrate, ethanol, paraldehyde, salicylates, scopolamine

Constricted pupils
Barbiturates, chloral hydrate, morphine, propoxyphene

Diaphoresis
Alcohol, fluoride, insulin, physostigmine

Diarrhea, nausea, vomiting
Alcohol (ethanol, methanol, ethylene glycol), cardiac glycosides, heavy metals (lead, arsenic), morphine and its analogs, salicylates

Dilated pupils
Alcohol, amphetamines, belladonna alkaloids (such as atropine and scopolamine), botulinum toxin, cocaine, cyanide, ephedrine, glutethimide, meperidine, parasympathomimetics

Dry mouth
Antihistamines, belladonna alkaloids, botulinum toxin, morphine, phenothiazines, tricyclic antidepressants

Extrapyramidal tremor
Phenothiazines

Hematemesis
Fluoride, mercuric chloride, phosphorus, salicylates

Kussmaul respirations
Ethanol, ethylene glycol, methanol, salicylates

Partial or total blindness
Methanol

Pink skin
Atropine (flushed, dry skin), carbon monoxide, cyanide, phenothiazines

Seizures
Alcohol (ethanol, methanol, ethylene glycol), amphetamines, carbon monoxide, cholinesterase inhibitors, hydrocarbons, phenothiazines, propoxyphene, salicylates, strychnine

What tests tell you
- Toxicology studies (including drug screens) of poison levels in the mouth, vomitus, urine, stool, or blood, or on the victim's hands or clothing, confirm the diagnosis. If possible, have the family or patient bring the container holding the poison to the ED for comparable study.
- In inhalation poisoning, chest X-rays may show aspiration pneumonia; for petroleum distillate inhalation, X-rays may show pulmonary infiltrates or edema. Abdominal X-rays may reveal iron pills or other radiopaque substances.
- ABG analysis, serum electrolyte levels, and CBC are used to evaluate oxygenation, ventilation, and the metabolic status of seriously poisoned patients.

What to do

- Contact Poison Control for specific treatment modalities and antidotes. Provide information directly from the containers when possible.
- Initial treatment includes emergency resuscitation, support of the patient's ABCs, and prevention of further poison absorption. Secondary treatment consists of continuing supportive or symptomatic care and, when possible, administration of a specific antidote.
- A poisoning victim who exhibits altered LOC routinely receives oxygen, glucose, and naloxone (Narcan). Activated charcoal is effective in eliminating many toxic substances. Specific treatment depends on the poison.
- Carefully monitor vital signs and LOC. If necessary, begin CPR.
- Depending on the poison, prevent further absorption by administering activated charcoal, inducing emesis, or by administering gastric lavage and cathartics (magnesium sulfate). The treatment's effectiveness depends on the speed of absorption and the time elapsed between ingestion and removal.

Emesis nemesis

- Never induce emesis if corrosive acid poisoning is suspected, if the patient is unconscious or has seizures, or if the gag reflex is impaired, even in a conscious patient. Instead, neutralize the poison by instilling the appropriate antidote by an NG tube. Common antidotes include milk, magnesium salts (milk of magnesia), activated charcoal, or other chelating agents, such as deferoxamine and edetate disodium.
- When possible, add the antidote to water or juice.
- To perform gastric lavage, instill 30 mL of fluid by NG tube and then aspirate the liquid; repeat until the aspirate is clear. Save vomitus and aspirate for analysis. (To prevent aspiration in the unconscious patient, an ET tube should be in place before lavage.)

Enter the IV

- If several hours have passed since the patient ingested the poison, use large quantities of IV fluids to force the poison through the kidneys to be excreted. The kind of fluid used depends on the patient's acid–base balance, cardiovascular status, and the flow rate necessary for effective diuresis of poison.
- If ingested poisoning is severe and requires peritoneal dialysis or hemodialysis, assist as necessary.

Give the patient some air

- To prevent further absorption of inhaled poison, remove the patient to fresh or uncontaminated air. Provide supplemental oxygen and, if needed, intubation. To prevent further absorption from skin contamination, remove the clothing covering the contaminated skin and immediately flush the area with large amounts of water.
- If the patient has severe pain, give analgesics as ordered; frequently monitor fluid intake and output, vital signs, and LOC.
- Keep the patient warm and provide support in a quiet environment.
- If the poison was ingested intentionally, obtain a psychiatric consultation and refer for counseling to help prevent future suicide attempts.

Quick quiz

1.   An adult patient brought to the ED has partial- and full-thickness burn injuries to the anterior chest, anterior abdomen, and entire right arm. Using the rule of nines, which percentage of total BSA does the nurse calculate has been affected?
   A.   18%
   B.   27%
   C.   45%
   D.   50%

Answer: B. The anterior chest and abdomen constitute 18% of the BSA, and the entire right arm is 9%, for a total of 27%.

2.   A patient admitted to the ED is suspected of taking an overdose of atropine. Which assessment data does the nurse anticipate?
   A.   Kussmaul respirations
   B.   Diarrhea and nausea and vomiting
   C.   Hot, dry skin and dilated pupils
   D.   Extrapyramidal tremors

Answer: C. A patient who has overdosed on atropine will have hot, dry skin and dilated pupils.

3.   How does the nurse document the type of hypothermia for a patient who has a core body temperature of 80° F (26.7° C)?
   A.   Low
   B.   Mild
   C.   Moderate
   D.   Severe

Answer: D. Severe hypothermia is a core body temperature of less than 82.4° F (<28° C).

4.   A patient who is unconscious is brought to the ED with a very strong wintergreen odor to the breath. What does the nurse anticipate may have been ingested?
   A.   Ethanol
   B.   Acetone
   C.   Methyl salicylates
   D.   Cyanide

Answer: C. If a patient has ingested methyl salicylates, the breath will have a wintergreen odor.

Scoring

 If you answered all four questions correctly, stop and smell the roses! You're quite erudite when it comes to environmental emergencies.

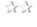 If you answered three questions correctly, breathe in the smell of success! Hopefully, lightning will strike again for you in the next chapter.

 If you answered fewer than three questions correctly, don't let it rain on your parade. Review the chapter again and give it another try.

Selected references

Centers for Disease Control and Prevention. (2018a). *Heat cramps.* Retrieved from https://www.cdc.gov/niosh/topics/heatstress/heatrelillness.html#_Heat_Cramps

Centers for Disease Control and Prevention. (2018b). *Heat exhaustion.* Retrieved from https://www.cdc.gov/niosh/topics/heatstress/heatrelillness.html#_Heat_Exhaustion

Centers for Disease Control and Prevention. (2018c). *Heat rash.* Retrieved from https://www.cdc.gov/niosh/topics/heatstress/heatrelillness.html#_Heat_Rash

Centers for Disease Control and Prevention. (2018d). *Heat stress.* Retrieved from https://www.cdc.gov/niosh/topics/heatstress/default.html

Centers for Disease Control and Prevention. (2018e). *Heat stroke.* Retrieved from https://www.cdc.gov/niosh/topics/heatstress/heatrelillness.html#_Heat_Stroke

Centers for Disease Control and Prevention. (2018f). *Heat syncope.* Retrieved from https://www.cdc.gov/niosh/topics/heatstress/heatrelillness.html#_Heat_Syncope

Centers for Disease Control and Prevention. (2018g). *Preventing dog bites.* Retrieved from https://www.cdc.gov/features/dog-bite-prevention/

Freer, L., Handford, C., & Imray, C. H. E. (2016). Frostbite. In P. S. Auerbach, T. A. Cushing, & N. S. Harris (Eds.), *Auerbach's wilderness medicine* (7th ed., pp. 197–221). Philadelphia, PA: Elsevier.

Ignatavicius, D., Workman, M., & Rebar, C. (2018). *Medical-surgical nursing: Concepts for interprofessional collaborative care* (9th ed.). St. Louis, MO: Elsevier.

Saqe-Rockoff, A., Schubert, F. D., Ciardiello, A., et al. (2018). Improving thermoregulation for trauma patients in the emergency department: An evidence-based practice project. *Journal of Trauma Nursing, 25*(1), 14–20. doi:10.1097/JTN.0000000000000336

Zafren, K., & Crawford Mechem, C. (2018). *Accidental hypothermia in adults.* Retrieved from https://www.uptodate.com/contents/accidental-hypothermia-in-adults

Chapter 13

Mass casualty and disaster

Just the facts

In this chapter, you'll learn:

- ◆ types of disasters
- ◆ elements of disaster preparedness
- ◆ components of the National Preparedness Goal and the National Response Framework
- ◆ elements of an Incident Command Center and Hospital Incident Command System
- ◆ the nurse's role in mass casualty and disaster nursing
- ◆ functions of triage and tagging.

Introduction to mass casualty and disaster nursing

As the largest sector of the health care workforce, there is no question that nurses are an essential part of response to any type of disasters. Disasters are defined as an event causing damage or destruction and that interrupt the everyday life of a community. Disasters are often catastrophic events that result in many casualties overwhelming a community and taxing the health care resources within. As such, disasters are measured by their impact to health and health services and are categorized as natural or man-made.

Mass casualty incident (MCI) is a term that is often used to specifically describe an event in which medical resources are overwhelmed by a disaster or incident. Large emergency departments can handle multiple surges of patients with fewer depleted resources, whereas a surge of 20 patients may overwhelm a smaller rural emergency department.

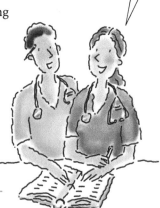

Nurses are often on the front line when caring for people who have been affected by a disaster.

Types of disasters

To best prepare to care for people affected by disasters, nurses benefit from understanding what constitutes the types of disasters.

Natural disasters

Natural disasters are caused by natural or environmental forces. These occur worldwide. All natural disasters are atmospheric, hydrologic, or geologic in nature and are classified into earthquakes, hurricanes, tornados, floods, or fires (Holleran et al., 2018). Almost all areas of the United States have experienced some form of a natural disaster, and all are vulnerable to experiencing one in the future.

Man-made disasters

Man-made disasters, just like they sound, are caused by mankind. They are accidental or intentional human-generated events, which can further be divided into the categories of complex emergencies, technologic disasters, and terrorism.

Complex emergencies result from war, civil strife, or other political conflict, causing severe property damage and/or human casualties. Technologic disasters include incidents that originate from human activities such as manufacturing, transportation, storage, and use of hazardous materials. Of the many definitions that can be found on terrorism, none are universally accepted. For purposes of this publication, terrorism refers to intentional, criminal, or malicious acts. Weapons of mass destruction (WMDs) are associated with terrorism and include the use of chemical, biological, radiological, nuclear, and explosive (CBRNE) agents along with arson, incendiary, armed attacks, industrial sabotage, and cyber terrorism.

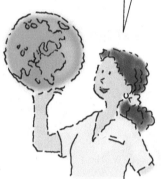

Weather events can be responsible for natural disasters.

Natural vs. man-made disasters

Natural and man-made disasters can be measured by the impact they have to life and property. Natural events are often referred to "acts of God" or situations where people have little control, whereas preparation, maintenance, security, and planning can mitigate the impact or outcome of a man-made disaster.

Disaster preparedness

History of disaster preparedness can be traced back before the birth of the United States. Early on, natural disasters that caused wide impact resulted in congressional acts to provide relief. This practice led to the Congressional Act of 1803, the first piece of disaster legislation, which provided assistance to Portsmouth, New Hampshire, after a devastating fire. Additional legislation was passed from the 1950s to 1980s strengthening the US government's ability to provide aid and recovery to those impacted by disasters, most notably the Robert T. Stafford Disaster Relief and Emergency Assistance Act.

The terrorist attacks on the New York City Twin Towers and the Pentagon in Washington, District of Columbia, on September 11, 2001, highlighted new and expounding threats giving rise to a new heightened level of preparedness: the Homeland Security Act of 2002 (Federal Emergency Management Agency [FEMA], 2002). Since then, additional strategies have been deployed on how agencies including local, state, federal, and private sector partners, including the health care sector, can prepare for and provide a unified domestic response to terrorist attacks, natural disasters, and other catastrophic events (FEMA, 2011; GMVEMS, 2018).

National Preparedness Goal

Today's National Preparedness Goal is to have "a secure and resilient nation with the capabilities required across the whole community to prevent, protect against, mitigate, respond to, and recover from the threats and hazards that pose the greatest risk" to the United States (FEMA, 2018; FEMA, 2019). Five Core Competencies of the National Preparedness Goal include (FEMA, 2018):

1. **Prevention**: Prevent, avoid, or stop an imminent, threatened, or actual act of terrorism.
2. **Protection**: Protect our citizens, residents, visitors, and assets against the greatest threats and hazards in a manner that allows our interests, aspirations, and way of life to thrive.
3. **Mitigation**: Reduce the loss of life and property by lessening the impact of future disasters.
4. **Response**: Respond quickly to save lives, protect property and the environment, and meet basic human needs in the aftermath of a catastrophic incident.
5. **Recovery**: Recover through a focus on the timely restoration, strengthening, and revitalization of infrastructure, housing, and a sustainable economy as well as the health, social, cultural, historic, and environmental fabric of communities affected by a catastrophic incident. (See *Core capabilities*, page 532.)

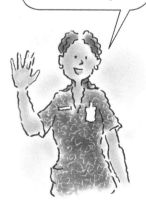

Remember, the Five Core Competencies of the National Preparedness Goal are Prevention, Protection, Mitigation, Response, and Recovery.

The National Preparedness System

The National Preparedness System (NPS) states that preparedness is a shared responsibility and follows a whole community approach to being prepared for all types of disasters in order to achieve the National Preparedness Goal. The whole community is composed of individuals, communities, private and nonprofit sectors, faith-based organizations, and all governments (local, regional/metropolitan, state, tribal, territorial, insular area, and federal). The NPS integrates efforts throughout the Core Competencies (Prevention, Protection, Mitigation, Response, and Recovery) to keep our nation secure and resilient (FEMA, 2016).

Core capabilities

Prevention	Protection	Mitigation	Response	Recovery
Planning				
Public information and warning				
Operational coordination				
Intelligence and information sharing		Community resilience	Infrastructure systems	
Interdiction and disruption		Long-term vulnerability reduction	Critical transportation	Economic recovery
Screening, search, and detection			Environmental response/health and safety	Health and social services
Forensics and attribution	Access control and identify verification	Risk and disaster resilience assessment	Fatality management services	Housing
	Cybersecurity	Threats and hazards identification	Fire management and suppression	Natural and cultural resources
	Physical protective measures		Logistics and supply chain management	
	Risk management for protection programs and activities		Mass care services	
	Supply chain integrity and security		Mass search and rescue operations	
			On-scene security, protection, and law enforcement	
			Operational communications	
			Public health, healthcare, and emergency medical services	
			Situational assessment	

Adapted from U.S. Department of Homeland Security. (2016). *National response framework.* Retrieved from https://www.fema.gov /media-library-data/1466014682982-9bcf8245ba4c60c120aa915abe74e15d/National_Response_Framework3rd.pdf

National Response Framework

The National Response Framework (NRF) is part of the NPS. It serves as a guide to how the whole community responds to all types of disasters and emergencies. This framework is a doctrine that is always in effect and describes how the nation responds to incidents. Built to be scalable, flexible, and adaptable, the concepts within this framework align key roles and responsibilities across the nation. Specific authorities and best practices

Core capabilities and critical tasks

	Objective	Critical tasks
Public health, healthcare, and emergency medical services	Provide lifesaving medical treatment via Emergency Medical Services and related operations and avoid additional disease and injury by providing targeted public health, medical, and behavioral health support, and products to all affected populations.	• Deliver medical countermeasures to exposed populations. • Complete triage and initial stabilization of illness or casualties and begin definitive care for those likely to benefit from care and survive. Develop public health interventions to maintain and improve the health of individuals placed at risk due to disruptions in healthcare and societal support networks. • Return medical surge resources to pre-incident levels, complete health assessments, and identify recovery processes.
Situational assessment	Provide all decision makers with decision-relevant information regarding the nature and extent of the hazard, any cascading effects, and the status of the response.	• Deliver information sufficient to inform decision making regarding immediate lifesaving and life-sustaining activities, and engage governmental, private, and civic sector resources within and outside of the affected area to meet basic human needs and stabilize the incident. • Deliver enhanced information to reinforce ongoing lifesaving and life-sustaining activities, and engage governmental, private, and civic sector resources within and outside of the affected area to meet basic human needs, stabilize the incident, and facilitate the integration of recovery activities.

Adapted from U.S. Department of Homeland Security. (2016). *National response framework*. Retrieved from https://www.fema.gov/media-library-data/1466014682982-9bcf8245ba4c60c120aa915abe74e15d/National_Response_Framework3rd.pdf

for managing incidents, ranging from the most serious local disasters to large-scale terrorist attacks or catastrophic natural disasters, are identified.

Within the NRF exist Core Capabilities and Critical Tasks—areas that are required to address threats and hazards (FEMA, 2016). Health care falls under Core Capability 14. The Public Health, Healthcare, and Emergency Medical Services' objective is to "provide lifesaving medical treatment via Emergency Medical Services and related operations and avoid additional disease and injury by providing targeted public health, medical, and behavioral health support, and products to all affected populations" (FEMA, 2016). (See *Core capabilities and critical tasks*.)

Emergency Support Functions (ESFs) are the ways in which resources are bundled and managed to deliver the Core Capabilities (FEMA, 2016). Health care is ESF 8, which is coordinated by the U.S. Department of Health & Human Services. Under ESF 8, functions include but are not limited to (FEMA, 2016):

- public health
- medical surge support including patient movement
- behavioral health services
- mass fatality management.

National Incident Management System

A coordinated response to incidents requires that all sectors work together with a common operating picture to ensure best outcomes. The NRF is built on the National Incident Management System (NIMS), a system that guides all levels of government, nongovernmental organizations, and the private sector to work together to prevent, protect against, mitigate, respond to, and recover from incidents (FEMA, 2017). NIMS, which applies to all incident from motor vehicle accidents to catastrophic disasters, provides a unified system with common vocabulary, systems, and processes to successfully deliver the capabilities described within the system.

Incident Command System

One of the operational systems within NIMS is the Incident Command System (ICS). ICS was developed in the 1970s and has gone through multiple revisions. It acts as a standardized management tool for meeting the demands of large or small incidents. The ICS is an organizational structure consisting of five major functional areas: command, operations, planning, logistics, and finance/administration. Each of these areas works together to provide management of the incident. The incident commander has authority over an incident. He or she delegates authority to the other command staff (consisting of the public information officer, safety officer, and liaison officer and four section chiefs [operations, planning, logistics, and finance/administration]) as needed. Section chiefs establish branches, groups, divisions, or units. The ICS coordinates the efforts of the response agencies to successfully prevent, protect, mitigate, and/or recover from the incident.

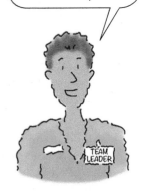

Experienced nurses may be called upon to function as a leader during an incidence response.

Key roles of the ICS include:

- **The incident commander**: This individual does not fall under the general or command staff. He or she is responsible for the overall incident management, including the establishment of incident objectives, and the approval of all actions and requests. In larger incidents that span multiple jurisdictions, authority and responsibility are divided into a unified command where agency executives or administrators collectively develop incident objectives and strategies.
- **Command staff**: The command staff consist of the public information officer, safety officer, and liaison officer. Command staff positions assign responsibility to general staff for key activities to meet the incident objectives.
- **General staff**: The general staff are responsible for carrying out the functional elements of the incident command structure. The general staff consist of operations, planning, logistics, and finance/administration sections.

Hospital Incident Command System (HICS)

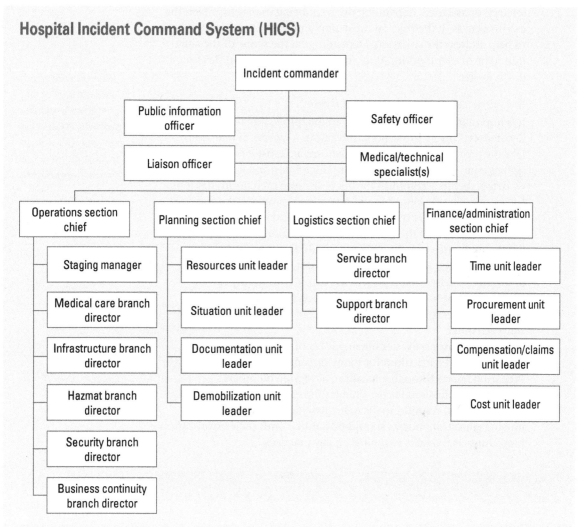

Adapted from Emergency Medical Services Authority of California. (2014). *Hospital Incident Command System guidebook.* Retrieved from https://emsa.ca.gov/wp-content/uploads/sites/71/2017/09/HICS_Guidebook_2014_11.pdf

Hospital Incident Command System

In the early 1970s, wildfires in California highlighted the need to have a system in place to manage complex events. The culmination of local, state, and federal agencies, speaking different languages with different expectations, came to be known as the Hospital Incident Command System (HICS). (See *Hospital Incident Command System (HICS).*)

The primary objective in an HICS (or any ICS) is that one person must be responsible. A singular leader must maintain control for directing and managing the event or situation. The individual may be selected or assigned, depending on event being managed. Given the expansiveness of the role, an incident commander has an entire team to help address the situation. Depending on the scope of the situation, type of event, or duration, the size of that team can flex up or down in size.

Interprofessional approach to disasters

It is important to note the need for an interprofessional approach to disaster prevention, protection, mitigation, response, and recovery. Like the professional makeup of the hospital, disaster response professionals come from a variety of health disciplines, and it is essential to work together to accomplish the goals. Because each health discipline has its own specific language and operational protocol, the National Preparedness Goal, NRF, and incident command structure work together to ensure that there is a common operational language. This highlights the need for the different health disciplines to be educated and trained together well before disaster strikes. Participating in disaster exercises that represent the whole community is one way to enable community stakeholders to test and validate plans and capabilities while learning to work alongside each other.

> Nurses work as an integral part of the interprofessional team during disaster prevention, protection, mitigation, response, and recovery efforts.

For this reason, disaster nursing is becoming part of the standard curriculum for many nursing programs. Preparing nurses through education, alongside members of the interprofessional team, enables nurses to better prepare for and respond to disasters. Beyond basic disaster nursing education, nurses should be familiar with their organization's procedures as it relates to their everyday practices.

Workplace and individual nurse preparation for disaster

Workplace preparation

Workplaces, particularly hospitals, should have a hazard vulnerability analysis (HVA). This document serves as a needs assessment and is a systematic approach to identifying hazards that may impact the demand for, or the ability to provide, services in time of a disaster (California Hospital Association's Hospital Preparedness Program, 2017). Risks associated with each type of hazard are analyzed on the HVA to prioritize planning, mitigation, response, and recovery initiatives (California Hospital Association's Hospital Preparedness Program, 2017). Community partners and emergency response agencies should be involved in the HVA. (See *Hazard and vulnerability assessment tool.*)

Hazard and vulnerability assessment tool

Human related events

		Severity = (magnitude − mitigation)						
	Probability	**Human impact**	**Property impact**	**Business impact**	**Preparedness**	**Internal response**	**External response**	**Risk**
Event	Likelihood this will occur	Possibility of death injury	Physical losses and damages	Interuption of services	Preplanning	Time, effectiveness, resources	Community/ mutual aid staff and supplies	Relative threat*
Score	0 = n/a 1 = Low 2 = Moderate 3 = High	0 = n/a 1 = Low 2 = Moderate 3 = High	0 = n/a 1 = Low 2 = Moderate 3 = High	0 = n/a 1 = Low 2 = Moderate 3 = High	0 = n/a 1 = High 2 = Moderate 3 = Low or none	0 = n/a 1 = High 2 = Moderate 3 = Low or none	0 = n/a 1 = High 2 = Moderate 3 = Low or none	0–100%
Mass casualty incident (trauma)								0%
Mass casualty incident (medical/ infectious)								0%
Terrorism, biological								0%
VIP situation								0%
Infant abduction								0%
Hostage situation								0%
Civil disturbance								0%
Labor action								0%
Forensic admission								0%
Bomb threat								0%
Average	**0.00**	**0.00**	**0.00**	**0.00**	**0.00**	**0.00**	**0.00**	**0%**

*Threat increases with percentage.

Risk = probability * severity		
0.00	0.00	0.00

Adapted from California Hospital Association. *Hazard vulnerability analysis.* Retrieved from https://www.calhospitalprepare.org /hazard-vulnerability-analysis

---

Individual nurse preparedness

Nurses play an integral role in disasters. For this reason, it is essential that each individual nurse is personally prepared to play a part in meeting the National Preparedness Goal in the time of a crisis. Being prepared as a nursing professional means having a personal emergency plan to ensure that family and personal needs are taken care of during a disaster response. When planning, consider the types of disasters that could affect the area you live and work in. Plans should be tailored toward the most likely incidents that could occur to ensure that the specific needs and responsibilities of daily living are met. Simple family emergency plans can easily be found online at www.ready.gov and include simple forms to plan for communications, family needs, and even pet care. Plans should be made specifically for child care, medication availability, and documents that should be readily available to take (e.g., birth certificates, passports, proof of insurance) if evacuation from an area is mandatory.

Questions are often raised about legal, ethical, and professional duties of first responders, including nurses, during times of disaster. At a minimum, nurses have an ethical duty to help care for and protect their patients. They also have a duty to take care of themselves (American Nurses Association, 2017). This can be taxing work because disasters situations can make responders feel unsafe and unsure about the care they are providing. Questions about how to get to the hospital safely, risk of disease or exposure, care of family members at home, or the stability and security of the facility are examples of things to be considered when thinking about responding during a disaster. There are also times that a nurse must morally make a choice between duties, and each nurse must consider his or her own professional integrity when making choices (American Nurses Association, 2017). This is a key part of disaster planning and preparedness (American Nurses Association, 2017).

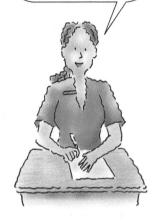

It is important for me to make a personal emergency plan and to keep it in place at all times.

Triage

During a mass casualty, resources are overwhelmed by a surge of casualties. The goal during this surge is to do the most good for the most number of patients. Nurses are often directly involved in the process of triage: identifying people that most need assistance and to what degree that assistance is needed.

Triage started during times of war by the Baron Dominique Jean Larrey, Napoleon's chief surgeon. The word "triage" is derived from the French word *trier*, which means to sort. By sorting the sickest or most injured from the individuals with minor needs, patients with survivable but life-threatening injuries can be treated before those with less threatening injuries. Triage is used daily in an emergency department or urgent care setting. Daily triage is a standardized process using a standardized approach based of clinical judgment ensuring patient care is prioritized by acuity. Daily triage can be stretched during acute incidents or ongoing medical crisis such as influenza.

Disaster triage is defined by the resources being depleted and the system being overwhelmed. When resources are depleted to the point that patients must be treated based on their chance of survival,

START adult triage

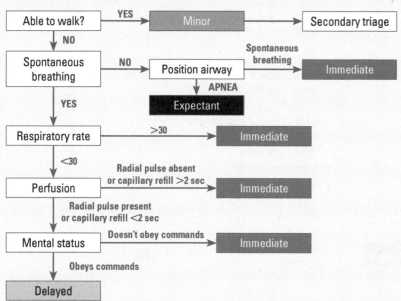

Triage categories

Expectant **Black triage tag color**
• Victim unlikely to survive given severity of injuries, level of available care, or both.
• Palliative care and pain relief should be provided.

Immediate **Red triage tag color**
• Victim can be helped by immediate intervention and transport
• Requires medical attention within minutes for survival (up to 60)
• Includes compromises to patient's Airway, Breathing, Circulation

Delayed **Yellow triage tag color**
• Victim's transport can be delayed
• Includes serious and potentially life-threatening injuries, but status not expected to deteriorate significantly over several hours

Minor **Green triage tag color**
• Victim with relatively minor injuries
• Status unlikely to deteriorate over days
• May be able to assist in own care: "walking wounded"

Adapted from U.S. Department of Health & Human Services. *Chemical hazards emergency medical management*. Retrieved from https://chemm.nlm.nih.gov/chemmimages/StartAdult TriageAlgorithm.gif

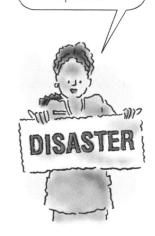

When performing triage during a mass casualty event, the nurse's goal is to do the most good for the most number of patients.

MCI/disaster triage needs to be used. There are multiple standardized triage systems that can be adopted for use, including simple triage and rapid treatment (START) and sort, assess, life-saving interventions, treatment, and/or transport (SALT). (See *START adult triage*, and *SALT mass casualty triage*, page 540.)

SALT mass casualty triage

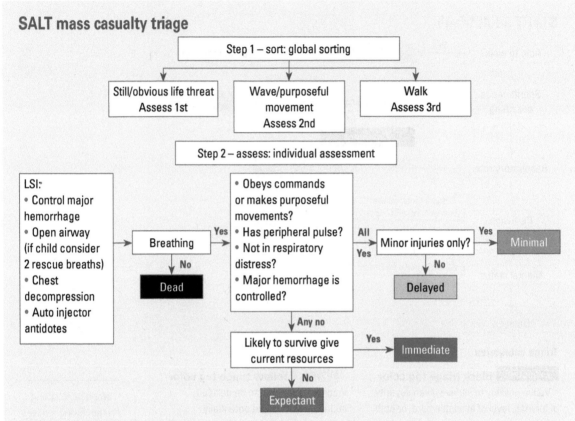

Adapted from U.S. Department of Health & Human Services. SALT mass casualty triage. Retrieved from https://umem.org/files/uploads/ems/2062899.png?471

The following categories describe how patients are triaged during an MCI/disaster according to START principles. Triage ribbons (tags) are often placed on patients to indicate their triage level. (See *First responder triage tags*.)

- **Minor/green**: Patients that are designated as minor/green patients are generally considered to be the "walking wounded." Their injuries or illness are not considered to be life-threatening. They only need basic medical care and can wait a considerable amount of time before receiving such care. (Examples of minor/green patients include those with injuries such as minor bleeding, cuts, and scratches.)
- **Urgent/yellow**: Urgent/yellow patients are often called delayed patients because their injuries or illness require treatment but are not immediately life-threatening. However, their condition does have a great potential for decompensation. (Example of urgent/yellow patients includes those with injuries to the spine or head, significant controlled bleeding, or orthopedic injuries with neurovascular compromise.)

First responder triage tags

Personal Property Receipt/
Evidence Tag

№ 304136

Destination _____
Via _____

№ 304136

TRIAGE
TAG

№ 304136

	Yes	No
Gross Decon	Yes	No
Secondary Decon	Yes	No
Solution		
Blunt Trauma		
Burn		
C-Spine		
Cardiac		
Crushing		
Fracture		
Laceration		
Penetrating Injury		

Age_____

☐ Male   ☐ Female

Other: _____

CONTAMINATED

№ 304136

VITAL SIGNS

Time	B/P	Pulse	Respiration

Time	Drug Solution	Dose

MORGUE
Pulseless/Non-Breathing

№ 304136

IMMEDIATE
Life Threatening Injury

№ 304136

DELAYED
Serious, Non Life Threatening

№ 304136

MINOR
Walking Wounded

№ 304136

- **Immediate/red**: Immediate/red patients often have immediate life-threatening conditions that are survivable with intervention and are considered the highest priority. The mnemonic "30-2-can-do" is a good way to determine who receives a red ribbon (Clarkson & Williams, 2018): Anyone with a respiratory rate *greater than 30*, an absent radial pulse or capillary refill greater than *2 seconds*, or is *unable to follow commands* should be triaged as immediate/red. (Another example of immediate/red patients includes those with uncontrolled hemorrhaging but still assessed to survive with intervention.)
- **Expectant/gray**: Patients who have injuries that are not likely to survive given the current resources are issued an expectant/gray ribbon. Expectant/gray patients should receive palliative care, such as pain medications, if time and resources allow. (Examples of expectant/gray patients include those with exposed brain matter, carotid artery hemorrhage, or burns totaling 90% of the total body surface area.)
- **Deceased/black**: Patients who have died should be marked with a deceased/black ribbon or a black and white striped tag.
- **Contaminated/orange**: An incident that involves hazardous materials requires that patients be decontaminated prior to entering the emergency department or any other part of the hospital. Those who have been exposed are issued a contaminated/orange ribbon. Once the decontamination is complete, the orange ribbon is removed.

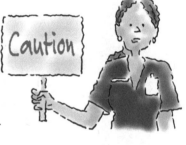

Anyone who is exposed to hazardous material gets an orange tag to indicate the need for decontamination.

Disaster recovery

Disaster recovery includes preplanning the quickest and most efficient ways to rebuild the infrastructure of a community after an incident. Incorporating recovery into disaster planning ensures that engaged community stakeholders are unifying efforts to increase the whole community's resilience toward the effects of a disaster. The National Disaster Recovery Framework (NDRF) is a component of the NPS and outlines the strategy and doctrine for how the whole community builds, sustains, and coordinates delivery of Recovery Core Capabilities identified in the National Preparedness Goal. There are eight guiding principles outlined in the NDRF that help to maximize the opportunity for achieving recovery success (FEMA, 2016). (See *Guiding principles*.) Disaster recovery in terms of health care is critical to most communities. In addition to the clinical health care needs of many communities, health care is a major economic driver that provides employment and economic sustainability.

Guiding principles

1. Individual and family empowerment
2. Leadership and local primacy
3. Pre-disaster recovery planning
4. Engaged partnerships inclusiveness
5. Unity of effort
6. Timeliness and flexibility
7. Resilience and sustainability
8. Psychological and emotional recovery

Quick quiz

1.   Which element of the National Preparedness Goal does the nurse identify that reduces the loss of life and property by lessening the impact of future disasters?
   A.   Prevention
   B.   Protection
   C.   Mitigation
   D.   Recovery

Answer: C. Mitigation involves reduction of the loss of life and property by lessening the impact of future disasters. Prevention encompasses preventing, avoiding, or stopping an imminent, threatened, or actual act of terrorism. Protection involves protection of individuals against great threats and hazards so that people can thrive. Recovery focuses on restoration following a disaster.

2.   What action is appropriate when a nurse engages in self-preparation prior to a disaster response? Select all that apply.
   A.   Plan for pet care.
   B.   Assess family needs.
   C.   Collect birth certificates.
   D.   Create a personal emergency plan.
   E.   Ensure that medications are refilled.

Answer: A, B, C, D, E. All of these actions should be undertaken to create a comprehensive self-preparation plan prior to a disaster response.

3.   Which triage ribbon will the nurse provide to a disaster victim who has ankle and wrist sprains and several small lacerations to the face?
   A.   Green
   B.   Yellow
   C.   Red
   D.   Gray

Answer: A. Green triage ribbons are assigned to victims who are considered to be "walking wounded." Their injuries or illness is not considered to be life-threatening, and they only need basic medical care. These individuals can wait a considerable amount of time before receiving such care. Yellow triage ribbons are given to people whose illness or injury may not constitute immediate treatment, yet their condition has a great potential for decompensation. Red triage tags are given to those who have immediate life threats. These people are considered the highest priority for medical intervention because they need immediate intervention, which should lead to their survival. Gray triage tags are assigned to victims who have injuries that are not likely to survive given the current resources.

4. What teaching will a disaster nursing expert provide to a group of new staff nurses regarding a mass casualty situation?
   A. "You do not have to help during a mass casualty situation."
   B. "The public information officer will direct you regarding what to do."
   C. "You can choose which nursing role you perform during the response."
   D. "Our role is to respond as quickly as possible to save as many lives as we can."

Answer: D. All members of the interprofessional team, including nurses, respond as quickly as possible during a mass casualty or disaster to save as many lives as possible. Nurses have an ethical duty to help during a mass casualty or disaster response. A public relations officer coordinates messages to the press and public but does not direct nurses. Nurses will be assigned roles within their respective scope of practice during the response; they do not choose which role to fulfill.

Scoring

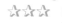 If you answered all four questions correctly, get up and cheer! You're a genius!

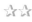 If you answered three questions correctly, pat yourself on the back! You're gearing up for success in understanding mass casualty and disaster information.

 If you answered fewer than three questions correctly, don't be sad. Just review the chapter and give it another go.

Selected references

American Nurses Association. (2017). *Who will be there? Ethics, the law, and a nurse's duty to respond in a disaster.* Retrieved from https://www.nursingworld.org/~4af058/globalassets/docs/ana/ethics/who-will-be-there_disaster-preparedness_2017.pdf

California Hospital Association's Hospital Preparedness Program. (2017). *Hazards vulnerability analysis.* Retrieved from https://www.calhospitalprepare.org/hazard-vulnerability-analysis

Clarkson, E., & Williams, M. (2018). *EMS, triage, mass casualty.* Retrieved from https://www.ncbi.nlm.nih.gov/books/NBK459369/

Emergency Medical Services Authority of California. (2014). *Hospital Incident Command System guidebook.* Retrieved from https://emsa.ca.gov/wp-content/uploads/sites/71/2017/09/HICS_Guidebook_2014_11.pdf

*Federal Emergency Management Agency. (2002). *State and local mitigation planning how-to guide: Integrating human-caused hazards.* Retrieved from https://www.fema.gov/media-library-data/20130726-1524-20490-4314/3howto7fwdintro.pdf

*Federal Emergency Management Agency. (2011). *Local mitigation plan review guide*. Retrieved from https://www.fema.gov/media-library-data/20130726-1809 -25045-7498/plan_review_guide_final_9_30_11.pdf

*Federal Emergency Management Agency. (2016). *National response framework* (3rd ed.). Washington, DC: U.S. Department of Homeland Security. Retrieved from https://www.fema.gov/media-library-data/1466014682982-9bcf8245ba4c60 c120aa915abe74e15d/National_Response_Framework3rd.pdf

Federal Emergency Management Agency. (2017). *National incident management system* (3rd ed.). Washington, DC: U.S. Department of Homeland Security. Retrieved from https://www.fema.gov/media-library-data/1508151197225-ced8c60378 c3936adb92c1a3ee6f6564/FINAL_NIMS_2017.pdf

Federal Emergency Management Agency. (2018). *National preparedness goal*. Retrieved from https://www.fema.gov/national-preparedness-goal

Federal Emergency Management Agency. (2019). *About the agency*. Retrieved from https://www.fema.gov/about-agency

Greater Miami Valley EMS Council. (2018). *GMVEMSC prehospital paramedic standing orders training manual*. Retrieved from https://www.gmvemsc.org/uploads /protocol/2018PMtrainingmanual.pdf

Holleran, R. S., Wolfe, A. C., & Frakes, M. A. (2018). *Patient transport: Principles & practice* (5th ed.). St. Louis, MO: Elsevier.

U.S. Department of Health & Human Services. *SALT mass casualty triage*. Retrieved from https://umem.org/files/uploads/ems/2062899.png?471

*Still current.

Chapter 14

Shock and multisystem trauma emergencies

Just the facts

In this chapter, you'll learn:

♦ emergency assessment of the patient experiencing shock and multisystem trauma

♦ diagnostic tests and procedures for shock and multisystem trauma

♦ shock disorders and multisystem trauma in the emergency department and their treatments.

Understanding shock and multisystem trauma emergencies

Shock and multisystem trauma are emergencies that can affect the control of every system in the body. Due to their wide-ranging effects, these conditions are commonly life-threatening.

Shock to the system

Shock is defined as inadequate tissue perfusion resulting in organ failure. It is associated with a complex cascade of events that if left untreated can progress to death due to complete cardiovascular collapse. In some cases, if the shock is severe enough, even with adequate treatment, it can still be fatal (i.e., septic shock, post-myocardial infarction [MI] cardiogenic shock). If recognized early, the majority of shock is reversible (Gaieski & Mikkelsen, 2018).

Inadequate tissue perfusion is a deficiency of the body's cells and tissues to receive or use adequate oxygenation. This results in a change of the body's natural energy producing aerobic metabolism cycle to an ineffective anaerobic metabolism. This leads to cellular death and organ failure. (See *Shock cell.*)

Shock cell

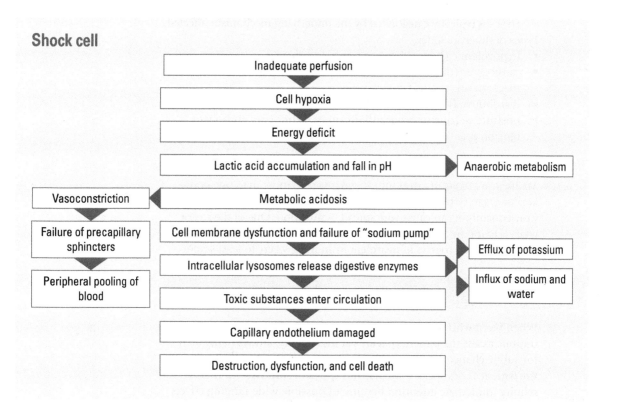

When you think of inadequate tissue perfusion, it is a helpful hint to think about supply and demand.

- Supply issues:
  - Respiratory issues can create inadequate gas exchange.
  - Cardiac issues may cause the heart to beat ineffectively causing a decrease in oxygen delivery.
  - Vascular issues can create a loss of intrinsic contractility to support the circulating blood volume (vasodilation) or pressure buildup in the blood vessels preventing delivery of blood volume.
  - Hematologic issues may not produce enough blood volume or hemoglobin (Hgb) to carry oxygen (anemia, hemorrhage, hypovolemia).
- Demand issues:
  - Oxygen may not be used appropriately by the cells.
  - Anxiety, pain, stress, and infection can cause an increase demand in the intracellular requirement for oxygen. Normally, the body can accommodate; however, if an individual is experiencing a trauma, the organ systems may not be able to meet the increased demand.

Shock is typically categorized by the underlying mechanism affected. Types of shock include:

- hypovolemic (hemorrhage or nonhemorrhagic)
- cardiogenic (due to intracardiac causes: arrhythmic, cardiomyopathy, mechanical)
- distributive (which includes neurogenic, septic, and anaphylactic)
- obstructive (due to extracardiac causes: pulmonary embolism, tension pneumothorax, pericardial tamponade).

Here, there, and everywhere

Multisystem trauma involves injury or damage to more than one body area or organ system from forces that disrupt the integrity of the systems. Consequently, it can cause widespread dysfunction. One of the major goals is to follow a systematic assessment strategy to address immediate life threats and progress in treatment from most severe to least severe.

Assessment

When faced with an emergency involving shock or multisystem trauma, assess the patient quickly yet thoroughly, always being alert for subtle changes that might indicate a potential deterioration in the patient's condition. Patients with shock or multisystem trauma require immediate attention because of possible wide-ranging effects on one or more body systems; prompt attention to the patient's vital functions is essential. Perform a primary and then a secondary assessment; you may need to intervene at any time.

When you've completed the assessment and the patient is stabilized, obtain a patient history. If you can't interview the patient because of the condition, gather history information from the medical record. In some cases, you may need to ask the patient's family or the emergency medical response team that transported him or her to the emergency department (ED).

Primary assessment: Use the alphabet

A primary survey consists of assessing the patient's **airway** (ensuring cervical spine immobilization), **breathing** (the patient may need ventilation), **circulation** (the patient may require large amounts of fluids, which may include blood products; cardiopulmonary resuscitation [CPR] may be required and possibly tourniquets applied to control massive hemorrhage from extremities), and **disability** (assess the patient's alertness and orientation and if the patient responds to voices or pain). The goal of the primary survey is to address immediate life threats (American College of Surgeons, 2018).

E: Expose/environmental controls

- Remove the patient's clothing to assess for obvious injuries or problems.
- Provide blankets or warming lights to prevent chilling.
- Use fluid warmers for mass transfusion or resuscitation.
- Room environment should be kept as warm as possible.

F: Full set of vital signs/focused adjuncts

- Obtain a complete set of vital signs.
- Anticipate the need for five interventions—pulse oximetry, cardiac monitoring, urinary catheterization, gastric intubation, and laboratory tests.
- Facilitate family presence.

Key point: If a patient's vital signs are not normalized by the end of the primary assessment (or sometimes called *survey*), progression to secondary assessment (survey) typically does not occur.

Secondary assessment

Secondary assessment involves a more in-depth evaluation of the patient's status after the ABCs have been maintained. Typically, this survey includes continued vital sign monitoring, history, head-to-toe physical examination, and inspection of the patient's posterior surfaces.

When the secondary assessment is complete, you can start on a more focused assessment of each body system. (See previous body system chapters for specific assessment information.)

G: Give comfort measures

- Provide verbal reassurance as warranted.
- Use touch to help alleviate anxiety and fear.
- Assess and manage pain.

H: History and head-to-toe assessment

- Complete a head-to-toe assessment.
- Observe for wounds, ecchymosis, deformities, and impaired movement or function.

I: Inspect posterior surfaces

This may be completed during primary assessment while conducting the survey during the disability and expose assessments (American College of Surgeons, 2018).

- Log roll the patient to the side.
- Inspect the posterior areas for wounds, bruising, and deformities.
- Palpate areas for tenderness and pain.
- Assist with rectal examination (tone assessment, Hemoccult or guaiac) (American College of Surgeons, 2018; Emergency Nurses Association, 2019).

Diagnostic tests

Numerous diagnostic tests may be performed, depending on the patient's underlying condition and overall status. Blood studies and radiologic and imaging studies are commonly performed.

Additional tests may be used based on facility policy and body area or systems affected. For example, angiography may be done to evaluate for vessel injury; more specifically, cerebral angiography may be used to evaluate cerebral blood flow. Cardiac monitoring and hemodynamic monitoring may be used to evaluate the patient's cardiac function and overall hemodynamic status.

Blood studies

Although specific blood studies may vary among facilities, some more common studies ordered for patients with shock or multisystem trauma include:

- complete blood count (CBC)
- electrolytes, blood urea nitrogen (BUN)/creatinine
- coagulation studies, such as prothrombin time (PT) and partial thromboplastin time (PTT)
- serum amylase, lipase
- liver function tests
- blood cultures (if infection suspected)
- serum lactate: Lactic acid is used as a marker to evaluate inadequate perfusion. When the body tissues and cells are hypoperfused, oxygen is not delivered to the cells and the body changes to anaerobic metabolism, which produces lactic acid (Rhodes et al., 2017).

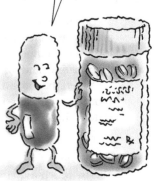

Some medications may influence blood test results, so be sure to check your patient's medication history.

Less common but important

In addition, arterial blood gas (ABG) analysis is commonly performed to evaluate the patient's acid–base balance. In trauma situations, a blood type and cross-match is done in anticipation of the need for a blood and blood products transfusion.

Practice pointers

- Tell the patient that the test requires a blood sample.
- Check the patient's medication history for medications that might influence test results.
- Check with your hospital lab; some blood tubes may be required to be placed on ice prior to running the test.

Radiologic and imaging studies

Specific radiologic and imaging studies completed for these patients depend on the underlying mechanism causing the shock and the body areas or organs affected by the trauma. The most common studies include X-rays of the chest, pelvis, cervical spine, thoracic and lumbar spine, and extremities. In addition, computed tomography (CT) scan of the head, chest, spine, and abdomen may be performed. Focused assessment with sonography for trauma (FAST) exam may be performed at the bedside. The FAST exam has widely replaced diagnostic peritoneal lavage.

The FAST exam or expanded FAST (eFAST) exam is used to assess key areas of potential intra-abdominal bleeding, pneumothorax, and pericardial tamponade (American College of Surgeons, 2018).

Practice pointers

- Prepare the patient for the X-ray or CT scan to be performed, including the reason for the study.
- Verify that the order includes pertinent history, such as trauma, and identifies sites of injury, tenderness, or pain.
- Make sure that all jewelry is removed from the patient.
- Confirm if they have any allergies to shellfish or iodine if receiving contrast.

Treatments

Treatments vary depending on the specific type of shock or the areas of injury with multisystem trauma. Common treatment measures include fluid resuscitation, blood transfusion therapy, drug therapy, and surgery.

Fluid resuscitation

The goal of fluid resuscitation is to have a balanced resuscitation approach, meaning the initial fluid of choice is a balanced salt solution such as lactated Ringer, Plasma-Lyte, or Normosol for the first 2 L. If the patient demonstrates a need for continued fluid resuscitation, implement the use of blood products as prescribed. Large infusions of normal saline have demonstrated acute kidney injury due to the large amounts of chloride and is not recommended (Semler et al., 2018).

Other treatments relate to the organ system affected. Oxygen therapy and ventilatory support may be required to ensure adequate respiratory function and oxygenation and treat respiratory-associated injuries.

Blood transfusion therapy

Blood transfusions treat decreased Hgb level and hematocrit (HCT). A whole blood transfusion replenishes the circulatory system's volume and oxygen-carrying capacity by increasing the mass of circulating red blood cells (RBCs). It's usually used in cases of hemorrhage.

- ABO compatibility: In general, type-specific blood is preferred when transfusing; however, often in the critically ill trauma patient, the blood type is unknown. For female patients who are of childbearing age, they must receive type O negative. This is done to avoid exposure of the Rh factor. For male patients, they can receive either type O negative or O positive. Type O is considered the "universal donor type," and type AB is considered the "universal recipient" (American College of Surgeons, 2018).

When to transfuse

Blood transfusion is not without risk. Even though blood is screened for major diseases such as hepatitis and HIV, there are still other risks and antibodies that can be transferred. Blood transfusion can also cause significant fluid overload and acute lung damage. Every effort should be made to avoid transfusion; however, if blood transfusion is needed, **do not delay**. Do not wait for the Hgb/HCT values to drop to significant levels to transfuse. It is important for the nurse to remember that there will be a delay between the patients bleeding and the reflection in the lab values. Be diligent in observing vital signs and serial assessments.

Most professional organizations indicate that the target threshold for transfusion is an Hgb between 7 and 8 g/dL and HCT of 21%. The one exception is for a patient demonstrating signs of acute MI and then the threshold rises to Hgb of 10 g/dL. This is called *restrictive transfusion* (Mirski et al., 2015).

Packed RBCs, a blood component from which 80% of the plasma has been removed, are transfused to restore the circulatory system's oxygen-carrying capacity. Packed RBCs are used when the patient has a normal blood volume to avoid possible fluid and circulatory overload (Sharma et al., 2011). (See *Guide to whole blood and cellular products*, pages 554 to 557.)

Whole blood and packed RBCs contain cellular debris, requiring in-line filtration during administration. There is new evidence from trials conducted by the U.S. military that suggests in the trauma patient population that whole blood transfusion may be the best option. Check with your facility to determine their protocol.

Washed packed RBCs, commonly used for patients previously sensitized to transfusions, are rinsed with a special solution that removes white blood cells (WBCs) and platelets, thus decreasing the chance of a transfusion reaction.

Refusin' transfusion

In some cases, a patient may refuse a blood transfusion. For example, a patient may refuse a blood transfusion due to religious beliefs. A competent adult has the right to refuse treatment. You may be able to use other treatment options if the patient refuses the blood transfusion, such as providing erythropoietin, iron, and folic acid supplements before and after surgery. Using available alternative treatments supports the patient's right of self-determination and honors his or her wishes. A court order requiring the patient to undergo transfusion therapy can be obtained when the patient's mental competency is questionable.

> Remember, the patient's right of self-determination means that he or she can choose to refuse a blood transfusion.

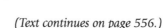

Nursing considerations

- Verify the health care provider's prescription and signed consent (during emergent situations, implied consent may be allowed).
- Obtain baseline vital signs and start an intravenous (IV) line if one isn't already started. Use a 20G or larger diameter catheter.
- Identify the patient and check the blood bag identification number, ABO blood group, Rh compatibility, and blood product expiration date. This step should be confirmed by another licensed professional. Follow your facility's policy for blood administration.
- Obtain the patient's vital signs after the first 15 minutes and then every 30 minutes (or according to your facility's policy) for the remainder of transfusion therapy.
- Record the date and time of the transfusion (time started and completed); the type and amount of transfusion product; the type and gauge of the catheter used for infusion; the patient's vital signs before, during, and after transfusion; a verification check of all identification data (including the names of individuals verifying the information); and the patient's response.
- Obtain follow-up laboratory tests as ordered to determine the effectiveness of therapy.
- For rapid blood replacement, use a pressure bag or rapid transfusion device if necessary. Be aware that excessive pressure may develop, leading to broken blood vessels and extravasation with hematoma and hemolysis of the infusing RBCs. Large-gauge IV catheters and central line introducers are preferred for rapid and pressured transfusions.
- If administering platelets or fresh frozen plasma, administer each unit immediately after obtaining it. Although some microaggregate filters can be used for up to 10 units of blood, always replace the filter and tubing if more than 1 hour elapses between transfusions. Document the patient's transfusion reaction and the treatment required (if any). When administering multiple units of blood products, use a blood warmer to avoid hypothermia.
- Notify the health care provider if the patient refuses the blood transfusion.

(Text continues on page 556.)

Guide to whole blood and cellular products

This chart lists blood components along with indications for their use and nursing considerations.

Blood component	Indications
Whole blood	
Complete (pure) blood	• To treat symptomatic chronic anemia • To prevent morbidity from anemia in patients at greatest risk for tissue hypoxia • To control active bleeding with signs and symptoms of hypovolemia • To aid preoperatively; hemoglobin less than 9 g/dL with possibility of major blood loss • To treat sickle cell disease
Packed red blood cells (RBCs)	
Same RBC mass as whole blood with 80% of the plasma removed	• To treat symptomatic chronic anemia • To prevent morbidity from anemia in patients at greatest risk for tissue hypoxia • To control active bleeding with signs and symptoms of hypovolemia • To aid preoperatively; hemoglobin less than 9 g/dL with possibility of major blood loss • To treat sickle cell disease
Leukocyte-reduced RBCs	
Same as packed RBCs except 70% of the leukocytes are removed	• The vast majority of RBCs transfused are now leukocyte reduced due to the risk of transfusion reaction (Silvergleid, 2017). • To treat symptomatic anemia • To prevent morbidity from anemia in patients at greatest risk for tissue hypoxia • To control active bleeding with signs and symptoms of hypovolemia • To aid preoperatively; hemoglobin less than 9 g/dL with possibility of major blood loss • To treat sickle cell disease • To prevent febrile reactions from leukocyte antibodies • To treat immunosuppressed patients • To restore RBCs to patients who have had two or more nonhemolytic febrile reactions
White blood cells (WBCs) (leukocytes)	
Whole blood with all the RBCs and 80% of the plasma removed	• To assist in treating sepsis that's unresponsive to antibiotics (especially if the patient has positive blood cultures or a persistent fever exceeding 101° F [38.3° C]) and accompanied by life-threatening granulocytopenia (granulocyte count less than 500/µL) or neutropenia

Nursing considerations

- Compatibility is ABO identical.
- Group A receives A; group B receives B; group AB receives AB; group O receives O. Rh type must match.
- Use blood administration tubing. You can infuse rapidly in emergencies, but adjust the rate to the patient's condition and the transfusion order and don't infuse over more than 4 hours.
- Whole blood is seldom administered other than in emergency situations because its components can be extracted and administered separately.
- Warm blood if giving a large quantity.
- Use only with normal saline.
- Monitor the patient's volume status for fluid overload.

- Compatibility: Group A receives A or O; group B receives B or O; group AB receives AB, A, B, or O; group O receives O. Rh type must match.
- Use blood administration tubing to infuse over more than 4 hours.
- Packed RBCs shouldn't be used for anemic conditions correctable by nutrition or drug therapy.
- Use only with normal saline.

- Compatibility: Group A receives A or O; group B receives B or O; group AB receives AB, A, B, or O; group O receives O. Rh type must match.
- Use blood administration tubing; may require a microaggregate filter (40-micron filter) for hard-spun, leukocyte-poor RBCs
- Cells expire 24 hours after washing.
- Leukocyte-reduced RBCs shouldn't be used for anemic conditions correctable by nutrition or drug therapy.

- Compatibility: Group A receives A or O; group B receives B or O; group AB receives AB, A, B, or O; group O receives O. Rh type must match. WBCs are preferably human leukocyte antigen (HLA)-compatible, although compatibility isn't necessary unless the patient is HLA-sensitized from previous transfusions.
- Use blood administration tubing. One unit daily is given for 4 to 6 days or until infection clears.
- WBC infusion may induce fever and chills. To prevent this reaction, the patient is premedicated with antihistamines, acetaminophen (Tylenol), or steroids. If fever occurs, give an antipyretic but don't stop the transfusion. Reduce the flow rate for the patient's comfort.
- Because reactions are common, administer slowly over 2 to 4 hours. Check the patient's vital signs and assess him every 15 minutes throughout the transfusion.
- Give the transfusion with antibiotics to treat infection.

(continued)

Guide to whole blood and cellular products *(continued)*

Blood component	Indications
Platelets	
Platelet sediment from RBCs or plasma	• To treat bleeding due to critically decreased circulating platelet counts or functionally abnormal platelets • To prevent bleeding due to thrombocytopenia • To treat a patient with a platelet count less than 50,000/μL before surgery or a major invasive procedure

Sharma, S., Sharma, P., & Tyler, L. N. (2011). Transfusion of blood and blood products: Indications and complications. *American Family Physician, 83*(6), 719–724.

Drug therapy

Drug therapy for shock and multisystem trauma varies depending on the patient's underlying condition. For example, antibiotics may be used to treat septic shock, whereas vasopressors may be considered to treat neurogenic or distributive shock.

In cases of shock and multisystem trauma, drugs are commonly required to support blood flow to the vital organs, such as the heart and brain. These drugs include:

- epinephrine (Adrenalin)
- vasopressin
- norepinephrine (Levophed)
- dopamine
- dobutamine
- milrinone
- calcium
- nitroglycerin
- sodium nitroprusside (Nitropress).

Surgery

Surgery also depends on the patient's underlying condition. For example, surgery may be indicated to repair a laceration of a wound or organ, repair a fracture, insert pins or a fixation device to stabilize bone, or incise and drain an abscess. Exploratory surgery may be necessary to identify the source of hemorrhage in a patient experiencing hypovolemic shock.

Nursing considerations

- Compatibility: ABO should be identical. Rh-negative recipients should receive Rh-negative platelets.
- Use a blood filter or leukocyte reduction filter. Don't use a microaggregate filter.
- Platelet transfusions aren't usually indicated for thrombocytopenic autoimmune thrombocytopenia or thrombocytopenia purpura unless the patient has a life-threatening hemorrhage.
- Patients with a history of platelet reaction require premedication with antipyretics and antihistamines.
- Use single-donor platelets if the patient has a need for repeated transfusions.

Common disorders

In the ED, you're likely to encounter patients with anaphylactic shock, cardiogenic shock, hypovolemic shock, neurogenic shock, septic shock, or multisystem trauma. Regardless of the disorder, your first priority is to ensure ABCs.

Anaphylactic shock

Anaphylactic shock, also called *anaphylaxis*, is an acute, potentially life-threatening type I (immediate) hypersensitivity reaction marked by the sudden onset of rapidly progressive *urticaria* (vascular swelling in skin accompanied by itching) and respiratory distress.

What causes it

Anaphylaxis usually results from ingestion of, or other systemic exposure to, sensitizing drugs or other substances. Such substances may include:

- serums (usually horse serum)
- vaccines
- allergen extracts
- enzymes, such as L-asparaginase
- hormones
- penicillin or other antibiotics (which induce anaphylaxis in 1 to 4 of every 10,000 patients treated, most likely after parenteral administration or prolonged therapy and in patients with an inherited tendency to food or drug allergy)
- sulfonamides

- local anesthetics
- salicylates
- polysaccharides
- diagnostic chemicals, such as sulfobromophthalein, sodium dehydrocholate, and radiographic contrast media
- food proteins, such as those in legumes, nuts, berries, seafood, and egg albumin
- food additives containing sulfite
- insect venom.

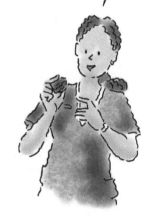

For some, it's a healthy snack; for others, it brings on an attack. In other words, nuts contain food proteins that cause anaphylaxis in some patients.

All about speed

With prompt recognition and treatment, the prognosis for anaphylaxis is good. However, a severe reaction may precipitate vascular collapse, leading to systemic shock and, sometimes, death. The reaction typically occurs within minutes but can occur up to 1 hour after exposure to an antigen.

How it happens

Anaphylaxis requires previous sensitization or exposure to the specific antigen, resulting in immunoglobulin (Ig) E production by plasma cells in the lymph nodes and enhancement by helper T cells. IgE antibodies then bind to basophils and membrane receptors on mast cells in connective tissue.

Here it comes again!

Upon exposure, IgM and IgG recognize the antigen and bind to it. Activated IgE on the basophils promotes the release of histamine, serotonin, and leukotrienes. An intensified response occurs as venule-weakening lesions form. Fluid then leaks into the cells, resulting in respiratory distress. Further deterioration occurs as the body's compensatory mechanisms fail to respond. (See *Understanding anaphylaxis*.)

What to look for

An anaphylactic reaction produces sudden physical distress within seconds or minutes after exposure to an allergen. A delayed or persistent reaction may occur up to 24 hours later. The severity of the reaction is inversely related to the interval between exposure to the allergen and the onset of symptoms. The patient, a relative, or another responsible person will report the patient's exposure to an antigen.

Immediately after exposure, the patient may report feelings of impending doom or fright, weakness, sweating, sneezing, dyspnea, nasal pruritus, and urticaria. The patient may appear extremely anxious. Keep in mind that the sooner signs and symptoms begin after exposure to the antigen, the more severe the anaphylaxis.

Understanding anaphylaxis

An anaphylactic reaction occurs after previous sensitization or exposure to a specific antigen. The sequence of events in anaphylaxis is described here.

Response to the antigen

Immunoglobulin (Ig) M and IgG recognize the antigen as a foreign substance and attach to it. Destruction of the antigen by the complement cascade begins but remains unfinished because of insufficient amounts of the protein catalyst or the antigen inhibits certain complement enzymes. The patient has no signs or symptoms at this stage.

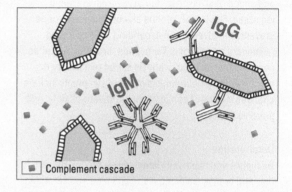

Released chemical mediators

The antigen's continued presence activates IgE on basophils. The activated IgE promotes the release of mediators, including histamine, serotonin, and leukotriene. The sudden release of histamine causes vasodilation and increases capillary permeability. The patient begins to have signs and symptoms, including sudden nasal congestion; itchy, watery eyes; flushing; sweating; weakness; and anxiety.

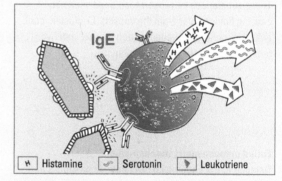

Intensified response

The activated IgE also stimulates mast cells in connective tissue along the venule walls to release more histamine and eosinophil chemotactic factor of anaphylaxis (ECF-A). These substances produce disruptive lesions that weaken the venules. Red, itchy skin; wheals; and swelling appear, and signs and symptoms worsen.

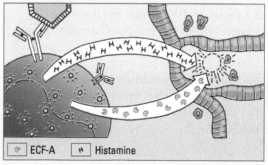

(continued)

Understanding anaphylaxis *(continued)*

Distress

In the lungs, histamine causes endothelial cells to burst and endothelial tissue to tear away from surrounding tissue. Fluids leak into the alveoli, and leukotriene prevents the alveoli from expanding, thus reducing pulmonary compliance. Tachypnea, crowing, use of accessory muscles, and cyanosis signal respiratory distress. Resulting neurologic signs and symptoms include changes in level of consciousness, severe anxiety, and possibly seizures.

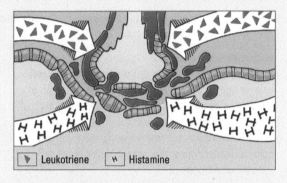

| ▶ Leukotriene | н Histamine |

Deterioration

Basophils and mast cells begin to release prostaglandins and bradykinin along with histamine and serotonin. These substances increase vascular permeability, causing fluids to leak from the vessels. Confusion; cool, pale skin; generalized edema; tachycardia; and hypotension signal rapid vascular collapse.

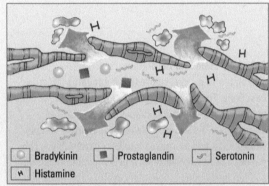

| ⊙ Bradykinin | ▪ Prostaglandin | ∿ Serotonin |
| н Histamine |

Failed compensatory mechanisms

Damage to the endothelial cells causes basophils and mast cells to release heparin. Additional substances are also released to neutralize the other mediators; eosinophils release arylsulfatase B to neutralize leukotriene, phospholipase D to neutralize heparin, and cyclic adenosine monophosphate and the prostaglandins E_1 and E_2 to increase the metabolic rate. These events can't reverse anaphylaxis. Hemorrhage, disseminated intravascular coagulation, and cardiopulmonary arrest result.

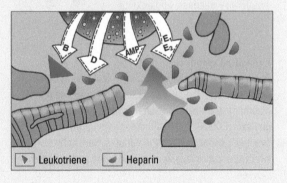

| ▶ Leukotriene | ◢ Heparin |

It's in the skin

On inspection, the patient's skin may display well-circumscribed, discrete cutaneous wheals with erythematous, raised, indented borders and blanched centers. They may coalesce to form giant hives. Angioedema may cause the patient to complain of a lump in his throat, or you may hear hoarseness or stridor. Wheezing, dyspnea, and complaints of chest tightness suggest bronchial obstruction. These signs and symptoms are early indications of impending airway compromise leading to respiratory failure.

Other effects may follow rapidly. The patient may report gastrointestinal (GI) and genitourinary effects, including severe stomach cramps, nausea, diarrhea, and urinary urgency and incontinence. Neurologic effects include dizziness, drowsiness, headache, restlessness, and seizures. Cardiovascular effects include hypotension, shock, and cardiac arrhythmias, which may precipitate vascular collapse if untreated.

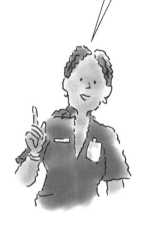

Remember, if your patient develops wheezing or dyspnea this is a sign that the airway is compromised. Alert the healthcare provider immediately!

What tests tell you

No single diagnostic test can identify anaphylaxis. It can be diagnosed by the rapid onset of severe respiratory or cardiovascular symptoms after ingestion or injection of a drug, vaccine, diagnostic agent, food, or food additive or after an insect sting. If these symptoms occur without a known allergic stimulus, other possible causes of shock (such as acute MI, status asthmaticus, or heart failure) must be ruled out.

These test results may provide some clues to the patient's risk for anaphylaxis:
- skin tests showing hypersensitivity to a specific allergen
- elevated serum IgE levels
- CBC with differential, total WBC elevation along with elevated eosinophil and basophil count.

How it's treated

Treatment focuses on maintaining a patent airway, ensuring adequate oxygenation, restoring vascular volume, and controlling and counteracting the effects of the chemical mediators released. Treatment includes:
- immediate administration of epinephrine (Adrenalin) 1:1,000 aqueous solution to reverse bronchoconstriction and cause vasoconstriction—intramuscularly, subcutaneously if the patient hasn't lost consciousness and is normotensive, or intravenously (1:10,000 concentration) if the reaction is severe (repeating dosage every 5 to 20 minutes as needed)
- endotracheal (ET) intubation and mechanical ventilation to maintain a patent airway, if compromised, occasionally emergent surgical airway via cricothyrotomy is performed
- oxygen therapy to increase tissue perfusion
- longer acting epinephrine, corticosteroids, and diphenhydramine (Benadryl) and famotidine (Pepcid)—histamine blockers—to

Giving epinephrine

When giving epinephrine to a patient with anaphylaxis, do the following:

• Check the patient's history for medication use. Epinephrine may be ineffective in patients taking beta-adrenergic blockers. Instead, anticipate administering glucagon as intravenous (IV) bolus as prescribed.

• When administering epinephrine intramuscularly or subcutaneously, expect to repeat after 5 to 10 minutes if no improvement is seen.

• Remember that IV administration of epinephrine is limited to profound, immediately life-threatening situations (such as the patient who is in shock or experiencing airway obstruction). In these cases, expect to give a dose intravenously over 5 minutes. If the patient is in cardiac arrest, give high-dose epinephrine IV push and repeat every 3 to 5 minutes.

• Important: Epinephrine concentration is different depending on the route of administration.

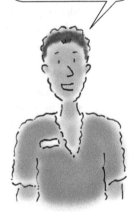

If a patient with anaphylaxis is in cardiac arrest, begin CPR right away.

decrease circulating histamine levels to reduce the allergic response (long-term management)

• albuterol (Proventil) nebulizer treatment
• volume expanders to maintain and restore circulating plasma volume
• IV vasopressors, such as norepinephrine (Levophed) and dopamine, to stabilize blood pressure
• CPR to treat cardiac arrest (De Bisschop & Bellou, 2012).

What to do

• Administer epinephrine as ordered. (See *Giving epinephrine.*)
• Assess the patient's ABCs. If the patient is in cardiac arrest, begin CPR and provide appropriate care.
• To reverse hypoxemia, administer supplemental oxygen as ordered at appropriate concentrations to maintain adequate pulse oximetry levels.
• Assess the patient's vital signs and respiratory status initially every 5 to 15 minutes and then less frequently as the patient's condition improves. Note continued evidence of hypotension and notify the health care provider immediately. Auscultate the lungs for decreased adventitious breath sounds.
• Be alert for decreased wheezing, which may signal an improvement in the patient's airflow. However, it could also indicate worsening of bronchoconstriction and obstruction. To determine what's happening, auscultate air movement throughout the lung fields. If decreased wheezing is a result of worsening bronchoconstriction, airflow will decrease.

Looking at ABG

- Observe for a positive response to oxygen therapy, such as improved breathing, color, pulse oximetry, and ABG values.
- Monitor oxygen saturation levels and ABG values for changes. Anticipate the need for ET intubation and mechanical ventilation if partial pressure of arterial oxygen (PaO_2) or supersaturated oxygen (SsO_2) continues to fall or partial pressure of arterial carbon dioxide ($PaCO_2$) rises.
- Expect ET intubation if the patient exhibits hoarseness, lingual edema, or posterior or oropharyngeal swelling. However, keep in mind that ET intubation may be difficult or impossible because it can result in increased laryngeal edema, bleeding, and further narrowing of the glottic opening. Fiber-optic ET intubation, needle cricothyrotomy (followed by transtracheal ventilation), or surgical cricothyrotomy may be necessary.
- Institute continuous cardiac monitoring to identify and treat arrhythmias as ordered.
- Assist with insertion of a central line placement if required. Monitor parameters at least every 15 to 30 minutes initially and then every hour as the patient's condition improves.

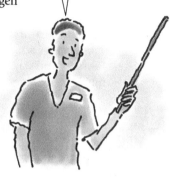

Watch the ABGs because falling PaO_2 means the patient may need intubation.

Eyeing the IV

- Begin IV or intraosseous (IO) fluid replacement therapy with crystalloids, such as lactated Ringer or normal saline solution, and colloids, such as albumin, as ordered. Monitor the patient's hemodynamic status for changes indicating improved cardiac output (CO).
- Assess the patient closely for signs and symptoms of fluid overload, such as crackles, S_3 heart sounds, jugular vein distention, and increases in hemodynamic parameters.
- If the patient doesn't respond to fluid replacement therapy, expect to administer vasopressors to raise blood pressure.
- Monitor intake and output closely, checking urine output every hour. Insert an indwelling urinary catheter as indicated and ordered to ensure accurate measurements. Notify the practitioner if urine output is less than 30 mL/hour.
- Administer additional pharmacotherapy as ordered, including antihistamines such as diphenhydramine, H_2 antagonists such as famotidine (Pepcid), inhaled beta-adrenergic agonists such as albuterol, and high-dose corticosteroids. Some health care providers will prescribe an anticholinergic such as ipratropium (Atrovent) for patients taking beta blockers, this will not work for acute wheezing due to its delayed onset of action.

Perfusion pointers

- Monitor level of consciousness (LOC) for changes indicating decreased cerebral perfusion. The first sign of altered tissue perfusion can be confusion or anxiety. It is important for the nurse to recognize these subtle changes.
- Evaluate peripheral tissue perfusion, including skin color, temperature, pulses, and capillary refill.
- Institute measures to control itching, such as cool compresses, avoidance of scratching, and using finger pads instead of nails.
- Reassure and stay with the patient; help the patient to relax as much as possible.

Cardiogenic shock in children

Although cardiogenic shock is uncommon in children, it may occur after cardiac surgery. It can also occur in children with acute arrhythmias, heart failure, or cardiomyopathy.

Cardiogenic shock

Sometimes called *pump failure*, cardiogenic shock is a condition of diminished CO that severely impairs tissue perfusion. Cardiogenic shock occurs as a serious complication in over 10% of patients who are hospitalized with acute MI (Kosaraju & Hai, 2019). (See *Cardiogenic shock in children.*)

Cardiogenic shock typically affects patients whose area of infarction involves 40% or more of left ventricular muscle mass; in such patients, mortality may exceed 85%. Most patients with cardiogenic shock die within 24 hours of onset. The prognosis for those who survive is poor.

What causes it

Cardiogenic shock can result from any condition that causes significant left ventricular dysfunction with reduced CO, such as MI (the most common cause), myocardial ischemia, papillary muscle dysfunction (rupture), pericardial tamponade, end-stage cardiomyopathy, and severe arrhythmias.

Other causes include myocarditis and depression of myocardial contractility after cardiac arrest and prolonged cardiac surgery. Mechanical abnormalities of the ventricle, such as acute mitral or aortic insufficiency or an acutely acquired ventricular septal defect or ventricular aneurysm, may also result in cardiogenic shock.

Blunt trauma to the chest can also result in cardiogenic shock due to myocardial stunning. Typically, it is the right ventricle involved due to the anatomical orientation of the heart.

How it happens

Regardless of the cause, left ventricular dysfunction initiates a series of compensatory mechanisms that increases heart rate, strengthens myocardial contractions, promotes sodium and water retention, and causes selective vasoconstriction. These mechanisms attempt to increase CO and maintain vital organ function.

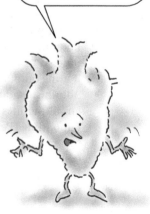

I feel so guilty—cardiogenic shock kills most patients within 24 hours of onset, and the prognosis for survivors is poor.

Stable but brief

However, these mechanisms also increase myocardial workload and oxygen consumption, thus reducing the heart's ability to pump blood, especially if the patient has myocardial ischemia. As CO falls, aortic and carotid baroreceptors activate sympathetic nervous responses. These compensatory responses further increase heart rate, left ventricular filling pressure, and peripheral resistance to flow in order to enhance venous return to the heart. These actions initially stabilize the patient but later cause deterioration with rising oxygen demands on the compromised myocardium.

CO cycle

These events constitute a vicious cycle of low CO, sympathetic compensation, myocardial ischemia, and even lower CO. Consequently, blood backs up, resulting in pulmonary edema. Eventually, CO falls and multisystem organ failure develops as the compensatory mechanisms fail to maintain perfusion.

What to look for

Typically, the patient's history includes a disorder (such as MI or cardiomyopathy) that severely decreases left ventricular function. A patient with underlying cardiac disease may complain of anginal pain because of decreased myocardial perfusion and oxygenation. Urine output is usually less than 20 mL/hour. Inspection typically reveals pale skin; decreased sensorium; and rapid, shallow respirations. Palpation of peripheral pulses may detect a rapid, thready pulse. The skin feels cold and clammy.

Auscultation of blood pressure usually discloses a mean arterial pressure (MAP) of less than 60 mm Hg and a narrowing pulse pressure. In a patient with chronic hypotension, the MAP may fall below 50 mm Hg before the patient exhibits signs of shock. Auscultation of the heart detects gallop rhythms, faint heart sounds, and, possibly (if shock results from rupture of the ventricular septum or papillary muscles), a holosystolic murmur (Gaieski & Mikkelsen, 2018).

Although many of these clinical features also occur in heart failure and other shock syndromes, they're usually more profound in cardiogenic shock.

Patients with pericardial tamponade may present with the typical findings associated with Beck triad: hypotension, jugular vein distension, and muffled heart tones.

Compensation clues

The patient's signs and symptoms may also provide clues to the stage of shock. For example, in the compensatory stage of shock, signs and symptoms may include:
- tachycardia and bounding pulse due to sympathetic stimulation
- restlessness and irritability related to cerebral hypoxia

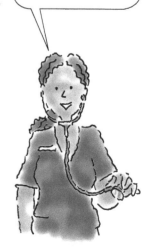

In a patient with chronic hypotension, mean arterial pressure may fall to less than 50 mm Hg before the patient exhibits signs of shock.

- tachypnea to compensate for hypoxia
- reduced urine output secondary to vasoconstriction
- cool, pale skin associated with vasoconstriction, sometimes mottling.

That's progress for ya

In the progressive stage of shock, signs and symptoms may include:
- hypotension as compensatory mechanisms begin to fail
- narrowed pulse pressure associated with reduced stroke volume
- weak, rapid, thready pulse caused by decreased CO
- shallow respirations as the patient weakens
- reduced urine output as poor renal perfusion continues
- cold, clammy skin caused by vasoconstriction
- cyanosis related to hypoxia.

No going back

In the irreversible stage, clinical findings may include:
- unconsciousness and absent reflexes caused by reduced cerebral perfusion, acid–base imbalance or electrolyte abnormalities, and elevated lactate acid levels
- rapidly falling blood pressure as decompensation occurs
- weak pulse caused by reduced CO
- slow, shallow, or Cheyne–Stokes respirations secondary to respiratory center depression
- hypoxia from pulmonary edema due to left ventricular failure
- anuria related to renal failure.

What tests tell you

- Pulmonary artery pressure (PAP) monitoring reveals increased PAP and pulmonary artery wedge pressure (PAWP), reflecting a rise in left ventricular end-diastolic pressure (preload) and heightened resistance to left ventricular emptying (afterload) caused by ineffective pumping and increased peripheral vascular resistance. Thermodilution catheterization reveals a reduced CO and cardiac index.
- Arterial pressure monitoring shows systolic arterial pressure less than 80 mm Hg caused by impaired ventricular ejection.
- ABG analysis may show metabolic and respiratory acidosis and hypoxia.
- Electrocardiography (ECG) demonstrates possible evidence of acute MI, ischemia, or ventricular aneurysm.
- Echocardiography determines left ventricular and right ventricular function and reveals valvular abnormalities.
- Serum enzyme measurements display elevated levels of creatine kinase (CK), lactate dehydrogenase (LD), aspartate aminotransferase, and alanine aminotransferase, which indicate MI or ischemia and suggest heart failure or shock. CK-MB and LD isoenzyme levels may confirm acute MI.

- Troponin levels (troponin I and troponin T) have become the preferred standard for detecting myocardial damage. They are the first levels to be elevated with MI.
- Lactic acid
- Prohormone brain natriuretic peptide (BNP)/BNP levels: BNP is a natural diuretic that the brain produces when the heart is overstretched. This level will rise as the heart failure worsens.
- Cardiac catheterization and echocardiography may reveal other conditions that can lead to pump dysfunction and failure, such as cardiac tamponade, papillary muscle infarct or rupture, ventricular septal rupture, pulmonary emboli, venous pooling, and hypovolemia.

How it's treated

Treatment aims to enhance cardiovascular status by increasing CO, improving myocardial perfusion, and decreasing cardiac workload with combinations of cardiovascular drugs and mechanically assisted techniques. These goals are accomplished by optimizing preload, decreasing afterload, increasing contractility, and optimizing heart rate.

Recommended IV drugs may include dopamine (a vasopressor that increases CO, blood pressure, and renal blood flow), milrinone or dobutamine (inotropic agents that increase myocardial contractility and increase CO), and norepinephrine (when a more potent vasoconstrictor is necessary).

Nitroglycerin or nitroprusside (vasodilators) may be used with a vasopressor to further improve CO by decreasing afterload and reducing preload. However, the patient must have adequate blood pressure to support nitroprusside therapy and must be monitored closely. Diuretics may also be used to reduce preload in the patient with fluid volume overload.

And just for good measure

Additional treatment measures for cardiogenic shock may include:
- thrombolytic therapy or coronary artery revascularization to restore coronary artery blood flow if cardiogenic shock is due to acute MI
- emergency surgery to repair papillary muscle rupture, ventricular septal defect, or coronary artery bypass surgery for emergent revascularization if either is the cause of cardiogenic shock
- mechanical support or devices used to support perfusion via artificial pumps and oxygenators such as extracorporeal membrane oxygenation (ECMO) or intra-aortic balloon pumps (IABPs) are being used earlier in treatment. There is a growing trend demonstrating utilization of these therapies early (such as in the ED) may lead to better outcomes.

What to do

- Begin IV infusions of normal saline solution or lactated Ringer solution using a large-bore (14G to 18G) catheter, which allows easier administration of later blood transfusions.
- Administer oxygen by face mask or artificial airway to ensure adequate tissue oxygenation. Adjust the oxygen flow rate to a higher or lower level, as blood gas measurements indicate. Many patients will need 100% oxygen, and some will require 5 to 15 cm H_2O of positive end-expiratory or continuous positive airway pressure ventilation.
- Monitor and record the patient's blood pressure, pulse, respiratory rate, and peripheral pulses every 1 to 5 minutes until the patient stabilizes.

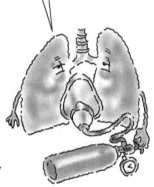

Administering oxygen by face mask ensures adequate tissue oxygenation.

Fascinating rhythm

- Monitor the patient's cardiac rhythm continuously. Systolic blood pressure less than 80 mm Hg usually results in inadequate coronary artery blood flow, cardiac ischemia, arrhythmias, and further complications of low CO. If blood pressure drops below 80 mm Hg, increase the oxygen flow rate and notify the practitioner immediately. A progressive drop in blood pressure accompanied by a thready pulse generally signals inadequate CO from reduced intravascular volume.
- Determine how much fluid to give by evaluating physical assessment findings, blood pressure, urine output, central venous pressure (CVP), or PAWP. (To increase accuracy, measure CVP at the level of the right atrium [phlebostatic axis] using the same reference point on the chest each time.) Whenever the fluid infusion rate is increased, watch for signs of fluid overload, such as an increase in CVP.
- Keep in mind that if the patient is hypovolemic, preload may need to be increased, which is typically accomplished with IV fluids. However, IV fluids must be given cautiously and increased gradually while hemodynamic parameters are closely monitored. In this situation, diuretics aren't given. Fluid boluses should be given incrementally in small volumes.

I'm going in

- Insert an indwelling urinary catheter if necessary to measure hourly urine output. If output is less than 30 mL/hour in adults, increase the fluid infusion rate but watch for signs of fluid overload such as an increase in CVP. Notify the practitioner if urine output doesn't improve.
- Administer a diuretic, such as furosemide (Lasix) or bumetanide, as ordered to decrease preload and improve stroke volume and CO.

- Monitor ABG values, CBC, and electrolyte levels. Expect to administer sodium bicarbonate by IV push if the patient demonstrates acidemia. Be aware that this is a temporizing effect. Reestablishing perfusion is the main goal. Administer electrolyte replacement therapy as ordered and indicated by laboratory test results.
- During therapy, assess skin color and temperature and note changes. Cold, clammy skin may be a sign of continuing peripheral vascular constriction, indicating progressive shock.
- Prepare the patient for possible emergency cardiac catheterization to determine eligibility for percutaneous transluminal coronary angioplasty or coronary artery bypass graft in an attempt to reperfuse areas with reversible injury patterns.

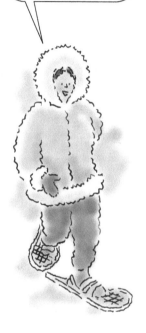

Cold, clammy skin is expected for me right now, but for a cardiogenic shock patient receiving therapy, it means the condition is progressing.

Hypovolemic shock

Hypovolemic shock most commonly results from acute blood loss—about 20% of total volume. Without sufficient blood or fluid replacement, it may cause irreversible damage to organs and systems.

What causes it

Massive volume loss may result from:
- GI bleeding
- internal or external hemorrhage, or any condition that reduces circulating intravascular volume or other body fluids, trauma
- intestinal obstruction
- peritonitis
- acute pancreatitis
- ascites
- dehydration from excessive perspiration, severe diarrhea, protracted vomiting, diabetes insipidus, diuresis, or inadequate fluid intake.

How it happens

Potentially life-threatening, hypovolemic shock stems from reduced intravascular blood volume, which leads to decreased CO and inadequate tissue perfusion. The subsequent tissue anoxia prompts a shift in cellular metabolism from aerobic to anaerobic pathways. This shift results in an accumulation of lactic acid, which produces metabolic acidosis.

Shock sequence

When compensatory mechanisms fail, hypovolemic shock occurs in this sequence:
1. Intravascular fluid volume decreases.
2. Venous return diminishes, which reduces preload and decreases stroke volume.

Estimating fluid loss

These assessment parameters indicate the severity of fluid loss.

Minimal fluid loss

Intravascular volume loss of 10% to 15% is regarded as minimal. Signs and symptoms include:
- slight tachycardia
- normal supine blood pressure
- positive postural vital signs, including a decrease in systolic blood pressure greater than or equal to 10 mm Hg or an increase in pulse rate greater than or equal to 20 beats per minute
- increased capillary refill time greater than or equal to 3 seconds
- urine output greater than or equal to 30 mL/hour
- cool, pale skin on arms and legs
- anxiety.

Moderate fluid loss

Intravascular volume loss of about 25% is regarded as moderate. Signs and symptoms include:
- rapid, thready pulse
- supine hypotension
- cool truncal skin
- urine output of 10 to 30 mL/hour
- severe thirst
- restlessness, confusion, or irritability.

Severe fluid loss

Intravascular volume loss of about 40% or more is regarded as severe. Signs and symptoms include:
- marked tachycardia
- marked hypotension
- weak or absent peripheral pulses
- cold, mottled, or cyanotic skin
- urine output less than 10 mL/hour
- unconsciousness.

(See *ATLS classification of hypovolemic shock.*)

3. CO is reduced.
4. MAP decreases.
5. Tissue perfusion is impaired.
6. Oxygen and nutrient delivery to cells decreases.
7. Multisystem organ failure occurs.

What to look for

The specific signs and symptoms exhibited by the patient depend on the amount of fluid loss. (See *Estimating fluid loss.*) Typically, the patient's history includes conditions that reduce blood volume, such as GI hemorrhage, trauma, or severe diarrhea and vomiting.

Assessment findings may include:
- pale skin
- decreased sensorium
- rapid, shallow respirations
- urine output less than 25 mL/hour
- rapid, thready peripheral pulses
- cold, clammy skin
- MAP less than 60 mm Hg and a narrowing pulse pressure
- decreased CVP, right atrial pressure, PAWP, and CO.

ATLS classification of hypovolemic shock

Class of hemorrhagic shock

	I	II	III	IV
Blood loss (mL)	Up to 750	750–1,500	1,500–2,000	>2,000
Blood loss (% blood volume)	Up to 15	15–30	30–40	>40
Pulse rate (per minute)	<100	100–120	120–140	>140
Blood pressure	Normal	Normal	Decreased	Decreased
Pulse pressure (mm Hg)	Normal or increased	Decreased	Decreased	Decreased
Respiratory rate (per minute)	14–20	20–30	30–40	>35
Urine output (mL/hour)	>30	20–30	5–15	Negligible
Central nervous system/ mental status	Slightly anxious	Mildly anxious	Anxious, confused	Confused, lethargic

What tests tell you

No single diagnostic test confirms hypovolemic shock, but these test results help support the diagnosis:
- low HCT
- decreased Hgb level
- decreased RBC and platelet counts
- elevated serum potassium, sodium, LD, creatinine, and BUN levels
- increased urine specific gravity (greater than 1.020) and urine osmolality
- urine sodium levels less than 50 mEq/L
- decreased urine creatinine levels
- decreased pH and PaO_2 and increased $PaCO_2$
- gastroscopy, X-rays, aspiration of gastric contents through a nasogastric tube, and tests for occult blood
- coagulation studies for coagulopathy from disseminated intravascular coagulation (DIC)
- elevated lactate level.

How it's treated

Emergency treatment relies on prompt, adequate fluid and blood replacement to restore intravascular volume, raise blood pressure, and maintain it above 80 mm Hg. Rapid infusion of normal saline or lactated Ringer solution and, possibly, albumin or other plasma expanders may expand volume adequately until whole blood can be matched. If hypovolemic shock is caused by massive bleeding,

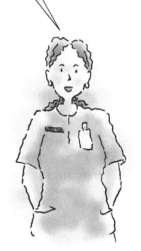

If urine specific gravity exceeds 1.020 while urine sodium levels fall to less than 50 mEq/L, your patient may have hypovolemic shock.

Ages and stages

Hypovolemic shock and children

Suspect hypovolemia in the infant or child who has a capillary refill longer than 2 seconds and accompanying history and signs of hypovolemic shock, such as tachycardia, altered level of consciousness, pale skin, lack of tears, and depressed fontanels.

Keep in mind that fluid replacement for an infant and a child is generally a crystalloid at a volume of 20 mL/kg of body weight in a fluid bolus. This bolus may be repeated for a total of three times while monitoring capillary refill as a response.

lactated Ringer solution is preferred for fluid replacement because it minimizes the risk of electrolyte imbalances.

Treatment may also include application (although controversial) of a pneumatic antishock garment, oxygen administration, control of bleeding, administration of dopamine or another inotropic drug, and surgery if appropriate.

What to do

- Ensure appropriate venous access. IO or central line access may be needed if unable to obtain adequate IV access in a short amount of time.
- Assess the patient for the extent of fluid loss and begin fluid replacement as ordered. (See *Hypovolemic shock and children*.)
- Obtain type and cross-match for blood component therapy.
- Assess the patient's ABCs.
- If the patient experiences cardiac or respiratory arrest, start CPR.
- Administer supplemental oxygen as ordered.
- Monitor the patient's oxygen saturation and ABG values for evidence of hypoxemia and anticipate the need for ET intubation and mechanical ventilation if the patient's respiratory status deteriorates.
- Place the patient in semi-Fowler position to maximize chest expansion.
- Keep the patient as quiet and comfortable as possible to minimize oxygen demands.
- Monitor the patient's vital signs, neurologic status, and cardiac rhythm continuously for such changes as cardiac arrhythmias and myocardial ischemia.

Capillary cues

- Observe the patient's skin color and check capillary refill.
- Notify the practitioner if capillary refill takes longer than 2 seconds. (See *When blood pressure drops*.)

Stay on the ball

When blood pressure drops

A drop below 80 mm Hg in systolic blood pressure usually signals inadequate cardiac output from reduced intravascular volume. Such a drop usually results in inadequate coronary artery blood flow, cardiac ischemia, arrhythmias, and other complications of low cardiac output. If the patient's systolic blood pressure drops below 80 mm Hg and the pulse is thready, increase the oxygen flow rate and notify the health care provider immediately. Prepare for fluid bolus. Be cognizant of other factors that may cause a stable, normal low blood pressure such as athletes or patients on beta blocker medications for heart failure (American College of Surgeons, 2018).

- Monitor hemodynamic parameters—including CVP, PAWP, and CO and cardiac input—as often as every 15 minutes to evaluate the patient's status and response to treatment.
- Monitor the patient's intake and output closely.
- Insert an indwelling urinary catheter and assess urine output hourly.

Watch for blood

- If bleeding from the GI tract is the suspected cause, check all stools, emesis, and gastric drainage for occult blood.
- If urine output falls below 30 mL/hour in an adult, expect to increase the IV fluid infusion rate but watch for signs of fluid overload such as elevated CVP.
- Notify the health care provider if urine output doesn't increase.
- Administer blood component therapy as prescribed; monitor serial Hgb values and HCT to evaluate the effects of treatment.
- Cautiously prepare for administration of dopamine or norepinephrine IV as prescribed to increase cardiac contractility and renal perfusion. If the cause is truly hypovolemic in nature, adding vasopressor medication will increase the demand and increase tissue hypoxia.
- Watch for signs of impending coagulopathy, such as petechiae, bruising, and bleeding or oozing from gums or venipuncture sites, and report them immediately. (See *Understanding DIC*, page 574.)
- Provide emotional support and reassurance as appropriate in the wake of massive fluid losses.
- Prepare the patient for surgery or interventional radiology as appropriate.

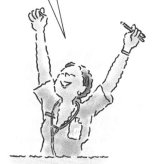

Stretch that chest! Putting the patient in semi-Fowler position maximizes chest expansion.

Neurogenic shock

In neurogenic shock, a temporary loss of autonomic function below the level of a spinal cord injury produces cardiovascular changes. Neurogenic shock is a type of distributive shock in which vasodilation causes a state of hypovolemia. It occurs most commonly from injuries at the spinal level of T6 or above.

What causes it

It may result from spinal cord injury: spinal anesthesia, vasomotor center depression, medications, or hypoglycemia.

How it happens

A loss of sympathetic vasoconstrictor tone in the vascular smooth muscle and reduced autonomic function lead to widespread arterial

Understanding DIC

Disseminated intravascular coagulation (DIC) can occur as a complication of hypovolemic shock. As a result, accelerated clotting occurs, causing small vessel occlusion resulting in organ necrosis due to the inability of perfusion to occur, depletion of circulating clotting factors and platelets, activation of the fibrinolytic system (rapid breaking down of clot), and consequent severe hemorrhage.

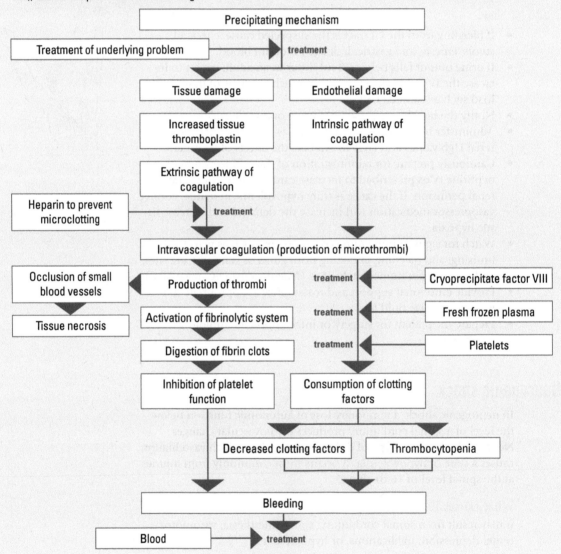

and venous vasodilation. Venous return is reduced as blood pools in the venous septum, leading to a drop in CO and hypotension.

What to look for

The neurogenic shock patient will display these signs and symptoms:
- hypotension
- bradycardia
- slow pulse
- warm, dry, and flushed skin
- hypothermia.

What tests tell you

Tests to determine neurogenic shock should include ABG to determine the degree of cardiopulmonary compensation, ECG to determine cardiac arrhythmias, and CT scan or magnetic resonance imaging to determine the extent of spinal injury.

How it's treated

Treatment goals include assessing ABCs, treating hypothermia, administering fluid resuscitation and vasoconstrictors to increase blood pressure, and administering agents to block vagal effects that cause bradycardia, such as atropine.

What to do

- Assess the patient's LOC.
- Assess the rate, depth, and pattern of respirations and auscultate breath sounds.
- Palpate for peripheral pulses and auscultate the apical heart rate.
- Assess the patient's vital signs, noting hypotension and bradycardia.
- Observe the patient for warm, dry skin.
- Obtain a blood sample for ABG analysis.
- Provide supplemental oxygen and prepare the patient for ET intubation and mechanical ventilation, as necessary.
- Initiate cardiac and hemodynamic monitoring.
- Treat hypothermia with a warming blanket.
- Insert an indwelling urinary catheter.
- Initiate and administer IV fluid resuscitation such as normal saline solution or lactated Ringer solution to increase intravascular volume and blood pressure.
- Administer medications such as vasopressors to increase blood pressure, blood products to increase intravascular volume, an osmotic diuretic such as mannitol if urine output is decreased to increase renal blood flow, and atropine or transcutaneous pacing to treat symptomatic bradycardia.

Septic shock

Septic shock is a type of distributive shock. It can occur in anyone with an infectious source that causes a syndromic response from the body. Those at highest risk are those who have impaired immunity (HIV positive individuals, transplant recipients, cancer patients) and older adults. Initially, low systemic vascular resistance and increased CO characterize septic shock. With progression to late sepsis, CO is decreased and complete vascular collapse occurs with multiple organ dysfunction. The disorder is thought to be a response to infections that release microbes or immune mediators, such as tumor necrosis factor (TNF) and interleukin-1.

The Surviving Sepsis Campaign creates guidelines for management of sepsis and septic shock. The last set of guidelines were released in 2016, with an updated addendum in 2018 (Levy et al., 2018; Rhodes et al., 2017).

In addition to the Surviving Sepsis Campaign, Sepsis-3, an international consensus for defining sepsis and septic shock was determined (Seymour et al., 2016). The purpose of the new definition is to prompt earlier recognition and treatment.

- Sepsis: life-threatening organ dysfunction caused by dysregulated host response to infection
- Septic shock: subset of sepsis with circulatory and cellular/metabolic dysfunction associated with higher risk of mortality

Sepsis-3 proposes use of the Sequential Organ Failure Assessment (SOFA) during the patient's hospitalization.

SOFA scoring is proposed for patients in the intensive care unit to estimate mortality rates and to prompt treatment changes. The initial baseline score is zero for patients with no previous organ dysfunction. A SOFA score of 2 or greater identified a 2- to 25-fold increased risk of dying compared with patients with a SOFA score less than 2.

For patients who present in the ED, in the ambulatory clinic, or in the hospital, a modified version of the SOFA scale referred to as the *quick SOFA* (qSOFA) is suggested. The qSOFA is used to prompt the nurse or health care provider to consider a diagnosis of sepsis in the patient and to conduct more thorough testing and/or aggressive treatment strategy (Rhodes et al., 2017). The qSOFA assesses the respiratory rate, mental status, and systolic blood pressure (Marik & Taeb, 2017).

What causes it

Any pathogenic organism can cause septic shock. Gram-negative bacteria, such as *Escherichia coli*, *Klebsiella pneumoniae*, *Serratia*, *Enterobacter*, and *Pseudomonas*, rank as the most common causes and account for up to 70% of all cases. Opportunistic fungi cause about 3% of cases. Rare causative organisms include mycobacteria and some viruses and protozoa.

> Gram-negative bacteria are the most common cause of septic shock.

How it happens

An immune response is triggered when bacteria release endotoxins. In response, macrophages secrete TNF and interleukins. These mediators in turn increase the release of platelet-activating factor (PAF), prostaglandins, leukotrienes, thromboxane A_2, kinins, and complement.

Truth about consequences

The consequences of this immune activity are vasodilation, increased capillary permeability, reduced systemic vascular resistance, microemboli, and an elevated CO. Endotoxins also stimulate the release of histamine, further increasing capillary permeability.

Moreover, myocardial depressant factor, TNF, PAF, and other factors depress myocardial function. CO falls, resulting in multisystem organ dysfunction syndrome. (See *Understanding MODS*, page 578.)

What to look for

The patient's history may include a disorder or treatment that causes immunosuppression or a history of invasive tests or treatments, surgery, or trauma. At onset, the patient may have fever and chills, although 20% of patients may be hypothermic. The patient's signs and symptoms will reflect the hyperdynamic (warm) phase of septic shock or the hypodynamic (cold) phase.

Hyper . . .

The hyperdynamic phase is characterized by:
- increased CO
- peripheral vasodilation
- decreased systemic vascular resistance
- altered LOC
- rapid, shallow respirations
- decreased urine output
- rapid, full, bounding pulse.

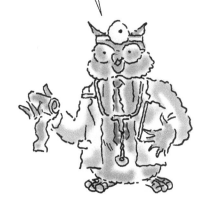

Any emergency nurse would be wise to look for these septic shock symptoms.

. . . or hypo

The hypodynamic phase is characterized by:
- decreased CO
- peripheral vasoconstriction
- increased systemic vascular resistance
- inadequate tissue perfusion
- pale, possibly cyanotic skin color
- mottling of extremities
- decreased LOC
- rapid, shallow respirations
- decreased or absent urine output
- absence of peripheral pulses or a rapid, weak, thready pulse

Understanding MODS

Multisystem organ dysfunction syndrome (MODS) is a condition that occurs when two or more organs or organ systems can't maintain homeostasis. Intervention is necessary to support and maintain organ function. MODS isn't an illness itself; rather, it's a manifestation of another progressive, underlying condition.

MODS develops when widespread systemic inflammation, a condition known as *systemic inflammatory response syndrome* (SIRS), overtaxes a patient's compensatory mechanisms. Infection, ischemia, trauma of any sort, reperfusion injury, or multisystem injury can trigger SIRS. If allowed to progress, SIRS can lead to organ inflammation and, ultimately, MODS.

Primary or secondary

Typically, MODS is classified as *primary* or *secondary*. In *primary MODS*, organ or organ system failure is due to a direct injury (such as trauma or a primary disorder) that usually involves the lungs, such as pneumonia, aspiration, near drowning, and pulmonary embolism. The organ failure can be positively linked to the direct injury. Typically, acute respiratory distress syndrome (ARDS) develops and progresses, leading to encephalopathy and coagulopathy from hepatic involvement. As the syndrome continues, other organ systems are affected.

In *secondary MODS*, organ or organ system failure is due to sepsis. Typically, the infection source isn't associated with the lungs. The most common infection sources include intra-abdominal sepsis, extensive blood loss, pancreatitis, or major vascular injuries. With secondary MODS, ARDS develops sooner and progressive involvement of other organs and organ systems occurs more rapidly.

Regardless of the type of MODS or triggering event, the overall underlying problem is inadequate perfusion.

Assessment findings

Assessment findings associated with MODS typically reveal an acutely ill patient with signs and symptoms associated with SIRS. SIRS is defined by:
- fever >100.4 ° F (38° C)
- hypothermia <96.8° F (36° C)

- tachycardia heart rate (HR) >90 beats per minute
- tachypnea respiratory rate (RR) >20 breaths per minute or partial pressure of arterial carbon dioxide ($Paco_2$) <32 mm Hg
- White blood cell (WBC) count >12,000/mm^3 or <4,000/mm^3 or the presence of >10% bands (immature neutrophils).

When two of these criteria are met, the condition is defined as SIRS. It is important to note that a patient can have severe SIRS and never have sepsis or a specific infectious source.

As SIRS progresses, findings reflect impaired perfusion of the tissues and organs, such as decreasing level of consciousness, respiratory depression, diminished bowel sounds, jaundice, oliguria, or anuria. *Pulmonary artery pressure* increases (due to pulmonary edema). Pulmonary artery wedge pressure increases and cardiac output decreases with the development of heart failure.

Organ dysfunction is determined by specific criteria. For example, pulmonary organ dysfunction is identified by the development of ARDS, requiring positive end-expiratory pressure greater than 10 cm H_2O and a fraction of inspired oxygen less than 0.5. Hepatic dysfunction is evidenced by jaundice with a serum bilirubin level of 8 to 10 mg/dL. An oliguria of less than 500 mL/day or an increasing serum creatinine level indicates mild renal system dysfunction, whereas the need for dialysis suggests severe organ involvement. Development of disseminated intravascular coagulation typically indicates severe hematologic system dysfunction.

Treatment

Treatment focuses on supporting respiratory and circulatory function by using mechanical ventilation, supplemental oxygen, hemodynamic monitoring, and fluid infusion to expand and maintain the intravascular compartment. Renal function is closely monitored, including hourly urine output measurements and serial laboratory tests to evaluate for trends indicating acute renal failure. Dialysis may ultimately be necessary.

Understanding MODS *(continued)*

Numerous drugs may be used:
- antimicrobial agents to treat underlying infection
- vasopressors, such as dopamine and norepinephrine
- isotonic crystalloid solutions, such as normal saline and lactated Ringer solutions, to expand the intravascular fluid spaces
- colloids, such as albumin, to help expand plasma volume without the added risk of causing fluid overload.

Some experimental agents are being used, such as antitumor necrosis factor, endotoxin, and anti–interleukin-1 antibodies. However, more evidence is needed to determine the effectiveness of these agents (Schmidt & Clardy, 2018).

Nursing care

Nursing care for the patient with MODS is primarily supportive. The patient is acutely ill and requires close, usually extensive, monitoring. Emotional support is also crucial because mortality for a patient with MODS is directly proportional to the number of organs or organ systems affected. For example, mortality is 85% when three organs are involved; it jumps to 95% when four organs are involved and up to 99% with five-organ involvement.

- cold, clammy skin
- hypotension, usually with a systolic pressure below 90 mm Hg or 50 to 80 mm Hg below the patient's previous level
- crackles or rhonchi if pulmonary congestion is present
- reduced or normal CVP.

What tests tell you

- Blood cultures are only seen positive in 50% of all cases of sepsis (Rhodes et al., 2017).
- CBC shows the presence or absence of anemia and leukopenia, severe or absent neutropenia, and (usually) the presence of thrombocytopenia.
- ABG studies may reveal metabolic acidosis, hypoxemia, and low $Paco_2$ that progress to increased $Paco_2$ (indicating respiratory acidosis).
- BUN and creatinine levels are increased, and creatinine clearance is decreased.
- PT, PTT, and bleeding time increase; platelets decrease; and fibrin split products increase.
- Chest X-rays reveal evidence of pneumonia (as the underlying infection) or acute respiratory distress syndrome (indicating progression of septic shock).
- ECG shows ST segment depression and inverted T waves.
- Amylase and lipase levels may show pancreatic insufficiency.
- Hepatic enzyme levels are elevated due to liver ischemia.
- Blood glucose levels are initially elevated and then decrease; goal is to maintain glucose levels less than 180 mg/dL.

- CT scan reveals abscesses or sources of possible infection.
- Serum lactate may indicate hypoperfusion. Resuscitation involves normalizing elevated serum lactate level (Rhodes et al., 2017).

How it's treated

Location and treatment of the underlying sepsis is essential to treating septic shock, including:

- removal of the source of infection, such as IV, intra-arterial, or urinary drainage catheters
- broad-spectrum, dual-agent antimicrobial therapy
- culture and sensitivity tests of urine and wound drainage
- source control surgery, if appropriate, to evacuate, debride infectious tissue; removal of infectious hardware such as infected orthopedic hardware
- reduction or discontinuation of immunosuppressive drug therapy
- possible granulocyte transfusions in patients with severe neutropenia
- oxygen therapy and mechanical ventilation if necessary
- colloid or crystalloid infusions
- administration of a vasopressor such as dopamine.

What to do

- Assess the patient's ABCs; monitor cardiopulmonary status closely.
- Administer supplemental oxygen as ordered.
- Monitor the patient's oxygen saturation and ABG values for evidence of hypoxemia and anticipate the need for ET intubation and mechanical ventilation if the patient's respiratory status deteriorates.
- Place the patient in semi-Fowler position to maximize chest expansion. Keep the patient as quiet and comfortable as possible to minimize oxygen demands.
- Monitor the patient's vital signs continuously for changes. Observe his skin color and check capillary refill. Notify the health care provider if capillary refill is longer than 2 seconds.

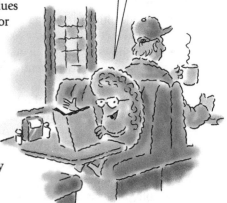

In a patient with septic shock, capillary refill shouldn't take longer than 2 seconds. I wish my "coffee-lary" refills were that quick!

Ups and downs

- Keep in mind that the patient's temperature is usually elevated in the early stages of septic shock and that shaking chills often occur. As the shock progresses, the temperature usually drops and the patient experiences diaphoresis.
- If the patient's systolic blood pressure drops below 80 mm Hg, increase the oxygen flow rate and notify the practitioner immediately. Alert the health care provider and increase the infusion rate if the patient experiences a progressive drop in blood pressure accompanied by a thready pulse.

- Remove IV, intra-arterial, or urinary drainage catheters and send them to the laboratory to culture for the presence of the causative organism (and prepare to reinsert or assist with reinsertion of new devices).
- Obtain blood cultures as ordered and begin antimicrobial therapy as ordered. Monitor the patient for possible adverse effects of therapy.
- Institute continuous cardiac monitoring to evaluate for possible arrhythmias, myocardial ischemia, or adverse effects of treatment.
- Monitor the patient's intake and output closely. Notify the health care provider if the urine output is less than 30 mL/hour.
- Administer IV fluid therapy as ordered, usually normal saline or lactated Ringer solution. Monitor hemodynamic parameters to determine the patient's response to therapy.

Overload alert!

- Be alert for signs and symptoms of possible fluid overload, such as dyspnea, tachypnea, crackles, peripheral edema, jugular vein distention, and increased PAP.
- Administer positive inotropic agents as prescribed.
- Institute infection control precautions; use strict aseptic technique for all invasive procedures.
- Monitor laboratory test results, especially coagulation studies and hepatic enzyme levels, for changes indicative of DIC and hepatic failure, respectively.
- Provide emotional support to the patient and family.
- Prepare the patient for surgery as appropriate.

Multisystem trauma

Trauma is a physical injury or wound that's inflicted by an external or violent act; it may be intentional or unintentional. Multisystem traumas involve injuries to more than one body area or organ and are the leading cause of death in people younger than age 45.

The type of trauma determines the extent of injury:
- *blunt trauma*—leaves the body intact
- *penetrating trauma*—disrupts the body surface
- *perforating trauma*—leaves entrance and exit wounds as an object passes through the body.

A patient experiencing multisystem trauma requires immediate action and a multidisciplinary team approach. The patient may have a head injury accompanied by chest and cardiac trauma, or have experienced a spinal cord injury along with numerous fractures and contusions to other body areas.

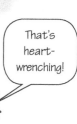

Did you know multisystem trauma is the leading cause of death for people younger than age 45?

I had no idea!

That's heart-wrenching!

What causes it

Trauma may be caused by weapons, automobile collision, physical confrontation, falls, explosions, or other unnatural occurrence to the body.

How it happens

Trauma typically creates wounds. Traumatic wounds include:
- *abrasion*—scraped skin, with partial loss of skin surface
- *laceration*—torn skin, causing jagged, irregular edges (severity of which depends on size, depth, and location)
- *puncture wound*—skin penetrated by a pointed object, such as a knife or glass fragment
- *traumatic amputation*—removal of part of the body (a limb or part of a limb).

What to look for

Assessment findings vary according to the type and extent of trauma. A conscious patient with multiple injuries may be able to help focus the assessment on areas that need immediate attention, such as difficulty breathing and neurologic symptoms.

Initially, the patient is assessed for life-threatening problems involving his ABCs. Monitor cardiac rhythm, initiate CPR, and administer drugs and electrical shock therapy (defibrillation and synchronized cardioversion) as appropriate for cardiac arrhythmias. After initially assessing and treating life-threatening conditions, perform a secondary assessment, including taking a history and performing a physical examination.

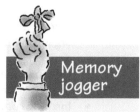

Memory jogger

To help remember what information to obtain during assessment of the trauma patient, use the acronym **SAMPLE**.

S—Signs and symptoms

A—Allergies

M—Medications

P—Past medical history

L—Last meal

E—Events leading to injury

Out of time

During an emergency, you won't have time to obtain all of the patient's history. Focus on the most important information, including:
- signs and symptoms related to the present condition
- allergies to drugs, foods, latex, or environmental factors
- medication history, including prescription and over-the-counter medications, herbs, and supplements
- past medical history
- last meal
- events leading to the injury or condition.

When the patient's condition is stabilized, fill in the other components of the normal health history. Remember to include a history of blood transfusions and tetanus immunization if the patient has an open wound. When the patient is stable, perform a body system examination according to your facility's policy and procedure. A thorough assessment helps systematically identify and correct problems and establishes a baseline for future comparison.

What tests tell you

The diagnostic tests performed are based on the body system affected by the trauma. For example, a patient with a blunt chest injury would require a chest X-ray to detect rib and sternal fractures, pneumothorax, flail chest, pulmonary contusion, and a lacerated or ruptured aorta. Angiography studies would also be performed with suspected aortic laceration or rupture. Diagnostic tests for a patient with head trauma may include a CT scan, a cervical spine X-ray, a skull X-ray, or an angiogram.

Some other diagnostic tests that may be performed on the patient with multisystem trauma include:

- ABG analysis to evaluate respiratory status and determine acidotic and alkalotic states
- CBC to indicate the amount of blood loss
- coagulation studies to evaluate clotting ability
- serum electrolyte levels to indicate the presence of electrolyte imbalances
- toxicology screening (drug and alcohol)
- type and screen for blood products.

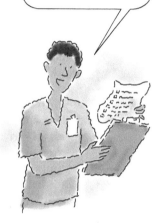

History of the patient is always important, but in multisystem trauma emergency cases, you'll have to settle for the abridged version.

How it's treated

Multisystem trauma care basics include:

- performing triage
- assessing and maintaining ABCs
- protecting the cervical spine
- assessing LOC
- preparing the patient for transport and possible surgery.

Six degrees of contamination

Management of traumatic wounds depends on the type of wound and degree of contamination. Treatment may include:

- controlling bleeding, usually by applying firm, direct pressure and elevating the extremity. If this fails to control the bleeding, tourniquets may be applied on an extremity or a clotting agent such as QuikClot can be used. QuikClot causes a mild chemical and thermal reaction to cause hemostasis (American College of Surgeons, 2018).
- cleaning the wound
- administering pain medication
- administering antibiotic therapy
- administering tetanus shot
- undergoing surgery.

Additional treatment is based on the body system that's affected by the trauma and the extent of injury. For example, treatment of a blunt chest injury may include maintaining a patent airway; providing adequate ventilation; maintaining fluid and electrolyte balance; and inserting a chest tube for pneumothorax, hemothorax, or tension pneumothorax.

What to do

- Assess the patient's ABCs and initiate emergency measures if necessary; administer supplemental oxygen as ordered.
- Immobilize the patient's head and neck with an immobilization device, sandbags, backboard, and tape. Assist with cervical spine X-rays. Monitor vital signs and note significant changes.
- Immobilize fractures.
- Monitor the patient's oxygen saturation and cardiac rhythm for arrhythmias.
- Assess the patient's neurologic status, including LOC and pupillary and motor response.
- Obtain blood studies, including type and cross-match.
- Insert two IV large-bore catheters (IO if unable to obtain IV access) and infuse normal saline or lactated Ringer solution.
- Quickly and carefully assess the patient for multiple injuries.
- Assess the patient's wounds and provide wound care as appropriate. Cover open wounds and control bleeding by applying pressure and elevating extremities.
- Assess for increased abdominal distention and increased diameter of extremities.
- Administer blood products as appropriate.
- Monitor the patient for signs of hypovolemic shock.
- Provide pain medication as appropriate.
- Provide reassurance to the patient and family.

Quick quiz

1. What's the highest priority when caring for a patient with hypovolemic shock?
    A. Assessing for dehydration
    B. Administering IV fluids
    C. Inserting a urinary catheter
    D. Obtaining a sample for CBC

Answer: B. Hypovolemic shock is an emergency that requires rapid infusion of IV fluids.

2. Which sign would lead the nurse to suspect that a patient is experiencing septic shock?
    A. Clear, watery sputum
    B. Severe hypertension
    C. Hypotension
    D. Polyuria

Answer: C. Hypotension—along with pale, possibly cyanotic skin; mottling of extremities; decreased LOC; rapid, shallow respirations; decreased or absent urine output; absence of peripheral pulses; or a rapid, weak pulse—is a sign of hypodynamic septic shock.

3.   Which nursing action is most appropriate when a cervical spine injury is suspected in a trauma patient?
   A.   Remove the cervical collar before attempting to open the airway.
   B.   Use the head-tilt, chin-lift maneuver to open the airway.
   C.   Turn the patient on his side to prevent aspiration.
   D.   Use the jaw-thrust maneuver to open the airway.

Answer: D. In a patient with a suspected cervical spine injury, the most appropriate way to open the airway is to use the jaw-thrust maneuver.

4.   Which drug would be used first for a patient with anaphylactic shock?
   A.   Epinephrine
   B.   Diphenhydramine
   C.   Albuterol
   D.   Prednisone

Answer: A. Immediate treatment for anaphylactic shock involves the administration of epinephrine to reverse bronchoconstriction. Later, corticosteroids, such as prednisone, diphenhydramine, and albuterol, may be given.

5.   Which sign would the nurse anticipate in a patient experiencing intravascular fluid volume loss of 10%?
   A.   Supine hypotension
   B.   Positive postural vital signs
   C.   Urine output less than 30 mL/hour
   D.   Cold, mottled skin

Answer: B. An intravascular fluid volume loss of approximately 10% is classified as minimal and would be manifested by positive postural vital signs, such as a decrease in systolic blood pressure greater than 10 mm Hg or an increase in pulse rate to greater than 20 beats per minute.

Scoring

 If you answered all five questions correctly, way to go! Your knowledge of this chapter's information is shockingly accurate!

If you answered three or four questions correctly, nice job! Treat yourself to a multisystem-pleasing rest before reviewing the chapter again.

If you answered fewer than three questions correctly, don't be shocked! Just review the material and try again.

Selected references

American College of Surgeons. (2018). *Advanced Trauma Life Support: Student course manual* (10th ed.). Chicago, IL: Author.

De Bisschop, M. B., & Bellou, A. (2012). Anaphylaxis. *Current Opinion in Critical Care, 18*(4), 308–317.

Emergency Nurses Association. (2019). *Trauma nursing course* (8th ed.). Des Plaines, IL: Author.

Gaieski, D., & Mikkelsen, M. (2018). *Definition, classification, etiology, and pathophysiology of shock in adults.* Retrieved from https://www.uptodate.com/contents/definition-classification-etiology-and-pathophysiology-of-shock-in-adults

Kosaraju, A., & Hai, O. (2019). *Cardiogenic shock.* Retrieved from https://www.ncbi.nlm.nih.gov/books/NBK482255/

Levy, M. M., Evans, L. E., & Rhodes, A. (2018). The Surviving Sepsis Campaign bundle: 2018 update. *Critical Care Medicine, 46*(6), 997–1000. doi:10.1097/CCM.0000000000003119

Marik, P., & Taeb, A. (2017). SIRS, qSOFA and new sepsis definition. *Journal of Thoracic Disease, 9*(4), 943–945. doi:10.21037/jtd.2017.03.125

Mirski, M. A., Frank, S. M., Kor, D. J., et al. (2015). Restrictive and liberal red cell transfusion strategies in adult patients: Reconciling clinical data with best practice. *Critical Care (London, England), 19*, 202.

Rhodes, A., Evans, L., Alhazzani, W., et al. (2017). Surviving Sepsis Campaign: International guidelines for management of sepsis and septic shock 2016. *Critical Care Medicine, 45*(3), 486–552.

Schmidt, G., & Clardy, P. (2018). *Investigational and ineffective therapies for sepsis.* Retrieved from https://www.uptodate.com/contents/investigational-and-ineffective-therapies-for-sepsis

Semler, M. W., Self, W. H., Wanderer, J. P., et al. (2018). Balanced crystalloids versus saline in critically ill adults. *The New England Journal of Medicine, 378*, 829–839.

Seymour, C. W., Liu, V. X., Iwashyna, T. J., et al. (2016). Assessment of clinical criteria for sepsis: For the Third International Consensus Definitions for Sepsis and Septic Shock (Sepsis-3). *JAMA, 315*(8), 762–774.

Sharma, S., Sharma, P., & Tyler, L. N. (2011). Transfusion of blood and blood products: Indications and complications. *American Family Physician, 83*(6), 719–724.

Silvergleid, A. (2017). *Leukoreduction to prevent complications of blood transfusion.* Retrieved from https://www.uptodate.com/contents/leukoreduction-to-prevent-complications-of-blood-transfusion

Appendices and index

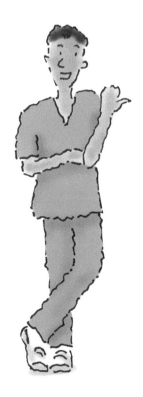

Practice makes perfect

1. The nurse is performing a primary survey on a patient who is suffering from multiple traumatic injuries. Which of the following is considered to be part of the primary survey?
    A. History and head to toe assessment
    B. Providing comfort measures
    C. Brief neurologic assessment
    D. Full set of vital signs

2. A 45-year-old patient arrives via ambulance with diaphoresis, shortness of breath, and chest pain. This patient should be prioritized into which category?
    A. Urgent
    B. Emergent
    C. Nonurgent
    D. Resuscitation

3. What does the mnemonic SAMPLE mean?
    A. Survey, assessment, monitor, past allergies, last bowel movement, events
    B. Subjective data, alarm, mean arterial pressure, postoperative vitals, last meal, evaluation
    C. Start assessment, action plan, morphine, plan of care, living situation, emesis
    D. Subjective data, allergies, medications, past medical history, last meal, events

4. What is one of the nurse educator's role in the emergency room?
    A. Acts as an administrative representative of the unit
    B. Uses excellent interpersonal skills
    C. Plans and implement patient care
    D. Makes medical diagnosis for triaging patients

5. Which patient requires enhanced therapeutic communication skills when the nurse is gathering a past and present sexual medical history? Select all that apply.
    A. 15-year-old female
    B. 30-year-old female
    C. 40-year-old bisexual
    D. 52-year-old male
    E. 60-year old female

6. A patient presents to the emergency department for the third time in 3 months with urinary urgency, frequency, and dysuria. Which condition will the nurse assess for when obtaining a medical history?
   A. Lupus erythematosus
   B. Diabetes mellitus
   C. Emphysema
   D. Crohn disease

7. Which teaching will the nurse provide to a patient who is preparing to undergo a computed tomography (CT) scan of the bladder?
   A. A full bladder is required for this test.
   B. The patient must be fasting for 12 hours prior to this scan.
   C. This test cannot be performed without a contrast medium.
   D. The patient will need to lie still and breathe normally during the procedure.

8. The nurse is caring for a patient with dehydration and multiple calcium crystals in the urinalysis. Which additional assessment finding does the nurse anticipate?
   A. Urine pH of 5
   B. Blood in urine
   C. Straw-colored urine
   D. Urine specific gravity of 1.020

9. Which condition does the nurse anticipate for a postpartum patient with a boggy uterus and laboratory findings including an elevated white blood cell (WBC) and erythrocyte sedimentation rate and a positive urine culture for *Staphylococcus*?
   A. Polycystic ovary syndrome (PCOS)
   B. Cervicitis
   C. Endometritis
   D. Salpingo-oophoritis

10. After attending football practice, a 17-year-old male presents to the emergency department with severe testicular pain for the past 2 hours. Which action will the nurse perform?
    A. Apply ice to the affected area.
    B. Administer fluids to increase hydration.
    C. Schedule the patient for immediate surgery.
    D. Gently elevate the scrotum to the symphysis pubis.

11. The nurse is caring for a patient whose right foot is hyperemic with edema. How will the nurse document this finding?
    A. First-degree frostbite
    B. Second-degree frostbite
    C. Third-degree frostbite
    D. Fourth-degree frostbite

12. The nurse is caring for a patient with moderate hypothermia. Which assessment finding does the nurse anticipate?
    A. Absence of palpable pulses
    B. Peripheral cyanosis
    C. Slurred speech
    D. Dilated pupils

13. How will the nurse care for a cat bite to a patient's hand? Select all that apply.
    A. Remove jewelry around the affected area.
    B. Assess for signs of infection.
    C. Irrigate the affected area with normal saline.
    D. Prepare the affected area for suturing.
    E. Teach to elevate the affected area.
    F. Administer measles, mumps, and rubella (MMR) vaccine as ordered.

14. When treating a patient with heat exhaustion, which nursing intervention is appropriate?
    A. Place several cubes of ice on the patient's temples.
    B. Apply cool water to the skin and fan with cool air.
    C. Use hypothermic blanket until temperature is 98.6° F (37° C).
    D. Administer medication as ordered to induce shivering.

15. A conscious patient who has ingested a corrosive acid presents to the emergency department. What is the appropriate nursing action?
    A. Induce vomiting to rid the body of the poison.
    B. Prepare to administer naloxone.
    C. Contact the Poison Control Center.
    D. Begin cardiopulmonary resuscitation (CPR).

16. The nurse is caring for a patient with a soft tissue facial injury. Which assessment finding does the nurse anticipate?
    A. Epidermal staining
    B. Wavy or watery vision
    C. Diplopia
    D. Change in hearing

17. When treating a patient with retinal detachment, which nursing intervention is appropriate?
    A. Maintain complete bed rest.
    B. Encourage fluids.
    C. Administer oxygen.
    D. Educate on deep breathing and coughing.

18. How will the nurse care for a patient with an emergent lower gastrointestinal bleed? Select all that apply.
    A. Monitor oxygen saturation levels.
    B. Assess cardiac and respiratory status every 15 minutes until patient is stabilized.
    C. Prepare to type and cross-match for blood.
    D. Administer a laxative.
    E. Provide emotional support to the patient.

19. The nurse is assessing a patient's abdomen and hears a harsh, grating sound like sandpaper over the patient's liver. How will the nurse document this finding?
    A. Hyperactive bowel sounds
    B. Systolic bruit
    C. Venous hum
    D. Friction rub

20. The nurse is caring for a patient with suspected retinal detachment who is reporting a sudden, painless vision loss. Which additional assessment finding does the nurse anticipate? Select all that apply.
    A. Wavy or watery vision
    B. Floaters
    C. Light flashes
    D. Auras around lights
    E. Epistaxis

21. A 25-year-old patient arrives to the emergency department with a sore throat and possible fever. This patient should be prioritized into which category?
    A. Urgent
    B. Emergent
    C. Nonurgent
    D. Resuscitation

22. The nurse is caring for a patient with a nasogastric tube connected to suction. Which action should the nurse take to assess the patient's bowel sounds?
    A. Clamp the nasogastric tube.
    B. Elevate the head of the bed 30 degrees.
    C. Use a Doppler.
    D. Palpate the abdomen.

23. The nurse is preparing a patient for a colonoscopy. Which medication should the nurse anticipate administering to the patient for sedation?
    A. Meloxicam
    B. Midazolam
    C. Metoprolol
    D. Montelukast

24. The health care provider has ordered aluminium hydroxide with magnesium hydroxide for a patient. The nurse should monitor for which adverse reaction?
    A. Migraines
    B. Hypomagnesemia
    C. Diarrhea
    D. Hypercalcemia

25. The nurse is reviewing a policy on ear irrigations for foreign objects in the ear canal. Which patient situation should be included in the policy as a contraindication for ear irrigation? Select all that apply.
    A. A patient aged 65 and older
    B. A patient aged 5 and younger
    C. A patient with a suspected ear infection
    D. A patient with a suspected vegetable in the ear canal
    E. A patient with a ruptured tympanic membrane

26. Which teaching will the nurse provide to a patient who presented with epistaxis and is being discharged from the emergency department?
    A. Sneeze through the nose with the mouth closed.
    B. Avoid using a humidifier in their home.
    C. Use cotton swabs to clear the nasal passages daily.
    D. Make an appointment to have the nasal packing removed.

27. Which color does the nurse identify that amniotic fluid will be if it is stained by meconium?
    A. Brown
    B. Yellow
    C. Green
    D. Red

28. What risk does the registered nurse identify for a neonate exposed to meconium?
    A. Aspiration
    B. Brain damage
    C. Decreased peristalsis
    D. Delay in achieving milestones

29. The nurse is preparing to care for a neonate who was exposed to meconium during the birth process. What is the appropriate nursing action?
    A. Suction the neonate's nose and then mouth.
    B. Prepare to transfer the neonate to the nursery.
    C. Assess the neonate's respiratory effort and heart rate.
    D. Facilitate the bonding process between the neonate and mother.

30. When caring for four patients in labor, which does the nurse identify as highest risk for experiencing a birth involving shoulder dystocia?
- A. 23 years old; 37 weeks pregnant; baby estimated to weigh 5 lb (2.44 kg), 6 oz
- B. 31 years old; 38 weeks pregnant; baby estimated to weigh 7 lb (3.21 kg), 1 oz
- C. 36 years old; 39 weeks pregnant; baby estimated to weigh 8 lb (3.89 kg), 9 oz
- D. 40 years old; 40 weeks pregnant; baby estimated to weigh 9 lb (4.52 kg), 15 oz

31. What is the appropriate nursing response when the patient with uterine rupture asks, "Can I ever have more children?"
- A. "Why are you afraid you will not have more babies?"
- B. "You will have no difficulty with future pregnancies."
- C. "Unfortunately, there is no chance you will be able to become pregnant again."
- D. "The provider will discuss a possible uterine repair or the need for hysterectomy."

32. The nurse is administering risperidone to a patient with bipolar disorder. What teaching should the nurse provide to the patient? Select all that apply.
- A. Get up slowly when moving from a lying or sitting position to a standing position.
- B. Inform your health care provider if you develop uncontrolled movements.
- C. Avoid alcoholic beverages.
- D. Do not stop taking this medication unless your health care provider tells you.
- E. Report symptoms of urinary burning, urine discoloration, or hematuria.

33. The nurse is caring for a patient with schizophrenia who is exhibiting agitation and anxiety. Which medication is the nurse most likely to administer?
- A. Loratadine
- B. Levothyroxine
- C. Lisinopril
- D. Lorazepam

34. A patient has been brought to the emergency department by a friend. The patient is unable to walk without help, is confused, has nausea with occasional vomiting, and has "blacked out" twice on the ride to the emergency department. Which blood alcohol content (BAC) results should the nurse anticipate?
    A. 0.11% to 0.20%
    B. 0.21% to 0.25%
    C. 0.26% to 0.40%
    D. >0.40%

35. The nurse is caring for a patient who has alcohol intoxication. Which intervention is the most appropriate?
    A. Restrict fluids to 500 mL daily.
    B. Administer mannitol intravenously.
    C. Use aspiration precautions.
    D. Prepare for endotracheal intubation.

36. A patient arrives to the emergency department presenting with circumoral cyanosis, difficulty to arouse, blood pressure of 86/54 mm Hg, pulse of 46 beats per minute, and pinpoint pupils. Which condition will the nurse assess for when obtaining a medical history?
    A. Opioid overdose
    B. Neuroleptic malignant syndrome
    C. Serotonin syndrome
    D. Medication-induced acute dystonia

37. Which anatomical location will the nurse auscultate to assess the mitral valve?
    A. Second intercostal space, left of the sternal border
    B. Second intercostal space, right of the sternal border
    C. Third intercostal space, left of the sternal border
    D. Fifth intercostal space, at the midclavicular line

38. What signs and symptoms will the nurse anticipate in a patient with left-sided heart failure? Select all that apply.
    A. Hepatomegaly
    B. Crackles in the lungs
    C. Dyspnea
    D. Pedal edema
    E. Orthopnea

39. How will the nurse assess for jugular venous distension?
    A. Have the patient lie flat and turn the head to the opposite direction of the jugular vein being assessed.
    B. Elevate the head of bed to 90 degrees and assess for pulsation of the jugular vein with the patient's head in a midline position.
    C. Position the patient supine with the head of bed elevated 30 to 45 degrees. Turn the patient's head slightly away from the nurse while assessing the jugular veins.
    D. Position the patient lying on the right side with the head of bed elevated 30 degrees and check for pulsation of the left jugular vein.

40. What assessment is the nurse conducting when palpating the patient's chest while asking the patient to say "ninety-nine" loudly?
    A. Vocal fremitus
    B. Tactile fremitus
    C. Bronchophony
    D. Whispered pectoriloquy

41. A 35-year-old woman who is 14 weeks pregnant and vomiting multiple times a day since the beginning of the pregnancy is at risk for which acid–base imbalance?
    A. Respiratory acidosis
    B. Respiratory alkalosis
    C. Metabolic acidosis
    D. Metabolic alkalosis

42. An emergency department nurse is providing discharge teaching for a patient with an acute asthma exacerbation who will be taking a course of oral prednisone over the next 2 weeks. What should the nurse teach the patient to report?
    A. Irritability
    B. Increased appetite
    C. Chills and rigors
    D. Acne

43. A patient arrives to the emergency department after being pulled from a fire with burns on the arms, neck, and torso. What is the priority nursing assessment?
    A. Skin integrity
    B. Airway
    C. Circulation
    D. Neurologic status

44. Which education will the nurse provide when teaching a patient about potential triggers for asthma? Select all that apply.
    A. Mold
    B. Anxiety
    C. Laughing
    D. Cold air
    E. Infection

45. Which of the following is *not* a priority in the primary survey of the trauma patient?
    A. Establishing an airway
    B. Providing a fluid bolus for hypotension
    C. Splinting a fracture
    D. Applying a tourniquet for arterial bleeding

46. What type of shock is reflected in the multisystem trauma patient with hypotension, bradycardia, warm torso, and cool extremities?
    A. Cardiogenic
    B. Hypovolemia
    C. Neurogenic
    D. Respiratory

47. What does the nurse recognize as the primary purpose of hospice?
    A. Allowing patients the opportunity to die at home
    B. Providing better quality of care than the family can alone
    C. Coordinating care for dying patients and their families
    D. Providing comfort and support for dying patients and their families

48. What does the nurse recognize as the primary purpose of palliative care?
    A. Improving the quality of life
    B. Providing care family cannot give
    C. Giving patients and families time to grieve
    D. Focusing on correcting disease processes

49. The nurse is assessing the neurologic status of a patient. Which assessment data requires immediate intervention?
    A. Fever
    B. Nausea
    C. Fatigue
    D. Lethargy

50. What does the nurse assess when using the Glasgow Coma Scale?
    A. Response to verbal, motor, and sensory stimulation
    B. Speech and orientation to situation
    C. Cognitive function
    D. Mood and affect

51. To assess the optic nerve (CN II), the nurse would use which tool?
    A. Penlight
    B. Snellen eye chart
    C. Cotton ball
    D. Tongue blade

52. The nurse instructs the patient to wrinkle the forehead and puff out the cheeks. These actions will allow the nurse to assess which cranial nerve?
    A. CN II
    B. CN V
    C. CN VII
    D. CN VIII

53. The nurse is caring for a patient who is scheduled to have a computed tomography (CT) angiography. Which lab value must be completed prior to the CT angiography?
    A. White blood cell count
    B. Hemoglobin and hematocrit
    C. Creatinine and blood urea nitrogen
    D. Red blood cell count

54. The nurse is caring for a patient with epilepsy. Which is a complication of seizures? Select all that apply.
    A. Anorexia
    B. Hypoxia
    C. Aspiration
    D. Injury
    E. Anxiety

55. The emergency department receives a patient immediately following a motor vehicle accident. The patient has muscle spasms in the back and neck that worsen with movement and reports a sensation of hot water running down the back. The nurse suspects which type of injury?
    A. Traumatic brain injury
    B. Spinal cord injury
    C. Contusion to the brain
    D. Subdural hematoma

56. The nurse is caring for a patient with spinal cord injury. Which nursing intervention is priority?
    A. Administer intravenous (IV) fluids for hypotension.
    B. Provide emotional support to the family.
    C. Monitor electrolytes and urinalysis.
    D. Insert nasogastric tube for intermittent suction.

57. The nurse is caring for a patient with a head injury following a motor vehicle accident. Which is the priority nursing action?
    A. Assess knees for bulge sign.
    B. Inspect skin for lacerations.
    C. Obtain cervical spine clearance.
    D. Palpate back and shoulders for injury.

58. How will the nurse document a patient's muscle strength who can complete range of motion (ROM) against gravity only?
    A. 1/5
    B. 2/5
    C. 3/5
    D. 4/5

59. What is the appropriate nursing response when a patient with knee edema asks, "What is an arthrocentesis?"
    A. "This is a joint puncture used to collect fluid."
    B. "Are you afraid of having an arthrocentesis done?"
    C. "The health care provider will discuss this procedure with you."
    D. "This procedure will determine whether you can undergo a magnetic resonance imaging."

60. Which patient should the nurse identify that cannot undergo a magnetic resonance imaging (MRI)?
    A. Patient with hearing aids
    B. Patient with bobby pins in the hair
    C. Patient with earrings and a necklace
    D. Patient with a residual piece of shrapnel in the arm

61. Which symptom does the nurse teach a patient to immediately report to the health care provider after application of a plaster cast to the arm?
    A. Swelling of the fingers
    B. Itching underneath the cast
    C. Capillary refill of <2 seconds
    D. The need for use of a sling

62. After a disaster occurs, a volunteer asks the nurse, "Who is in charge of the disaster response?" Who does the nurse identify?
    A. Safety officer
    B. Liaison office
    C. Incident commander
    D. Public information officer

63. After a disaster incident, which triage ribbon does the nurse assign to a patient with an ankle fracture and minor lacerations?
    A. Green
    B. Yellow
    C. Red
    D. Gray

64. What nursing action is appropriate for a patient who has been issued an orange ribbon via the triage process?
    A. Administer palliative medication.
    B. Escort to the decontamination zone.
    C. Flag down a transporter to transport to hospital.
    D. Reassure that treatment will come in the next few hours.

65. The nurse identifies that a patient flagged with a black and white striped ribbon means what?
    A. The patient has died.
    B. The patient does not speak English as a first language.
    C. The patient has been separated from a parent who is missing.
    D. The patient has been contaminated and requires decontamination.

66. The nurse is caring for a patient with an incomplete amputation of the thumb. Which assessment finding requires the nurse to immediately intervene?
    A. Pain of 5 on a 1 to 10 scale
    B. Dark red blood at site of injury
    C. Capillary refill in fingers of 4 seconds
    D. A portion of the thumb is still attached to the hand

67. A patient with a newly applied leg cast reports swelling and excruciating pain in the toes. Which nursing action is appropriate?
    A. Contact the health care provider.
    B. Elevate the extremity to return blood to the heart.
    C. Massage the affected area to increase blood supply.
    D. Reassure that this is a normal sensation that will dissipate.

68. What teaching will the nurse provide to a patient with an open compound fracture of the right lower extremity who had a tetanus immunization 6 years ago?
    A. "You are up-to-date on the tetanus immunization."
    B. "Tetanus boosters should be given every 5 years."
    C. "Immunization is not needed with this type of injury."
    D. "People only need to receive the tetanus shot once in a lifetime."

69. What technique will the nurse use to examine underneath the patient who has a possible spinal injury?
    A. Forego this assessment until the spine has been cleared of injury.
    B. Use logrolling technique with assistance of three other individuals.
    C. Ask the patient to help move self from one side of gurney to another.
    D. Raise patient's legs gently and observe area directly underneath buttocks.

70. What teaching will the nurse provide to a patient diagnosed with a third-degree ankle sprain?
    A. "The sprain will heal on its own, so just give it time."
    B. "Use heat for the first 24 to 48 hours and then switch to ice."
    C. "You may need to see an orthopedic specialist for evaluation."
    D. "Take acetaminophen three times daily to decrease inflammation."

Answers

1. Correct answer: C. Rationale: The primary survey begins with an assessment of airway, breathing, and circulation. Additional assessment parameters in the primary survey include neurologic status, designated as disability (D), and exposure and environment, designated as (E). The secondary survey includes a full set of vital signs, head to toe assessment, health history, and providing comfort.
Client needs category: Physiological integrity
Client needs subcategory: Physiological adaptation
Cognitive level: Knowledge

2. Correct answer: B. Rationale: According to the Emergency Nurses Association triage established guidelines, patients needing immediate nursing assessment and rapid treatment include those with head injuries, chest pain, stroke, asthma, and sexual assault injuries. These patients would be triaged as emergent. Patients triaged as urgent need quick attention but could wait up to 30 minutes before being treated. Patients triaged as nonurgent can wait up to 2 hours for assessment and treatment. Patients triaged as resuscitation need immediate nursing and medical attention such as those with cardiopulmonary arrest, major trauma, severe respiratory distress, and seizures.
Client needs category: Safe and effective care environment
Client needs subcategory: Management of care
Cognitive level: Comprehension

3. Correct answer: D. Rationale: The acronym SAMPLE is a mnemonic to help the nurse remember the types of information needed to obtain the patient's history: *S*ubjective data, *A*llergies, *M*edications, *P*ast medical history, *L*ast meal eaten, *E*vents/Environment leading to injury.
Client needs category: Physiological integrity
Client needs subcategory: Physiological adaptation
Cognitive level: Comprehension

4. Correct answer: B. Rationale: The role of a nurse educator is to use excellent interpersonal skills to ensure optimal performance and outcomes. In addition, other roles for the nurse educator include assessing patients' and families' learning needs, planning and implementing teaching strategies to meet those needs, evaluating the effectiveness of teaching, and educating peers and colleagues.
Client needs category: Safe and effective care environment
Client needs subcategory: Management of care
Cognitive level: Comprehension

5. Correct answers: A, C, and D. Rationale: Therapeutic communication is needed and should always be used with all patients. Enhanced therapeutic communication skills should be used with teenage girls due to possible feelings of shame or illegal activity. Older adult men may feel that sexual problems are a sign of decreased masculinity. Members of the LGBT community may be hesitant to discuss sexual history due to fear of judgment or misunderstanding.
Client needs category: Psychosocial integrity
Cognitive level: Comprehension

6. Correct answer: B. Rationale: Diabetes mellitus increases a patient's risk for urinary tract infections. Lupus, emphysema, and Crohn disease are not associated with increased risk for urinary tract infection.
Client needs category: Physiological integrity
Client needs subcategory: Physiological adaptation
Cognitive level: Comprehension

7. Correct answer: D. Rationale: The nurse will teach the patient to lie still and breathe normally during a CT scan of the bladder. A full bladder is not required for this test or does the patient need to be fasting, although food and fluid will be restricted once the test is ordered. A contrast medium can be used during CT scans but is not necessary for test completion.
Client needs category: Physiological integrity
Client needs subcategory: Physiological adaptation
Cognitive level: Application

8.   Correct answer: B. Rationale: A patient with dehydration and calcium crystals in the urine likely has kidney stones. The nurse anticipates bloody urine, a high specific gravity, darker discoloration to the urine, and a higher urine pH due to the calcium crystals.
Client needs category: Physiological integrity
Client needs subcategory: Physiological adaptation
Cognitive level: Application

9.   Correct answer: C. Rationale: Endometritis is frequently associated with postpartum or postabortion pelvic inflammatory disease. Other forms of pelvic inflammatory disease, such as cervicitis and salpingo-oophoritis, do not present with a boggy uterus. WBC count may also be normal in cervicitis. PCOS may present with Mittelschmerz pain following ovulation and is not associated with a boggy uterus.
Client needs category: Physiological integrity
Client needs subcategory: Physiological adaptation
Cognitive level: Application

10. Correct answer: D. Eliciting Prehn sign by slightly elevating the scrotum will cause increased pain with testicular torsion; this assessment action can assist the health care provider in making a diagnosis. Applying ice to the area could further reduce blood flow in a possibly already ischemic area. The presence of testicular torsion must be determined prior to considering surgery, and the patient should remain nothing by mouth (NPO) until the need for surgery is determined.
Client needs category: Physiological integrity
Client needs subcategory: Physiological Adaptation
Cognitive level: Application

11. Correct answer: A. Rationale: First-degree frostbite is characterized by hyperemic skin with edema at the affected area. Second-degree frostbite includes large blisters with clear or milky fluid and partial thickness necrosis. Third-degree frostbite includes small blisters with dark fluid. The area of the skin is cool, numb, nonblanchable, and blue or red. Fourth-degree frostbite involves full-thickness necrosis extending to the muscle and bone where the affected area is cold, numb, and without circulation.
Client needs category: Physiological integrity
Client needs subcategory: Physiological adaptation
Cognitive level: Application

12. Correct answer: B. Rationale: Peripheral cyanosis, muscle rigidity, and atrial arrhythmias are expected findings in patients with moderate hypothermia. Patients with mild hypothermia may have slurred speech or impaired judgment. Patients with severe hypothermia may have an absence of palpable pulses, dilated (or nonreactive) pupils, and rigor mortis–like findings.
Client needs category: Physiological integrity
Client needs subcategory: Physiological adaptation
Cognitive level: Application

13. Correct answers: A, B, C, and E. Rationale: When caring for a patient who has experienced a cat bite to the hand, the nurse will remove jewelry and clothing from the affected area, irrigate with normal saline, apply medication as ordered, teach to elevate the hand, and administer tetanus prophylaxis as ordered. The area will likely be left open (not sutured) to avoid closing bacteria in the puncture-like wounds. An MMR vaccination is inappropriate.
Client needs category: Physiological integrity
Client needs subcategory: Physiological adaptation
Cognitive level: Analysis

14. Correct answer: B. Rationale: When caring for a patient with moderate hyperthermia, the most effective way to cool the body is to apply cool water to the skin and then fan with cool air. Applying ice cubes directly on the skin compromises skin integrity. Use of a hypothermic blanket should be discontinued when the patient's temperature reaches 101° F (38.3° C) because hypothermia may develop. If medications are used, they will be indicated to control—not induce—shivering.
Client needs category: Physiological integrity
Client needs subcategory: Physiological adaptation
Cognitive level: Application

15. Correct answer: C. Rationale: The nurse will contact the Poison Control Center to receive instructions on the appropriate treatment approach. When caring for a conscious patient, neither naloxone nor CPR is indicated. The nurse should not induce vomiting because this could cause the corrosive substance to reenter the esophagus, causing further harm.
Client needs category: Physiological integrity
Client needs subcategory: Physiological adaptation
Cognitive level: Application

16. Correct answer: A. Rationale: Signs and symptoms associated with soft tissue facial injuries may include epidermal staining (friction injuries), evidence of skin opening or revealing teeth marks, intraoral deformities, and superficial to deep lacerations on any area of the face. Wavy or watery vision or hearing changes are not associated with soft facial injuries.
Client needs category: Physiological integrity
Client needs subcategory: Physiological adaptation
Cognitive level: Application

17. Correct answer: A. Rationale: When treating a patient with retinal detachment, the nurse should maintain complete bed rest and instruct the patient to restrict eye movements until surgical reattachment is performed. In addition, the nurse should urge the patient to avoid activities in bed that could increase intraocular pressure such as straining at stool, bending down, forceful coughing, sneezing, and vomiting. Encouraging fluids and administering oxygen are not typical interventions for retinal detachment.
Client needs category: Physiological integrity
Client needs subcategory: Physiological adaptation
Cognitive level: Application

18. Correct answers: A, B, C, and E. Rationale: The nurse caring for a patient coming to the emergency department with an emergent lower gastrointestinal bleed should take the following actions to ensure appropriate management and prevention of complication: Monitor oxygen saturation levels, assess cardiac and respiratory status every 15 minutes until patient is stabilized, prepare to type and cross-match for blood, and provide emotional support to the patient. Administering a laxative could cause further bleeding.
Client needs category: Physiological integrity
Client needs subcategory: Physiological adaptation
Cognitive level: Application

19. Correct answer: D. Rationale: A friction rub is a harsh, grating sound like two pieces of sandpaper rubbing against each other. The friction rub can be observed over the liver and spleen or lung areas. In the gastrointestinal system, a friction rub is caused by the inflammation of the peritoneal surface of the liver.
Client needs category: Physiological integrity
Client needs subcategory: Physiological adaptation
Cognitive level: Application

20. Correct answers: A, B, and C. Rationale. A patient with retinal detachment will exhibit the following signs and symptoms: a sudden, painless vision loss; wavy or watery vision; floaters; and light flashes. Auras around lights and epistaxis do not occur with retinal detachment.
Client needs category: Physiological integrity
Client needs subcategory: Physiological adaptation
Cognitive level: Application

21. Correct answer: C. Rationale: According to the Emergency Nurses Association triage established guidelines, patients with minor symptoms such as sore throat and menstrual cramps can wait up to 2 hours or possibly longer for an assessment and treatment. Patients requiring immediate nursing assessment and rapid treatment include those with head injuries, chest pain, stroke, asthma, and sexual assault injuries. These patients would be triaged as emergent. Patients triaged as urgent need quick attention but could wait up to 30 minutes before being treated. Patients triaged as resuscitation need immediate nursing and medical attention such as those with cardiopulmonary arrest, major trauma, severe respiratory distress, and seizures.
Client needs category: Safe and effective care environment
Client needs subcategory: Management of care
Cognitive level: Comprehension

22. Correct answer: A. Rationale: Before auscultating the abdomen of a patient with a nasogastric tube or other abdominal tube connected to suction, briefly clamp the tube or turn off the suction. Suction noises can obscure or mimic actual bowel sounds. The other answers are not necessary for auscultating the abdomen.
Client needs category: Health promotion and maintenance
Cognitive level: Application

23. Correct answer: B. Rationale: Midazolam injection is used for patient before surgery or procedures to illicit drowsiness and reduce anxiety. Meloxicam is used for pain and inflammation typically in patients with arthritis. Metoprolol is used to treat high blood pressure, angina, and heart failure. Montelukast is used to treat symptoms of asthma.
Client needs category: Physiological integrity
Client needs subcategory: Pharmacological and parenteral therapies
Cognitive level: Application

24. Correct answer: C. Rationale: Diarrhea is a common adverse reaction to aluminium hydroxide with magnesium hydroxide (Maalox). Hypermagnesemia can occur in patients with severe renal impairment. Migraines and hypercalcemia are not common adverse reactions for Maalox.
Client needs category: Physiological integrity
Client needs subcategory: Pharmacological and parenteral therapies
Cognitive level: Comprehension

25. Correct answers: B, C, D, and E. Ear irrigations are contraindicated in patients younger than 5 years old, with a ruptured tympanic membrane, with an ear infection, or with a vegetable or soft foreign body that would absorb water.
Client needs category: Physiological integrity
Client needs subcategory: Physiological adaptation
Cognitive level: Application

26. Correct answer: D. Rationale: For a patient presenting to the emergency department with epistaxis and being discharged, the nurse should teach the patient to sneeze with the mouth open; use a humidifier in the home; avoid inserting cotton swabs, tissues, or other objects in the nose; and to make an appointment to remove nasal packing and to follow up.
Client needs category: Physiological integrity
Client needs subcategory: Physiological adaptation
Cognitive level: Application

27. Correct answer: C. Rationale: Meconium is stool that a fetus passes before delivery, and it is green in color.
Client needs category: Physiological integrity
Client needs subcategory: Physiological adaptation
Cognitive level: Knowledge

28. Correct answer: A. Rationale: Aspiration of meconium by the neonate can lead to pneumonia; this is the highest risk factor for exposure to meconium; it is not related to the risk for brain damage, decreased peristalsis, or delay in milestone achievement.
Client needs category: Physiological integrity
Client needs subcategory: Physiological adaptation
Cognitive level: Comprehension

29. Correct answer: C. Rationale: The neonate exposed to meconium during the birth process is at risk for aspiration of stained amniotic fluid and, thus, pneumonia. The nurse will assess respiratory effort and heart rate and be prepared to follow the Neonatal Resuscitation Program (NRP) because this neonate is not stable enough to be

transferred to the nursery. The nurse would suction the mouth and then nose of the neonate. Facilitation of bonding is always important, yet the priority is to assess the neonate's respiratory effort and heart rate due to the risk involved with meconium exposure.
Client needs category: Physiological integrity
Client needs subcategory: Physiological adaptation
Cognitive level: Application

30. Correct answer: D. Rationale: Shoulder dystocia is a condition in which there is a complication in the anterior shoulder of the neonate passing under the pubic arch. It is uncommon yet happens more frequently when fetal size differs from the opening between the fetal shoulders and the pelvic inlet. The mother whose baby is estimated to be largest is at the highest risk for this condition.
Client needs category: Physiological integrity
Client needs subcategory: Physiological adaptation
Cognitive level: Application

31. Correct answer: D. Rationale: Uterine rupture may be able to be corrected as a laceration repair or may require hysterectomy. Until the provider has assessed the degree of damage, it is impossible to guarantee that a patient will or will not be able to become pregnant in the future. In this scenario, the accurate answer from the nurse involves objectively notifying the patient that the provider will discuss this situation with her, instead of providing false reassurance or false alarm. It is not appropriate to question the patient's concern by asking a "why" question.
Client needs category: Physiological integrity
Client needs subcategory: Physiological adaptation
Cognitive level: Application

32. Correct answers: A, B, C, and D. Rationale: Common side effects and precautions of risperidone include dizziness (change positions slowly), light-headedness, and tardive dyskinesia (uncontrolled movements involving the face, lips, arms, legs, and tongue). Alcohol may increase symptoms of dizziness. The medication should be taken regularly at the same time daily to ensure optimal benefit and should continue as prescribed. Urinary side effects have not been commonly reported with this medication.
Client needs category: Physiological integrity
Client needs subcategory: Physiological adaptation
Cognitive level: Application

33. Correct answer: D. Rationale: Lorazepam (Ativan) is an antianxiety agent that is the most commonly used benzodiazepine for short-term calming and sedation for patients with agitation. Loratadine is an antihistamine agent, levothyroxine is a thyroid hormone replacement agent, and lisinopril is an antihypertension agent.
Client needs category: Psychosocial integrity
Cognitive level: Application

34. Correct answer: B. Rationale: An individual exhibiting the inability to walk without assistance, confusion, dysphoric mood, nausea and vomiting, and possible blackouts has had approximately 4 to 6 drinks and may have a corresponding BAC of 0.21% to 0.25%. Lower BAC results typically have less severe symptoms, whereas higher BAC results have more severe symptoms including unconsciousness.
Client needs category: Physiological integrity
Client needs subcategory: Physiological adaptation
Cognitive level: Application

35. Correct answer: C. Rationale: An individual with alcohol intoxication may be unconscious and vomit. Measures to prevent aspiration need to be included in the plan of care to ensure a patent airway. Fluid replacement (intravenously) should be included in the plan of care to replace the volume lost by the diuretic effects of alcohol. Mannitol is not appropriate for alcohol intoxication treatment, and endotracheal intubation is usually indicated for opioid overdose.
Client needs category: Physiological integrity
Client needs subcategory: Physiological adaptation
Cognitive level: Application

36. Correct answer: A. Rationale: An individual with opioid overdose will present with signs and symptoms of suppressed respiratory function and breathing because opioids affect the part of the brain that regulates breathing. Signs and symptoms include pale clammy skin, limp body, nail bed and circumoral cyanosis, vomiting, mental confusion, difficulty to awaken or arouse, bradycardia, bradypnea, hypotension, and pinpoint pupils.
Client needs category: Physiological integrity
Client needs subcategory: Physiological adaptation
Cognitive level: Application

37. Correct answer: D. Rationale: The mitral valve can best be auscultated at the fifth intercostal space, at the midclavicular line.
Client needs category: Physiological integrity
Client needs subcategory: Physiological adaptation
Cognitive level: Knowledge

38. Correct answers: B, C, and E. Rationale: Early signs and symptoms of left-sided heart failure include fatigue, nonproductive cough, orthopnea, dyspnea, and paroxysmal dyspnea. As left-sided heart failure progresses, crackles are audible on auscultation, restlessness and agitation can develop, and hemoptysis and additional heart sounds (S_3, S_4) may occur. Hepatomegaly and pedal edema are associated with right-sided heart failure.
Client needs category: Physiological integrity
Client needs subcategory: Physiological adaptation
Cognitive level: Application

39. Correct answer: C. Rationale: The nurse will assess for jugular venous distension by positioning the patient supine with the head of the bed elevated 30 to 45 degrees. Turn the patient's head slightly away from the nurse while assessing the jugular vein. Normally, the highest pulsation takes place no more than 1½" (3.8 cm) above the sternal notch. If pulsations appear higher, it indicates elevation in central venous pressure (CVP) and jugular vein distention.
Client needs category: Physiological integrity
Client needs subcategory: Physiological adaptation
Cognitive level: Comprehension

40. Correct answer: B. Rationale: To check for tactile fremitus, place open palms on both sides of the patient's back. Ask the patient to repeat the word "ninety-nine" loud enough to produce palpable vibrations. Then palpate the front of the chest using the same hand positions.
Client needs category: Physiological integrity
Client needs subcategory: Physiological adaptation
Cognitive level: Understanding

41. Correct answer: D. Rationale: Excessive loss of hydrochloric acid due to prolonged vomiting can cause a deficit in hydrogen ions and could progress into metabolic alkalosis.
Client needs category: Physiological integrity
Client needs subcategory: Physiological adaptation
Cognitive level: Application

42. Correct answer: C. Rationale: The nurse should educate the patient to report any signs of infection including chills and rigors because they can be an indication of fever. Acne, increased appetite, and irritability are side effects of oral prednisone.
Client needs category: Physiological integrity
Client needs subcategory: Physiological adaptation
Cognitive level: Application

43. Correct answer: B. The patient's airway is always a priority in emergency situations but even more so in this situation due to the risk for airway compromise related to thermal inhalation.
Client needs category: Safe and effective care environment
Client needs subcategory: Management of care
Cognitive level: Application

44. Correct answers: A, B, C, D, and E. Rationale: All of these can be triggers for asthma. It is important that patients understand triggers for asthma as well as focus on their own specific triggers if they have been identified.
Client needs category: Physiological integrity
Client needs subcategory: Physiological adaptation
Cognitive level: Application

45. Correct answer: C. Rationale: The goal of the primary survey is to address immediate threats to life. Arterial bleeding, hypotension, and inadequate airway are all immediate threats that would be addressed in the primary survey. Splinting a fracture would occur during the secondary assessment.
Client needs category: Physiological integrity
Client needs subcategory: Physiological adaptation
Cognitive level: Application

46. Correct answer: C. Rationale: In neurogenic shock, a temporary loss of autonomic function below the level of a spinal cord injury produces cardiovascular changes. Neurogenic shock is a type of distributive shock in which vasodilation causes a state of hypovolemia. The neurogenic shock patient will display these signs and symptoms: hypotension; bradycardia; warm, dry, and flushed skin; and hypothermia.
Client needs category: Physiological integrity
Client needs subcategory: Physiological adaptation
Cognitive level: Application

47. Correct answer: D. Rationale: The primary purpose for hospice is to provide comfort and support for dying patients and their families.
Client needs category: Physiological integrity
Client needs subcategory: Basic care and comfort
Cognitive level: Knowledge

48. Correct answer: A. Rationale: The primary purpose of palliative care is to improve the quality of life.
Client needs category: Physiological integrity
Client needs subcategory: Basic care and comfort
Cognitive level: Knowledge

49. Correct answer: D. Rationale: Symptoms of a neurologic emergency include headache, visual disturbances, changes in loss of consciousness, motor disturbances, seizures, and lethargy. Neurologic emergencies require immediate nursing intervention.
Client needs category: Safe and effective care environment
Client needs subcategory: Management of care
Cognitive level: Analysis

50. Correct answer: A. Rationale: The Glasgow Coma Scale assesses a patient's ability to respond to verbal, motor, and sensory stimulation.
Client needs category: Physiological integrity
Client needs subcategory: Physiological adaptation
Cognitive level: Comprehension

51. Correct answer: B. Rationale: The nurse would assess visual acuity and visual field when assessing the optic nerve (CN II). To assess this, the nurse would use the Snellen eye chart.
Client needs category: Physiological integrity
Client needs subcategory: Physiological adaptation
Cognitive level: Application

52. Correct answer: C. Rationale: Wrinkling the forehead and puffing the cheeks allow the nurse to assess the motor function of the facial nerve (CN VII).
Client needs category: Physiological integrity
Client needs subcategory: Physiological adaptation
Cognitive level: Application

53. Correct answer: C. Rationale: A CT angiography requires the use of intravenous (IV) contrast, which is excreted through the urine. The serum creatinine and blood urea nitrogen should be evaluated prior to assess renal function.
Client needs category: Safe and effective care environment
Client needs subcategory: Management of care
Cognitive level: Analysis

54. Correct answers: B, C, D, and E. Rationale: Complications of seizures include hypoxia, aspiration, injury, and anxiety. Anorexia is loss of appetite, which is not a complication of seizures.
Client needs category: Physiological integrity
Client needs subcategory: Physiological adaptation
Cognitive level: Application

55. Correct answer: B. Rationale: The signs and symptoms reported by the patient indicate spinal cord injury.
Client needs category: Physiological integrity
Client needs subcategory: Physiological adaptation
Cognitive level: Application

56. Correct answer: A. Rationale: The priority intervention for a patient with spinal cord injury is to administer IV fluids for hypotension. The other interventions may be appropriate but are not the priority.
Client needs category: Physiological integrity
Client needs subcategory: Physiological adaptation
Cognitive level: Application

57. Correct answer: C. Rationale: The nurse will eventually perform all these actions, yet the priority is to ensure that the cervical spine has been cleared. The nurse can ensure that this is being undertaken by a health care provider and then proceed to inspect the skin, assess the knees, and palpate the back and shoulders.
Client needs category: Physiological integrity
Client needs subcategory: Physiological adaptation
Cognitive level: Analysis

58. Correct answer: C. Rationale: Muscle strength is graded on a 0 to 5 scale as follows:
- 5/5 = normal—patient moves joint through full ROM and against gravity with full resistance
- 4/5 = good—patient completes ROM against gravity with moderate resistance
- 3/5 = fair—patient completes ROM against gravity only
- 2/5 = poor—patient completes full ROM with gravity eliminated (passive motion)
- 1/5 = trace—patient's attempt at muscle contraction is palpable but without joint movement
- 0/5 = zero—there is no evidence of muscle contraction

This patient is able to complete ROM against gravity only, so the nurse will document 3/5 for muscle strength.
Client needs category: Physiological integrity
Client needs subcategory: Physiological adaptation
Cognitive level: Application

59. Correct answer: A. Rationale: It is important for the nurse to give accurate information when a patient asks a question. The nurse factually will answer that arthrocentesis is a joint puncture used to collect fluid. It is presumptuous to assume the patient is fearful of the test, and the nurse should not automatically defer all questions to the health care provider. Arthrocentesis is used to assess fluid for infection and other types of conditions; it is not used to determine whether a patient can undergo a magnetic resonance imaging.
Client needs category: Physiological integrity
Client needs subcategory: Physiological adaptation
Cognitive level: Application

60. Correct answer: D. Rationale: Patients with any type of metal in or on their body cannot undergo an MRI because the magnetic forces are so strong that they may cause dislodging. Hearing aids, bobby pins, and jewelry can be removed immediately prior to having an MRI, but residual shrapnel would preclude a patient from having an MRI until it was surgically removed.
Client needs category: Physiological integrity
Client needs subcategory: Physiological adaptation
Cognitive level: Application

61. Correct answer: A. Rationale: Swelling of the fingers can be an indication that the cast is applied too tightly; this must be reported to the health care provider. Itching underneath the cast, a capillary re-fill of <2 seconds, and the need to use a sling are all normal findings that do not need to be reported.
Client needs category: Physiological integrity
Client needs subcategory: Physiological adaptation
Cognitive level: Application

62. Correct answer: C. Rationale: The incident commander is in charge of all operations during a disaster response. All other positions report upward to the incident commander.
Client needs category: Physiological integrity
Client needs subcategory: Physiological adaptation
Cognitive level: Understanding

63. Correct answer: B. Rationale: Yellow ribbons indicate that a patient has physiologically stable injuries. These individuals need treatment because their injuries could result in decompensation, but they do not need treatment as fast as a patient with a red ribbon who needs immediate intervention in order to survive. Green ribbons are assigned to patients who have illnesses or injuries that are not life-threatening and that only need basic medical care that can come hours later. Gray ribbons are assigned to patients who should receive palliative care if time and resources allow because their injuries are likely not survivable.
Client needs category: Physiological integrity
Client needs subcategory: Physiological adaptation
Cognitive level: Application

64. Correct answer: B. Rationale: Orange ribbons are given to individuals who require decontamination prior to entering the emergency department or other area of treatment. This patient should be escorted to the decontamination area. Someone with a gray ribbon requires palliative medication if resources permit. Someone with a yellow or red ribbon requires transport to the hospital. Someone with a green ribbon will receive treatment, but it may be several hours later.
Client needs category: Physiological integrity
Client needs subcategory: Physiological adaptation
Cognitive level: Application

65. Correct answer: A. Rationale: Patients who have been given a black or black and white striped ribbon have died. All other answers are incorrect.
Client needs category: Physiological integrity
Client needs subcategory: Physiological adaptation
Cognitive level: Knowledge

66. Correct answer: C. Rationale: Absence of distal pulses or capillary refill of more than 3 seconds requires the nurse to intervene because perfusion has been interrupted. Pain is expected, and a 5 on a scale of 1 to 10 is not the worse pain imaginable. Dark red blood indicates a venous injury, not an arterial injury. In an incomplete amputation, it is expected that a portion of the injured body part will still be attached.
Client needs category: Physiological integrity
Client needs subcategory: Physiological adaptation
Cognitive level: Knowledge

67. Correct answer: A. Rationale: Compartment syndrome is an orthopedic emergency. Symptoms include swelling, paresthesia, pain out of proportion to the injury, and diminished pulse (a late sign). The cast needs to be immediately removed, so the health care provider should be contacted right away. Elevating the extremity or massaging the area will not correct the problem. This is not a normal sensation after cast application.
Client needs category: Physiological integrity
Client needs subcategory: Physiological adaptation
Cognitive level: Application

68. Correct answer: B. Rationale: Tetanus boosters should be given every 5 years per the Centers for Disease Control and Prevention (2018). It is not a lifetime vaccination. The patient's booster is not up-to-date. Because of the mechanism of injury and the length of time since the patient's last booster, an immunization is necessary.
Client needs category: Health promotion and maintenance
Cognitive level: Application

69. Correct answer: B. Rationale: A patient with a possible spinal injury should only be logrolled with the assistance of three people to keep the spine immobilized in complete alignment. It is important to assess for any bleeding underneath the patient by logrolling, and the visual assessment of the spine can be completed during this procedure as well. The patient should not be asked to help move or should the patient's legs be raised because this can compromise the position of the spine.
Client needs category: Physiological integrity
Client needs subcategory: Physiological adaptation
Cognitive level: Application

70. Correct answer: C. Rationale: A third-degree sprain may need further evaluation by a specialist because ongoing evaluation and treatment may be necessary for healing. This type of sprain needs analgesia, rest, ice, and elevation, and the patient will likely need crutches or a knee scooter to ambulate. Ice is always applied for the first 24 to 48 hours to decrease swelling and then heat can be applied for comfort. Acetaminophen does not reduce swelling; the patient will likely be prescribed a nonsteroidal anti-inflammatory drug for this purpose.
Client needs category: Physiological integrity
Client needs subcategory: Physiological adaptation
Cognitive level: Application

Glossary

abduct: move away from the midline of the body; opposite of *adduct*

adduct: move toward the midline of the body; opposite of *abduct*

advance directives: written legal documents that identify a person's advance wishes regarding health care if that person is unable to make decisions

agonist: drug that binds to a receptor to elicit a physiologic response

alveolus: in the lung, a small saclike dilation of the terminal bronchioles

anaerobic: oxygen not required for growth

angina: pain felt in the chest region; typically associated with a heart attack

anion: ion with a negative electrical charge

anorexia: loss of appetite

antagonist: drug that binds to a receptor but doesn't produce a response or blocks the response at the receptor

anterior: front or *ventral*; the opposite of *posterior* or *dorsal*

antibody: immunoglobulin produced by the body in response to exposure to a specific foreign substance (antigen)

antigen: foreign substance that causes antibody formation when introduced into the body

anuria: urine output of less than 100 mL in 24 hours

aphasia: language disorder characterized by difficulty expressing or comprehending speech

apnea: cessation of breathing

apraxia: inability to perform coordinated movements, even though no motor deficit is present

arthrosis: joint or articulation

ascites: accumulation of fluid in the abdominal cavity

assessment: first step in the nursing process that involves data gathering

ataxia: uncoordinated actions when voluntary muscle movements are attempted

atrophy: wasting away

automaticity: ability of the heart to generate its own electrical impulse

avulsion fracture: fracture that occurs when a joint capsule, ligament, tendon, or muscle is pulled from a bone

axonal injury: diffuse brain injury that usually results from tension and shearing forces

Battle sign: bruising immediately behind the ear that usually indicates a fracture of the posterior portion of the skull

Biot respirations: respirations that are rapid and deep and alternate with abrupt periods of apnea

blepharitis: inflammation of the eyelids

body mechanics: use of body positioning or movement to prevent or correct problems related to activity or immobility

borborygmi: loud sounds produced by the normal movement of air through the intestines

bradycardia: abnormally slow heart rate; usually less than 60 beats per minute

bradypnea: abnormally slow respiratory rate; usually less than 10 breaths per minute

bruit: abnormal sound heard over peripheral vessels that indicates turbulent blood flow

buccal: pertaining to the cheek

bursa: fluid-filled sac in the joint lined with synovial membrane

capillary: microscopic blood vessel that links arterioles with venules

cardiac cycle: period from the beginning of one heartbeat to the beginning of the next; includes two phases: systole and diastole

carpal: pertaining to the wrist

cartilage: connective supporting tissue occurring mainly in the joints, thorax, larynx, trachea, nose, and ear

celiac: pertaining to the abdomen

central nervous system: one of the two main divisions of the nervous system; consists of the brain and spinal cord

cognition: thinking and awareness

colloid: fluid containing starches or proteins

consciousness: state involving full awareness and ability to respond to stimuli

contralateral: on the opposite side; opposite of *ipsilateral*

coronary: pertaining to the heart or its arteries

cortex: outer part of an internal organ; the opposite of *medulla*

costal: pertaining to the ribs

crackles: intermittent, nonmusical, crackling breath sounds that are caused by collapsed or fluid-filled alveoli popping open

crepitus: noise or vibration produced by rubbing together irregular cartilage surfaces or broken ends of a bone; also the sound heard when air in subcutaneous tissue is palpated

cutaneous: pertaining to the skin

cyanosis: bluish discoloration of the skin or mucous membranes

debridement: removal of dead tissue or foreign material from a wound

dehiscence: separation of a wound's edges

deltoid: shaped like a triangle (as in the deltoid muscle)

dermis: skin layer beneath the epidermis

diaphragm: membrane that separates one part from another; the muscular partition separating the thorax and abdomen

diastole: resting portion of the cardiac cycle where the coronary arteries are filling with blood and the ventricles are relaxed

distal: far from the point of origin or attachment; the opposite of *proximal*

diuresis: formation and excretion of large amounts of urine

dorsal: pertaining to the back or posterior; the opposite of *ventral* or *anterior*

dysarthria: speech defect commonly related to a motor deficit of the tongue or speech muscles

dysphagia: difficulty swallowing

dyspnea: difficult or labored breathing

edema: accumulation of fluid in soft tissues

empathy: process of putting oneself into the feelings of another

endocardium: interior lining of the heart

endocrine: pertaining to secretion into the blood or lymph rather than into a duct; the opposite of *exocrine*

endometrium: inner mucosal lining of the uterus

epidermis: outermost layer of the skin

epiphyseal growth plate: the cartilage between the epiphysis and metaphysis of long bones that permits growth

epiphysis: the two expanded ends of a long bone

Erb point: auscultatory point on the precordium at the third intercostal space to the left of the sternum

evisceration: internal organ protrusion through an opening in a wound

exocrine: pertaining to secretion; the opposite of *endocrine*

exophthalmos: abnormal protrusion of the eyeball

fistula: abnormal opening between organs or between an organ and body surface

flaccidity: decrease in muscle tone that causes muscle to become weak or flabby

fluid wave: rippling across the abdomen during percussion; indicative of the presence of ascites

fremitus: palpable vibration that results from air passing through the bronchopulmonary system and transmitting vibrations to the chest wall

gastric lavage: instillation of solution into the stomach and subsequent withdrawal to remove stomach contents

glomerulus: compact cluster; the capillaries of the kidney

hematuria: blood in the urine

hemoglobin: protein found in red blood cells that contains iron

hemoptysis: blood in the sputum

hordeolum: inflammation of the sebaceous gland of the eyelid; also called *stye*

hydrocele: accumulation of serous fluid in a saclike structure such as the testis

hyperopia: defect in vision that allows a person to see objects clearly at a distance but not at close range; also called *farsightedness*

hyperresonance: increased resonance produced by percussion

hypertonic: having a greater concentration than body fluid

hypotonic: having a lesser concentration than body fluid

hypoxemia: state in which the blood contains a lower than normal amount of oxygen

hypoxia: state in which the tissues have a decreased amount of oxygen

infarction: death of tissue due to ischemia

inferior: lower; the opposite of *superior*

infiltration: seepage or leakage of fluid into the tissues

informed consent: legal document that a patient or legal guardian signs giving permission for a procedure after the patient has demonstrated understanding of the procedure

ipsilateral: on the same side; opposite of *contralateral*

ischemia: insufficient blood supply to a part

isotonic: having the same concentration as body fluid

Korotkoff sounds: sounds heard when auscultating blood pressure denoting systolic and diastolic pressures

laceration: wound caused by tearing of the tissues

lacrimal: pertaining to tears

lateral: pertaining to the side; the opposite of *medial*

lethargy: slowed responses, sluggish speech, and slowed mental and motor processes in a person oriented to time, place, and person

living will: advance directive that states the medical care that a person would want or refuse should the person be unable to give consent or refusal

lumbar: pertaining to the area of the back between the thorax and the pelvis

maceration: tissue softening as a result of excessive moisture

manubrium: upper part of the sternum

meatus: opening or passageway

medial: pertaining to the middle; opposite of *lateral*

metaphysis: the flared portion of a long bone just above the epiphysis

myocardium: thick, contractile layer of muscle cells that forms the heart wall

nephron: structural and functional unit of the kidney

neutropenia: decreased number of neutrophils

neutrophil: white blood cell that removes and destroys bacteria, cellular debris, and solid particles

Nitrazine paper: treated paper used to detect pH and determine the presence of amniotic fluid

nociceptors: nerve endings that respond to noxious stimuli

olfactory: pertaining to the sense of smell

oliguria: urine output of less than 500 mL in 24 hours

ophthalmic: pertaining to the eye

pectoral: pertaining to the chest or breast

percussion: use of tapping on a body surface with fingers

pericardium: fibroserous sac that surrounds the heart and the origin of the great vessels

peristalsis: movement through the intestines

phrenic: pertaining to the diaphragm

plantar: pertaining to the sole

pleura: thin, serous membrane that encloses the lung

plexus: network of nerves, lymphatic vessels, or veins

popliteal: pertaining to the back of the knee

posterior: back or dorsal; the opposite of *anterior* or *ventral*

pronate: to turn the hand or forearm so that the palm faces down or back; opposite of *supinate*

proximal: situated nearest the center of the body; opposite of *distal*

pruritus: itching

pulse deficit: difference between the apical and radial pulse rates

pulse pressure: difference between the systolic blood pressure and diastolic blood pressure readings

purulent: pus producing or pus containing

range of motion: extent to which a person can move joints or muscles

sanguineous: referring to or containing blood

serosanguineous: containing blood and serum

spasticity: sudden, involuntary increase in muscle tone or contractions

sprain: complete or incomplete tear in the supporting ligaments surrounding a joint

station: relationship of the presenting part to the ischial spines

strain: injury to the muscle or tendinous attachment

striated: marked with parallel lines, such as striated (skeletal) muscle

subcutaneous: related to the tissue layer under the dermis

sublingual: under the tongue

superior: higher; opposite of *inferior*

supinate: to turn the palm or forearm upward; the opposite of *pronate*

systole: period of ventricular contraction

tachycardia: rapid heart rate; usually more than 100 beats per minute

tachypnea: rapid respiratory rate, usually more than 20 breaths per minute

tendon: band of fibrous connective tissue that attaches a muscle to a bone

transducer: external mechanical device that translates one physical quantity to another, most commonly seen in capturing fetal heart rates and transmitting and recording the value onto a fetal monitor

Valsalva maneuver: forceful exhalation with a closed glottis; bearing down

ventral: pertaining to the front or *anterior*, the opposite of *dorsal* or *posterior*

ventricle: small cavity, such as one of several in the brain or one of the two lower chambers of the heart

viscera: internal organs

xiphoid: sword shaped; the lower portion of the sternum

Index

Note: i refers to an illustration; t refers to a table.

Note: i refers to an illustration; t refers to a table.

Note: i refers to an illustration; t refers to a table.

Note: i refers to an illustration; t refers to a table.

Note: i refers to an illustration; t refers to a table.

Note: i refers to an illustration; t refers to a table.

Note: i refers to an illustration; t refers to a table.

Note: i refers to an illustration; t refers to a table.

Note: i refers to an illustration; t refers to a table.

Note: i refers to an illustration; t refers to a table.

Note: i refers to an illustration; t refers to a table.

Note: i refers to an illustration; t refers to a table.